Handbook of Dialysis Therapy

Handbook of Dialysis Therapy

Editor: Sean Eastwood

FOSTER ACADEMICS

www.fosteracademics.com

www.fosteracademics.com

FOSTER ACADEMICS

Cataloging-in-Publication Data

Handbook of dialysis therapy / edited by Sean Eastwood.
p. cm.
Includes bibliographical references and index.
ISBN 978-1-63242-861-5
1. Hemodialysis. 2. Dialysis. 3. Blood--Filtration. 4. Therapeutics. I. Eastwood, Sean.
RC901.7.H45 H36 2019
617.461 059--dc23

Foster Academics,
118-35 Queens Blvd., Suite 400,
Forest Hills, NY 11375, USA

ISBN 978-1-63242-861-5 (Hardback)

Printed and bound in China.

Contents

Preface

This book has been a concerted effort by a group of academicians, researchers and scientists, who have contributed their research works for the realization of the book. This book has materialized in the wake of emerging advancements and innovations in this field. Therefore, the need of the hour was to compile all the required researches and disseminate the knowledge to a broad spectrum of people comprising of students, researchers and specialists of the field.

The process of removing excess water, toxins and solutes from the body of those whose kidneys are no longer able to naturally perform these functions is called dialysis. It is usually done in patients with acute kidney injury or end-stage kidney disease. It can act as a temporary relief measure in patients awaiting kidney transplant, and as a permanent measure in cases in which transplant is not possible. The primary types of dialysis include hemodialysis, peritoneal dialysis and hemofiltration. Hemodiafiltration and intestinal dialysis are its secondary types. This book brings forth some of the most innovative concepts and elucidates the unexplored aspects of dialysis therapy. It covers in detail some existing theories and innovative concepts revolving around dialysis therapy. This book includes contributions of experts and scientists, which will provide innovative insights into the subject.

At the end of the preface, I would like to thank the authors for their brilliant chapters and the publisher for guiding us all-through the making of the book till its final stage. Also, I would like to thank my family for providing the support and encouragement throughout my academic career and research projects.

Editor

Comparison of the Impact of High-Flux Dialysis on Mortality in Hemodialysis Patients with and without Residual Renal Function

Hyung Wook Kim[1,7], Su-Hyun Kim[2], Young Ok Kim[1], Dong Chan Jin[1], Ho Chul Song[1], Euy Jin Choi[1], Yong-Lim Kim[3], Yon-Su Kim[4], Shin-Wook Kang[5], Nam-Ho Kim[6], Chul Woo Yang[1], Yong Kyun Kim[1,8]*]

1 Department of Internal Medicine, College of Medicine, The Catholic University of Korea, Seoul, Korea, **2** Department of Internal Medicine, College of Medicine, Chung-Ang University, Seoul, Korea, **3** Department of Internal Medicine, Kyungpook National University School of Medicine, Daegu, Korea, **4** Department of Internal Medicine, College of Medicine, Seoul National University, Seoul, Korea, **5** Department of Internal Medicine, College of Medicine, Yonsei University, Seoul, Korea, **6** Department of Internal Medicine, Chonnam National University Medical School, Gwangju, Korea, **7** St. Vincent's Hospital, Suwon, Korea, **8** MRC for Cell Death Disease Research Center, The Catholic University of Korea, Seoul, Korea

Abstract

Background: The effect of flux membranes on mortality in hemodialysis (HD) patients is controversial. Residual renal function (RRF) has shown to not only be as a predictor of mortality but also a contributor to β2-microglobulin clearance in HD patients. Our study aimed to determine the interaction of residual renal function with dialyzer membrane flux on mortality in HD patients.

Methods: HD Patients were included from the Clinical Research Center registry for End Stage Renal Disease, a prospective observational cohort study in Korea. Cox proportional hazards regression models were used to study the association between use of high-flux dialysis membranes and all-cause mortality with RRF and without RRF. The primary outcome was all-cause mortality.

Results: This study included 893 patients with 24 h-residual urine volume ≥100 ml (569 and 324 dialyzed using low-flux and high-flux dialysis membranes, respectively) and 913 patients with 24 h-residual urine volume <100 ml (570 and 343 dialyzed using low-flux and high-flux dialysis membranes, respectively). After a median follow-up period of 31 months, mortality was not significantly different between the high and low-flux groups in patients with 24 h-residual urine volume ≥100 ml (HR 0.86, 95% CI, 0.38–1.95, $P = 0.723$). In patients with 24 h-residual urine volume <100 ml, HD using high-flux dialysis membrane was associated with decreased mortality compared to HD using low-flux dialysis membrane in multivariate analysis (HR 0.40, 95% CI, 0.21–0.78, $P = 0.007$).

Conclusions: Our data showed that HD using high-flux dialysis membranes had a survival benefit in patients with 24 h-residual urine volume <100 ml, but not in patients with 24 h-residual urine volume ≥100 ml. These findings suggest that high-flux dialysis rather than low-flux dialysis might be considered in HD patients without RRF.

Editor: Martin H. de Borst, University Medical Center Groningen and University of Groningen, Netherlands

Funding: This work was supported by a grant of the Korea Healthcare Technology R & D Project, Ministry of Health and Welfare, Republic of Korea (HI10C2020). The funders had no role in study design, data collection and analysis, decision to publish, or preparation of the manuscript.

Competing Interests: The authors have declared that no competing interests exist.

* E-mail: drkimyk@catholic.ac.kr

Introduction

Patients with End-stage renal disease (ESRD) undergoing maintenance hemodialysis (HD) have a high risk of morbidity and mortality [1]. Therefore, the most effective and best-tolerated HD treatment may improve clinical outcomes in this patient population [2]. In particular, the dialyzer used in HD treatment is one of the important determinants of the effectiveness of dialysis. HD using high-flux dialysis membrane can clear more middle molecular weight uremic toxins such as β2-microglobulin than HD using low-flux dialysis membrane because of its higher porosity [3].

Despite the beneficial effects of middle-molecule removal by high-flux dialysis, the effects of dialyzer membrane flux on mortality are controversial. A number of observational studies have suggested that HD using high-flux dialysis membrane results in improved outcomes compared with low-flux dialysis [4–7]. However, two large randomized clinical trials, the HEMO study and the European Membrane Permeability Outcome (MPO) study, showed no significant survival difference between HD using high-flux dialysis membrane and HD using low-flux dialysis membrane [8,9]. This discrepancy may be due to differences in the populations studied or study design.

Residual renal function is known to be an important determinant of serum β2-microglobulin level and a contributor of β2-microglobulin clearance in patients with HD [10,11]. In patients with greater residual renal function, the beneficial effects of β2-microglobulin removal by high-flux dialysis may not be apparent. Therefore, it may be postulated that the beneficial effect of high-flux dialysis on mortality may be different between patients with different degrees of residual renal function.

This study aimed to determine the interaction of residual renal function with dialyzer membrane flux on mortality in patients enrolled in the Clinical Research Center (CRC) registry for ESRD cohort which is an observational prospective cohort study conducted in Korea.

Materials and Methods

Study Population

All patients included in this study were enrolled in the CRC registry for ESRD. This is an ongoing observational prospective cohort study patients with ESRD from 31 medical centers in Korea. The cohort started in April 2009 and included adult (>18 years of age) dialysis patients. A total 3,067 patients undergoing HD were enrolled in this cohort. For the present study, we excluded patients for whom information about the dialysis membrane used or 24 h-urine volume was not available (n = 1,261). So, 1,806 patients were included in the final analysis.

Demographic and clinical data were collected at the time of enrollment. Assessment of dialysis characteristics and measurements of health were done every 6 months until follow-up was complete. Dates and causes of mortality were reported throughout the follow-up period.

Ethics

The study was approved by the institutional review board at each center [The Catholic University of Korea, Bucheon St. Mary's Hospital; The Catholic University of Korea, Incheon St. Mary's Hospital; The Catholic University of Korea, Seoul St. Mary's Hospital; The Catholic University of Korea, St. Mary's Hospital; The Catholic University of Korea, St. Vincent's Hospital; The Catholic University of Korea, Uijeongbu St. Mary's Hospital; Cheju Halla General Hospital; Chonbuk National University Hospital; Chonnam National University Hospital; Chung-Ang University Medical Center; Chungbuk National University Hospital; Chungnam National University Hospital; Dong-A University Medical Center; Ehwa Womens University Medical Center; Fatima Hospital, Daegu; Gachon University Gil Medical Center; Inje University Pusan Paik Hospital; Kyungpook National University Hospital; Kwandong University College of Medicine, Myongji Hospital; National Health Insurance Corporation Ilsan Hospital; National Medical Center; Pusan National University Hospital; Samsung Medical Center, Seoul; Seoul Metropolitan Government, Seoul National University, Boramae Medical Center; Seoul National University Hospital; Seoul National University, Bundang Hospital; Yeungnam University Medical Center; Yonsei University, Severance Hospital; Yonsei University, Gangnam Severance Hospital; Ulsan University Hospital; Wonju Christian Hospital (in alphabetical order)] and performed in accordance to the Declaration of Helsinki. Written informed consent was obtained from all patients.

Clinical and Dialysis Parameters

In the CRC registry for ESRD study, baseline demographic and clinical data including age, sex, body mass index (BMI), type of dialysis membrane, primary causes of ESRD, comorbidities (cardiovascular disease and DM), laboratory values, and therapeutic characteristics were recorded. Cardiovascular disease was defined as the presence of coronary artery disease, congestive heart failure, peripheral vascular disease, cerebrovascular disease, or atrial fibrillation. Serum hemoglobin, serum albumin, serum creatinine, blood urea nitrogen, serum potassium and serum total cholesterol (TC) were measured. The single-pool Kt/V (spKt/V) was determined by two-point urea modeling based on the intradialytic reduction in blood urea and intradialytic weight loss. Timed 24 h urine collection was performed during the interdialytic intervals at the time of enrollment and 24 h-urine volume was recorded. Zero- residual renal function was operationally defined as having 24 h-urine volume <100 ml. Patients were grouped as having zero- residual renal function or non-zero residual renal function. To estimate the residual glomerular filtration rate, residual renal clearance (ml/min) was calculated as the mean of the creatinine clearance and urea clearance in patients with 24 h-urine volume ≥100 ml [12].

In order to analyze the effects of the dialysis membrane type on mortality in patients with zero- and non-zero residual renal function, the patients were further divided into high-flux and low-flux dialysis groups according to the type of dialysis membrane used. High-flux dialysis was defined as an ultrafiltration coefficient of ≥20 ml/mm Hg per hour and a sieving coefficient for β2-microglobulin >0.6. Low-flux dialysis was defined as an ultrafiltration coefficient of ≤10 ml/mm Hg per hour and a sieving coefficient for β2-microglobulin = 0 [9].

A total of 21 types of low-flux dialyzer and 26 types of high-flux dialyzers were used in this study. The most common low-flux dialyzer was the Gambro polyflux 14L (used in 34.2% of cases) and the most common high-flux dialyzer was the Gambro polyflux 170H (used in 18.9% of cases). All of the dialysis membrane materials were synthetic membranes in the high-flux dialyzer group, whereas 99.0% contained synthetic membranes and 1.0% contained substituted cellulose membranes in low-flux dialyzer group. All dialysis sessions were performed without reuse of the dialyzers. All dialysate solutions were bicarbonate-based. Dialysate complied with the criteria adopted by the European Best Practice Guidelines [13] and the ultrapure dialysates were used in all patients using high-flux dialyzer.

Outcomes

The clinical outcome of this study was all-cause mortality. For each death, the principal investigator at that given institution completed a form that included cause of death according to the CRC registry for ESRD study classification.

Statistical Analyses

Data with continuous variables and normal distribution are presented as means ± SD, and those without normal distribution are presented as the median with ranges as appropriate for the type of variable. Student's t-tests, Mann–Whitney U tests, one-way ANOVA tests and Kruskal-Wallis tests were used to determine the differences in continuous variables. Categorical variables are presented as percentages. Pearson's chi-square test or Fisher's exact test were used to determine the differences in categorical variables.

Absolute mortality rates were calculated per 100 person-years of follow-up. The survival curves were estimated using the Kaplan–Meier method and compared by the log-rank tests between the high- and low-flux dialysis groups. The Cox proportional hazard regression model was used to calculate hazard ratio (HR) with 95% confidence interval (CI) for all-cause mortality. Analyses were adjusted for potential confounders including age, gender, use of high-flux membrane, BMI, diabetes mellitus, cardiovascular disease, primary cause of ESRD, duration of dialysis therapy, systolic blood pressure (BP), diastolic BP, hemoglobin, serum albumin, serum β2-microglobulin, serum TC, type of vascular access, residual renal clearance, and spKt/V. A value of $P<0.05$ was considered to be statistically significant. All statistical analyses were performed using SPSS 11.5 software (Chicago, IL, USA).

Results

Patients Characteristics

A total of 893 patients with 24 h-residual urine volume ≥ 100 ml and 913 patients with 24 h-residual urine volume < 100 ml were included in this study. Table 1 shows the baseline characteristics of participants.

In the patients with 24 h-residual urine volume ≥100 ml, 64% (569 of 893) patients were dialyzed using low-flux dialysis membranes and 36% (324 of 893) were dialyzed using high-flux dialysis membranes. The high-flux group had a higher prevalence of cardiovascular diseases and lower serum β2-microglobulin levels than the low-flux group. Arteriovenous fistula as the vascular access was more used in high-flux group and catheter was more used in low-flux group. There was no significant difference in rate of arteriovenous graft use between the high- and the low-flux groups. There were no significant differences in age, gender, BMI, prevalence of diabetes mellitus, primary cause of ESRD, duration of dialysis therapy, systolic BP, diastolic BP, serum hemoglobin levels, serum albumin levels, serum TC levels, 24-h urine volume, residual renal clearance and spKt/V between the high- and the low-flux groups.

In the patients with 24 h-residual urine volume <100 ml, 62% (570 of 913) were dialyzed using low-flux dialysis membranes and 38% (343 of 913) were dialyzed using high-flux dialysis membranes. The high-flux group was younger and had a lower prevalence of diabetes mellitus. Diabetes mellitus as a primary cause of ESRD was more prevalent in lower flux group. The high-flux group had a longer duration of dialysis therapy, higher serum albumin levels and lower spKt/V than the low-flux group. Arteriovenous fistula as the vascular access was more used in high-flux group and catheter was more used in low-flux group. There was no significant difference in rate of arteriovenous graft use between the high- and the low-flux groups. There were no

Table 1. Baseline characteristics of the study populations.

Characteristics	24 h-residual urine volume ≥100 ml (n = 893)			24 h-residual urine volume <100 ml (n = 913)		
	Low-Flux (n = 569)	High-Flux (n = 324)	p	Low-Flux (n = 570)	High-Flux (n = 343)	p
Age (years)	59±14	58±13	0.504	59±13	57±13	0.027
Male, n (%)	338 (9.4)	205 (63.3)	0.255	331 (58.1)	184 (53.6)	0.192
Body mass index (kg/m^2)	23.0±3.7	22.6±3.1	0.082	22.6±3.3	22.2±3.5	0.137
Comorbidities						
Diabetes mellitus, n (%)	303 (53.3)	192 (59.3)	0.108	339 (59.5)	165 (48.1)	0.001
Cardiovascular diseases, n (%)	207 (36.4)	144 (44.4)	0.029	253 (44.4)	146 (42.6)	0.865
Causes of ESRD, n (%)			0.059			0.001
Diabetes mellitus	302 (53.1)	189 (58.3)		300 (52.6)	150 (43.7)	
Glomerulonephritis	89 (15.6)	40 (12.3)		83 (14.6)	49 (14.3)	
Renal vascular disease	99 (17.4)	44 (13.6)		74 (13.0)	48 (22.7)	
Others/unknown	79 (13.9)	51 (15.7)		113 (19.8)	66 (19.2)	
Duration of dialysis therapy (months)	0 (0–3)	0 (0–7)	0.114	17 (0–53)	46 (17–84)	<0.001
Measurement before dialysis						
Systolic BP (mmHg)	141±24	143±25	0.233	142±21	143±20	0.438
Diastolic BP (mmHg)	77±14	76±14	0.278	79±13	80±12	0.073
Hemoglobin (g/dl)	9.0±1.7	9.2±1.7	0.060	10.1±1.5	10.3±1.4	0.071
Serum albumin (g/dl)	3.5±0.6	3.4±0.6	0.067	3.7±0.6	3.9±0.5	<0.001
Serum TC (mg/dl)	154±43	154±47	0.988	158±44	155±37	0.275
Serum β2-microglobulin (mg/L)	22.2 (17.2–29.3)	20.3 (15.4–26.2)	0.011	34.4 (23.0–44.9)	30.0 (24.0–44.3)	0.788
Vascular access			<0.001			<0.001
Arteriovenous fistula, n (%)	174 (30.9)	139 (43.6)		330 (58.8)	247 (74.2)	
Arteriovenous graft, n (%)	49 (8.7)	35 (11.0)		98 (17.5)	47 (14.1)	
Catheter, n (%)	340 (60.4)	145 (45.5)		133 (23.7)	39 (11.7)	
24 h-urine volume (ml)	900 (518–1300)	810 (465–1300)	0.285	0 (0–0)	0 (0–0)	0.829
Residual renal clearance (ml/min)	2.9 (1.4–5.2)	2.7 (1.4–4.2)	0.062	-	-	
spKt/V	1.43±0.66	1.46±0.44	0.539	1.52±0.39	1.35±0.78	0.001

Data are expressed as mean ± SD or medians (interquartile percentile) or numbers (percentages).
Abbreviations: ESRD, end-stage renal disease; BP, blood pressure; TC, total cholesterol; Kt/V: K, dialyzer clearance; t, time; V, volume of water a patient's body contains.

significant differences in gender, BMI, prevalence of cardiovascular diseases, systolic BP, diastolic BP, serum hemoglobin levels, serum TC levels, serum β2-microglobulin level and 24-h urine volume between the high- and the low-flux groups.

Effect of Membrane Flux on All-cause Mortality

The median follow-up period was 31 months (interquartile range, 13–40 months). Total of 170 deaths occurred during the follow-up period. Cardiovascular diseases were the leading cause of death (32.9% of all deaths). Table 2 shows the causes of death in each group. The distribution of causes of death was not significantly different between high- and low-flux groups in patients with 24 h-residual urine volume ≥100 ml or in patients with 24 h-residual urine volume <100 ml ($p = 0.239$ and $p = 0.938$, respectively).

In patients with 24 h-residual urine volume ≥100 ml, 197 patients left the study during the follow-up period for reasons other than death, including 38 patients who received kidney transplantation, 81 patients who transferred to a nonparticipating hospital, 44 patients who refused further participation and 34 for unspecified reasons. There were 69 deaths in this group during the follow-up period. The leading cause of death was cardiovascular diseases (36.2% of all deaths) (Table 2). The absolute mortality rate during the follow-up period was 4.2 deaths per 100 person-years. In univariate Cox regression analysis, use of high-flux membrane was not associated with mortality (HR 1.08, 95% CI, 0.66–1.76, $P = 0.765$). Figure 1A shows the Kaplan-Meier plot for all-cause mortality in the high- and the low-flux groups for the patients with 24 h-residual urine volume ≥100 ml. As shown, there was no significant difference in survival between the high-flux group and the low-flux group ($P = 0.764$ by log-rank test). After adjustment for demographics, comorbid conditions, and laboratory data, the adjusted HR for mortality in the high-flux group was 0.86 (95% CI, 0.38–1.95, $P = 0.723$), implying the mortality was not significantly different between the high- and the low-flux groups in the patients with 24 h-residual urine volume ≥ 100 ml (Table 3).

In patients with 24 h-residual urine volume <100 ml, 174 patients left the study during the follow-up period for reasons other than death, including 51 patients who received kidney transplantation, 78 patients who transferred to a nonparticipating hospital, 21 patients who refused further participation and 24 for unspecified reasons. There were a total of 101 deaths in this group during the follow-up period. The leading causes of death were cardiovascular diseases (30.7% of all deaths) and infectious diseases (30.7%of all deaths) (Table 2). The absolute mortality rate during the follow-up period was 4.2 deaths per 100 person-years. In univariate Cox regression analysis, the high-flux group was significantly associated with reduced mortality (HR 0.53, 95% CI, 0.34–0.83, $P = 0.005$). Figure 1B shows the Kaplan-Meier plot for all-cause mortality in the high- and the low-flux groups in patients with 24 h-residual urine volume <100 ml. Survival was increased in the high-flux group compared to the low-flux group ($P = 0.005$ by log-rank test). Even after adjustment for demographics, comorbid conditions, and laboratory data, the adjusted HR for mortality in the high-flux group was 0.40 (95% CI, 0.21–0.78, $P = 0.007$), implying that the high-flux group had a risk of death that was 60% lower than the low-flux group in patients with 24 h-residual urine volume <100 ml (Table 3).

Discussion

The major findings of this study were that HD using high-flux dialysis membrane was associated with decreased mortality compared to HD using low-flux dialysis membrane in patients with 24 h-residual urine volume <100 ml, whereas there was no significant difference in mortality between the high- and the low-flux dialysis group in patients with 24 h-residual urine volume ≥ 100 ml. These data suggest that high-flux dialysis impacts survival differently according to residual renal function and that high-flux dialysis is superior to low-flux dialysis in patients without residual renal function.

Residual renal function is associated with improved survival and clinical outcomes such as hospitalization, nutrition, anemia, and serum phosphorous control in HD patients [14–16]. Furthermore, residual renal function is a strong predictor of serum β2-microglobulin levels, since the kidney is the primary organ for the clearance of β2-microglobulin [11]. In this study, serum β2-microglobulin levels were significantly higher in patients with 24 h-residual urine volume <100 ml (31 mg/L, interquartile range, 23–45 mg/L) than in those with 24 h-residual urine volume ≥100 ml (21 mg/L, interquartile range, 16–28 mg/L) ($p<0.001$) (data not shown). A previous study also reported that increment of residual renal function was associated with a decrease in serum β2-microglobulin levels in dependent of years on dialysis [11]. Therefore, the beneficial effects of high-flux dialysis by clearance of middle molecules such as β2-microglobulin on clinical outcomes may be overshadowed by residual renal function in HD patients. Thus, it could be postulated that the beneficial effect of high-flux dialysis may be more apparent in patients with lesser residual renal function.

The HEMO study showed that there was no statistically significant interaction between baseline residual renal function and the type of flux intervention with respect to all-cause mortality although there was a trend towards decreased mortality in patients with lesser residual renal function [17]. They reported that all-

Table 2. Causes of deaths in each group.

	24 h-residual urine volume ≥100 ml		24 h-residual urine volume <100 ml	
	Low-Flux (44 deaths)	**High-Flux (25 deaths)**	**Low-Flux (75 deaths)**	**High-Flux (26 deaths)**
Cardiovascular diseases including cerebrovascular diseases, n (%)	13 (29.5)	12 (48.0)	23 (30.7)	8 (30.8)
Infectious diseases, n (%)	14 (31.8)	2 (8.0)	24 (32.0)	7 (26.9)
Malignancy, n (%)	2 (4.5)	1 (4.0)	7 (9.3)	2 (7.7)
Others, n	15 (34.1)	10 (40.0)	21 (28.0)	9 (34.6)

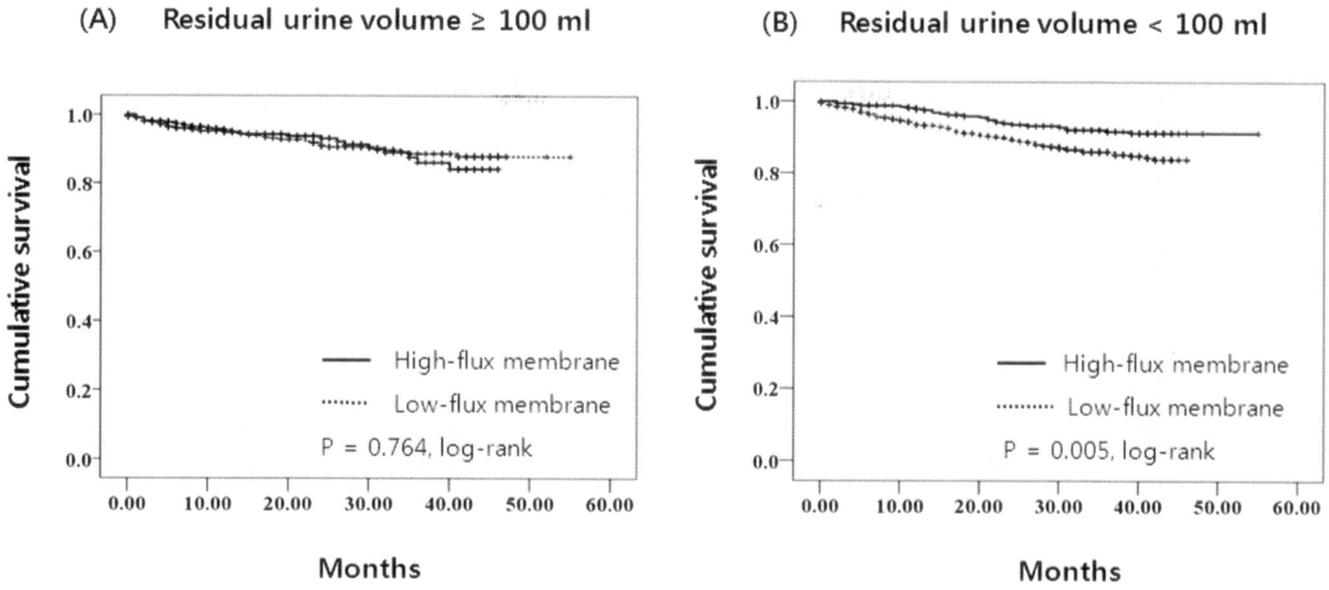

Figure 1. Kaplan-Meier survival curve for mortality in (A) patients with 24 h-residual urine volume ≥100 ml (P = 0.764 by log-rank test) and in (B) patients with 24 h-residual urine volume <100 ml (P = 0.005 by log-rank test).

cause mortality rates were not significantly different between patients with residual urea clearance ≤0.24 ml/min and those with residual urea clearance >0.24 ml/min (P = 0.24) [17], which is not consistent with our results. There are a number of possible explanations for this discrepancy.

First, it should be noted that the HEMO study only included patients with residual urea clearance <1.5 ml/min/35L of urea. Because the impact of high-flux dialysis on mortality may be less apparent in patients with greater residual renal function, the exclusion of patients with greater residual renal function may be a

Table 3. Multivariate Cox regression analysis of mortality in study populations.

	24 h-residual urine volume ≥100 ml			24 h-residual urine volume <100 ml		
	HR	**95% CI**	**P**	**HR**	**95% CI**	**P**
High-flux membrane (versus low-flux)	0.86	0.38–1.95	0.723	0.40	0.21–0.78	0.007
Age (1-yearincrement)	1.09	1.05–1.14	<0.001	1.04	1.01–1.07	0.005
Male (versus female)	0.72	0.32–1.64	0.431	0.86	0.45–1.62	0.633
BMI (per increment of 1 kg/m^2)	0.98	0.87–1.10	0.743	0.95	0.86–1.05	0.325
Comorbidities						
Diabetes mellitus (versus none)	0.85	0.12–5.88	0.869	2.19	0.73–6.57	0.162
Cardiovascular diseases (versus none)	1.54	0.74–3.22	0.250	1.28	0.69–2.36	0.437
Causes of ESRD						
Diabetes mellitus (versus non diabetes mellitus)	1.32	0.19–9.23	0.78	2.01	0.71–5.89	0.183
Systolic BP (per increment of 10 mmHg)	1.00	0.98–1.02	0.998	1.01	0.99–1.03	0.276
Diastolic BP (per increment of 10 mmHg)	1.02	0.98–1.06	0.385	1.00	0.97–1.04	0.858
Hemoglobin (per increment of 1 g/dl)	0.86	0.67–1.11	0.256	1.05	0.85–1.30	0.645
Serum albumin (per increment of 1 g/dl)	0.41	0.20–0.82	0.012	0.81	0.41–1.61	0.552
Serum β2-microglobulin ((per increment of 1 mg/L)	1.00	1.00–1.00	0.801	1.00	0.99–1.01	0.769
Serum TC (per increment of 10 mg/dl)	1.00	0.99–1.01	0.993	1.00	0.99–1.01	0.686
Residual renal clearance (per increment of 1 ml/min)	1.10	0.97–1.25	0.131			
spKt/V	1.15	0.51–2.62	0.735	0.57	0.31–1.04	0.067

Multivariate model includes age, gender, use of high-flux membrane, BMI, diabetes mellitus, cardiovascular disease, causes of ESRD, duration of dialysis therapy, systolic BP, diastolic BP, hemoglobin, serum albumin, serum β2-microglobulin, serum TC, type of vascular access, residual renal clearance and spKt/V.
Abbreviations: BMI, body mass index; HR, hazard ratio; TC, total cholesterol.

confounding factor in comparing the impact of high-flux dialysis on mortality according to residual renal function.

Additionally, the HEMO study included HD patients in which dialyzers were reused. Although the relationship between reuse of the dialyzer and effectiveness of removal of middle molecules has been controversial, reuse of dialyzers may be associated with structural damage of the membrane and a reduced permeability to middle molecules [18,19]. Therefore, reuse of dialyzer also may be a confounder to determine the impact of dialyzer membrane flux on mortality.

Another large randomized controlled trial, the MPO study, showed that there was no significant difference in mortality between high- and low-flux dialysis in the whole cohort [9]. In subgroup analysis, the MPO study showed a survival benefit with high-flux dialysis in patients with serum albumin level ≤4 mg/dl, while there was no significant difference in mortality between high- and low-flux dialysis in patients with serum albumin level > 4 mg/dl. Data on interaction between residual renal function and the type of flux intervention with respect to all-cause mortality were not shown in the MPO study. However, the MPO study provides some interesting clues on the impact of residual renal function on the relationship between high flux dialysis and mortality. First, patients with serum albumin level ≤4 mg/dl in the MPO study had longer duration of follow-up than the patients with serum albumin level >4 mg/dl because the study protocol was amended during the course of the study [9]. The longer duration of follow-up in patients with serum albumin level ≤ 4 mg/dl may explain the relationship between survival benefit with high-flux dialysis and residual renal function. Long duration of dialysis may cause accumulation of toxic middle molecules and decrease residual renal function to remove them. Therefore, in the MPO study, the patients with serum albumin level ≤4 mg/dl could have benefited more from the removal of toxic middle molecules with high-flux dialysis than the patients with serum albumin level >4 mg/dl because of the longer follow up. Second, the survival benefit of high-flux dialysis in the patients with serum albumin level ≤4 mg/dl was evident only after about 12 months of follow-up period, possibly when the residual renal function was lost. These findings of the MPO study therefore support the results of our study.

Our findings have a number of clinical implications. The European Best Practice Guideline (EBPG) relating to dialyzer membrane permeability recommends that the use of synthetic high-flux membranes should be considered to delay long-term complications of HD therapy [20]. The EBPG suggests the specific indication for high-flux dialysis to reduce dialysis-related amyloidosis, to improve control of hyperphosphatemia, to reduce the increased cardiovascular risk, and to improve control of anemia [20]. Our findings support the evidence for use of high-flux dialysis membrane and further contribute to the indications established for high-flux dialysis therapy in HD patients without residual renal function.

Our study has several limitations. First, the design of our study was not a randomized, controlled study but rather was a prospective observational study. The prescription of the dialyzer might be influenced by the results of previous study for the membrane flux on mortality such as MPO study. Accordingly, some baseline characteristics between the high-flux dialysis group and low-flux dialysis group differed in our study, indicating potential selection bias. In addition, the median follow-up period of 31 months was relatively short. Finally, despite the multicenter nature of the study, our cohort consisted of solely Korean patients. Therefore, it is uncertain whether our results can be generalized to other ethnic groups with HD treatment.

In conclusion, we found that HD using high-flux dialysis membranes had survival benefit in patients with 24 h-residual urine volume <100 ml, but not in patients with 24 h-residual urine volume ≥100 ml. These findings suggest that dialyzer membrane flux impacts survival differently according to residual renal function. Thus, high-flux dialysis rather than low-flux dialysis might be considered in HD patients without residual renal function.

Acknowledgments

We thank the study coordinators Hye Young Lim, Nam Hee Kim, Mi Joung Moon, Hwa Young Lee, Mi Joung Kwon, Su Yeon An, Su Joung Oh and Hye Young Kwak for contribution to this study.

Author Contributions

Conceived and designed the experiments: YKK CWY. Performed the experiments: HWK SHK YKK YOK DCJ HCS EJC. Analyzed the data: HWK YKK CWY. Contributed reagents/materials/analysis tools: SHK YKK YOK DCJ YLK YSK SWK NHK CWY. Wrote the paper: HWK YKK.

References

1. Yoshino M, Kuhlmann MK, Kotanko P, Greenwood RN, et al. (2006) International differences in dialysis mortality reflect background general population atherosclerotic cardiovascular mortality. J Am Soc Nephrol 17: 3510–3519.
2. Ward RA (2011) Do clinical outcomes in chronic hemodialysis depend on the choice of a dialyzer? Semin Dial 24: 65–71.
3. DiRaimondo CR, Pollak VE (1989) Beta 2-microglobulin kinetics in maintenance hemodialysis: a comparison of conventional and high-flux dialyzers and the effects of dialyzer reuse. Am J Kidney Dis 13: 390–395.
4. Hornberger JC, Chernew M, Petersen J, Garber AM (1992) A multivariate analysis of mortality and hospital admissions with high-flux dialysis. J Am Soc Nephrol 3: 1227–1237.
5. Port FK, Wolfe RA, Hulbert-Shearon TE, Daugirdas JT, Agodoa LY, et al. (2001) Mortality risk by hemodialyzer reuse practice and dialyzer membrane characteristics: results from the usrds dialysis morbidity and mortality study. Am J Kidney Dis 37: 276–286.
6. Chauveau P, Nguyen H, Combe C, Chêne G, Azar R, et al. (2005) Dialyzer membrane permeability and survival in hemodialysis patients. Am J Kidney Dis 45: 565–571.
7. Krane V, Krieter DH, Olschewski M, März W, Mann JF, et al. (2007) Dialyzer membrane characteristics and outcome of patients with type 2 diabetes on maintenance hemodialysis. Am J Kidney Dis 49: 267–275.
8. Eknoyan G, Beck GJ, Cheung AK, Daugirdas JT, Greene T, et al. (2002) Effect of dialysis dose and membrane flux in maintenance hemodialysis. N Engl J Med 347: 2010–2019.
9. Locatelli F, Martin-Malo A, Hannedouche T, Loureiro A, Papadimitriou M, et al. (2009) Effect of membrane permeability on survival of hemodialysis patients. J Am Soc Nephrol 20: 645–654.
10. McCarthy JT, Williams AW, Johnson WJ (1994) Serum beta 2-microglobulin concentration in dialysis patients: importance of intrinsic renal function. J Lab Clin Med 123: 495–505.
11. Cheung AK, Rocco MV, Yan G, Leypoldt JK, Levin NW, et al. (2006) Serum beta-2 microglobulin levels predict mortality in dialysis patients: results of the HEMO study. J Am Soc Nephrol 17: 546–555.
12. Peritoneal Dialysis Adequacy 2006 Work Group. (2006) Clinical practice guidelines for peritoneal adequacy, update 2006. Am J Kidney Dis 48 Suppl 1: S91–97.
13. Ward RA (2004) Ultrapure dialysate. Semin Dial. 17: 489–497.
14. Shemin D, Bostom AG, Laliberty P, Dworkin LD (2001) Residual renal function and mortality risk in hemodialysis patients. Am J Kidney Dis 38: 85–90.
15. Vilar E, Wellsted D, Chandna SM, Greenwood RN, Farrington K (2009) Residual renal function improves outcome in incremental haemodialysis despite reduced dialysis dose. Nephrol Dial Transplant 24: 2502–2510.
16. van der Wal WM, Noordzij M, Dekker FW, Boeschoten EW, Krediet RT, et al. (2011) Full loss of residual renal function causes higher mortality in dialysis

patients; findings from a marginal structural model. Nephrol Dial Transplant 2011: 2978–2983.
17. Cheung AK, Levin NW, Greene T, Agodoa L, Bailey J, et al. (2003) Effects of high-flux hemodialysis on clinical outcomes: results of the HEMO study. J Am Soc Nephrol 14: 3251–3263.
18. Matos JP, André MB, Rembold SM, Caldeira FE, Lugon JR (2000) Effects of dialyzer reuse on the permeability of low-flux membranes. Am J Kidney Dis 35: 839–844.
19. Cheung AK, Agodoa LY, Daugirdas JT, Depner TA, Gotch FA, et al. (1999) Effects of hemodialyzer reuse on clearances of urea and beta2-microglobulin. The Hemodialysis (HEMO) Study Group. J Am Soc Nephrol 10: 117–127.
20. Tattersall J, Canaud B, Heimburger O, Pedrini L, Schneditz D, et al. (2010) High-flux or low-flux dialysis: a position statement following publication of the Membrane Permeability Outcome study. Nephrol Dial Transplant 25: 1230–1232.

2

Physical, Cognitive and Emotional Factors Contributing to Quality of Life, Functional Health and Participation in Community Dwelling in Chronic Kidney Disease

Ulla K. Seidel[1], Janine Gronewold[1], Michaela Volsek[2], Olga Todica[1], Andreas Kribben[2], Heike Bruck[2], Dirk M. Hermann[1]*

1 Department of Neurology, University Hospital Essen, Essen, Germany, **2** Department of Nephrology, University Hospital Essen, Essen, Germany

Abstract

Background: Quality of life (QoL) impairment is a well-known consequence of chronic kidney disease (CKD). The factors influencing QoL and late life functional health are poorly examined.

Methods: Using questionnaires combined with neuropsychological examinations, we prospectively evaluated physical, cognitive, and emotional factors influencing QoL, functional health and participation in community dwelling in 119 patients with CKD stages 3–5 including hemodialysis (61.5±15.7years; 63% men) and 54 control patients of the same age without CKD but with similar cardiovascular risk profile.

Results: Compared with control patients, CKD patients showed impairment of the physical component of QoL and overall function, assessed by the SF-36 and LLFDI, whereas disability, assessed by LLFDI, was selectively impaired in CKD patients on hemodialysis. Multivariable linear regressions (forced entry) confirmed earlier findings that CKD stage ($\beta = -0.24$; $p = 0.012$) and depression ($\beta = -0.30$; $p = 0.009$) predicted the QoL physical component. Hitherto unknown, CKD stage ($\beta = -0.23$; $p = 0.007$), cognition ($\beta = 0.20$; $p = 0.018$), and depression ($\beta = -0.51$; <0.001) predicted disability assessed by the LLFDI, while age ($\beta = -0.20$; $p = 0.023$), male gender ($B = 5.01$; $p = 0.004$), CKD stage ($\beta = -0.23$; $p = 0.005$), stroke history ($B = -9.00$; $p = 0.034$), and depression ($\beta = -0.41$; $p < 0.001$) predicted overall function. Interestingly, functional health deficits, cognitive disturbances, depression, and anxiety were evident almost only in CKD patients with coronary heart disease (found in 34.2% of CKD patients). The physical component of QoL and functional health decreased with age and depressive symptoms, and increased with cognitive abilities.

Conclusions: In CKD, QoL, functional health, and participation in community dwelling are influenced by physical, cognitive, and emotional factors, most prominently in coronary heart disease patients.

Editor: Christoph Kleinschnitz, Julius-Maximilians-Universität Würzburg, Germany

Funding: This work was supported by the Federal Ministry of Education and Research (BMBF/NGFN 01GR0807), the Heinz Nixdorf Foundation, and Dr. Werner Jackstädt Foundation. The funders had no role in study design, data collection and analysis, decision to publish, or preparation of the manuscript.

Competing Interests: The authors have declared that no competing interests exist.

* E-mail: dirk.hermann@uk-essen.de

Introduction

Chronic kidney disease (CKD) is a worldwide growing health problem that is found in 23–35% of adults above 64 years [1]. Quality of life (QoL) is reduced in this population [2]. The underlying reasons are largely unknown. A better understanding is important, because QoL is closely linked to patient morbidity and mortality [3]. QoL is also frequently used as outcome measure in CKD treatment studies [3]. In CKD patients requiring dialysis, QoL has previously been associated with compliance to dialysis, hospitalization and survival [4–6].

CKD patients exhibit high loads of vascular risk factors and co-morbidities [7–9], compromising QoL in this patient group [10]. As a matter of fact, vascular diseases are not the only factors influencing QoL in CKD: CKD patients frequently present with cognitive deficits and depressive symptoms [9]. Depressive symptoms have frequently been studied in stage 5D patients on dialysis, where they predisposed to QoL impairment [11–14], but less often in earlier stages of CKD [15–17]. Whether and how cognitive performance affects QoL in CKD was hitherto unknown.

For the evaluation of late life functioning, assessments of functional health and participation in community dwelling are widely used in health services research [18,19]. In age-related diseases, the Late Life Function and Disability Instrument (LLFDI), which consists of a disability and overall function dimension that can be broken down into various subscales, is particularly well validated [20,21]. Together with the Medical Outcomes Study Short Form-36 (SF-36) health survey [22] and a detailed neuropsychological examination, this tool allows particularly thorough QoL investigations.

Considering the lack of a comprehensive study that examined the effect of physical, cognitive and emotional factors on QoL, functional health and participation in community dwelling, we prospectively studied 119 patients with CKD stages 3–5 and 5D, which we compared with a control group consisting of 54 control patients without CKD, but with similar age and vascular risk profile. In these subjects, we investigated QoL and late life functional health using the SF-36 and LLFDI questionnaires, and performed a detailed neuropsychological examination, in which we evaluated the patients' cognitive performance.

Methods

Ethics Statement

This study was approved by the ethics committee of the faculty of medicine at the University of Duisburg-Essen (08-3817). All participants enrolled in the study provided written informed consent.

Participants

The New Tools for the Prevention of Cardiovascular Disease in CKD study (NTCVD) is a prospective study analyzing the effects of risk factors and markers of cardiovascular disease in patients with CKD [23]. 119 patients with CKD stages 3–5 (according to K/DOQI-classification) [24] including hemodialysis were recruited together with 54 control patients with similar cardiovascular risk profile but without CKD at the Department of Nephrology at the University Hospital Essen with the help of local physicians. 30 of 119 patients had CKD stage 3A (45≤estimated glomerular filtration rate [eGFR]<60 ml/min/1.73m^2), 21 had CKD stage 3B (30≤eGFR<45 ml/min/1.73m^2), 21 had CKD stage 4 (15≤ eGFR<30 ml/min/1.73m^2), 12 had CKD stage 5 not requiring hemodialysis (eGFR<15 ml/min/1.73m^2) and 35 had CKD stage 5D requiring hemodialysis (any eGFR). All patients underwent a standardized interview to collect demographic data and a medical history, followed by a physical examination, laboratory analyses and neuropsychological testing. All patients completed standardized questionnaires to assess quality of life, functional health and participation in community dwelling, and mood disturbances.

Medical History and Laboratory Tests

The detailed medical history included information about the onset and treatment of CKD, known cardiovascular risk factors, associated illnesses (specifically coronary heart disease (CHD), myocardial infarct, stroke, transient ischemic attack (TIA), peripheral artery disease (PAD)), and current medications. Blood and urine samples were collected, in which the stage of CKD and vascular risk profile were evaluated in addition to routine blood parameters. eGFR was calculated using the modification of diet in renal disease formula (MDRD). Education was assessed by evaluating the highest academic degree and patient years of school education.

Standardized Questionnaires

Three standardized self-report questionnaires were completed:

(1) QoL was assessed using the SF-36 health survey [22]. The SF-36 consists of two summary scores, the physical component score and mental component score, that are broken down in eight subscales ('physical function', 'physical role', 'bodily pain', 'general health perceptions', 'mental health', 'emotional role', 'social function', 'vitality'). Raw values of all summary scales were transformed into standardized 0–100 scales. Higher scores indicate better QoL or less impairment for each domain.

(2) Functional health and participation in community dwelling was evaluated by the LLFDI [20,21]. The LLFDI consists of a total disability component score, composed of two summary scales, the disability dimension and overall function. The disability dimension is broken down in frequency of performance (measuring social and personal role domains) and limitation in capability (measuring instrumental and management role domains). The function component assesses overall function in three subcategories (upper extremity, basic lower extremity and advanced lower extremity). All items are scored on a 5-point ordinal scale. Component scores range from 0–100, higher scores indicating less impairment. Raw scores were transferred in scaled scores by summing up subscale relevant items.

(3) Depression and anxiety were examined using the Hospital Anxiety and Depression Scale (HADS) [25]. The HADS is a 14-item questionnaire, of which 7 items each examine depressive and anxiety symptoms on a 4-point scale. As such, scores from 0–21 points are obtained for both subscales, higher scores indicating higher symptom prevalence. In accordance with Zigmond and Snaith (1983) [25], categories were formed with 0–7 points being interpreted as normal, 8–10 points as borderline finding, and ≥11 points as suggestive for depression or anxiety.

Neuropsychological Assessment

Participants were examined with a battery of ten standardized tests, namely (a) the revised Wechsler memory scale (subtests digit and block span, forward and backward; assessment of verbal and spatial short-term and working memory) [26], (b) the trail making test (TMT) part A (assessment of information processing speed) [27], (c) the trail making test part B (assessment of executive flexibility) [27], (d) the Stroop test (assessment of executive flexibility) [28], (e) the Regensburg word fluency test (subtests 'animals' and 's-words'; assessment of lexical and semantical word fluency) [29] and (f) the Rey-Osterrieth complex figure test (copy task, assessment of visuo-constructive function) [30]. For CKD patients, z-scores were calculated for all ten neuropsychological tests based on norm values generated in the control cohort [9]. A global cognitive performance variable was formed by computing mean values of these z-scores. This global cognitive performance variable was used for further analyses. To rule out major confounders of cognitive performance as a consequence of patient tremor, the Whiget tremor rating scale was used. Examiners were not notified about the medical condition of the participants by the recruiting staff.

Statistical Analysis

Continuous data are expressed as mean±SD for normally and median (Q1;Q3) for non-normally distributed variables, categorical data as counts (%). For continuous data, group differences between control patients and all CKD patients were calculated with unpaired two-tailed t-tests (normally distributed data) or Mann-Whitney tests (non-normally distributed data). To compare control patients with CKD patients with or without dialysis, (a) one-way analyses of variance (ANOVA) followed by Bonferroni (equal variances) or Games-Howell (unequal variances) post-hoc tests (normally distributed continuous data) and (b) Kruskall-Wallis tests followed by Mann-Whitney tests with Bonferroni corrections for multiple testing (non-normally distributed continuous data) were used. Categorical data were evaluated by chi-square or Fisher tests. Predictors of QoL, functional health and participation in community dwelling, and depression were analyzed using univariate and multivariable linear regressions (forced entry strategy). In the regression studies, SD values were used as unit for determining β values. All comparisons were performed with SPSS 19 for Windows (SPSS Inc., Chicago, IL).

Results

Study Cohort

The characteristics of the NTCVD cohort are summarized in Table 1. CKD patients in this study had a mean age of 61.5±15.7 years, with a predominance of men (63%) in the sample. As described before [9], the age and gender profile did not differ from control patients. Compared with patients belonging to CKD stages 3–5 that did not receive renal replacement therapy, patients with CKD stage 5D on hemodialysis were younger and slightly (though not significantly) more often men. Education assessed as highest academic degree did not differ between groups, although CKD stage 3–5 patients not requiring dialysis had significantly less years of school education than control patients. Handedness did not differ between groups. CKD patients showed higher Whiget tremor scores for the left hand (median (Q1;Q3) = 0 (0;2)) compared with control patients (0 (0;0)).

Medical History and Laboratory Findings

Medical history and laboratory findings are also shown in Table 1. As expected, CKD patients exhibited a high prevalence of CHD or myocardial infarcts (34.2%) and PAD (10.2%). Only 5.9% reported strokes or TIAs. The prevalence of cardiovascular diseases did not differ between control patients, CKD stage 3–5 patients not receiving hemodialysis, and CKD stage 5D patients receiving hemodialysis. Stroke prevalence was higher in CKD stage 3–5 patients (8.4%) than in control (0%) and stage 5D (0%) patients. Hemoglobin (Hb) was lower in CKD stage 3–5 (12.5±1.7 g/dl) and stage 5D (12.5±1.6 g/dl) patients than in control patients (14.1±1.3 g/dl). Creatinine was elevated in CKD, more strongly in stage 5D (median (Q1;Q3) = 5.9 (4.4;8.1) mg/dl) than stage 3–5 (1.8 (1.3;3.2) mg/dl; control patients: 1.1 (0.9;1.2) mg/dl). Mean eGFR in the CKD group not requiring dialysis was 35.2±16.0 ml/min/1.73 m^2, compared with 70.9±9.6 ml/min/1.73 m^2 in control patients.

Cognition and Mood

Neuropsychological test results, depression and anxiety scores are also shown in Table 1. As previously shown [9], global cognitive performance, evaluated by z-scores as mean of ten neuropsychological tests, was worse in CKD stage 3–5 (−0.56±0.81) and stage 5D (−0.46±0.90) than in control (0.0±0.58) patients. 30.3% of CKD patients had a poor cognitive performance that was more than one standard deviation below controls.

Mean depression and anxiety scores, evaluated by HADS, did not significantly differ between control patients and CKD groups. Yet, stage 5D patients receiving hemodialysis had a higher prevalence of depressive symptoms (31.4% with HADS score≥11), than control patients (5.6%) and CKD stage 3–5 patients not receiving hemodialysis (8.3%). The prevalence of anxiety symptoms did not significantly differ between groups.

Quality of Life

In the SF-36 questionnaire, stage 3–5 (40.7±11.3) and stage 5D (40.5±10.3) patients showed a significant lower physical component score than control patients (47.4±11.2) (Table 2). The mental component score did not differ between groups. In the physical component, CKD patients showed impairments in physical function, physical role and general health. In the mental component, CKD patients revealed impairments in social function. In the latter score, stage 5D patients had significant lower values than stage 3–5 patients not requiring dialysis.

Functional Health and Participation in Community Dwelling

CKD patients had worse scores in the LLFDI disability dimension (62.3±9.9) and overall function (60.1±12.8) scales than control patients (disability dimension: 67.0±7.5, overall function: 68.3±8.3), which was evident in all subscales except in the social role domain (Table 2). In general, CKD stage 3–5 patients not on hemodialysis did not differ from stage 5D patients on hemodialysis, except for the personal role domain, in which stage 5D patients exhibited lower scores.

Predictors for Quality of Life: Role of Medical Conditions

To evaluate QoL predictors, univariate and multivariable linear regressions were computed for the whole cohort using a variety of models in which demographic factors (age, gender, education), CKD-related factors (CKD stage, hemoglobin), vascular diseases (CHD/myocardial infarct, stroke/TIA, PAD), cognitive performance, depression and anxiety were inserted in different combinations (Table 3). In univariate regressions, the factors age (β = −0.22; p = 0.005), education (β = 0.18; p = 0.020), CKD stage (β = −0.21; p = 0.006), CHD/myocardial infarct (B = −3.83; p = 0.041), PAD (B = −7.22; p = 0.030), cognitive performance (β = 0.26; p = 0.001) depression (β = −0.36; p<0.001) and anxiety (β = −0.21; p = 0.001) were predictors of the physical component of QoL, while the factors CHD/myocardial infarct (B = −4.12; p = 0.020), depression (β = −0.62; p<0.001) and anxiety (β = −0.68 per SD; p<0.001) were predictors of the mental component of QoL.

In multivariable regressions (forced entry strategy), the physical component of QoL was predicted by the factors age (β = −0.23; p = 0.018) and CKD stage (β = −0.30; p = 0.002) (model 2 in Table 3, which contains demographic factors, CKD-related factors and vascular diseases), the latter of which disappeared, while depression became predictive (β = −0.30; p = 0.009), when cognitive performance, depression and anxiety were inserted into the regression analysis (full model 3 in Table 3). The mental component of QoL was predicted by the factors depression (β = −0.35; p<0.001) and anxiety (β = −0.45; p<0.001) only (full model 3 in Table 3).

Predictors of Functional Health and Participation in Community Dwelling: Role of Medical Conditions

Since impairments in daily life activities have an impact on QoL in other medical conditions [31], we next examined predictors of functional health and participation in community dwelling using the LLFDI disability dimension and overall function summary scores with the same univariate and multivariable linear regression models as above (Table 4). In univariate regressions, the factors age (β = −0.22; p = 0.007), male gender (B = −3.85; p = 0.018), CKD stage (β = −0.27; p = 0.001), CHD/myocardial infarct (B = −4.46; p = 0.007), cognitive performance (β = 0.39; p<0.001), depression (β = −0.58; p<0.001) and anxiety (β = −0.33; p<0.001) predicted the disability dimension of the LLFDI (in which higher scores indicate better health), whereas the factors age (β = −0.29; p< 0.001), education (β = 0.16; p = 0.037), CKD stage (β = −0.25; p = 0.001), hemoglobin (β = 0.17; p = 0.025), CHD/myocardial infarct (B = −5.78; p = 0.002), stroke/TIA (B = −12.79; p = 0.012), PAD (B = −9.27; p = 0.007), cognitive performance (β = 0.36; p<

Table 1. Characteristics of control patients and CKD patients, the latter also split into patients not requiring and requiring hemodialysis.

	Controls (n = 54)	CKD all (all, n = 119)	CKD stages 3–5 (n = 84)	CKD stage 5D (n = 35)
Age (years)	62.3±10.1	61.5±15.7	64.5±13.5	54.6±18.4†
Gender (male)	40 (74.1)	75 (63.0)	48 (57.1)	27 (77.1)
Highest academic degree				
No degree	1 (1.9)	10 (8.4)	8 (9.5)	2 (5.7)
Secondary School	40 (74.1)	94 (79.0)	66 (78.6)	28 (80.0)
Baccalaureate	7 (13.0)	9 (7.6)	5 (6.0)	4 (11.4)
University degree	6 (11.1)	6 (5.0)	5 (6.0)	1 (2.9)
Education (years of school)	10 (8;10)	9 (8;10)*	8 (8;10)*	9 (8;10)
Handedness (right hand)	45 (83.3)	99 (83.2)	67 (79.8)	32 (91.4)
Tremor right hand (score)	0 (0;0)	0 (0;1)	0 (0;1)	0 (0;1)
Tremor left hand (score)	0 (0;0)	0 (0;2)*	0 (0;2)*	0 (0;3)*
CHD/myocardial infarct	22 (40.7)	40 (34.2)	25 (30.5)	15 (42.9)
PAD	2 (3.7)	12 (10.2)	7 (8.4)	5 (14.3)
Stroke/TIA	0	7 (5.9)*	7 (8.4)	0†
Hemoglobin (g/dl)	14.1±1.3	12.5±1.7*	12.5±1.6*	12.5±1.9*
Creatinine (mg/dl)	1.1±0.2	3.6±2.7*	2.5±1.9*	6.2±2.3*†
eGFR (ml/min/1.73m²)	70.9±9.6	28.2±17.6*	35.2±16.0*	n.a.
Time since first dialysis (months)	n.a.	n.a	n.a.	21.0 (5.3;42.4)
Time since last dialysis (hours)	n.a.	n.a	n.a.	28.0 (22.5;35.5)
Cognitive Performance (mean z-scores)	0.00±0.58	−0.53±0.84*	−0.56±0.81*	−0.46±0.90*
Cognitive Impairment (more than 1 z-score below controls)	Reference	36 (30.3)*	26 (31.0)*	10 (28.6)*
HADS-depression scale (mean score)	5.0 (2.0;6.5)	4.0 (2.0;8.0)	4.0 (2.0;7.0)	6.0 (2.0;13.0)
HADS-depression scale (score ≥11)	3 (5.6)	18 (15.1)	7 (8.3)	11 (31.4)*†
HADS-anxiety scale (mean score)	5.0 (3.0;8.0)	5.0 (2.0;7.0)	5.0 (2.0;7.0)	6.0 (4.0;12.0)
HADS-anxiety scale (score ≥11)	7 (13.0)	19 (16.0)	10 (11.9)	9 (25.7)

Data are means ± SD for normally distributed continuous data or median (Q1;Q3) for non-normally distributed continuous data, categorical data are presented as n (%). Continuous data were evaluated by unpaired two-tailed t-tests for comparisons between control patients and all CKD patients. Continuous data were evaluated by oneway ANOVA followed by Bonferroni or Games-Howell (in case of non-equal variances) tests (normally distributed data) or Kruskall-Wallis followed by Mann-Whitney tests (non-normally distributed data) for comparisons between control patients, CKD patients requiring hemodialysis and CKD patients not requiring hemodialysis. Categorical data were evaluated by chi-square or Fisher exact tests.
*p<0.05 compared with control patients,
†p<0.05 compared with CKD patients not requiring hemodialysis. CHD, coronary heart disease; CKD, chronic kidney disease; eGFR, estimated glomerular filtration rate; ESRD, end stage renal disease; HADS, Hospital Anxiety and Depression Scale; PAD, peripheral artery disease; TIA, transient ischemic attack.

0.001), depression (β = −0.48; p<0.001) and anxiety (β = −0.26; p = 0.001) predicted overall function.

In multivariable regressions, the factors age (β = −0.22 per SD; p = 0.021), CKD stage (β = −0.37; p<0.001) and CHD/myocardial infarct (B = −4.04; p = 0.018) predicted the LLFDI disability dimension, whereas age (β = −0.29; p = 0.001), male gender (B = 3.77; p = 0.047), CKD stage (β = −0.32; p<0.001), CHD/myocardial infarct (B = −5.54; p = 0.005) and stroke/TIA (B = −9.45; p = 0.044) predicted overall function (model 2 in Table 4, which contains demographic factors, CKD-related factors and vascular diseases). When cognitive performance, depression and anxiety were included into multivariable regression analyses (model 3 in Table 4), CHD/myocardial infarct did not predict the disability dimension and overall function any more. Instead, cognitive performance (β = 0.20; p = 0.018) and depression (β = −0.51; p<0.001) (disability dimension) or depression (β = −0.41; p<0.001) (overall function) became predictive.

Predictors of Quality of Life in CKD: Role of Functional Health and Participation in Community Dwelling

To evaluate how functional health and participation in community dwelling influenced QoL in CKD patients, univariate and multivariable linear regressions were again evaluated, in which demographic factors, CKD-related factors (both as above) and LLFDI scores were inserted (Table 5). In univariate regressions, the factors age (β = −0.22; p = 0.005), CKD stage (β = −0.21; p = 0.006), disability dimension (β = 0.56; p<0.001), overall function (β = 0.80; p<0.001), cognitive performance (β = 0.26; p<0.001), depression (β = −0.38 per SD; p<0.001) and anxiety (β = −0.21; p = 0.008) predicted the physical component of QoL that was assessed by the SF-36, whereas the factors disability dimension (β = 0.35; p<0.001), overall function (β = 0.21; p = 0.001), depression (β = −0.62; p<0.001) and anxiety (β = −0.68; p<0.001) predicted the mental component of QoL.

In multivariable regressions, the factor overall function (β = 0.78; p<0.001) was the only predictor of the physical

Table 2. Quality of life data of control subjects and CKD patients, the latter also split into patients not requiring and requiring hemodialysis.

	Controls (n = 54)	CKD all (n = 119)	CKD stages 3–5 (n = 84)	CKD stage 5D (n = 35)
SF-36: Physical Component	47.4±11.2	40.6±11.0*	40.7±11.3*	40.5±10.3*
SF-36: Physical Function	90.0 (70.0;96.3)	67.5 (41.9;90.0)*	67.5 (40.0;90.0)*	62.5 (45.0;90.0)*
SF-36: Role Physical	100.0 (50.0;100.0)	75.0 (0;100.0)*	75.0 (0;100.0)*	62.5 (0;100.0)*
SF-36: Bodily Pain	82.0 (41.0;100.0)	74.0 (41.0;100.0)	74.0 (51.0;100)	67.0 (31.0;100.0)
SF-36: General Health	61.0±22.9	46.3±19.9*	48.4±18.5*	41.2±22.3*
SF-36: Mental Component	49.9±10.7	49.4±11.0	51.1±9.3	45.3±13.6
SF-36: Mental Health	76.0 (59.0;88.0)	73.5 (55.6;88.0)	76.0 (57.0;88.0)	68.0 (36.0;84.0)
SF-36: Role Emotional	100.0 (66.7;100.0)	100.0 (66.7;100.0)	100.0 (66.7;100.0)	100.0 (0;100.0)
SF-36: Social Function	100.0 (75.0;100.0)	87.5 (56.3;100.0)*	87.5 (62.5;100.0)*	62.5 (50.0;100.0)*†
SF-36: Vitality	58.7±17.7	52.7±21.4	54.2±20.1	48.9±24.1
LLFDI: Disability Component	135.2±13.6	121.4±21.4*	122.9±20.1*	118.3±24.0*
LLFDI: Disability Dimension	67.0±7.5	62.3±9.9*	63.5±9.3	59.7±10.9*
LLFDI: Frequency of Performance	30.5±4.0	28.7±5.0*	29.1±4.8	27.6±5.1*
LLFDI: Social Role Domain	13.2±2.7	12.2±3.1	12.3±3.1	12.1±3.0
LLFDI: Personal Role Domain	17.3±2.2	16.5±2.9*	16.9±2.8	15.5±2.9*†
LLFDI: Limitation in Capability	38.0 (35.0;40.0)	36.0 (29.0;40.0)*	36.0 (30.0;40.0)	34.5 (27.0;37.8)*
LLFDI: Instrumental Role Domain	19.0 (17.5;20.0)	18.0 (15.0;20.0)*	18.0 (14.5;20.0)	17.0 (15.0;20.0)
LLFDI: Management Role Domain	19.0 (19.0;20.0)	18.0 (15.0;20.0)*	19.0 (16.0;20.0)*	17.2 (12.3;20.0)*
LLFDI: Overall Function	68.3±8.3	60.1±12.8*	60.9±12.0*	58.2±14.6*
LLFDI: Upper Extremity	25.0 (24.0;25.0)	24.0 (20.0;25.0)*	24.0 (21.0;25.0)*	23.0 (19.0;25.0)*
LLFDI: Basic Lower Extremity	29.0 (27.0;30.0)	27.0 (22;30.0)*	27.0 (23.0;30.0)*	26.0 (20.0;30.0)*
LLFDI: Advanced Lower Extremity	17.0 (14.0;19.0)	14.0 (9.0;18.0)*	14.0 (9.0;18.0)*	14.0 (8.0;18.0)*

Data are means ± SD for normally distributed data or median (Q1;Q3) for non-normally distributed data. Data were evaluated by unpaired two-tailed t-tests for comparisons between control patients and all CKD patients. Data were evaluated by oneway ANOVA followed by Bonferroni or Games-Howell (non-equal variances) tests (normally distributed data) or Kruskall-Wallis followed by Mann-Whitney tests (non-normally distributed data) for comparisons between control subjects, CKD patients requiring hemodialysis and CKD patients not requiring hemodialysis.
*$p<0.05$ compared with control subjects,
†$p<0.05$ compared with CKD patients not requiring hemodialysis. CKD, chronic kidney disease; ESRD, end stage renal disease; LLFDI, Late-Life Function and Disability Instrument; SF-36, 36-Item Short Form Health Survey.

component of QoL, while the factors cognitive performance ($\beta=0.17$; $p=0.035$), depression ($\beta=-0.34$; $p=0.001$) and anxiety ($\beta=0.44$; $p<0.001$) predicted the mental component (model 1 in Table 5). When inserting subscales of overall function into the regression analysis, basic lower extremity ($\beta=0.42$; $p<0.001$) and advanced lower extremity ($\beta=0.50$; $p<0.001$) function predicted the physical component (model 3 in Table 5).

Predictors of Depressive Symptoms in CKD: Role of Medical Conditions

In view of the eminent effect of depression on QoL in CKD, we subsequently analyzed predictors of depressive symptoms in CKD patients using univariate and multivariable linear regressions, in which demographic factors, CKD-related factors, vascular diseases and cognitive performance (all as above) were inserted (Table 6). In univariate regressions, the factors CKD stage ($\beta=0.18$; $p=0.017$), CHD/myocardial infarct ($B=2.22$; $p=0.001$) and cognitive performance ($\beta=-0.19$; $p=0.012$) were predictors of depressive symptoms as evaluated by the HADS depression scale, whereas in multivariable regressions the factor CHD/myocardial infarct alone ($B=1.77$; $p=0.018$) predicted depressive symptoms (full model 3 in Table 6).

Predictors of Depressive Symptoms in CKD: Role of Functional Health and Participation in Community Dwelling

To evaluate how functional health and participation in community dwelling affect depression in CKD, we finally analyzed predictors of depressive symptoms using univariate and multivariable linear regressions, in which demographic factors, CKD-related factors and LLFDI scores (all as above) were included (Table 7). In univariate regressions, the factors CKD stage ($\beta=0.18$ per SD; $p=0.017$), disability dimension ($\beta=-0.58$; $p<0.001$), overall function ($\beta=-0.50$; $p<0.001$) and cognitive performance ($\beta=-0.10$; $p=0.012$) predicted depressive symptoms, whereas in multivariable regressions, the factors disability dimension ($\beta=-0.45$; $p<0.001$), overall function ($\beta=-0.21$; $p=0.036$) and cognitive performance ($\beta=0.05$; $p=0.036$) predicted depressive symptoms (model 1 in Table 7). Further analyses revealed that both frequency of performance ($\beta=-0.33$; $p<0.001$) and limitation in capability ($\beta=-0.35$; $p<0.001$) influenced depressive symptoms within the disability dimension (model 2 in Table 7), whereas upper extremity function ($\beta=-0.22$; $p=0.025$) influenced depressive symptoms in the overall function dimension (model 3 in Table 7).

Table 3. Predictors for Quality of life in all patients: Role of medical conditions.

	Physical Component								Mental Component							
	Univariate		Model 1		Model 2		Model 3		Univariate		Model 1		Model 2		Model 3	
	B or β	p	B or β	p	B or β	p	B or β	p	B or β	p	B or β	p	B or β	p	B or β	p
Age	−0.22	**0.005**	−0.29	**0.001**	−0.23	**0.018**	−0.17	0.100	0.04	0.639	0.03	0.736	0.05	0.624	0.07	0.387
Gender (male vs. female)	0.22	0.910	1.06	0.574	1.66	0.410	2.84	0.151	−1.65	0.369	−1.04	0.588	−0.21	0.918	0.79	0.589
Education	0.18	**0.020**	0.08	0.292	0.04	0.650	0.84	0.401	0.03	0.746	0.04	0.674	0.04	0.677	−0.07	0.295
CKD stage	−0.21	**0.006**	−0.31	**0.001**	−0.30	**0.002**	−0.24	**0.012**	−0.10	0.237	−0.13	0.184	−0.01	0.344	0.02	0.818
Hemoglobin	0.10	0.217	0.01	0.951	0.01	0.961	−0.01	0.974	−0.04	0.659	−0.09	0.324	−0.06	0.544	0.00	0.978
CHD/myocardial infarct (yes vs. no)	3.83	**0.041**	–	–	3.53	0.089	1.83	0.369	4.12	**0.020**	–	–	3,87	0.066	0.75	0.619
Stroke/TIA (yes vs. no)	7.18	0.104	–	–	4.26	0.340	3.39	0.434	0.15	0.971	–	–	1,32	0.770	0.12	0.969
PAD (yes vs. no)	7.22	**0.030**	–	–	1.61	0.649	1.28	0.705	−2.36	0.456	–	–	−3,48	0.332	−3.69	0.143
Cognitive performance	0.26	**0.001**	–	–	–	–	0.06	0.558	0.15	0.065	–	–	–	–	0.09	0.214
HADS-depression scale	−0.36	**<0.001**	–	–	–	–	−0.30	**0.009**	−0.62	**<0.001**	–	–	–	–	−0.35	**<0.001**
HADS-anxiety scale	−0.21	**<0.001**	–	–	–	–	0.01	0.922	−0.68	**<0.001**	–	–	–	–	−0.45	**<0.001**

Effect of Age, Cognition and Depression on Quality of Life and Related Outcome Measures

To elucidate how age, cognition and depression influenced quality of life and related outcome measures, we stratified the data based on age categories (≤55 years, 55<x≤70 years, >70 years), cognitive performance terciles (<−0.620 z-scores, −0.620≤x<−0.016 z-scores, ≥−0.016 z-scores) and HADS depression categories (<7 points, 7≤x<11 points, ≥11 points). These analyses showed that the physical component of QoL, overall function of the LLFDI and cognitive performance decreased with increasing age, while the mental component of QoL, the disability dimension of the LLFDI, depression and anxiety did not change with age (Fig. 1A). The physical component of QoL, the disability dimension of the LLFDI and the overall function dimension of the LLFDI increased with cognitive capabilities, whereas depression scores were higher in subjects with low than intermediate cognitive function (Fig. 1B). Both the physical and mental component of QoL and the disability and overall function dimension of the LLFDI decreased with increasing depression scores, as did anxiety (Fig. 1C).

Effect of CHD/myocardial Infarcts on Quality of Life and Related Outcome Measures

To elucidate how the presence of CHD or myocardial infarcts modified quality of life related outcome measures, we compared patients with and without CHD/myocardial infarcts in their history. These studies showed that while the mental component of QoL, the disability dimension of the LLFDI, the overall function dimension of the LLFDI and cognition were reduced in CKD patients with CHD/myocardial infarcts (most strongly and in case of the disability dimension significant only in CKD stage 5D patients), depression was increased in stage 5D patients with CHD/myocardial infarcts (Fig. 2A). Notably, the latter relationships were not at all noticed in CKD patients not exhibiting CHD/myocardial infarcts in their history (Fig. 2B). These CKD patients did not reveal a reduced mental component of QoL or a reduced disability dimension of the LLFDI, and they did not exhibit an impaired cognitive performance or an increased depression score.

Discussion

We for the first time provide a comprehensive analysis of physical, cognitive and emotional factors influencing QoL, functional health and participation in community dwelling using a cohort of 119 patients with CKD stages 3–5 (including stage 5D requiring hemodialysis) that we compared with 54 control patients of the same age with similar cardiovascular risk profile without CKD. As such, we confirmed previous findings that the physical component of QoL, which is impaired both in CKD stage 3–5 and stage 5D patients, is predicted by CKD stage and depressive symptoms, furthermore showing that the disability dimension of functional health and participation in community dwelling, which assesses socially defined life tasks as part of the LLFDI, is in addition influenced by cognitive performance. Age, male gender, CKD stage, stroke history and depression are predictors of overall function, which measures the ability to perform discrete actions and activities without assistance within the LLFDI. Functional health deficits, cognitive and emotional disturbances were found mainly in CKD patients suffering from CHD, thus further corroborating the close relationship between physical factors, cognition and emotion and health-related QoL in CKD.

Our observation that QoL is reduced in the physical, but not mental domain, is well in line with previous studies

Table 4. Predictors for functional health and participation in community dwelling in all patients: Role of medical conditions.

	Disability Dimension								Overall Function							
	Univariate		Model 1		Model 2		Model 3		Univariate		Model 1		Model 2		Model 3	
	B or β	p	B or β	p	B or β	p	B or β	p	B or β	p	B or β	p	B or β	p	B or β	p
Age	−0.22	**0.007**	−0.31	**<0.001**	−0.22	**0.021**	−0.07	0.414	−0.29	**<0.001**	−0.39	**<0.001**	−0.29	**0.001**	−0.20	**0.023**
Gender (male vs. female)	−3.85	**0.018**	−2.94	0.062	−2.76	0.084	−1,30	0.340	1.29	0.515	2.18	0.244	3.77	**0.047**	5,01	**0.004**
Education	0.09	0.276	−0.03	0.711	−0.06	0.453	−0.07	0.388	0.16	**0.037**	0.02	0.763	−0.01	0.920	−0.01	0.873
CKD stage	−0.27	**0.001**	−0.34	**<0.001**	−0.37	**<0.001**	−0.23	**0.007**	−0.25	**0.001**	−0.31	**<0.001**	−0.32	**<0.001**	−0.23	**0.005**
Hemoglobin	0.10	0.223	0.01	0.909	−0.01	0.956	−0.01	0.941	0.17	**0.025**	0.08	0.313	0.04	0.635	0.03	0.714
CHD/myocardial infarct (yes vs. no)	−4.46	**0.005**	–	–	−4.04	**0.018**	−1,81	0.144	−5.78	**0.002**	–	–	−5.54	**0.005**	−3,12	0.089
Stroke/TIA (no vs. yes)	7.65	0.054	–	–	−6.62	0.081	−5,78	0.071	12.79	**0.012**	–	–	−9.45	**0.044**	−9,00	**0.034**
PAD (yes vs. no)	−2.81	0.295	–	–	3.51	0.200	3,37	0.214	−9.27	**0.007**	–	–	−1.90	0.572	−2,06	0.499
Cognitive performance	0.39	**<0.001**	–	–	–	–	0.20	**0.018**	0.36	**<0.001**	–	–	–	–	0.11	0.168
HADS-depression scale	−0.58	**<0.001**	–	–	–	–	−0.51	**<0.001**	−0.48	**<0.001**	–	–	–	–	−0.41	**<0.001**
HADS-anxiety scale	−0.33	**<0.001**	–	–	–	–	0.05	0.635	−0.26	**0.001**	–	–	–	–	0.02	0.821

For the adjusted models, linear regressions were calculated using a forced entry strategy. Model 1: Age, gender, education, CKD stage, hemoglobin. Model 2: Age, gender, education, CKD stage, hemoglobin, CHD or myocardial infarct, stroke or TIA, PAD. Model 3: Age, gender, education, CKD stage, hemoglobin, CHD or myocardial infarct, stroke or TIA, PAD, global cognitive performance, depression and anxiety. CHD, coronary heart disease; CKD, chronic kidney disease; HADS, Hospital Anxiety and Depression Scale; LLFDI, Late-Life Function and Disability Instrument; PAD, peripheral artery disease; SF-36, 36-Item Short Form Health Survey.

Table 5. Predictors for quality of life in all patients: Role of functional health and participation in community dwelling.

	Physical Component								Mental Component							
	Univariate		Model 1		Model 2		Model 3		Univariate		Model 1		Model 2		Model 3	
	B or β	p	B or β	p	B or β	p	B or β	p	B or β	p	B or β	p	B or β	p	B or β	p
Age	−0.22	**0.005**	−0.03	0.699	−0.20	**0.031**	−0.04	0.472	0.04	0.639	0.105	0.200	0.13	0.111	0.07	0.368
Gender (male vs. female)	0.22	0.910	−0.02	0.988	3.60	0.057	0.37	0.752	−1.65	0.369	0.935	0.530	0.10	0.946	1.13	0.431
Education	0.18	0.202	0.09	0.127	0.12	0.127	0.09	0.081	0.03	0.746	−0.081	0.232	−0.09	0.187	−0.10	0.138
CKD stage	−0.21	**0.006**	−0.08	0.152	−0.17	**0.027**	−0.07	0.145	−0.09	0.237	0.032	0.642	0.04	0.561	0.01	0.845
LLFDI:Disability Dimension	0.56	**<0.001**	0.05	0.545	–	–	–	–	0.35	**<0.001**	0.049	0.592	–	–	–	–
LLFDI:Frequency of Performance	0.37	**<0.001**	–	–	0.19	**0.050**	–	–	0.28	**<0.001**	–	–	−0.05	0.573	–	–
LLFDI:Limitation in Capability	0.55	**<0.001**	–	–	0.34	**<0.001**	–	–	0.31	**<0.001**	–	–	0.04	0.640	–	–
LLFDI:Overall Function	0.80	**<0.001**	0.78	**<0.001**	–	–	–	–	0.21	**0.001**	−0.094	0.279	–	–	–	–
LLFDI:Upper Extremity	0.53	**<0.001**	–	–	–	–	−0.07	0.288	0.19	**0.016**	–	–	–	–	−0.10	0.245
LLFDI:Basic Lower Extremity	0.76	**<0.001**	–	–	–	–	0.42	**<0.001**	0.19	**0.014**	–	–	–	–	0.02	0.881

For the adjusted models, linear regressions were calculated using a forced entry strategy. Model 1: Age, gender, education, CKD stage, Disability Dimension, Overall Function, depression, anxiety and global cognitive performance. Model 2: Age, gender, education, CKD stage, Frequency of Performance, Limitation in Capability, depression, anxiety and global cognitive performance 3: Age, gender, education, CKD stage, Upper Extremity, Basic Lower Extremity, Advanced Lower Extremity, depression, anxiety and global cognitive performance. CKD, chronic kidney disease; HADS, Hospital Anxiety and Depression Scale; LLFD, Late-Life Function and Disability Instrument; SF-36, 36-Item Short Form Health Survey.

Table 6. Disease relevant predictors for depressive symptoms in all patients.

	HADS-depression scale							
	Univariat		Model 1		Model 2		Model 3	
	B or β	p	B or β	p	B or β	p	B or β	p
Age	0.10	0.188	0.16	0.068	0.11	0.267	0.06	0.548
Gender (male vs. female)	1.28	0.050	1.06	0.115	0.79	0.264	0.68	0.341
Education	−0.04	0.621	0.01	0.869	0.03	0.708	0.04	0.688
CKD stage	0.18	**0.017**	0.22	**0.013**	0.18	0.061	0.153	0.114
Hemoglobin	−0.05	0.511	0.00	0.960	−0.01	0.267	−0.01	0.958
CHD/myocardial infarct (yes vs. no)	−2.22	**0.001**	-	-	−1.89	**0.011**	−1.77	**0.018**
Stroke/TIA (yes vs. no)	−0.01	0.903	-	-	−0.21	0.897	0.02	0.990
PAD (yes vs. no)	−1.17	0.303	-	-	0.01	0.992	−0.01	0.995
Cognitive Performance	−0.19	**0.012**	-	-	-	-	−0.10	0.328

For the adjusted models, linear regressions were calculated using a forced entry strategy. Model 1: Age, gender, education, CKD stage, hemoglobin. Model 2: Age, gender, education CKD stage, hemoglobin, CHD or myocardial infarct, stroke or TIA, PAD. Model 3: Age, gender, education, CKD stage, CHD or myocardial infarct, stroke or TIA, PAD, global cognitive performance. CHD, coronary heart disease; CKD, chronic kidney disease; HADS, Hospital Anxiety and Depression Scale; PAD, peripheral artery disease; TIA, transient ischemic attack.

[11,13,15,16,32–34]. Interestingly, stage 3–5 and stage 5D patients did not differ to major extent in the physical component of QoL and the overall function dimension of functional health and participation in community dwelling. In case of QoL assessments, patients with advanced (stages 4 and 5) CKD not requiring dialysis previously exhibited either slightly better [15] or comparable [32] QoL scores than stage 5D patients on dialysis. Differences in the constitution of CKD cohorts and dialysis protocols may account for diverging findings in the past. Systematic analyses of functional health and participation in community dwelling have not yet been performed in CKD patients. For assessments of daily life activities, the Karnofsky score has mainly been used in the past [11,34]. The Karnofsky score has been developed for the evaluation of chemotherapies in oncology patients [35]. Unlike the LLFDI, the Karnofsky score represents a rough scale of independence stages ranging from 0 to 100% that does not provide more differentiated insights into late life function and disabilities.

Linear regressions revealed that CHD and myocardial infarcts were the most important predictors both for the disability dimension and overall function dimension of the LLFDI in addition to age and CKD stage, when age, gender, education, CKD stage, hemoglobin and vascular diseases were inserted into a multivariable analysis. Interestingly, CHD and myocardial infarcts did not continue to be predictive for both functional health scales any more, when cognitive performance, depression and anxiety were included into the regression analyses. Thus, depression and - in case of the disability dimension - cognition and anxiety were identified as predictors of functional health and participation in community dwelling. That CHD and myocardial infarcts indeed potently influenced functional health in CKD was confirmed in subsequent studies showing that the mental component of QoL, the disability dimension of the LLFDI, overall function of the LLFDI and cognitive performance decreased with progressive CKD severity in patients suffering from CHD, but not in those without. Moreover, depression and anxiety were selectively increased in CKD stage 5D patients suffering from CHD. That cardiovascular diseases are major factors influencing QoL in CKD has previously been shown [24,36]. In addition to earlier studies, we herein demonstrate that CHD modifies cognitive performance, depression and anxiety in CKD patients. We have previously reported that the inflammation marker fibrinogen predicts cognitive performance in CKD patients in multivariable regression analyses [9]. Whether inflammation associated with CHD is responsible for CKD-related QoL and functional health deficits remains to be shown.

Our observation of a link between CHD, functional health and QoL argues in favor of the so-called 'concept of loss', upon which the loss of physical strength and social activities contributes to depression that in turn compromises QoL [37]. In that study, patients with CKD were characterized using a so-called Kidney Disease Loss Scale that aimed to identify the most severe individual-defined losses and subsequently evaluated grief responses associated with these losses. That depression is highly prevalent in CKD and that it contributes to QoL deficits, is well established [32,37–40]. Although the link between physical deficits and depression is plausible, assessments of overall function in our study revealed that upper extremity deficits were particularly associated with depressive symptoms, whereas lower extremity deficits were associated with reduced QoL. Our observations suggest that physical conditions may affect depression and QoL in different ways.

It is known that the physical component of QoL decreases with age [32,33,41,42] and depressive symptoms [32,36] in CKD. In

Table 7. Predictors for depressive symptoms in all patients: Role of functional health and participation in community dwelling.

HADS-depression scale	Univariate		Model 1		Model 2		Model 3	
	B or β	p	B or β	p	B or β	p	B or β	p
Age	0.10	0.188	−0.05	0.584	−0.00	0.986	−0.05	0.617
Gender (male vs. female)	1.28	0.050	0.71	0.267	0.23	0.742	1.61	**0.010**
Education	−0.04	0.621	−0.01	0.863	−0.02	0.764	0.01	0.855
CKD stage	0.18	**0.017**	−0.01	0.949	0.02	0.804	0.04	0.656
LLFDI:Disability Dimension	−0.58	**<0.001**	−0.45	**<0.001**	–	–	–	–
LLFDI:Frequency of Performance	−0.48	**<0.001**	–	–	−0.33	**<0.001**	–	–
LLFDI:Limitation in Capability	−0.48	**<0.001**	–	–	−0.35	**<0.001**	–	–
LLFDI:Overall Function	−0.50	**<0.001**	−0.21	**0.036**	–	–	–	–
LLFDI:Upper Extremity	−0.41	**<0.001**	–	–	–	–	−0.22	**0.025**
LLFDI:Basic Lower Extremity	−0.46	**<0.001**	–	–	–	–	−0.17	0.190
LLFDI:Advanced Lower Extremity	−0.41	**<0.001**	–	–	–	–	−0.16	0.149
Global cognitive performance	−0.10	**0.012**	0.05	**0.036**	0.05	0.553	−0.02	0.836

For the adjusted models, linear regressions were calculated using a forced entry strategy. Model 1: Age, gender, education, CKD stage, Disability Dimension, Overall Function and global cognitive performance. Model 2: Age, gender, education, CKD stage, Frequency of Performance, Limitation in Capability and global cognitive performance. Model 3: Age, gender, education, CKD stage, Upper Extremity, Basic Lower Extremity, Advanced Lower Extremity and global cognitive performance. CKD, chronic kidney disease; HADS, Hospital Anxiety and Depression Scale; LLFD, Late-Life Function and Disability Instrument.

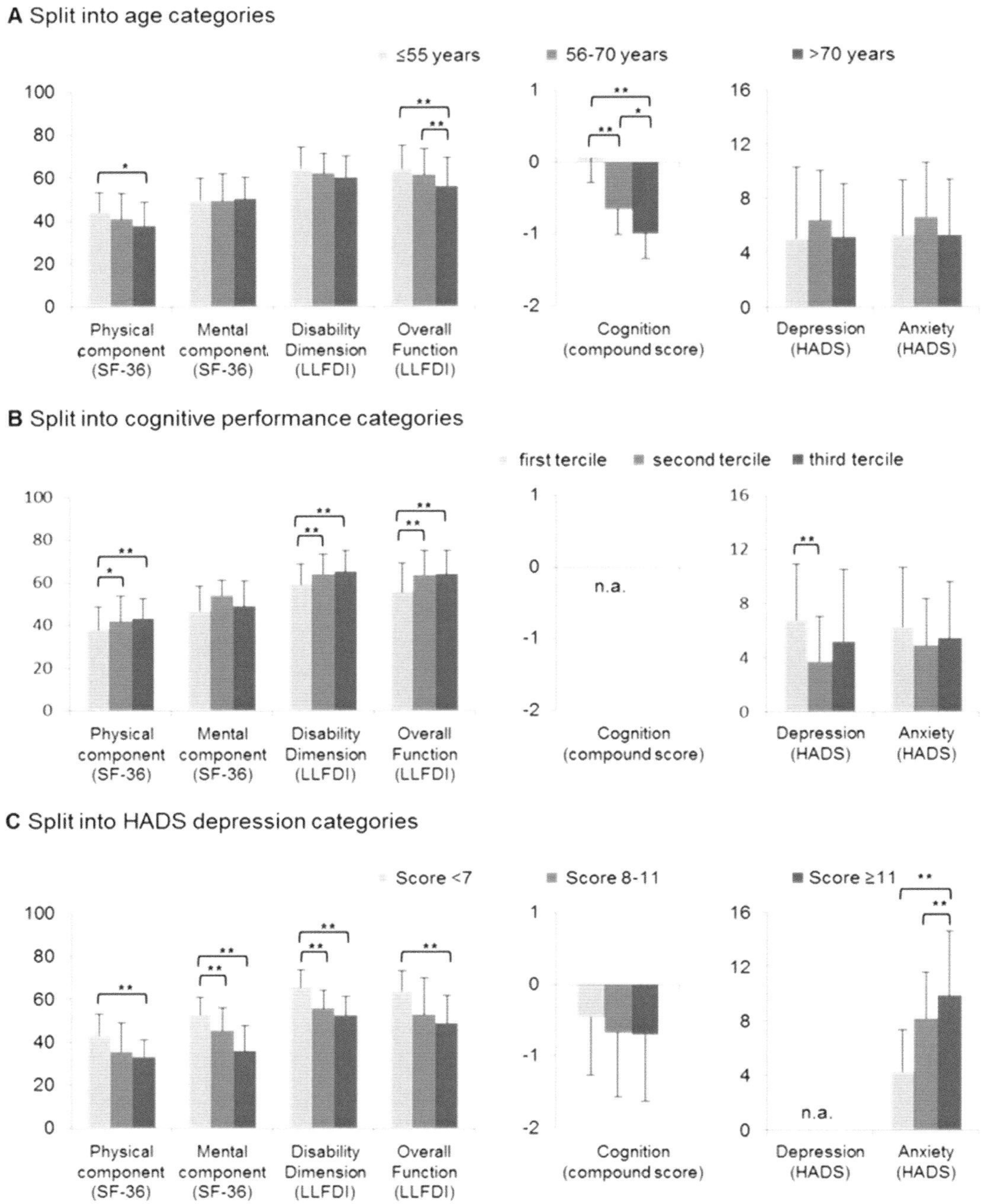

Figure 1. Quality of life, functional health and participation in community dwelling, cognition, depression and anxiety: Role of age, cognition and depressive symptoms. Note that (A) QoL, functional health and participation in community dwelling, and cognitive performance decrease with age. (B) Patients with higher cognitive performance show better physical abilities. Patients with (C) higher depression scores show impairment in QoL and functional health. Data are means and standard deviations. Significance was evaluated by one-way ANOVA followed by Bonferroni (equal variances) or Games-Howell (non-equal variances) tests (in case of normally distributed data) or Kruskall-Wallis followed by Mann-Whitney tests with Bonferroni corrections (in case of non-normally distributed data). $^*p<0.05/^{**}p<0.01$. Cognitive compound score represents z-scores (calculated based on norm values generated in the control cohort), which cover ten neuropsychological tests. First tercile: <-0.620 z-scores, second tercile: $-0.620\leq x<-0.016$ z-scores, third tercile: ≥-0.016 z-scores. CKD, chronic kidney disease; HADS, Hospital Anxiety and Depression Scale; LLFDI, Late-Life Function and Disability Instrument; SF-36, 36-Item Short Form Health Survey.

line with these findings, our studies revealed that the QoL physical component and overall function of the LLFDI decreased with age and depressive symptoms. Interestingly and hitherto unknown, not only age and depressive symptoms, but also cognitive performance were found to modify health-related QoL. Thus, the physical component of QoL, the disability dimension of the LLFDI and the

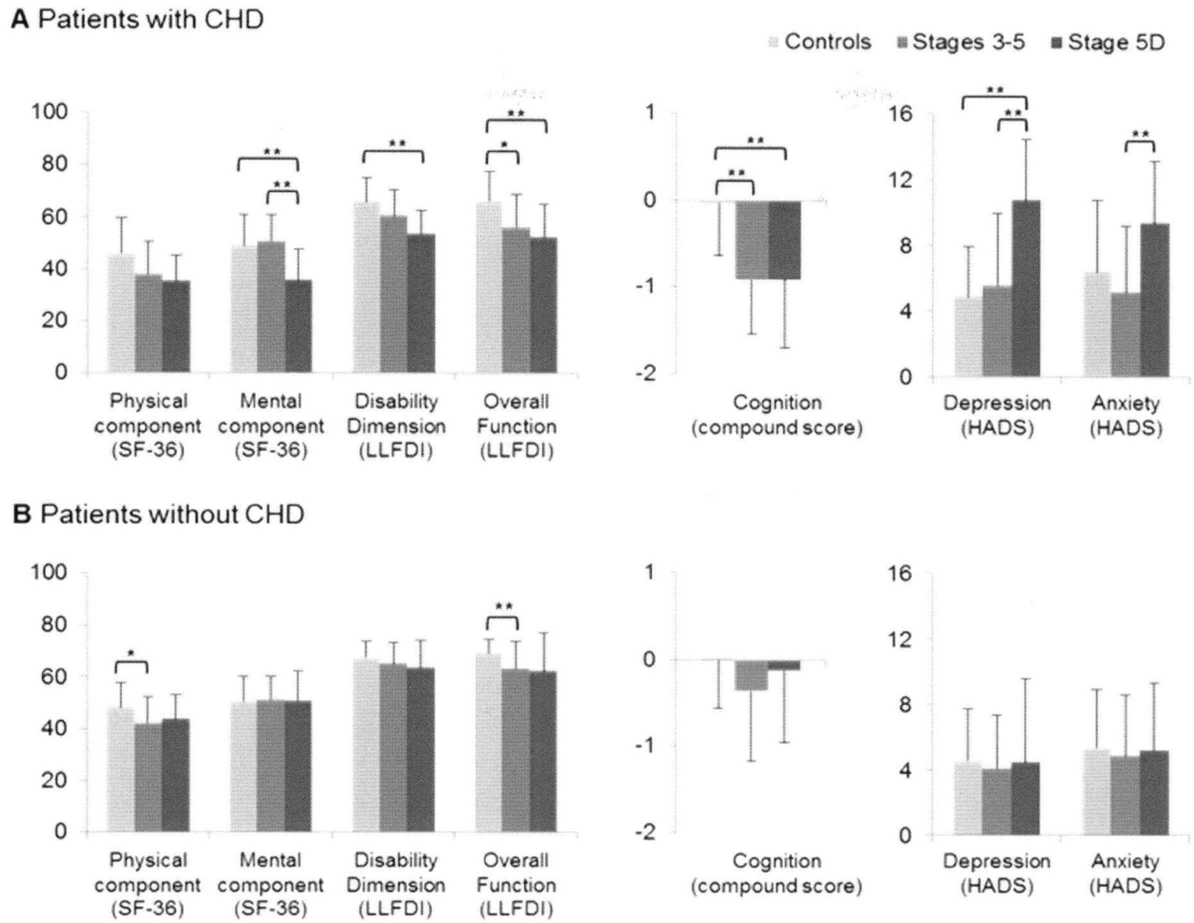

Figure 2. Quality of life, functional health and participation in community dwelling, cognition, depression and anxiety: Role of CKD and CHD. Note that compared with control patients, CKD patients with CHD show impairment in all domains except the physical component of the SF-36. Such impairment is almost absent in patients without CHD. Data are means and standard deviations. Significance was evaluated by one-way ANOVA followed by Bonferroni (equal variances) or Games-Howell (non-equal variances) tests (in case of normally distributed data) or Kruskall-Wallis followed by Mann-Whitney tests with Bonferroni corrections (in case of non-normally distributed data). *$p<0.05$/**$p<0.01$. Cognitive compound score represents z-scores (calculated based on norm values generated in the control cohort), which cover ten neuropsychological tests. CHD, coronary heart disease; CKD, chronic kidney disease; HADS, Hospital Anxiety and Depression Scale; LLFDI, Late-Life Function and Disability Instrument; SF-36, 36-Item Short Form Health Survey.

overall function dimension of the LLFDI increased with cognitive performance. An obvious strength of this study is the recruitment of an own control group of patients without CKD with similar cardiovascular risk profile. In fact, all except three [10,43,44] previous studies used healthy control subjects for evaluating QoL in CKD. Given that this cross-sectional study establishes associations and not causal relationships, longitudinal studies are urgently needed for evaluating the role of physical, cognitive and emotional factors in CKD.

Acknowledgments

We thank Gisela Behrendt for administrative and technical support.

Author Contributions

Conceived and designed the experiments: OT AK HB DMH. Performed the experiments: UKS JG OT MV HB. Analyzed the data: UKS JG DMH. Contributed reagents/materials/analysis tools: AK DMH. Wrote the paper: UKS JG DMH.

References

1. Zhang QL, Rothenbacher D (2008) Prevalence of chronic kidney disease in population-based studies: systematic review. BMC Public Health 8: 117.
2. Avramovic M, Stefanovic V (2012) Health-related quality of life in different stages of renal failure. Artif Organs 36: 581–589.
3. Lopes AA, Bragg-Gresham JL, Satayathum S, McCullough K, Pifer T, et al. (2003) Health-related quality of life and associated outcomes among hemodialysis patients of different ethnicities in the United States: The Dialysis Outcomes and Practice Patterns Study (DOPPS). Am J Kidney Dis 41: 605–615.
4. DeOreo PB (1997) Hemodialysis patient-assessed functional health status predicts continued survival, hospitalization, and dialysis attendance compliance. Am J Kidney Dis 30: 204–212.
5. Lowrie EG, Curtin RB, Lepain N, Schatell D (2003) Medical outcomes study short form-36: a consistent and powerful predictor of morbidity and mortality in dialysis patients. Am J Kidney Disease 41: 1286–1292.
6. Mapes DL, Lopes AA, Satayathum S, McCullough KP, Goodkin DA, et al. (2003) Health-related quality of life as a predictor of mortality and hospitalization: the Dialysis Outcomes and Practice Pattern Study (DOPPS). Kidney Int 64: 339–349.
7. U.S. Renal Data System (2003) Excerpts from the USRDS 2002 Annual Data Report. Atlas of end-stage renal disease in the United States. Am J Kidney Dis 41 (4 Suppl 2): v-ix, S7–S254.

8. Baber U, Auguste U (2013) Patients with chronic kidney disease/diabetes mellitus: the high-risk profile in acute coronary syndrome. Curr Cardiol Rep 15: 386.
9. Seidel UK, Gronewold J, Volsek M, Todica O, Kribben A, et al. (2013) The prevalence, severity, and association with HbA1c and fibrinogen of cognitive impairment in chronic kidney disease. Kidney Int. doi: 10.1038/ki.2013.366.
10. Odden MC, Whooley MA, Shlipak MG (2006) Depression, stress, and quality of life in persons with chronic kidney disease: The Heart and Soul Study. Nephron Clin Pract 103: c1–7.
11. McClellan WM, Anson C, Birkeli K, Tuttle E (1991) Functional status and quality of life: predictors of early mortality among patients entering treatment for end-stage renal disease. J Clin Epidemiol 44: 83–89.
12. Gokal R (1993) Quality of life in patients undergoing renal replacement therapy. Kidney Int Suppl 40: S23–27.
13. Kalantar-Zadeh K, Kopple JD, Block G, Humphreys MH (2001) Association among SF36 quality of life measures and nutrition, hospitalization, and mortality in hemodialysis. J Am Soc Nephrol 12: 2797–2806.
14. Watnick S, Kirwin P, Mahnensmith R, Concato J (2003) The prevalence and treatment of depression among patients starting dialysis. Am J Kidney Dis 41: 105–110.
15. Perlman RL, Finkelstein FO, Liu L, Roys E, Kiser M, et al. (2005) Quality of life in chronic kidney disease (CKD): a cross-sectional analysis in the Renal Research Institute-CKD Study. Am J Kidney Dis 45: 658–666.
16. Mendelssohn DC, Mujais SK, Soroka SD, Brouillette J, Takano T, et al. (2009) A prospective evaluation of renal replacement therapy modality eligibility. Nephrol Dial Transplant 24: 555–561.
17. Abdel-Kader K, Myaskovsky L, Karpov I, Shah J, Hess R, et al. (2009) Individual quality of life in chronic kidney disease: influence of age and dialysis modality. Clin J Am Soc Nephrol 4: 711–718.
18. Ouellette MM, LeBrasseur NK, Bean JF, Phillips E, Stein J, et al. (2004) High-intensity resistance training improves muscle strength, self-reported function, and disability in long-term stroke survivors. Stroke 35: 1404–1409.
19. Lowe SS, Watanabe SM, Baracos VE, Courneya KS (2013) Home-based functional walking program for advanced cancer patients receiving palliative care: a case series. BMC Palliat Care 12(1): 22.
20. Jette AM, Haley SM, Coster WJ, Kooyoomjian JT, Levenson S, et al. (2002) Late Life function and disability instrument: I. Development and evaluation of the disability component. J Gerontol A Biol Si Med Sci 57: M209–216.
21. Haley SM, Jette AM, Coster WJ, Kooyoomjian JT, Levenson S, et al. (2002) Late Life function and disability instrument: II. Development and evaluation of the function component. J Gerontol A Biol Si Med Sci 57: M217–222.
22. Bullinger M, Kirchberger I (1998) SF-36 Fragebogen zum Gesundheitszustand. Göttingen, Germany: Hogrefe.
23. Salem S, Bruck H, Bahlmann FH, Peter M, Passlick-Deetjen J, et al. (2012) Relationship between magnesium and clinical biomarkers on inhibition of vascular calcification. Am J Nephrol 35: 31–39.
24. National Kidney Foundation (2002) K/DOQI clinical practice guidelines for chronic kidney disease: evaluation, classification, and stratification. Am J Kidney Dis 39: S1–266.
25. Zigmond AS, Snaith RP (1983) The hospital anxiety and depression scale. Acta Psychiatr Scand 67: 361–370.
26. Härting C, Markowitsch HJ, Neufeld U, Calabrese P, Deisinger J, et al. (2000) Wechsler Gedächtnistest – Revidierte Fassung (WMS-R). Göttingen, Germany: Hans Huber Verlag.
27. Reitan RM (1992) Trail Making Test. Tucson, AZ: Reitan Neuropsychology Laboratory.
28. Bäumler G (1985) Farbe-Wort-Interferenz-Test nach J. R. Stroop (FWIT). Göttingen, Germany: Hogrefe, Verlag für Psychologie.
29. Aschenbrenner S, Tucha O, Lange KW (2000) Regensburger Wortflüssigkeits-Test. Göttingen, Germany: Hogrefe, Verlag für Psychologie.
30. Russ M (2002) Rey Complex Figure Test. Anleitung für die Anwendung im Frankfurter Neuropsychologischen Testprofil (FNTP). Available: www.fntp.de/mediapool/80/807841/data/CFT_Scoring.pdf. Accessed December 4, 2013.
31. Karp JF, Skidmore E, Lotz M, Lenze E, Dew MA, et al. (2009) Use of the late-life function and disability instrument to assess disability in major depression. J Am Geriatr Soc 57: 1612–1619.
32. Abdel-Kader K, Unruh ML, Weisbord SD (2009) Symptom burden, depression, and quality of life in chronic and endstage kidney disease. Clin J Am Soc Nephrol 4: 1057–1064.
33. Pagels AA, Söderkvist BK, Medin C, Hylander B, Heiwe S (2012) Health-related quality of life in different stages of chronic kidney disease and at initiation of dialysis treatment. Health Qual Life Outcomes 10: 71.
34. Cruz MC, Andrade C, Urrutia M, Draibe S, Nogueira-Martins LA, et al. (2011) Quality of life in patients with chronic kidney disease. Clinics (Sao Paulo) 66: 991–995.
35. Karnofsky DA, Burchenal JH (1949) The clinical evaluation of chemotherapeutic agents in cancer. In: MacLeod CM, ed. Evaluation of chemotherapeutic agents. New York: Columbia University Press 196.
36. Mujais SK, Story K, Brouillette J, Takano T, Soroka S, et al. (2009) Health-related quality of life in CKD patients: correlates and evolution over time. Clin J Am Soc Nephrol 4: 1293–1301.
37. Chan R, Brooks R, Erlich J, Chow J, Suranyi M (2009) The effects of kidney-disease-related loss on long-term dialysis patients depression and quality of life: positive affect as mediator. Clin J Am Soc Nephrol 4: 160–167.
38. Montinaro V, Iaffaldano GP, Granata PP, Porcelli P, Todarello O, et al. (2010) Emotional symptoms, quality of life and cytokine profile in hemodialysis patients. Clin Nephrol 73: 36–43.
39. Feng L, Yap KB, Ng TP (2013) Depressive symptoms in older adults with chronic kidney disease: mortality, quality of life outcomes, and correlates. Am J Geriatr Psychiatry 21: 570–579.
40. Lee YL, Kim MS, Cho S, Kim SR (2013) Association of depression and anxiety with reduced quality of life in patients with predialysis chronic kidney disease. Int J Clin Pract 67: 363–368.
41. Gyamlani G, Basu A, Geraci S, Lee F, Moxey M, et al. (2011) Depression, screening and quality of life in chronic kidney disease. Am J Med Sci 342: 186–191.
42. Kimmel PL, Peterson RA, Weihs KL, Simmens SJ, Boyle DH, et al. (1995) Behavioral compliance with dialysis prescription in hemodialysis patients. J Am Soc Nephrol 5: 1826–1834.
43. Hedayati SS, Jiang W, O'Conner CM, Kuchibhatla M, Krishnan KR, et al. (2004) The association between depression and chronic kidney disease and mortality among patients hospitalized with congestive heart failure. Am J Kidney Dis 44: 207–215.
44. Condé SA, Fernandes N, Santos FR, Chouab A, Mota MM, et al. (2010) Cognitive decline, depression and quality of life in patients at different stages of chronic kidney disease. J Bras Nefrol 32: 242–248.

Epidemiology and Mortality of Liver Abscess in End-Stage Renal Disease Dialysis Patients

Chon-Seng Hong[1], Kun-Ming Chung[2], Po-Chang Huang[3], Jhi-Joung Wang[4*¶], Chun-Ming Yang[5], Chin-Chen Chu[4], Chung-Ching Chio[6], Fu-Lin Chang[7], Chih-Chiang Chien[8,9*¶]

1 Department of Internal Medicine, Chi-Mei Medical Center, Tainan, Taiwan, **2** Department of General Medicine, Chi-Mei Medical Center, Tainan, Taiwan, **3** Department of Orthopedics Medicine, Chi-Mei Medical Center, Taiwan, **4** Department of Medical Research, Chi-Mei Medical Center, Tainan, Taiwan, **5** Department of Neurology, Chi-Mei Medical Center, Tainan, Taiwan, **6** Department of Neurological Surgery, Chi-Mei Medical Center, Tainan, Taiwan, **7** Department of Pharmaceutical Science and Technology, Chung Hwa University of Medical Technology, Tainan, Taiwan, **8** Department of Nephrology, Chi-Mei Medical Center, Tainan, Taiwan, **9** Department of Food Nutrition, Chung Hwa University of Medical Technology, Tainan, Taiwan

Abstract

Background and Objectives: To determine the incidence rates and mortality of liver abscess in ESRD patients on dialysis.

Design, Setting, Participants, & Measurements: Using Taiwan's National Health Insurance Research Database, we collected data from all ESRD patients who initiated dialysis between 2000 and 2006. Patients were followed until death, end of dialysis, or December 31, 2008. Predictors of liver abscess and mortality were identified using Cox models.

Results: Of the 53,249 incident dialysis patients identified, 447 were diagnosed as having liver abscesses during the follow-up period (224/100,000 person-years). The cumulative incidence rate of liver abscess was 0.3%, 1.1%, and 1.5% at 1 year, 5 years, and 7 years, respectively. Elderly patients and patients on peritoneal dialysis had higher incidence rates. The baseline comorbidities of diabetes mellitus, polycystic kidney disease, malignancy, chronic liver disease, biliary tract disease, or alcoholism predicted development of liver abscess. Overall in-hospital mortality was 10.1%.

Conclusions: The incidence of liver abscess is high among ESRD dialysis patients. In addition to the well known risk factors of liver abscess, two other important risk factors, peritoneal dialysis and polycystic kidney disease, were found to predict liver abscess in ESRD dialysis patients.

Editor: Li-Min Huang, National Taiwan University Hospital, Taiwan

Funding: This study was supported by grants CMFHR10242 from Chi Mei Hospital and NHRI-NHIRD-99182 from the National Health Research Institutes in Taiwan. The funders had no role in study design, data collection and analysis, decision to publish, or preparation of the manuscript.

Competing Interests: The authors have declared that no competing interests exist.

* E-mail: ccchien58@yahoo.com.tw (C-C. Chien); 400002@mail.chimei.org.tw (JJW)

These authors contributed equally to this work.

¶ These authors also contributed equally to this work.

Introduction

Liver abscess is associated with significant morbidity, mortality, and increased consumption of healthcare resources [1–3]. Several studies [1–4] report the incidence of liver abscess to be 1.1–3.3 per 100,000 person-years in general Western populations. Liver abscess, which is highly endemic in Taiwan, has an incidence of 11.5–17.5 per 100,000 person-years [5]. Additionally, renal failure is a significant risk factor for liver abscess [5].

The precise incidence of liver abscess has not been investigated in end-stage renal disease (ESRD) dialysis patients. ESRD patients are known to be at increased risk of infectious diseases [6,7], and associated with high mortality [8,9]. Liver abscess is the most common extra-renal abscess among this population [10]. One study from a general population [5] reported that patients with renal disease had three times the risk of liver abscess compared to general population. Yang et al. [11] reported in a hospital-based study using retrospective chart review, that 27 of 20,676 admitted patients with ESRD had liver abscess. However, no any longitudinal cohort study have investigated the precise incidence of liver abscess in ESRD dialysis patients.

Although the global prevalence and incidence of ESRD dialysis patients has recently increased markedly [12,13], there are no published epidemiological data on subject of increased risked of liver abscess using a national cohort of dialysis patients. Nearly half of ESRD patients have DM. In addition, they are characteristically older in age and at increased risk of infectious diseases. We hypothesized that this patient population would have a high incidence of liver abscess. To find out, we used a national cohort longitudinal follow-up design to calculate the incidence of this disease in ESRD patients receiving dialysis. We trapped a large data set, Taiwan's National Health Insurance Research Database

(NHIRD), to perform a nationwide investigation of the epidemiology, incidence, and mortality of liver abscess in ESRD dialysis patients.

Methods

Database

For this study, we retrieved ambulatory care claims, all inpatient claims, and the updated registry for all ESRD patients receiving dialysis from 1998 to 2008. Data was collected from Taiwan's NHIRD provided by Taiwan's National Health Insurance (NHI), a compulsory universal health insurance program which has covered the healthcare costs of all of Taiwan's residents except of prison inmates since 1995. The program requires all medical institutions to use standard computerized claim documents for reimbursement of medical expenses. Patients with end-stage renal disease (ESRD) are eligible for every type of renal replacement therapy without any charge, and all their expenses are covered by NHI. The NHIRD contains nearly all (99%) inpatient and outpatient medical benefit claims for the 23 million residents of Taiwan, and has been used extensively in various studies [14–17]. This database provides a great deal of information, including gender, birth date, dates of admission and discharge, the medical institutions providing the services, the ICD-9-CM (International Classification of Diseases, 9th Revision, Clinical Modification) diagnostic and procedure codes (up to five each), and encrypted outcomes. NHIRD is released with de-identified secondary data for public research purposes. All personal identification information on files connected with the present study was scrambled using surrogate identification numbers to ensure patient confidentiality. The Bureau of National Health Insurance approves the application (NHRI-NHIRD-99182), and the institutional review board of Chi-Mei Medical Center waived the need for approval.

Patient Selection and Definition

This longitudinal cohort study selected adult ESRD patients (≥ 18 years old) on maintenance dialysis who began renal replacement therapy between January 1, 2000, and December 31, 2006. ESRD patients on maintenance dialysis were defined as having undergone dialysis for more than 90 days. Patients who had undergone renal transplantation before beginning dialysis were excluded. Patients were followed-up from the first reported date of dialysis to the date of death, end of dialysis, or December 31, 2008. The data of 53,249 incident dialysis patients were analyzed.

We linked study subjects to their inpatient claim data to identify the first episode of liver abscess. Cases were selected by using the following criteria: the 3 primary discharge diagnoses included liver abscess (ICD-9-CM 572.0). A total of 447 patients were diagnosed with liver abscess during the follow-up period.

Demographic and Comorbid Variables

We linked to the diagnostic codes through the inpatient and outpatient claims databases of the NHIRD. We collected survival status, date of death, patient demographics, and baseline comorbidities. Baseline comorbidities, which were diabetes mellitus (DM), polycystic kidney disease (PCKD), malignancy, chronic liver disease (CLD), biliary tract disease, and alcoholism, are important factors affecting episodes of liver abscess [1–5,11] and were assessed at the start of dialysis.

Statistical Analysis

The incidence of newly diagnosed liver abscess was expressed as the number of cases of liver abscess per 100,000 person-years. Parametric Pearson's chi square test was used to compare each variable in the groups of patients with and without liver abscess. Age was entered as a categorical variable (18–44, 45–64, and 65 years or older). Significance was set at $p<0.05$. The cumulative proportion of patients with liver abscess and of survivors after liver abscess were calculated using the Kaplan-Meier method. The log rank test was used to analyze significance. Cox proportional hazards models were used to identify the risk factors of liver abscess and mortality after liver abscess. Hazard ratios (HRs) and 95% confidence intervals (CIs) were derived from Cox proportional hazards models. Cox models met the assumption of proportionality of risks. To adjust for potential confounding in the relationship between comorbidities and the risk of mortality, multivariate analyses were used to model to all-cause mortality. The Statistical Package for Social Sciences for Windows 17.0 (SPSS Inc; Chicago, IL, USA) was used for all statistical analyses.

Results

Demographics and Clinical Characteristics

A total 53249 adult incident dialysis patients were enrolled in this study. Of these patients, 447 patients (224/100,000 person-years) had liver abscess during the follow-up period (Table 1). Elderly patients had higher incidence of liver abscesses. Only 0.5% of the patients 18–44 years old and 0.9% of those ≥65 years old had liver abscess ($p = 0.003$). Patients with liver abscess tended to have more comorbidities than those without it. Many more patients with liver abscess than without it had DM, PCKD, malignancy, CLD, biliary tract disease, and alcoholism. Mean in-hospital stays was 22.74±17.56 days. During the study period, there were 211 and 18,612 deaths in patients with and without liver abscess group, respectively.

Cumulative Incidence and Risk Factors for Liver Abscess

The cumulative incidence rates of liver abscess in ESRD dialysis patients were 0.3% at one year, 0.7% at three years, 1.1% at five years, and 1.5% at seven years (Figure 1). After multivariate adjustment, no significant difference was found between male and female patients (Table 2). Patients ≥65 years had more than twice the incidence of liver abscess than those 18–44 years old (HR 2.33, 95% CI: 1.64–3.32). Patients on hemodialysis (HD) had a lower rate of liver abscess than those on peritoneal dialysis (PD) (HR 0.66, 95% CI: 0.46–0.93). Additionally, the following predicted a higher incidence of liver abscess: DM (HR 1.72, 95% CI: 1.41–2.09), PCKD (HR 1.99, 95% CI: 1.09–3.64), malignancy (HR 1.81, 95% CI: 1.32–2.49), CLD (HR 1.76, 95% CI: 1.44–2.17), biliary tract disease (HR 4.21, 95% CI: 2.36–7.51) or alcoholism (HR 2.617, 95% CI: 1.28–5.37).

Cumulative Survival Rate and Risk Factors for All-cause-mortality

Overall in-hospital mortality of liver abscess was 10.14% (Figure 2). Survival curves after liver abscess were stratified by those with and without liver abscess. For the control group (patients without liver abscess), patients' age, sex, mode of dialysis and comorbidities were matched to the liver abscess group. Patients with DM had a 64% higher risk of long-term death after liver abscess (HR 1.64, 95% CI: 1.19–2.25) than those without DM (Table 3). Additionally, having CLD was also associated with significantly higher long-term mortality after liver abscess (HR 1.62, 95% CI: 1.17–2.25).

Table 1. Patient characteristics and association with (n = 447) and without (n = 52802) liver abscess among end-stage renal disease dialysis patients.

	Without LA	(n = 52,802)	With LA	(n = 447)	P
	n	(%)	n	(%)	
Sex					0.283
Female	27242	(99.1)	242	(0.9)	
Male	25560	(99.2)	205	(0.8)	
Age (years)					0.003
18–44	7421	(99.5)	39	(0.5)	
45–64	23125	(99.2)	197	(0.8)	
≥65	22256	(99.1)	211	(0.9)	
Dialysis modality					0.55
PD	3749	(99.1)	35	(0.9)	
HD	49053	(99.2)	412	(0.8)	
Diabetic mellitus					<0.001
No	26896	(99.3)	190	(0.7)	
Yes	25906	(99)	257	(1)	
Coronary artery disease					0.864
No	40462	(99.2)	341	(0.8)	
Yes	12340	(99.1)	106	(0.9)	
Cerebrovascular disease					0.027
No	46245	(99.2)	376	(0.8)	
Yes	6557	(98.9)	71	(1.1)	
Chronic obstructive lung disease					0.299
No	47779	(99.2)	398	(0.8)	
Yes	5023	(99)	49	(1)	
Malignancy					0.03
No	49520	(99.2)	404	(0.8)	
Yes	3282	(98.7)	43	(1.3)	
Polycystic kidney disease					0.084
No	52026	(99.2)	436	(0.8)	
Yes	776	(98.6)	11	(1.4)	
Chronic liver disease					<0.001
No	41935	(99.3)	306	(0.7)	
Yes	10867	(98.7)	141	(1.3)	
Biliary tract disease					<0.001
No	52525	(99.2)	435	(0.8)	
Yes	277	(95.8)	12	(4.2)	
Alcoholism					0.001
No	52484	(99.2)	439	(0.8)	
Yes	318	(97.5)	8	(2.5)	
Death	18612	(35.4)	211	(47.3)	<0.001

Data are n (%) unless otherwise indicated. LA: liver abscess. PD: Peritoneal dialysis; HD: Hemodialysis.

Discussion

This study represents the first nationwide population-based epidemiological study to investigate the incidence of liver abscess in chronic dialysis patients. ESRD patients receiving dialysis had a significantly higher incidence of liver abscess than general population. In addition to the well-known risk factors of liver abscess, this study was the first to report both peritoneal dialysis and polycystic kidney disease to be important risk factors for liver abscess in ESRD dialysis patients.

ESRD patients receiving dialysis have a significantly higher incidence of liver abscess. Previous studies [1–4] report an annual incidence of liver abscess to be about 1.1–3.3 per 100,000 person-years in general populations in Denmark, Canada, and the United States (Table 4). In Taiwan, Tsai et al. [5] reported that incidence to be 17.59 per 100,000

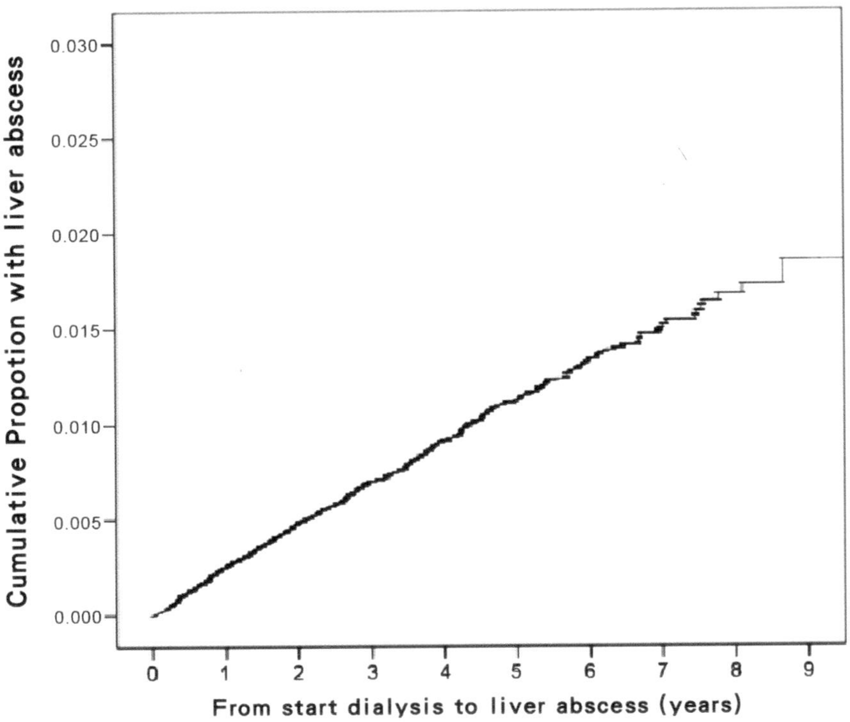

Number at risk 53249 47335 40528 30049 21463 14740 9523 5470 2257 47

Figure 1. Cumulative proportion of liver abscess in end-stage renal disease dialysis patients.

person-years. *Klebsiella pneumoniae* liver abscess is an endemic health problem in the East Asia and is emerging as a global disease [18]. In Taiwan, *Klebsiella pneumoniae* is the primary pathogen and DM is a major predisposing factor of liver abscess [5]. Renal disease is also a strong risk factor of liver abscess. Neutrophil dysfunction and the risk of infection are higher in ESRD dialysis patients than in the general population [6,7]. This study found that ESRD patients receiving dialysis to have much higher incidence of liver abscess, around 224 per 100,000 person-years. Diabetic nephropathy is the leading cause of ESRD, accounting for 40–50% of patients on maintenance dialysis [16]. Therefore, it is no surprise that the incidence of liver abscess was found to be high among chronic dialysis patients.

Besides the well-known risk factors in general population, this study found PCKD and PD to be as significant risk factors for liver abscess among ESRD dialysis patients. One study reported that 83% of PCKD between the ages of 15 and 46 years have hepatic cysts [19], entities associated with significant risk for liver abscess formation [20,21]. Patients with PCKD in this study had nearly twice the risk of liver abscess than those without it. Dialysis modality was found to be an important risk factor. The most frequent infective complication of PD is peritonitis. Because intra-abdominal infection like bowel leakage or peritonitis is a major cause of liver abscess formation, it is reasonable to speculate that patients on PD have a higher risk of liver abscess than those on HD. Further studies are needed at next step to evaluate the mechanism underlying the development of liver abscess in PD patients based on the result of this study.

The in-hospital mortality in ESRD in this study (10.14%) was similar to that in the general Taiwanese population (10.9%) reported by Tsai et al. [5]. Because liver abscess is mostly an acute illness, the determinant factors for short-term mortality are always the severity of the acute illness and immediate

Table 2. Risk factor for liver abscess after initiation of dialysis in end-stage renal disease dialysis patients (n = 53,249).

Factors	Univariate HR (95% CI)	Multivariate HR (95% CI)
Sex (Male vs. Female)	0.954 (0.792–1.149)	0.922 (0.764–1.112)
Age (years)		
<45 (Referent)	1	1
45–64	1.826 (1.295–2.575)*	1.577 (1.110–2.240)*
≥65	2.597 (1.842–3.662)*	2.333 (1.638–3.323)*
Dialysis modality (HD vs. PD)	0.899 (0.637–1.270)	0.656 (0.461–0.932)*
Comorbidities		
Diabetic mellitus (yes vs. no)	1.711 (1.416–2.066)*	1.718 (1.414–2.087)*
PCKD (yes vs. no)	1.620 (0.890–2.947)	1.987 (1.086–3.636)*
Malignancy (yes vs. no)	1.978 (1.444–2.709)*	1.809 (1.316–2.486)*
Chronic liver disease (yes vs. no)	1.784 (1.461–2.178)*	1.764 (1.436–2.165)*
Biliary tract disease (yes vs. no)	5.680 (3.201–10.08)*	4.211 (2.362–7.508)*
Alcoholism (yes vs. no)	3.827 (1.901–7.701)*	2.617 (1.277–5.365)*

*HR adjusted for sex, age, dialysis modality, diabetic mellitus, polycystic kidney. disease, malignancy, chronic liver disease, biliary tract disease and alcoholism.
*HR: Hazard ratio; CI: Confidence interval; PD: Peritoneal dialysis; HD: Hemodialysis; PCKD: polycystic kidney disease.

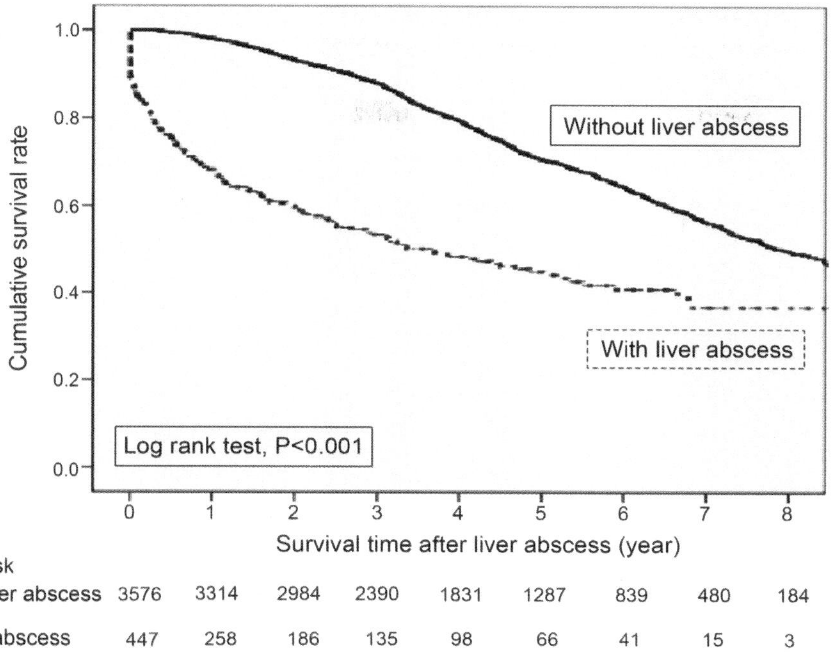

Figure 2. Overall survival curves after liver abscess in end-stage renal disease dialysis patients stratified by with and without liver abscess. For the control group (patients without liver abscess), patients' age, sex, mode of dialysis and comorbidities were matched to the liver abscess group.

therapy. In Taiwan, medical resource is very popular and sound. The medical expensed for patients with ESRD are covered by the National Health Insurance program. Drainage of liver abscess can be performed in most hospitals in Taiwan, especially for patients found to be refractory to antibiotic treatment. Thus, the average short term mortality rate between

Table 3. Risk factor for long-term mortality after liver abscess in end-stage renal disease dialysis patients (n = 447).

Factors	Univariate analysis	Multivariate analysis
	HR (95% CI)	HR (95% CI)
Sex (Male vs. Female)	1.083 (0.825–1.422)	1.082 (0.820–1.427)
Age (years)		
<45 (referent)	1	1
45–64	1.111 (0.552–2.236)	0.965 (0.465–2.000)
≥65	2.125 (1.082–4.172)*	1.975 (0.971–4.008)
Dialysis modality (HD vs. PD)	1.721 (0.912–3.249)	1.461 (0.764–2.795)
Comorbidities		
Diabetic Mellitus (yes vs. no)	1.545 (1.156–2.065)*	1.639 (1.193–2.252)*
Coronary artery disease (yes vs. no)	1.325 (0.981–1.789)	1.166 (0.840–1.618)
Cerebrovascular disease (yes vs. no)	1.354 (0.959–1.913)	1.149 (0.804–1.642)
COPD (yes vs. no)	0.877 (0.558–1.377)	0.832 (0.526–1.316)
Malignancy (yes vs. no)	1.377 (0.906–2.092)	1.093 (0.702–1.704)
PCKD (yes vs. no)	0.345 (0.086–1.389)	0.533 (0.129–2.195)
Chronic liver disease (yes vs. no)	0.929 (0.112–7.677)	1.622 (1.170–2.249)*
Biliary tract disease (yes vs. no)	2.016 (0.992–4.094)	1.729 (0.836–3.587)
Alcoholism (yes vs. no)	1.540 (0.570–4.157)	1.834 (0.632–5.322)

*HR adjusted for sex, age, dialysis modalities, diabetic mellitus, congestive heart failure, coronary artery disease, cerebrovascular accident, chronic obstructive pulmonary disease, polycystic kidney disease, malignancy, chronic liver disease, biliary tract disease and alcoholism.
*HR: Hazard ratio; CI: Confidence interval; PD: Peritoneal dialysis; HD: Hemodialysis; COPD: chronic obstructive pulmonary disease; PCKD: polycystic kidney disease.
*$P<0.05$.

Table 4. Incidence, risk factors, and in-hospital mortality from liver abscess in different study population.

Author	Country	Study population	Annual incidence (n/100,000)	Risk factor for LA	In-hospital mortality (%)
Hansen et al.[6]	Demark	County - based	1.1	DM, alcoholism	6
		General population	/100,000 general population		
Mølle et al.[7]	Demark	Nationwide-based	23.3		Alcoholic cirrhosis: 38.5%
		Liver cirrhosis population	/100,000 Liver cirrhosis		Non - alcoholic cirrhosis: 62.5%
Kaplan et al.[8]	Canada	City - based	2.3	Older age, DM, caner	10
		General population	/100,000 general population	men, liver tansplantation,	
Meddings et al.[9]	United States	Nationwide - based	3.6		6
		General population	/100,000 General population		
Tsai et al.[10]	Taiwan	Nationwide - based	11.5~17.5	DM, cancer,	10.9
		General population	/100,000 general population	renal disease, pneumonia	
Yang et al.[11]	Taiwan	Hospital - based	NA	DM	33.3
		ESRD population	(Chart review)		
This study	Taiwan	Nationwide - based	224.9	PD, Older age, DM,	10.14
		ESRD population	/100,000 ESRD population	biliary tract disease	
				alcoholism, PCKD	

DM: diabetes mellitus; PCKD: polycystic kidney disease.

patient with and without ESRD is similar. Yang et al. [11], performing a study in a referral hospital (National Taiwan University Hospital) for the most seriously ill patients in Taiwan, reported that the mortality rate for liver abscess among ESRD patients to be 33.3%, much higher than the result reported in the current study based on nationwide and representative data. Thus, it is reasonable to speculate that in-hospital mortality due to liver abscess among ESRD patients would probably be high if acute treatment is performed in referral hospitals reserved for seriously ill patients.

Although the in-hospital death from liver abscess is most often acute, long-term mortality in our study population was often related to their ESRD status and baseline comorbidities, mostly DM and CLD. This study found DM to be an independent predictor of long-term mortality from liver abscess in ESRD dialysis patients. ESRD dialysis patients with DM generally have multiple comorbidities and have a higher risk of death [22–27]. Taiwan is an endemic area of chronic hepatitis because of a high prevalence of virus hepatitis B and C infection. Only few previous studies showed that the CLD to be an independent predictor of mortality. Liu et al. used United States Renal Data System to demonstrate liver disease is independent predictors of mortality (Relative risk 1.21, 95%CI: 1.15–1.27) [28]. Chien et al. further used Taiwan National Health Insurance Database [16] to report a high prevalence rate of liver cirrhosis among ESRD patients, and showed that liver cirrhosis is an important predictor of mortality in dialysis patients (HR 1.472, 95% CI: 1.329–1.634). ESRD patients with PCKD is a different disease entity from those without PCKD, who also frequently have DM, hypertension, glomerulonephritis and cardiovascular disease. ESRD patients with PCKD on dialysis have a significantly longer survival rate than those without PCKD [29–31]. We further analyzed the differences between ESRD patients with and without PCKD in our database. We also found that patients with PCKD tended to have less comorbidities than those without it. Only 13.2%, 16.5%, and 13.2% of patients with PCKD had DM, coronary artery disease, and heart failure, respectively. However, 49.7%, 23.5%, and 25.7% of patients without PCKD had DM, coronary artery disease, and heart failure, respectively. Perrone et al. [28], using data from the United States Renal Data System, found a lower mortality rate in PCKD dialysis patients than in nondiabetic dialysis patients. Zeier et al. [29] presumed that such an improvement may be a result of better hemoglobin levels on cardiac function.

This study has several limitations. First, similar to other studies using administrative data, our study has the problem of unmeasured confounders. Second, the comorbidities were identified based on claims data and ICD-9-CM diagnosis codes, some of which might have been incorrect. Third, our study lacked specific data on nutritional status, microbiology and biochemical data, as well as socioeconomic characteristics. The lack of microbiological data limited the interpretation of the impact of these findings in the settings. Finally, it is better to obtain more information when comparing ESRD patients with liver abscess to patients with liver abscess but no ESRD. However, our database (NHRI-NHIRD-99182) only included ESRD patients receiving dialysis, but no non-ESRD subjects for comparison. Thus, we were unable to use the current database to compare ESRD patients with liver abscess to patients with liver abscess but without ESRD.

In conclusion, there is a high incidence of liver abscess in ESRD dialysis patients, especially patients ≥ 65 years, receiving PD, and those with a history of DM, PCKD, malignancy, CLD, biliary tract disease, or alcoholism. More attention should be paid to awareness of liver abscess when treating these high-risk patients.

Author Contributions

Conceived and designed the experiments: CSH KMC C.C. Chien. Performed the experiments: CSH KMC JJW C.C. Chu C.C. Chio C.C. Chien. Analyzed the data: CSH KMC JJW PCH CMY FLC C.C. Chu C.C. Chio C.C. Chien. Contributed reagents/materials/analysis tools: C.C. Chien. Wrote the paper: CSH C.C. Chien.

References

1. Hansen PS, Schønheyder HC (1998) Pyogenic hepatic abscess. A 10-year population-based retrospective study. APMIS 106: 396–402.
2. Mølle I, Thulstrup AM, Vilstrup H, Sørensen HT (2001) Increased risk and case fatality rate of pyogenic liver abscess in patients with liver cirrhosis: a nationwide study in Denmark. Gut 48: 260–263.
3. Kaplan GG, Gregson DB, Laupland KB (2004) Population-based study of the epidemiology of and the risk factors for pyogenic liver abscess. Clin Gastroenterol Hepatol 2: 1032–1038.
4. Meddings L, Myers RP, Hubbard J, Shaheen AA, Laupland KB, et al. (2010) A population-based study of pyogenic liver abscesses in the United States: incidence, mortality, and temporal trends. Am J Gastroenterol 105: 117–124.
5. Tsai FC, Huang YT, Chang LY, Wang JT (2008) Pyogenic liver abscess as endemic disease, Taiwan. Emerg Infect Dis 14: 1592–1600.
6. Chonchol M (2006) Neutrophil dysfunction and infection risk in end-stage renal disease. Semin Dial 19: 291–296.
7. Vanholder R, Ringoir S (1993) Infectious morbidity and defects of phagocytic function in end-stage renal disease: a review. J Am Soc Nephrol 3: 1541–1554.
8. Gabriel R (1984) Morbidity and mortality of long-term haemodialysis: a review. J R Soc Med 77: 595–601.
9. Collins AJ, Foley RN, Gilbertson DT, Chen SC (2009) The state of chronic kidney disease, ESRD, and morbidity and mortality in the first year of dialysis. Clin J Am Soc Nephrol (Suppl 1): S5–S11.
10. Chuang FR, Lee CH, Chen JB, Cheng YF, Yang BY (2002) Extra-renal abscess in chronic hemodialysis patients. Ren Fail 24: 511–521.
11. Yang YF, Wang HJ, Kan WC, Kuo HL, Huang CC (2006) Pyogenic liver abscess in ESRD patients undergoing maintenance dialysis therapy. Am J Kidney Dis 47: 856–861.
12. United States Renal Data System (2009) Excerpts from the USRDS 2009 annual data report: atlas of end-stage renal disease in the United States. Available: http://www.usrds.org. Accessed 2011 August 25.
13. Yang WC, Hwang SJ, Taiwan Society of Nephrology (2008) Incidence, prevalence and mortality trends of dialysis end-stage renal disease in Taiwan from 1990 to 2001: the impact of national health insurance. Nephrol Dial Transplant 23: 3977–3982.
14. Chen HA, Wang JJ, Chou CT, Chien CC, Chu CC, et al. (2011) Predictors of longterm mortality in patients with and without systemic lupus erythematosus on maintenance dialysis: a comparative study. J Rheumatol 38: 2390–2394.
15. Chien CC, Yen CS, Wang JJ, Chen HA, Chou MT, et al. (2012) Reverse epidemiology of hypertension-mortality associations in hemodialysis patients: a long-term population-based study. Am J Hypertens 25: 900–906.
16. Chien CC, Wang JJ, Sun YM, Sun DP, Sheu MJ, et al. (2012) Long-term survival and predictors for mortality among dialysis patients in an endemic area for chronic liver disease: a national cohort study in Taiwan. BMC Nephrol 13: 43.
17. Chou MT, Wang JJ, Sun YM, Sheu MJ, Chu CC, et al. (2013) Epidemiology and mortality among dialysis patients with acute coronary syndrome: Taiwan National Cohort Study. Int J Cardiol 167: 2719–2723.
18. Siu LK, Yeh KM, Lin JC, Fung CP, Chang FY (2012) Klebsiella pneumoniae liver abscess: a new invasive syndrome. Lancet Infect Dis 12: 881–887.
19. Bae KT, Zhu F, Chapman AB, Torres VE, Grantham JJ, et al. (2006) Magnetic resonance imaging evaluation of hepatic cysts in early autosomal-dominant polycystic kidney disease: the Consortium for Radiologic Imaging Studies of Polycystic Kidney Disease cohort. Clin J Am Soc Nephrol 1: 64–69.
20. Telenti A, Torres VE, Gross JB Jr, Van Scoy RE, Brown ML, et al. (1990) Hepatic cyst infection in autosomal dominant polycystic kidney disease. Mayo Clin Proc 65: 933–942.
21. Cigarrán S, Neches C, Lamas JM, García-Trio G, Alonso M, et al. (2008) A case report of a pyogenic liver abscess caused by Fusobacterium nucleatum in a patient with autosomal dominant polycystic kidney disease undergoing hemodialysis. Ther Apher Dial 12: 91–95.
22. Lee KT, Wong SR, Sheen PC (2001) Pyogenic liver abscess: an audit of 10 years' experience and analysis of risk factors. Dig Surg 18: 459–465.
23. Chen SC, Lee YT, Lai KC, Cheng KS, Jeng LB, et al. (2006) Risk factors for developing metastatic infection from pyogenic liver abscesses. Swiss Med Wkly 136: 119–126.
24. United States Renal Data System (2010) Excerpts from the USRDS 2009 annual data report: Atlas of end-stage renal disease in the United States. Am J Kidney Dis (Suppl 1): S1–S420.
25. Wolfe RA, Gaylin DS, Port FK, Held PJ, Wood CL (1992) Using USRDS generated mortality tables to compare local ESRD mortality rates to national rates. Kidney Int 42: 991–996.
26. United States Renal Data System (2006) Excerpts from the USRDS 2005 annual data report: Atlas of end-stage renal disease in the United States. Am J Kidney Dis (Suppl 1): S1–S286.
27. Tien KJ, Lin ZZ, Chio CC, Wang JJ, Chu CC, et al (2013) Epidemiology and Mortality of New-Onset Diabetes Mellitus After Dialysis: Taiwan national cohort study. Diabetes Care 36: 3027–3032.
28. Liu J, Huang Z, Gilbertson DT, Foley RN, Collins AJ (2010) An improved comorbidity index for outcome analyses among dialysis patients. Kidney Int 77: 141–151.
29. Lee PW, Chien CC, Yang WC, Wang JJ, Lin CC (2013) Epidemiology and mortality in dialysis patients with and without polycystic kidney disease: a national study in Taiwan. J Nephrol 26: 755–762.
30. Perrone RD, Ruthazer R, Terrin NC (2001) Survival after end-stage renal disease in autosomal dominant polycystic kidney disease: contribution of extrarenal complications to mortality. Am J Kidney Dis 38: 777–784.
31. Zeier M, Jones E, Ritz E (1996) Autosomal dominant polycystic kidney disease—the patient on renal replacement therapy. Nephrol Dial Transplant 11 Suppl 6: 18–20.

4

Elevated Serum Interleukin-18 Level Is Associated with All-Cause Mortality in Stable Hemodialysis Patients Independently of Cardiac Dysfunction

Yen-Wen Liu[1], Chi-Ting Su[2], Yu-Tzu Chang[3], Wei-Chuan Tsai[1], Yu-Ru Su[4], Saprina P. H. Wang[5], Chun-Shin Yang[6], Liang-Miin Tsai[1], Jyh-Hong Chen[1], Junne-Ming Sung[3]*

1 Division of Cardiology, Department of Internal Medicine, National Cheng Kung University Hospital, College of Medicine, National Cheng Kung University, Tainan, Taiwan, **2** Division of Nephrology, Department of Internal Medicine, National Taiwan University Hospital Yun-Lin Branch, Yun-Lin, Taiwan, **3** Division of Nephrology, Department of Internal Medicine, National Cheng Kung University Hospital, College of Medicine, National Cheng Kung University, Tainan, Taiwan, **4** Department of Statistics, National Cheng Kung University, Tainan, Taiwan, **5** Graduate Institute of Biomedical Engineering, National Cheng Kung University, Tainan, Taiwan, **6** Division of Nephrology, Department of Internal Medicine, Catholic Fu-An Hospital, Yun-Lin, Taiwan

Abstract

Background: High circulating interleukin (IL)-18 level predicts a higher hospitalization rate among dialysis patients, possibly through cardiovascular mechanisms; however, whether higher IL-18 level is associated with mortality in dialysis patients is less clear. In addition, its impacts on left ventricular (LV) function are also unknown. We conducted a cohort study to examine the impacts of IL-18 level on LV function and prognosis among clinically stable hemodialysis patients.

Methods: Clinically stable patients undergoing maintenance hemodialysis (≥3 months) were prospectively enrolled from December 2008 to January 2009, and were followed up for 31 months. The enrolled patients (41% male, 66.4±10.9 years of age) received 2-dimensional echocardiography and myocardial deformation (strain) analysis, including LV peak systolic longitudinal strain (GLS) and circumferential strain (CS). Laboratory measurements were also performed. Cox regression analysis was used to investigate prognostic factors.

Results: Seventy-five patients were stratified into 2 groups by the median value of IL-18 (654.2 pg/ml). Between these 2 groups, there was no significant difference in baseline characteristics including LV ejection fraction. The high IL-18 group had a worse LV systolic function as demonstrated by reduced GLS and CS. Seventeen patients (22.7%) died during the follow-up period. Multivariate Cox regression analysis showed that low serum albumin, the presence of hypertension, high serum IL-18, and less negative GLS (>−15%) were independently associated with all-cause mortality. No significant interaction between IL-18 and less negative GLS was noted in the final Cox model.

Conclusion: Hemodialysis patients with high IL-18 levels tend to have worse LV systolic function and higher mortality rate. However, elevated serum IL-18 level is predictive of poor prognosis among stable hemodialysis patients, independently of LV dysfunction. This suggests an additional value of IL-18 to echocardiographic study in predicting all-cause mortality, and IL-18 may be helpful in early risk stratification of hemodialysis patients.

Editor: Matthias Stuber, Centre Hospitalier Universitaire Vaudois, Switzerland

Funding: This study was supported by the National Science Council (NSC), Executive Yuan,Taipei, Taiwan: Grants NSC 98-2314-B-006-051 and 101-2314-B-006-035. The funders had no role in study design, data collection and analysis, decision to publish, or preparation of the manuscript.

Competing Interests: The authors have declared that no competing interests exist.

* E-mail: jmsung@mail.ncku.edu.tw

Introduction

End-stage renal disease (ESRD) is notorious for high mortality, and cardiovascular disease is the leading cause of morbidity and mortality [1–3]. Thus, early cardiovascular risk stratification and understanding the mechanism(s) are important issues in managing dialysis patients, and they may enable early identification of high-risk patients and optimizing therapeutic interventions. Increased circulating levels of pro-inflammatory cytokines, such as C-reactive protein (CRP), interleukin (IL)-6 and 18, can be detected among ESRD patients. The increased pro-inflammatory cytokines play a crucial role in chronic inflammation, and are associated with cardiovascular events and poor outcomes in dialysis patients [4–7]. Among the inflammatory cytokines, elevated IL-18 level was shown to be associated with higher future hospitalization rate in dialysis patients, possibly, through cardiovascular mechanisms [7,8]. Evidence from the experimental and clinical studies emerge that the expression of IL-18 is intimately related to atherosclerotic plaque progression and vulnerability [9–12]. Furthermore, over-expression of IL-18 was reported to lead to aggravated cardiac remodeling in animals [13], and daily administration of IL-18 may cause myocardial dysfunction in healthy mice [14]. Thus, it is suggested that IL-18 possibly causes LV dysfunction indirectly by aggravating coronary atherosclerosis or directly by acting on cardiomyocytes to induce myocardial dysfunction [11–14]. Increased levels of circulating IL-18 have proved to be a strong and independent predictor of cardiovascular death in patients with coronary artery disease (CAD) [15]. However, whether a higher IL-18 level is associated with mortality and whether IL-18 is useful for early risk stratification in dialysis patients are still unclear.

Cardiac structural and functional abnormalities are associated with high cardiovascular and all-cause mortality among ESRD patients, and cardiovascular abnormalities can be used for risk stratification of hemodialysis patients. [16–18]. To explore the role of IL-18 in all-cause mortality, the relationships between the serum IL-18 level and outcome-related cardiac structural and functional abnormalities should be clarified. Left ventricular (LV) function in ESRD patients has been studied extensively by conventional echocardiographic parameters, e.g. LV ejection fraction (LVEF). However, these measurements are semi-quantitative and are insensitive in the early detection of subtly deteriorating cardiac function [19]. Two-dimensional speckle-tracking echocardiography (STE) with myocardial deformation analysis (2D strain analysis) is an objective and reproducible modality that is more sensitive than conventional echocardiographic study for assessing subtle LV dysfunction, and it is especially true for evaluating the systolic function [20–22]. LV peak systolic longitudinal strain (GLS) (or circumferential strain [CS]) is the ratio of the maximal change in myocardial longitudinal (or circumferential length) in systole to the original length. During systole, LV myocardium in the longitudinal and circumferential directions shortens, so GLS and CS are represented by a negative value. More negative of GLS or CS values refer to better LV systolic function. Importantly, less negative GLS has been proven to be a more sensitive and powerful predictor of all-cause mortality than LVEF in general population [23]. Furthermore, our recent study indicated an additional value of GLS to conventional echocardiography in predicting all-cause and cardiac mortality in stable hemodialysis patients with preserved LVEF (LVEF≥50%) [24]. To date, the impact of elevated IL-18 on LV function is not well studied in ESRD patients receiving maintenance hemodialysis. In the current studies, we aimed to investigate the association between IL-18 levels and LV function using 2D strain analysis and to assess the outcome predictive effects of IL-18 in clinically stable hemodialysis patients.

Materials and Methods

Ethics Statement

The study adhered to the Declaration of Helsinki. The study protocol was approved by the Human Research and Ethics Committee of the National Cheng Kung University Hospital (IRB number: ER-98-073). All the enrolled patients provided written informed consent.

Study Design

As previously described [24,25], from December 2008 to January 2009, we prospectively enrolled adult ESRD patients (≥ 18 years old) receiving maintenance hemodialysis program, 4 hours/day, three times a week for more than 3 months, from two community hospitals in Yun-Lin, Taiwan: the National Cheng Kung University Hospital Dou-Liou Branch, and the Catholic Fu-An Hospital. The exclusion criteria are as follows: (1) severe valvular heart disease (including mitral/aortic regurgitation or stenosis); (2) recent infection; (3) hospitalization due to an active episode of decompensated heart failure (HF) presenting with pulmonary edema (≥NYHA FC III) or acute coronary syndrome in recent 3 months; (4) atrial fibrillation; (5) refusing blood tests; and (6) poor echocardiographic image quality.

Upon enrollment, clinical information on co-morbidities, medical history, and current cardiovascular medication were obtained by careful review of each patient's medical record and a self-reported questionnaire. Patients' compliance with regards to prescribed medication was reliably ascertained. Additionally, the adequacy of dialysis was evaluated based on the recommendations of the Kidney/Disease Outcome Quality Initiative (KDOQI). The enrolled patient medical records during the follow-up period (31 months, from December 2008 to June 2011) were carefully reviewed, and all the participants were assured to receive adequate clearance of dialysis.

Laboratory Measurements

Blood was collected just before the midweek dialysis session in the same week when echocardiographic study was performed. Serum was stored at −80°C until analysis and thawed to measure the levels of high-sensitivity C-reactive protein (hsCRP, BN II analyzer; Dade Behring, Glasgow, DE), IL-6 (chemiluminescent sandwich ELISA, Quantikine Human IL-6; R&D Systems Inc., Minneapolis, MN, USA), IL-18 (Sandwich ELISA, R&D Inc., Minneapolis, MN, USA), and procollagen type I C-terminal peptide (PICP, Takara Bio Inc., Otsu, Shiga, Japan) [24,25]. Serum cholesterol, triglyceride, calcium, phosphate, and albumin were measured using an automatic analyzer.

Echocardiographic Measurements

All patients were examined in the left lateral decubitus position by one well-trained cardiologist (YWL, with 10 years' experience with echocardiographic examination) using a commercially available ultrasound system with a 3.5 MHz probe (Vivid-i, GE Healthcare, Horten, Norway). As previously described, two-dimensional STE and tissue Doppler imaging (TDI) were obtained [21,22,24,25]. All hemodialysis patients received an echocardiographic examination during the halfway point of the hemodialysis session (the second or third hour of each session) [22]. According to the recommendation of the American Society of Echocardiography (ASE) [26,27], we measured LV mass index, volume, and LVEF, left atrial volume index. Using pulsed-wave Doppler, we measured the peak early (E)-wave and late (A)-wave velocities of the mitral inflow.

The pulse TDI of the mitral annulus movement was acquired from the apical 4-chamber view when a sample volume was placed first at the septal side and then at the lateral side of the mitral annulus. To obtain the peak systolic (s′) and early diastolic (e′) velocities, we measured 3 end-expiratory beats and averaged these values for further analysis. We used the average e′ velocity acquired from the septal and lateral sides of mitral annulus to calculate ratio of the mitral inflow E velocity to e′ velocity (average $E/e' = E/[(e'_{septal}+e'_{lateral})/2]$). We acquired 2D gray-scale images in the 3 standard apical views (i.e. apical 4-chamber, apical 2-chamber, and apical 3-chamber) for 3 cardiac cycles and stored digitally with a frame rate of 50–90 frames/second for subsequent off-line analysis.

Inferior vena cava (IVC) diameter measurement in ESRD patients

To evaluate the fluid status of ESRD patients, we measured IVC diameter twice at the end of expiration in a subxiphoid location and just proximal to the junction of the hepatic veins that lie approximately 0.5 to 3.0 cm proximal to the ostium of the right atium [22,28–30]. The average value of the measured end-

Table 1. Baseline demographic characteristic of hemodialysis (HD) patients.

	Total (n = 75)	IL-18 <654.2 pg/ml (n = 38)	IL-18 ≥654.2 pg/ml (n = 37)	p^*
Age (years)	66.4±10.9	66.4±11.1	66.4±10.9	0.97
Male, n (%)	31 (41%)	16 (42%)	15 (41%)	0.89
BMI (kg/m^2)	21.9±2.8	21.8±3.1	22.0±2.5	0.76
Heart Rate (beats/minute)	77.1±12.1	76.8±13.3	77.5±10.9	0.81
SBP (mmHg)	146.1±16.0	145.3±16.4	147.0±15.9	0.65
DBP (mmHg)	76.9±8.5	75.9±7.1	77.9±9.6	0.30
HD duration (years)‡	6.1±5.1	5.0±3.7	7.4±6.2	0.24
Kt/V	1.70±0.24	1.74±0.26	1.67±0.21	0.22
IDWG (%)	5.2±1.8	4.9±1.5	5.5±2.1	0.18
Concomitant diseases, number (%)				
Prevalent CAD	30 (40%)	12 (32%)	17 (46%)	0.20
Heart failure under control	12 (16%)	5 (13%)	7 (19%)	0.50
Diabetes mellitus	38 (51%)	18 (47%)	20 (54%)	0.56
Hypertension	64 (85%)	32 (84%)	32 (86%)	0.78
Hyperlipidemia	20 (27%)	11 (29%)	9 (24%)	0.65
LV hypertrophy	60 (80%)	29 (76%)	31 (84%)	0.67
Chronic hepatitis	38 (51%)	14 (37%)	24 (65%)	0.02
Cardiovascular drugs, number (%)				
CCB	41 (55%)	20 (53%)	21 (57%)	0.72
β-Blockade	34 (45%)	17 (45%)	17 (46%)	0.92
ACEIs/ARBs	42 (56%)	21 (55%)	21 (57%)	0.90
Statin	12 (16%)	5 (13%)	7 (19%)	0.50
Serum biochemistry study				
Calcium (mg/dL)	9.2±0.8	9.3±0.8	9.1±0.8	0.45
Phosphate (mg/dL)	4.5±1.3	4.5±1.3	4.5±1.4	0.87
Albumin (g/dL)	3.3±0.3	3.4±0.3	3.3±0.4	0.17
Cholesterol (mg/dL)	167.2±38.6	169.6±36.6	164.8±40.8	0.60
Triglyceride (mg/dL)‡	143.9±114.0	156.4±144.7	131.3±71.4	0.91
IL-6 (pg/ml)‡	20.1±59.5	27.3±81.9	12.2±9.0	0.76
IL-18 (pg/ml)‡	949.1±750.0	731.6±550.5	1172.4±862.3	<0.001
hsCRP (mg/dL)‡	1.0±1.5	0.5±0.5	1.5±2.0	0.03
PICP (ng/ml)	878.5±382.5	842.8±356.8	917.4±410.3	0.41

Abbreviations: ACEI, angiotensin-converting enzyme inhibitor; ARB, angiotensin II-receptor blocker; BMI, body mass index; CAD, coronary artery disease; CCB, calcium channel blocker; DBP, diastolic blood pressure; hsCRP, high-sensitivity C-reactive protein; IDWG, inter-dialytic weight gain; IL, interleukin; LV, left ventricular; PICP procollagen type I C-terminal peptide.; SBP, systolic blood pressure.

Continuous data are expressed as mean ± SD.

‡Non-normal distributed continuous data.

* *p* value by Student's *t*-test for normal distributed continuous data, nonparametric Mann-Whitney U test for non-normal distributed continuous data, and chi-square test or Fisher's exact test for categorical variables.

expiratory IVC diameter was defined as IVCe. It has been reported that IVCe>1.53 cm is a marker of hypervolemia in ESRD patients [22,30].

Echocardiographic Analysis

Off-line 2D strain analysis was performed using automated function imaging software (EchoPAC work station, BT09, GE Healthcare, Israel). Peak systolic longitudinal strain was automatically obtained from the 3 standard apical views. The average peak systolic longitudinal strain value from the 3 apical views was regarded as GLS [21,22,24]. Six LV segments on the para-sternal short-axis view at the mid-papillary level were examined to obtain the circumferential strain in systole and the average of the circumferential strain of these six segments was defined as CS [21,24].

Because the hemodialysis patients received echocardiographic examinations during dialysis in the study, we performed echocardiography twice (during hemodialysis and on a non-dialysis day) for 10 of these patients to explore whether hemodialysis per se affects GLS. There was no significant difference in GLS during hemodialysis versus a non-dialysis day (−17.0±5.8% *vs.* −16.6±5.8%, respectively; $p = 0.87$). In addition, the Bland-Altman analysis revealed no systemic bias of GLS between intra- and inter-observer agreements [24].

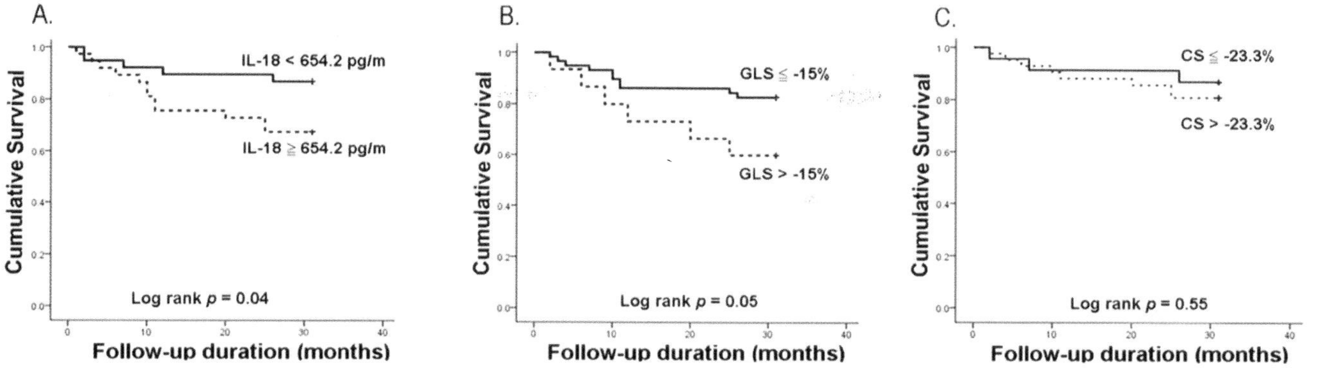

Figure 1. Kaplan-Meier survival curves of all-cause mortality in clinically stable hemodialysis patients using the cutoff values of interleukin (IL)-18 (A), left ventricular global peak systolic longitudinal strain (GLS) (B), and circumferential strain (C).

Statistical Analysis

Continuous data were presented as mean ± standard deviation. Dichotomous data were presented as numbers and percentages. The differences in continuous variables were evaluated using Student's *t*-test, or Mann-Whitney U test when the data did not follow normal distributions. Chi-square test or Fisher's exact test was used for comparing categorical variables. Kaplan-Meier method with log-rank test was used to compare survival rates between strata. The relationships among continuous variables were evaluated using Pearson correlation analysis or Spearman's correlation analysis when the data did not follow normal distributions. The uni- and multi-variate Cox regression analyses were used to examine the risk factors of all-cause mortality. A $p <$ 0.05 was considered statistically significant, and all statistical analyses were made using the SPSS (Statistical Package for the Social Sciences) software (version 17.0, SPSS Inc, Chicago, IL, USA).

Results

Clinical Characteristics

In total, 109 ESRD patients undergoing maintenance hemodialysis were eligible for this study. Patients were subsequently excluded because of old age (≥80 years, n = 3), atrial fibrillation (n = 4), recent infarction (n = 1), decompensated HF within 3 months (n = 5), severe valvular heart disease (n = 2), or inadequate

Table 2. Echocardiographic study results of stable hemodialysis patients.

	Total (n = 75)	IL-18 <654.2 pg/ml (n = 38)	IL-18 ≥654.2 pg/ml (n = 37)	p^*
Traditional parameters				
LV EDVi (ml/m^2)‡	73.6±25.8	72.4±23.6	74.5±27.7	0.78
LV mass index (gm/m^2)‡	153.2±58.1	153.5±61.3	152.8±49.5	0.46
LV EF (%)‡	62.9±8.8	63.6±8.6	62.1±9.1	0.68
E velocity (cm/sec)	80.0±29.6	74.8±27.7	85.8±31.0	0.13
E/A	0.82±0.40	0.87±0.50	0.75±0.22	0.19
LAVi (ml/m^2)	34.8±8.1	32.9±8.3	36.3±7.8	0.16
IVCe diameter (cm)	1.27±0.31	1.26±0.26	1.29±0.36	0.70
Tissue Doppler imaging parameters				
s' (cm/sec)	8.3±2.2	8.5±2.2	8.0±2.2	0.32
Average e' (cm/sec)	4.8±1.4	4.8±1.3	4.8±1.4	0.88
Average E/e'	17.5±9.1	17.0±10.5	18.1±7.4	0.63
Two-dimensional strain analysis				
GLS (%)	−17.8±3.9	−18.7±4.1	−16.8±3.4	0.03
LSRs (sec^{-1})	−0.97±0.22	−1.00±0.22	−0.92±0.22	0.13
Circumferential strain (%)	−20.6±6.3	−22.1±6.2	−18.8±6.0	0.03
CSRs (sec^{-1})	−1.90±0.65	−1.91±0.49	−1.88±0.80	0.85

Abbreviations: CSRs, systolic circumferential strain rate; EDVi, end-diastolic volume index; EF, ejection fraction; E/e', early transmitral velocity to tissue Doppler mitral annular early diastolic velocity ratio; GLS, global left ventricular peak systolic longitudinal strain; IVCe, end-expiratory inferior vena cava diameter; LAVi, left atrial volume index; LSRs, systolic longitudinal strain rate; LV, left ventricular; s', peak systolic mitral annular velocity.
Data are expressed as mean ± SD.
‡Non-normal distributed continuous data.
* p value by Student's *t*-test for normal distributed continuous data and nonparametric Mann-Whitney U test for non-normal distributed continuous data.

Table 3. Baseline demographic characteristic of hemodialysis patients with left ventricular global peak systolic longitudinal strain (GLS)≤−15% or GLS>−15%.

	GLS≤−15% (n = 59)	GLS>−15% (n = 16)	*p*
Age (years)	67.0±10.5	64.1±12.6	0.40
Male, n (%)	22 (54%)	9 (56%)	0.17
BMI (kg/m^2)*	22.0±2.9	21.4±2.5	0.61*
Heart Rate (beats/minute)	77.3±11.8	76.1±14.1	0.78
SBP (mmHg)	147.1±15.1	142.6±19.1	0.41
DBP (mmHg)	77.1±8.2	76.2±9.6	0.75
Hemodialysis duration (years)*	6.3±5.2	5.0±4.6	0.36*
Kt/V	1.72±0.22	1.64±0.31	0.43
IDWG (%)	5.1±1.9	5.4±1.4	0.54
Prevalent CAD	16 (27%)	13 (82%)	<0.01
Heart failure under control	4 (7%)	8 (50%)	<0.01
Diabetes mellitus	29 (49%)	9 (56%)	0.62
Hypertension	51 (86%)	32 (82%)	0.69
Hyperlipidemia	18 (31%)	2 (13%)	0.21
LV hypertrophy	50 (85%)	15 (94%)	>0.99
LV EDVi (ml/m^2)	70.1±18.4	84.6±40.7	0.23
LV mass index (gm/m^2)*	139.1±31.0	201.1±95.0	<0.01*
LV EF (%)	65.0±6.5	55.4±11.6	<0.01
E/A	0.78±0.37	0.96±0.46	0.17
LAVi (ml/m^2)	33.3±7.7	41.6±6.8	0.01
IVCe diameter (cm)	1.21±0.23	1.50±0.44	0.03
s′ (cm/sec)	8.7±1.9	6.7±2.6	0.01
Average e′ (cm/sec)	5.0±1.3	4.0±1.3	0.01
Average E/e′*	16.3±8.0	21.9±11.6	0.03*
PICP (ng/ml)	877.0±394.2	883.9±349.3	0.95

Abbreviations: BMI, body mass index; CAD, coronary artery disease; DBP, diastolic blood pressure; EDVi, end-diastolic volume index; EF, ejection fraction; E/e′, early transmitral velocity to tissue Doppler mitral annular early diastolic velocity ratio; GLS, global left ventricular peak systolic longitudinal strain; IDWG, inter-dialytic weight gain; IVCe, end-expiratory inferior vena cava diameter; Kt/V, dialysis clearance; LAVi, left atrial volume index; LSRs, systolic longitudinal strain rate; LV, left ventricular; PICP procollagen type I C-terminal peptide; SBP, systolic blood pressure; s′, peak systolic mitral annular velocity.
Data are expressed as mean ± standard deviation or number (%).
* *P* values were calculated by nonparametric Mann-Whitney U test.

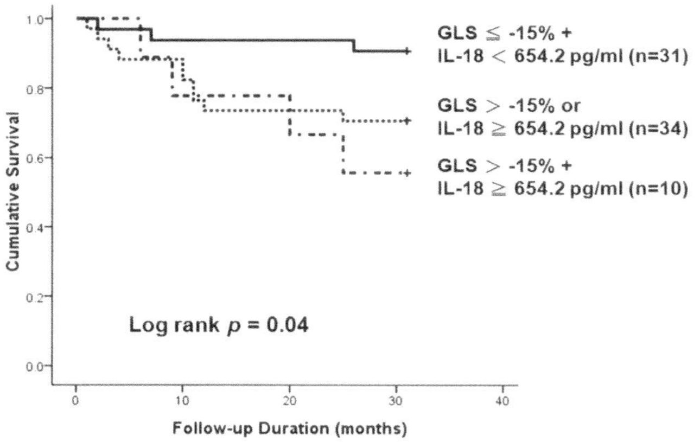

Figure 2. Kaplan-Meier survival curves of all-cause mortality in clinically stable hemodialysis patients using the cutoff values of interleukin (IL)-18 and left ventricular global peak systolic longitudinal strain (GLS). Clinically stable hemodialysis patients with high IL-18 levels (≥667 pg/ml) and less negative GLS (>−15%) had the worst prognosis.

image quality for analysis (n = 6). Thirteen patients were subsequently excluded due to missing data of IL-18 (because of insufficient volumes of stored serum in theses 13 patients for assaying IL-18 levels); thus, there were 75 patients entering the final statistic analyses. There was no significant difference, except for modest difference of cholesterol and triglyceride levels, between the baseline clinical characteristics of patients included in final analyses and those of 19 excluded patients (6 with inadequate echocardiographic images and 13 with missing IL-18 data). Furthermore, there was no significant difference in echocardiographic parameters between patients included in final analyses and 13 excluded because of missing IL-18 data. All enrolled patients presented with anuria. Based on the recommendations of the KDOQI, they all received adequate hemodialysis (average Kt/V [an indicator of dialysis adequacy; K, urea clearance; T, dialysis time; V, urea distribution volume] was 1.71±0.24; and cardiothoracic ratio on chest X-ray was 48±5%).

Since the distribution of IL-18 levels was skewed to the right (skewness = 2.14), we defined the median concentrations of IL-18 (654.2 pg/ml) as the cut-off values. According to this cutoff, the enrolled patients were stratified into two groups: (1) high IL-18

Table 4. Univariate Cox regression analysis of factors in relation to all-cause mortality.

Variables	All-Cause Mortality	
	HR (95% C.I.)	*p* value
Gender, male	0.60 (0.23–1.56)	0.29
Age (years)	1.05 (1.002–1.10)	0.04
Prevalent HF	1.19 (0.34–4.15)	0.78
Prevalent CAD	2.76 (1.05–7.27)	0.04
Hypertension	3.67 (1.35–9.97)	0.01
Diabetes mellitus	1.89 (0.70–5.12)	0.21
LV hypertrophy	0.31 (0.09–1.10)	0.07
Hyperlipidemia	0.54 (0.16–1.87)	0.33
Chronic hepatitis	1.87 (0.69–5.05)	0.22
Hemodialysis duration (years)	0.97 (0.86–1.09)	0.59
Kt/V	0.47 (0.05–4.24)	0.50
IDWG (%)	1.02 (0.79–1.33)	0.86
Heart rate (beats/minute)	0.99 (0.95–1.04)	0.75
CCB prescription	0.54 (0.21–1.43)	0.22
β-blockade prescription	0.63 (0.23–1.70)	0.36
ACEIs/ARBs prescription	0.29 (0.10–1.18)	0.12
Statin prescription	0.66 (0.15–2.89)	0.58
Serum Albumin (g/dL)	0.07 (0.01–0.36)	0.002
Serum hs-CRP (mg/dL)	1.25 (0.92–1.49)	0.11
Serum IL-6 (pg/ml)	0.99 (0.94–1.05)	0.83
Serum IL-18 (pg/ml)	1.001 (1.00–1.001)	0.007
Serum PICP (ng/ml)	1.00 (0.99–1.002)	0.62
Serum Ca * P	0.98(0.95–1.02)	0.35
LV mass index (gm/m^2)	1.00 (0.99–1.01)	0.98
LV EF (%)	0.99 (0.94–1.05)	0.84
LAVi (ml/m^2)	1.03 (0.96–1.10)	0.47
Average E/e′	0.99 (0.93–1.06)	0.75
GLS (%)	1.09 (0.95–1.24)	0.23
LSRs (sec^{-1})	1.66 (0.16–17.42)	0.67
Circumferential strain (%)	1.06 (0.96–1.16)	0.25
Systolic circumferential strain rate (sec^{-1})	1.09 (0.43–2.78)	0.85
Increased IL-18 level (≥654.2 pg/ml)	2.71 (1.01–7.70)	0.04
Less negative GLS (>−15%)	2.61 (0.95–7.18)	0.05
Less negative Circumferential strain (>−23.3%)	1.50 (0.40–5.65)	0.55

Abbreviations: ACEI, angiotensin-converting enzyme inhibitor; ARB, angiotensin II-receptor blocker; CAD, coronary artery disease; CCB, calcium channel blocker; hsCRP, high-sensitivity C-reactive protein; IDWG, inter-dialytic weight gain; IL, interleukin; Kt/V, dialysis clearance; LV, left ventricular; PICP procollagen type I C-terminal peptide; EF, ejection fraction; E/e′, early transmitral velocity to tissue Doppler mitral annular early diastolic velocity ratio; GLS, global left ventricular peak systolic longitudinal strain; LAVi, left atrial volume index; LSRs, systolic longitudinal strain rate; LSRe, early diastolic longitudinal strain rate.

group (IL-18 ≥654.2 pg/ml, n = 37) with IL-18 values of 1479.5±753.5 pg/ml; and (2) low IL-18 group (IL-18 < 654.2 pg/ml, n = 38) with IL-18 values of 432.6±131.2 pg/ml. There was no significant difference of demographic data, concomitant diseases (except chronic hepatitis), medication(s), and blood biochemical test results between these two groups (Table 1).

Follow-up outcome

The enrolled patients were followed up for 26.4±9.4 months (range 1 to 31 months). No patient was lost during the follow-up period. Seventeen patients (22.7%) died, including eight from cardiovascular death, six from infections, and three from liver diseases. Importantly, the high IL-18 group had a worse prognosis (mortality rate: high IL-18 group *vs.* low IL-18 group: 32.4% *vs.* 13.2%, $p = 0.046$, Figure 1A).

Evaluation of Volume Status

In this study, LVEDVi (LV end-diastolic volume index) and IVCe were measured to assess the patients' volume status. There was no significant difference in either LVEDVi or IVCe between the two groups (Table 2), and the IVCe was not engorged in either group. These data indicated that the patients included in these two groups were not hypervolemic.

Evaluation of Cardiac Function

Based on the diagnostic criteria of LV hypertrophy [26], most of the enrolled patients had LV hypertrophy (Tables 1 and 2). There were 4 patients with reduced LVEF (<50%) in the high IL-18 group and 2 in the low IL-18 group. No significant difference of LVEF or s′ existed between these two groups. Nevertheless, the high IL-18 group had less negative GLS and CS, indicating worse LV systolic function (Table 2), and this difference might suggest that subclinical LV systolic dysfunction may partially contribute to a worse prognosis in clinically stable hemodialysis patients with high IL-18 levels. In addition, most of the enrolled patients in both groups had LV diastolic dysfunction, presenting with reverse E/A ratio, high average E/e′ values, and increased PICP levels, indicating the presence of increased LV filling pressure [25].

Because GLS might be affected by the intravascular volume status or blood pressure, we evaluated patient characteristics by stratifying the patients into two groups (GLS≤−15% vs. GLS>−15%, Table 3). There was no significant difference in either blood pressure or hypertension prevalence, nor were these two patient groups hypervolemic.

Prognostic predictors

Kaplan-Meier survival curve revealed that the high IL-18 group had higher all-cause mortality rate (Figure 1A). Recently, we proved that less negative GLS (GLS>−15%) is a prognostic predictor in clinically stable hemodialysis patients with preserved LVEF [24]. However, the cutoff of CS to evaluate its prognostic role in hemodialysis patients is still unknown. Based on a recent meta-analysis study regarding the normal value of CS [31], we defined the CS cutoff point as −23.3%. Using the cutoffs of GLS (−15%) and CS (−23.3%), we demonstrated that GLS ($p = 0.05$, nearly significant), but not CS ($p = 0.55$), might provide prognostic information (Figure 1B and 1C). Furthermore, patients with both a high IL-18 level and less negative GLS had the highest all-cause mortality rate (Figure 2), suggesting that the combination of IL-18 and GLS may be a more powerful prognostic predictor. However, these data cannot exclude the possible interaction between IL-18 level and GLS measurement to all-cause mortality in stable hemodialysis patients.

Subsequently, using univariate Cox regression analysis, we found several potential factors associated with the risk of all-cause mortality, including old age, prevalent CAD, hypertension, low serum albumin level, and increased serum IL-18 concentrations, and less negative GLS (all $p<0.05$ except for the reduced GLS [$p = 0.05$, marginal significance], Table 4). We then performed correlation analyses between different parameters of potential

Table 5. Correlation study between different parameters.

	Albumin	IL-18	hsCRP	Ca*P	HD duration (years)	
GLS	Pearson/Spearman's* Correlation	−0.174	0.196*	0.199*	−0.089	−0.191*
	p value	0.15	0.10*	0.09*	0.46	0.13*
CS	Pearson/Spearman's* Correlation	−0.217	0.239*	0.188*	−0.021	−0.140*
	p value	0.09	0.07*	0.14*	0.87	0.30*
Albumin	Pearson/Spearman's* Correlation		−0.196*	−0.549*	0.197	−0.061*
	p value		0.10*	<0.01*	0.10	0.63*
IL-18	Pearson/Spearman's* Correlation	−0.196*		0.281*	0.027*	0.218*
	p value	0.10*		0.02*	0.82*	0.08*
hsCRP	Pearson/Spearman's* Correlation	−0.549*	0.281*		0.013*	0.192*
	p value	<0.01*	0.02*		0.91*	0.13*
Ca*P	Pearson/Spearman's* Correlation	0.197	0.027*	0.013*		0.100*
	p value	0.10	0.82*	0.91*		0.43*

Abbreviations: CS, circumferential strain; GLS, Global left ventricular peak systolic longitudinal strain; HD, hemodialysis; hsCRP, high-sensitivity C-reactive protein; IL, interleukin.
* The non-normal distributed data were analyzed by Spearman's correlation analysis.

prognostic factors and found a modest correlation between IL-18 and hsCRP levels, and a moderate correlation between hsCRP and albumin levels (Table 5). We then conducted 5 multivariate Cox regression models to determine independent prognostic predictors of all-cause mortality. For the stable hemodialysis patients, decreased albumin level, hypertension, increased serum IL-18 level, and less negative GLS were the independent prognostic predictors (Table 6). Furthermore, no significant interaction between serum IL-18 levels and less negative GLS were noted in terms of all-cause mortality ($p = 0.74$). Receiver operating characteristic curve analysis revealed that using a combination of GLS and IL-18 may facilitate risk stratification for the outcomes (Figure 3).

Discussion

In this prospective cohort study, we demonstrated for the first time that hemodialysis patients with high serum IL-18 concentrations had worse LV systolic function, represented as less negative GLS and CS (Table 2), and higher all-cause mortality (Figure 1A) compared with patients with low IL-18 levels. However, increased IL-18 levels predicted higher all-cause mortality in clinically stable hemodialysis patients, independently of LV dysfunction (Tables 4 and 6). Furthermore, we highlighted the concomitant application of GLS and IL-18 for better prognostic risk assessment in clinically stable hemodialysis patients (Table 6 and Figure 3).

Chiang et al. [7] reported that serum IL-18 level is a strong predictor of hospitalization in hemodialysis patients; however, serum IL-18 did not predict future mortality in hemodialysis patients in their studies. The follow-up period in their study was 12 months, which may be too short when evaluating mortality (only 10.8% in their study). On the contrary, the follow-up period in our study was 31months (26.4±9.4 months in the enrolled patients) with 22.7% mortality, and we showed that increased IL-18 levels predicted all-cause mortality in stable hemodialysis patients.

Malnutrition-inflammation-atherosclerosis (MIA) syndrome has been shown to be a powerful prognostic indicator in hemodialysis patients [32,33]. Although albumin has been proven to be a strong predictor of mortality in ESRD patients [34,35], the correlation between albumin and pro-inflammatory cytokines levels is still under debate [7,33]. Our data showed that that there was no significant difference in albumin levels between the low and high IL-18 groups; however, a significant difference was noted in the hsCRP levels (Table 1). Furthermore, IL-18 levels, as a continuous

Table 6. Multivariate Cox regression analysis for all-cause mortality in stable hemodialysis patients.

	Model 1		Model 2		Model 3		Model 4		Model 5	
Covariates	**HR (95% CI)**	***p***	**HR (95% CI)**	***p***	**HR (95% CI)**	***p***	**HR (95% CI)**	***p***	**HR (95% CI)**	***p***
Age	1.003 (0.95–1.06)	0.91	1.01 (0.96–1.07)	0.6	1.02 (0.97–1.07)	0.43	1.02 (0.97–1.09)	0.44	1.04 (0.98–1.09)	0.2
Serum albumin	0.06 (0.01–0.32)	0.001	0.11 (0.02–0.53)	0.006	0.08 (0.02–0.39)	0.002	0.2 (0.04–0.95)	0.04	0.13 (0.03–0.64)	0.01
Prevalent CAD	2.54 (0.91–7.05)	0.07	–	–	–	–	–	–	–	–
Hypertension	–	–	3.31 (1.11–9.82)	0.03	3.78 (1.29–11.12)	0.02	4.59 (1.46–14.4)	0.01	4.70 (1.56–14.13)	0.01
Less negative GLS(>−15%)	–	–	–	–	–	–	3.55 (1.18–10.7)	0.02	4.15 (1.31–13.21)	0.01
Serum IL-18	–	–	–	–	1.001 (1.00–1.001)	0.02	–	–	1.001 (1.00–1.001)	0.01

Abbreviations: CAD, coronary artery disease; CI, confidence interval; GLS, global left ventricular peak systolic longitudinal strain; HR, hazard ratio; IL, interleukin.
–, not enrolled.

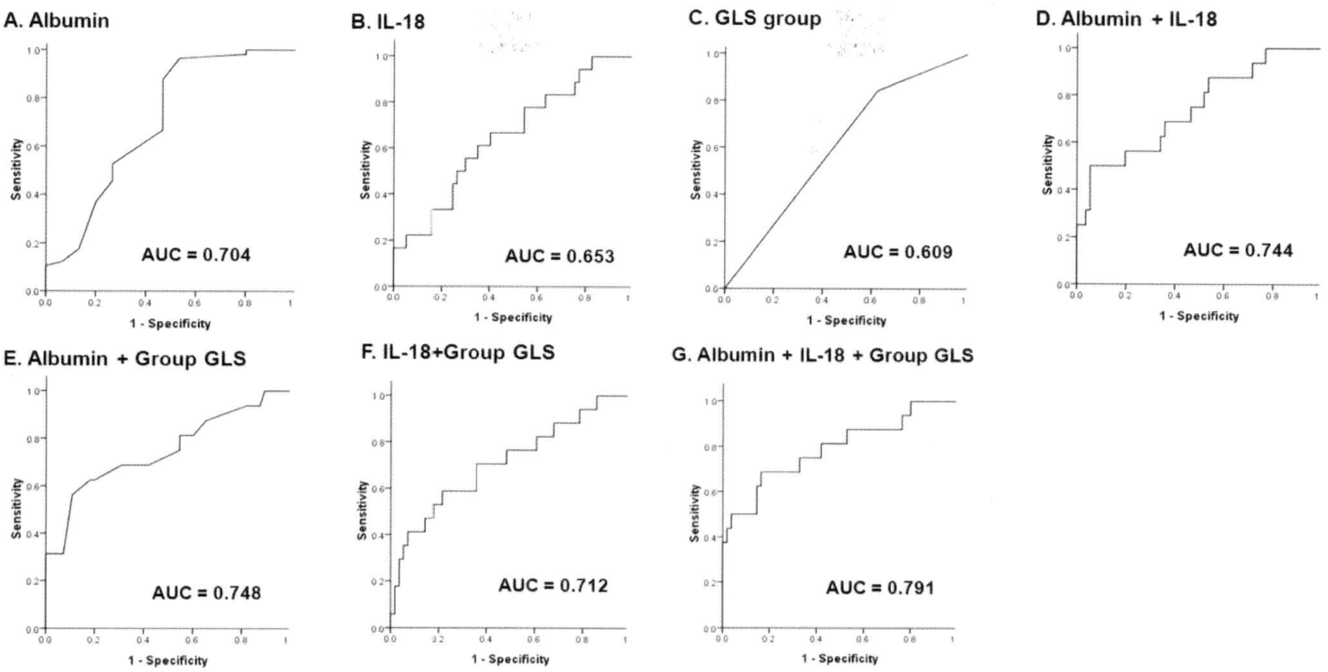

Figure 3. Receiver operating characteristic (ROC) curve of the ability of serum albumin (A), serum interleukin (IL)-18 (B), left ventricular global peak systolic longitudinal strain (GLS) group (C), the 2-combination parameters (D–F), and the 3-combination parameter (G) to predict all-cause mortality in clinical stable hemodialysis patients.

variable, showed modest correlations with hsCRP levels (Table 4), suggesting that IL-18 may play a role in the MIA syndrome of ESRD patients.

Compared with healthy subjects, ESRD patients commonly have elevated IL-18 levels, which might represent of a subclinical-inflammation state in stable HD patients [7,8]. Both uremic milieus and dialysis-related factors (such as bio-incompatibility with the dialyzer or chronic endotoxin exposure) may contribute to the high IL-18 levels [7]. There might be a connection between IL-18 levels and chronic hepatitis in stable hemodialysis patients (IL-18 levels with *vs.* without hepatitis: 1172.39±862.28 *vs.* 731.64±550.49 pg/ml, $p = 0.01$). However, chronic hepatitis is not a prognostic predictor (Table 4).

IL-18 is a middle-molecule and protein-bound uremic toxin, which is difficult to remove by any of the currently available dialytic strategies [36]. Uremic toxins affect many organs, including cardiovascular systems. It is speculated that IL-18 may cause LV dysfunction indirectly by aggravating coronary atherosclerosis or directly by acting on cardiomyocytes to induce myocardial remodeling [11-14]. For the vascular effects, IL-18 may stimulate Th1 cells to secrete interferon-γ [9], which plays a pivotal role in inflammation-related vascular injury [10] and intimal atherosclerotic plaque formation and its instability [11]. Clinical observations revealed associations between higher serum concentrations of IL-18 and the carotid intima-media thickness (IMT) [37] and also with poor outcome of CAD patients [15]. For the cardiac effects, IL-18 has been demonstrated to induce cardiac systolic and diastolic dysfunction *in vivo* [13,14]. There were several possible mechanisms of IL-18 involved myocardial injury. IL-18 may enhance activation of Myeloid Differentiation 88 and IL-1R associated kinase pathways, then up-regulate nuclear factor-κB (NF-κB) and p38 mitogen-activated protein kinases, and finally result in myocardial dysfunction [38–40]. Furthermore, after myocardial injury, IL-18 may induce apoptosis by inducing cytokines release and up-regulating either extrinsic death receptor signaling or intrinsic mitochondrial control pathway [41–43]. Furthermore, IL-18 was demonstrated to stimulate phosphatidylinositol 3-kinase-Akt pathway, followed by activating NF-κB and expressing transcription factor GATA4 and atrial natriuretic peptide [44,45].

In the present study, most of the hemodialysis patients had LV hypertrophy, high average E/e′ values, and increased PICP levels that were compatible with cardiac fibrosis and diastolic dysfunction [25]. However, both the high and low IL-18 groups had diastolic dysfunction, increased LV filling pressure, and similar severity of cardiac fibrosis, suggesting that IL-18 may not be a major risk factor for LV diastolic dysfunction in hemodialysis patients.

It should be noted that although hemodialysis patients with high IL-18 level tend to have worse LV systolic function compared with patients with low IL-18 levels, there was no significant linear correlation between IL-18 levels and GLS. This finding suggests other factors may play a significant role in systolic dysfunction in hemodialysis patients. There are many potential risk factors other than IL-18 for LV systolic dysfunction in hemodialysis patients, such as hypertension, hyperlipidemia, endothelial dysfunction, oxidative stress, insulin resistance, hemodialysis-related myocardial stunning, intra-dialytic hypotension, hypervolemia and positive sodium balance, high oxidative stress status, abnormalities of mineral metabolism with low 1,25-dihydroxyvitamin D and high parathyroid hormone levels, and high indoxyl sulfate level [41]. Besides, we found that those patients with less negative GLS ($>-15\%$) suffered from background HF and/or CAD more often than patients with more negative GLS ($\leq -15\%$). Since multi-variate Cox regression analyses showed that neither CAD nor HF was an independent prognostic predictor in our studied patients, and there is no large difference among hazard ratios of GLS in different models (including CAD and/or HF or not) (Table S1), the prognostic impact of GLS may not be attributable to the background CAD and/or HF. In this study, we clearly demonstrated that both elevated IL-18 levels and less negative GLS predict all-cause mortality independently in stable hemodialysis patients, suggesting the possibility that different mechanisms increase mortality in these two conditions. The reasons for this finding are currently unknown; however, we speculated that high IL-18 levels might result in atherosclerotic plaque progression and increased vulnerability of coronary or other arteries, which might lead to increased mortality. In contrast, less negative GLS is a marker of subclinical LV dysfunction which may progress to overt HF and result in high mortality. This speculation is based on the fact that there has been no human study demonstrating the association between high IL-18 level and HF-related mortality, although animal studies have suggested that high IL-18 may cause LV systolic and diastolic dysfunction. Nevertheless, further studies are needed to delineate this issue.

There were several limitations regarding this study that are worth noting. First, the number of enrolled patients was limited, so this study does not have enough power to explore the association between serum IL-18 levels and all-cause mortality in greater details. For example, we could not explore the role of cardiac troponin T in this association. In addition, we cannot analyze the impact of IL-18 on cause-specific mortality, such as cardiovascular mortality and infection-related mortality. With the current sample size, however, we have enough statistical power to detect the effects of IL-18 on all-cause mortality already, and therefore the finding was statistically significant. Nevertheless, a study with larger sample size to evaluate more predictors simultaneously in the future may help confirm our findings. Second, some hemodialysis patients had severe valvular heart diseases, atrial fibrillation, or poor echocardiographic image quality, which excluded the possibility of GLS analysis. Third, we recognized that although this study was cohort observational study, the laboratory tests and echocardiographic study were performed once in the start of the study. We could not conclude whether longitudinal laboratory tests and echocardiographic study might improve their predictive powers. Fourth, we did not measure brain natriuretic peptide levels. Last, we did not have the IL-18 data for the healthy subjects.

Conclusions

Hemodialysis patients with high IL-18 level tend to have worse LV systolic function and a higher mortality rate compared with patients with lower IL-18 levels. However, both elevated IL-18 and less negative GLS are independent prognostic predictors in stable hemodialysis patients. The combination of GLS and IL-18 may facilitate risk stratification for the outcomes and inform clinical decision making in stable hemodialysis patients. Further studies for developing strategies to treat hemodialysis patients who have increased IL-18 and/or less negative GLS are warranted.

Author Contributions

Conceived and designed the experiments: YWL CTS YTC WCT LMT JHC JMS. Performed the experiments: YWL WCT SPHW CTS CSY. Analyzed the data: YWL YTC YRS JMS. Wrote the manuscript: YWL JMS. Performed the echocardiogram studies and 2D strain analysis; YWL. Collected the patients' data: YWL CTS SPHW CSY.

References

1. Wen CP, Cheng TY, Tsai MK, Chang YC, Chan HT, et al. (2008) All-cause mortality attributable to chronic kidney disease: a prospective cohort study based on 462 293 adults in Taiwan. Lancet 371:2173–2182.
2. deFilippi C, Wasserman S, Rosanio S, Tiblier E, Sperger H, et al. (2003) Cardiac troponin T and C-reactive protein for predicting prognosis, coronary atherosclerosis, and cardiomyopathy in patients undergoing long-term hemodialysis. JAMA 290:353–359.
3. Yang WC, Hwang SJ (2008) Incidence, prevalence and mortality trends of dialysis end-stage renal disease in Taiwan from 1990 to 2001: the impact of national health insurance. Nephrol Dial Transplant 23:3977–3982.
4. Wong CK, Szeto CC, Chan MH, Leung CB, Li PK,et al. (2007) Elevation of pro-inflammatory cytokines, C-reactive protein and cardiac troponin T in chronic renal failure patients on dialysis. Immunol Invest 36:47–57.
5. Zoccali C, Tripepi G, Mallamaci F (2006) Dissecting inflammation in ESRD: do cytokines and C-reactive protein have a complementary prognostic value for mortality in dialysis patients? J Am Soc Nephrol 17 (Suppl 3):S169–S173.
6. Tripepi G, Mallamaci F, Zoccali C (2005) Inflammation markers, adhesion molecules, and all-cause and cardiovascular mortality in patients with ESRD: searching for the best risk marker by multivariate modeling. J Am Soc Nephrol 16 (Suppl 1):S83–S88.
7. Chiang CK, Hsu SP, Pai MF, Peng YS, Ho TI, et al. (2004) Interleukin-18 is a strong predictor of hospitalization in haemodialysis patients. Nephrol Dial Transplant 19:2810–2815.
8. Yano A, Nakao K, Sarai A, Akagi S, Kihara T, et al. (2005) Elevated serum interleukin-18 levels might reflect the high risk of hospitalization in patients on peritoneal dialysis. Nephrology (Carlton) 10:576–582.
9. Mallat Z, Corbaz A, Scoazec A, Besnard S, Lesèche G, et al. (2001) Expression of interleukin-18 in human atherosclerotic plaques and relation to plaque instability. Circulation 104:1598–1603.
10. Whitman SC, Ravisankar P, Daugherty A (2002) Interleukin-18 enhances atherosclerosis in apolipoprotein E(−/−) mice through release of interferon gamma. Circ Res 90:E34–E38.
11. Gerdes N, Sukhova GK, Libby P, Reynolds RS, Young JL, et al. (2002) Expression of interleukin (IL)-18 and functional IL-18 receptor on human vascular endothelial cells, smooth muscle cells, and macrophages: implications for atherogenesis. J Exp Med 195:245–257.
12. Blankenberg S, Luc G, Ducimetière P, Arveiler D, Ferrières J, et al. (2003) Interleukin-18 and the risk of coronary heart disease in European men: the Prospective Epidemiological Study of Myocardial Infarction (PRIME). Circulation 108:2453–2459.
13. Xing SS, Bi XP, Tan HW, Zhang Y, Xing QC, et al. (2010) Overexpression of interleukin-18 aggravates cardiac fibrosis and diastolic dysfunction in fructose-fed rats. Mol Med 16:465–470.
14. Woldbaek PR, Sande JB, Stromme TA, Lunde PK, Djurovic S, et al. (2005) Daily administration of interleukin-18 causes myocardial dysfunction in healthy mice. Am J Physiol Heart Circ Physiol.;289:H708–H714.
15. Blankenberg S, Tiret L, Bickel C, Peetz D, Cambien F, et al. (2002) Interleukin-18 is a strong predictor of cardiovascular death in stable and unstable angina. Circulation 106:24–30.
16. Wang AY, Lam CW, Yu CM, Wang M, Chan IH, et al. (2006) Troponin T, left ventricular mass, and function are excellent predictors of cardiovascular congestion in peritoneal dialysis. Kidney Int 70:444–452.
17. Sharma R, Gaze DC, Pellerin D, Mehta RL, Gregson H, et al. (2006) Cardiac structural and functional abnormalities in end stage renal disease patients with elevated cardiac troponin T. Heart 92:804–809.
18. Goicoechea M, de Vinuesa SG, Gomez-Campdera F, Luno J (2005) Predictive cardiovascular risk factors in patients with chronic kidney disease (CKD). Kidney Int Suppl 93:S35–S38.
19. Edwards NC, Hirth A, Ferro CJ, Townend JN, Steeds RP (2008) Subclinical abnormalities of left ventricular myocardial deformation in early-stage chronic kidney disease: the precursor of uremic cardiomyopathy? J Am Soc Echocardiogr 21:1293–1298.
20. Wang J, Khoury DS, Yue Y, Torre-Amione G, Nagueh SF (2008) Preserved left ventricular twist and circumferential deformation, but depressed longitudinal and radial deformation in patients with diastolic heart failure. Eur Heart J 29:1283–1289.
21. Liu YW, Tsai WC, Su CT, Lin CC, Chen JH (2009) Evidence of left ventricular systolic dysfunction detected by automated function imaging in patients with heart failure and preserved left ventricular ejection fraction. J Card Fail 15:782–789.

22. Liu YW, Su CT, Huang YY, Yang CS, Huang JW, et al. (2011) Left ventricular systolic strain in chronic kidney disease and hemodialysis patients. Am J Nephrol 33:84–90.
23. Stanton T, Leano R, Marwick TH (2009) Prediction of all-cause mortality from global longitudinal speckle strain: comparison with ejection fraction and wall motion scoring. Circ Cardiovasc Imaging 2:356–364.
24. Liu YW, Su CT, Sung JM, Wang SP, Su YR, et al. (2013) Association of left ventricular longitudinal strain with mortality among stable hemodialysis patients with preserved left ventricular ejection fraction. Clin J Am Soc Nephrol 26:1564–1574.
25. Su CT, Liu YW, Lin JW, Chen SI, Yang CS, et al. (2012) Increased Procollagen Type I C-Terminal Peptide Levels Indicate Diastolic Dysfunction in End-Stage Renal Disease Patients Undergoing Maintenance Dialysis Therapy. J Am Soc Echocardiogr 25:895–901.
26. Lang RM, Bierig M, Devereux RB, Flachskampf FA, Foster E, et al. (2005) Recommendations for chamber quantification: a report from the American Society of Echocardiography's Guidelines and Standards Committee and the Chamber Quantification Writing Group, developed in conjunction with the European Association of Echocardiography, a branch of the European Society of Cardiology. J Am Soc Echocardiogr 18:1440–1463.
27. Nagueh SF, Appleton CP, Gillebert TC, Marino PN, Oh JK, et al. (2009) Recommendations for the evaluation of left ventricular diastolic function by echocardiography. J Am Soc Echocardiogr 22:107–133.
28. Yashiro M, Kamata T, Yamadori N, Tomita M, Muso E (2007) Evaluation of markers to estimate volume status in hemodialysis patients: atrial natriuretic peptide, inferior vena cava diameter, blood volume changes and filtration coefficients of microvasculature. Ther Apher Dial 11:131–137.
29. Rudski LG, Lai WW, Afilalo J, Hua L, Handschumacher MD, et al. (2010) Guidelines for the echocardiographic assessment of the right heart in adults: a report from the American Society of Echocardiography endorsed by the European Association of Echocardiography, a registered branch of the European Society of Cardiology, and the Canadian Society of Echocardiography. J Am Soc Echocardiogr 23:685–713; quiz 786–788.
30. Ando Y, Yanagiba S, Asano Y (1995) The inferior vena cava diameter as a marker of dry weight in chronic hemodialyzed patients. Artif Organs 19:1237–1242.
31. Yingchoncharoen T, Agarwal S, Popović ZB, Marwick TH (2013) Normal ranges of left ventricular strain: a meta-analysis. J Am Soc Ehocardiogr 26:185–191.
32. Akdag I, Yilmaz Y, Kahvecioglu S, Bolca N, Ercan I, et al. (2008) Clinical value of the malnutrition-inflammation-atherosclerosis syndrome for long-term prediction of cardiovascular mortality in patients with end-stage renal disease: a 5-year prospective study. Nephron Clin Pract 108:c99–c105.
33. Owen WF, Jr., Lew NL, Liu Y, Lowrie EG, Lazarus JM (1993) The urea reduction ratio and serum albumin concentration as predictors of mortality in patients undergoing hemodialysis. N Engl J Med 329:1001–1006.
34. Leavey SF, Strawderman RL, Jones CA, Port FK, Held PJ (1998) Simple nutritional indicators as independent predictors of mortality in hemodialysis patients. Am J Kidney Dis 31:997–1006.
35. Ikizler TA, Wingard RL, Harvell J, Shyr Y, Hakim RM (1999) Association of morbidity with markers of nutrition and inflammation in chronic hemodialysis patients: a prospective study. Kidney Int 55:1945–1951.
36. Vanholder R, Van Laecke S, Glorieux G (2008) What is new in uremic toxicity? Pediatr Nephrol 23:1211–1221.
37. Yamagami H, Kitagawa K, Hoshi T, Furukado S, Hougaku H, et al. (2005) Associations of serum IL-18 levels with carotid intima-media thickness. Arterioscler Thromb Vasc Biol 25:1458–1462.
38. Wang M, Markel T, Crisostomo P, Herring C, Meldrum KK, et al. (2007) Deficiency of TNFR1 protects myocardium through SOCS3 and IL-6 but not p38 MAPK or IL-1beta. Am J Physiol Heart Circ Physiol 292:H1694–H1699.
39. Adachi O, Kawai T, Takeda K, Matsumoto M, Tsutsui H, et al. (1998) Targeted disruption of the MyD88 gene results in loss of IL-1- and IL-18-mediated function. Immunity 9:143–150.
40. Cain BS, Meldrum DR, Dinarello CA, Meng X, Joo KS, et al. (1999) Tumor necrosis factor-alpha and interleukin-1beta synergistically depress human myocardial function. Crit Care Med 27:1309–1318.
41. Li S, Jiao X, Tao L, Liu H, Cao Y, et al. (2007) Tumor necrosis factor-alpha in mechanic trauma plasma mediates cardiomyocyte apoptosis. Am J Physiol Heart Circ Physiol 293:H1847–H1852.
42. Liao X, Liu JM, Du L, Tang A, Shang Y, et al. (2006) Nitric oxide signaling in stretch-induced apoptosis of neonatal rat cardiomyocytes. FASEB J 20:1883–1885.
43. Konopleva M, Zhao S, Xie Z, Segall H, Younes A, et al. (1999) Apoptosis. Molecules and mechanisms. Adv Exp Med Biol 457:217–236.
44. Reddy VS, Harskamp RE, van Ginkel MW, Calhoon J, Baisden CE, et al. (2008) Interleukin-18 stimulates fibronectin expression in primary human cardiac fibroblasts via PI3K-Akt-dependent NF-kappaB activation. J Cell Physiol 215:697–707.
45. Chandrasekar B, Mummidi S, Claycomb WC, Mestril R, Nemer M (2005) Interleukin-18 is a pro-hypertrophic cytokine that acts through a phosphatidylinositol 3-kinase-phosphoinositide-dependent kinase-1-Akt-GATA4 signaling pathway in cardiomyocytes. J Biol Chem 280:4553–4567.

5

Relative Survival of Peritoneal Dialysis and Haemodialysis Patients: Effect of Cohort and Mode of Dialysis Initiation

James G. Heaf[1]*, Sonja Wehberg[2]

1 Department of Nephrology B, Copenhagen University Hospital at Herlev, Herlev, Denmark, 2 Department of Epidemiology, Odense University Hospital, Odense, Denmark

Abstract

Introduction: Epidemiological studies consistently show an initial survival advantage for PD patients compared to HD. It has recently been suggested that this is due to the fact that many HD patients are referred late, and start dialysis on an acute, in-patient basis. The present study was performed to investigate (1) whether, and if so, how, PD and HD prognosis had changed in recent years, (2) whether a potential survival advantage of PD versus HD is constant over dialysis duration, and (3) whether differences in prognosis could be explained by patient age, renal diagnosis of diabetic nephropathy, or mode of dialysis initiation.

Patients and Methods: 12095 patients starting dialysis therapy between 1990 and 2010 in Denmark were studied. Prognosis was assessed according to initial dialysis modality on an intention-to-treat basis, censored for transplantation. Results were adjusted for age, sex, renal diagnosis, Charlson Comorbidity Index (CCI), and mode of dialysis initiation.

Results: Overall adjusted prognosis improved by 34% (HD 30%, PD 42%). PD prognosis relative to HD improved, and was 16% better at the end of the period. Final PD prognosis improved consistently from 1990–99 to 2000–10 in all subgroups. PD was associated with a significant initial survival advantage, both overall and for all subgroups For the latter cohort, overall PD prognosis was better than HD for the first 4 years, after which it was insignificantly worse. The initial survival advantage was also present in a subgroup analysis of patients with early & routine ESRD initiation.

Conclusions: Dialysis survival has increased during the past 20 years. PD survival since 2000 has been better than HD, overall and for all subgroups. The difference in survival is not explained by mode of dialysis initiation.

Editor: Emmanuel A. Burdmann, University of Sao Paulo Medical School, Brazil

Funding: There are no current funding sources for this study.

Competing Interests: The authors have read the journal's policy and have the following conflicts. James Heaf has received travel funding and lecture fees from Baxter and Fresenius, and a research grant from Fresenius. This does not alter the authors' adherence to all the PLOS ONE policies on sharing data and materials.

* E-mail: heaf@dadlnet.dk

Introduction

The relative survival of end stage renal disease (ESRD) patients treated with peritoneal dialysis (PD) and hemodialysis (HD) has received much epidemiological interest in recent years [1–25]. Most studies [1,2,5,8–11,14,15,20,22,25] show a relative survival advantage for patients receiving PD lasting 1–2 years after dialysis initiation. Results in the long term differ, some showing identical survival [1,20,22,25] and others [4,6–10,15,19] showing poorer survival on PD.

This consensus has recently been challenged. The ANZA [19] study showed poorer survival for PD patients than a comparison group of center-HD and home-HD patients, Another paper by Quinn et al. [22] studied a subgroup of patients with early and routine referral to a nephrologist, i.e. the group that is most likely to have made an informed choice between the two therapies, and not have it forced upon them. In this group there was no survival difference between the two groups. The suspicion arises that the initial survival disadvantage of HD patients could be due to mode of ESRD initiation, with associated acute morbidity, that may be unrecorded in registry studies.

The Danish Nephrology Registry (DNR) is a prospective, national, incident registry of all patients receiving active ESRD therapy. It was established on 1.1.1990, and has a data completeness of >99% [26]. The present study was performed to answer the following questions:

(1) Has there been any change in the relative survival of PD versus HD since 1990?
(2) Is the (potential) survival advantage of PD versus HD constant over dialysis duration?
(3) How is PD prognosis in subgroups of patients with diabetic nephropathy, patients older than 65 years, and patients with an early (>90 days before ESRD) and routine ESRD initiation.

Patients and Methods

Patients

All patients resident in Denmark, and thus possessing a national identity number, starting active treatment with dialysis for ESRD between 1.1.1990 and 31.12.2010 were included in the study. Patients receiving a preemptive transplant were not included. Data were extracted from the following databases:

1) The Danish Nephrology Registry (DNR) contains data from all patients starting active treatment in Denmark. A patient is regarded as having ESRD if (a) the nephrologist considers him/her to have ESRD on the day of first active treatment or

Table 1. Patient characteristics N (%) and hazard ratios (HR) together with 95%-confidence intervals (CI) for factors.

Factor Dialysis modality[1]	HD	PD	All	Model 1: HR (CI)	Model 2: HR (CI)
	8273 (68)	3822 (32)	12095 (100)	.89 (.84–.93)	.87 (.83–.92)**
Cohort				**	**
1990–94	1099 (13)	748 (20)	1847 (15)	1 (ref)	1 (ref)
1995–99	1877 (23)	792 (21)	2669 (22)	.85 (.79–.91)**	.86 (.80–.93)*
2000–04	2482 (30)	1022 (27)	3504 (29)	.7 (.65–.75)**	.76 (.70–.81)**
2005–10	2815 (34)	1260 (33)	4075 (34)	.59 (.54–.64)**	.66 (.61–.72)**
Age				**	
0–59	2961 (36)	1962 (51)	4923 (41)	1 (ref)	
60–69	2158 (26)	975 (26)	3133 (26)	1.88 (1.76–2.01)**	
70–79	2337 (28)	697 (18)	3034 (25)	2.7 (2.52–2.89)**	
>=80	817 (10)	188 (5)	1005 (8)	3.62 (3.3–3.97)**	
Age>=65	4335 (52)	1344 (35)	5679 (47)		2.09 (1.99–2.20)**
Female Sex	3045 (37)	1449 (38)	4494 (37)	.98 (.94–1.03)	.99 (.94–1.04)
Renal Diagnosis				**	
Unknown	1931 (23)	852 (22)	2783 (23)	1 (ref)	
Glomerulonephritis (GN)	846 (10)	590 (15)	1436 (12)	.76 (.69–.84)**	
Chronic interstitial (CIN)	996 (12)	390 (10)	1386 (12)	.92 (.85–1)	
Polycystic	504 (6)	356 (9)	860 (7)	.73 (.66–.82)**	
Hypertensive	961 (12)	430 (11)	1391 (11)	.99 (.91–1.07)	
Type 1 DM	824 (10)	632 (17)	1456 (12)	1.57 (1.44–1.71)**	
Type 2 DM	998 (12)	284 (7)	1282 (11)	1.41 (1.30–1.52)**	
Renal Cancer	136 (2)	19 (0.5)	155 (1)	1.13 (.90–1.42)	
Myeloma	207 (3)	32 (0.8)	239 (2)	2.08 (1.75–2.47)**	
Amyloidosis	71 (0.9)	41 (1)	112 (0.9)	2.11 (1.64–2.73)**	
Systemic GN	97 (1)	52 (1)	149 (1)	.98 (.76–1.26)	
Vasculitis	377 (5)	70 (2)	447 (4)	.83 (.72–.96)*	
HUS/TTP[2]	40 (0.5)	15 (0.4)	55 (0.5)	.49 (.29–.81)*	
Other	285 (3)	59 (2)	344 (3)	.97 (.83–1.13)	
DM diagnosis	1822 (22)	916 (24)	2738 (23)		1.51 (1.43–1.6)**
Comorbidity				**	**
0	2837 (34)	1941 (51)	4778 (40)	1 (ref)	1 (ref)
1–2	3623 (44)	1423 (37)	5046 (42)	1.6 (1.51–1.69)**	1.69 (1.6–1.79)**
>2	1813 (22)	458 (12)	2271 (19)	2.3 (2.14–2.46)**	2.52 (2.35–2.7)**
ESRD Initiation				**	**
Early & Routine	2145 (26)	1419 (37)	3564 (29)	.91 (.86–.96)*	.89 (.84–.94)**
Late & Acute	2138 (26)	648 (17)	2786 (23)	1.1 (1.03–1.16)*	1.12 (1.05–1.19)**
Other	3990 (48)	1755 (46)	5745 (47)	1 (ref)	1 (ref)

Corresponding significant *p*-values are presented as.
*: $p<.05$;
**:$p<.001$.
For definition of models see methods section.
[1]:HD is the reference category;
[2]: Hemolytic Uremic Syndrome/ThrombocoticThrombocytopenic Purpura.

Table 2. Prognosis according to cohort and modality.

Within one year:

Cohort	Modality	N	Dead without change of modality (within 1 year)		LTF[1] without change		Transplantation		Change of modality, later death		Change without subsequent death		Unchanged after 1 year	
			N	%	N	%	N	%	N	%	N	%	N	%
90-94	HD	1099	221	20.1	0	0	112	10.2	18	1.6	145	13.2	603	54.9
95-99		1877	446	23.8	2	.1	92	4.9	19	1	172	9.2	1146	61.1
00-04		2482	590	23.8	1	0	71	2.9	29	1.2	138	5.6	1653	66.6
05-10		2815	557	19.8	348	12.4	63	2.2	22	.8	160	5.7	1665	59.1
90-94	PD	748	59	7.9	0	0	103	13.8	28	3.7	121	16.2	437	58.4
95-99		792	66	8.3	0	0	82	10.4	34	4.3	107	13.5	503	63.5
00-04		1022	81	7.9	0	0	78	7.6	26	2.5	156	15.3	681	66.6
05-10		1260	98	7.8	154	12.2	117	9.3	25	2	174	13.8	692	54.9
Within 5 years														
90-94	HD	1099	529	48.1	0	0	231	21	85	7.7	99	9	155	14.1
95-99		1877	1048	55.8	2	.1	256	13.6	103	5.5	112	6	356	19
00-04		2482	1512	60.9	1	0	221	8.9	94	3.8	101	4.1	553	22.3
05-10		2815	1163	41.3	1157	41.1	165	5.9	70	2.5	136	4.8	124	4.4
90-94	PD	748	231	30.9	0	0	194	25.9	137	18.3	134	17.9	52	7
95-99		792	206	26	0	0	174	22	175	22.1	154	19.4	83	10.5
00-04		1022	285	27.9	0	0	231	22.6	161	15.8	219	21.4	126	12.3
05-10		1260	244	19.4	394	31.3	226	17.9	114	9	256	20.3	26	2.1
Within 10 years														
90-94	HD	1099	625	56.9	0	0	247	22.5	107	9.7	79	7.2	41	3.7
95-99		1877	1259	67.1	2	.1	296	15.8	142	7.6	79	4.2	99	5.3
00-04		2482	1766	71.2	216	8.7	259	10.4	127	5.1	75	3	39	1.6
05-10		2815	1177	41.8	1262	44.8	169	6	70	2.5	137	4.9		
90-94	PD	748	254	34	0	0	196	26.2	193	25.8	99	13.2	6	.8
95-99		792	238	30.1	0	0	184	23.2	249	31.4	112	14.1	9	1.1
00-04		1022	331	32.4	37	3.6	238	23.3	240	23.5	173	16.9	3	.3
05-10		1260	246	19.5	415	32.9	227	18	116	9.2	256	20.3		

[1]: Lost to Follow-up.

Table 3. Cohort and mortality.

Cohort	HD	PD	Relative Mortality PD/HD
1990–94	1 (ref)	.95 (.85–1.06)	.95 (.85–1.06)
1995–1999	.88 (.8–.97)	.8 (.72–.89)	.9 (.82–1)
2000–04	.79 (.72–.86)	.66 (.59–.74)	.84 (.77–.92)
2005–10	.7 (.63–.77)	.56 (.49–.63)	.80 (.71–.89)

Adjusted hazard ratio (CI) based on a Cox regression model with interaction term between dialysis modality and cohort. Overall hazard ratio for PD versus HD was .8 (.71–.89). Overall p-value for interaction term was 0.11 (not significant).

later; (b) a renal transplant is performed; (c) there is some doubt regarding the reversibility of the uraemia (e.g. crescentic glomerulonephritis, acute tubulointerstitial nephropathy), but the patient has received at least 90 days of dialysis. Patients were included if (a) their first ESRD therapy was between 1.1.1990 and 31.12.2010; (b) their first ESRD therapy was PD or HD. The following data was extracted: patient age, sex, renal diagnosis, initial therapy (PD/HD), therapy at 90 days, and all changes of therapy. Renal diagnosis was classified as unknown, glomerulonephritis, chronic interstitial nephritis (including chronic pyelonephritis and post-renal uremia), polycystic kidneys, hypertensive nephropathy, Type 1 diabetic nephropathy, type 2 diabetic nephropathy, renal cancer, myeloma, amyloidosis, systemic glomerulonephritis, vasculitis, hæmolytic uremic syndrome/thrombotic thrombocytopenic purpura (HUS/TTP) and other. This is a multicenter study covering all 15 dialysis centres in the country and their satellite units.

2) Discharge diagnoses for all admissions to public hospitals in Denmark between 1977–2010 were extracted from the National Patient Registry (LPR). A modified Charlson Comorbidity Index (CCI) [27] at ESRD was calculated, removing the contribution of the original categories based on diabetes and renal disease from the score calculation. Our CCI takes into account the presence of the following comorbid conditions: previous myocardial infarction (AMI), cardiac insufficiency, peripheral atherosclerosis, cerebrovascular disease, dementia, chronic lung disease, collagenosis, stomach ulcer, liver disease, hemiplegia, cancer, leukemia, lymphoma, liver failure, metastatic disease, AIDS [28]. Since hospital care is public in Denmark, the coverage of this database is essentially 100% [29,30].

3) Details of patient referral were extracted from LPR. The date of first consultation at a specialist nephrology department was registered. Referrals were classified as early if the first consultation was >90 days before ESRD and late if it was <91 days. Therapy initiation was acute if the first ESRD therapy was as an in-patient and routine if it was as an out-patient. Patients were grouped as either Early & Routine (E&R), Late & Acute (L&A), and other. The LPR has registered referral dates and consultation dates for all in-patient and out-patient referrals and has been comprehensive since 1992. Data for the years 1990–1991 was incomplete.

Methods and statistical analysis

Since most modality changes are from PD to HD, and are associated with increased mortality after change, an "as treated" model is unsuitable for this subject. Patient survival was therefore assessed on an intention-to-treat basis - only the first dialysis course was evaluated - using Cox regression models with robust variance estimation as a safeguard against misspecification. All patients were followed until either death, renal transplant or lost-to-follow-up (LTF) (censoring date 1.1.2011). Model 1 included first dialysis modality (PD, HD), cohort (according to date of dialysis initiation: 1990–1994, 1995–1999, 2000–2004, 2005–2010) patient age at date of dialysis initiation (categorized into 0-, 60-, 70- and 80-), sex, renal diagnosis, CCI (categorized into 0, 1–2, > = 3) and type of ESRD initiation (early & routine, late & acute, other). For

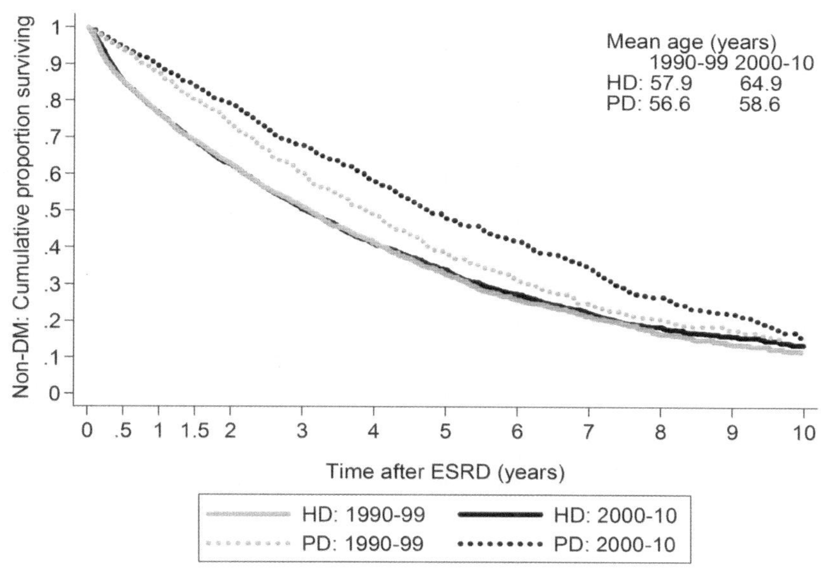

Figure 1. Patient Survival based on Kaplan-Meier curves, stratified for Modality and Cohort. Non-DM.

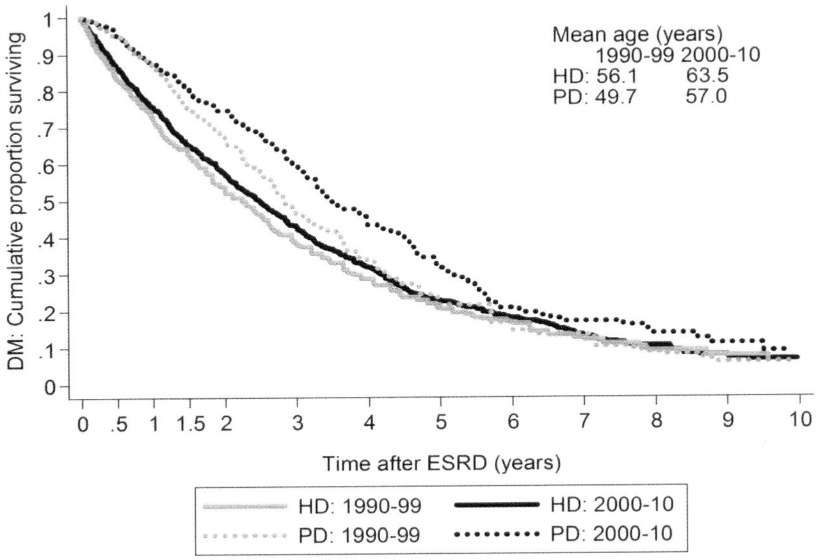

Figure 2. Patient Survival based on Kaplan-Meier curves, stratified for Modality and Cohort. DM.

model 2, age was substituted by the binary age >= 65 years (yes/no), and renal diagnosis was substituted by binary DM diagnosis (yes/no), i.e. patients with and without diabetic nephropathy.

To explore the development of relative survival PD/HD Prior over cohorts, an interaction term for cohort and dialysis modality was subsequently added to model 2.

To study the effect of dialysis duration (since date of dialysis initiation) on the estimated relative survival PD versus HD, a piecewise Cox regression analysis was fitted independently for the following time periods: 0–6, 6–12, 12–18, 18–24, 24–36, 36–48 and >48 months, adjusted for covariates as in model 2 but stratified for cohort (1990–99, 2000–10). Additionally, the time-dependent hazard ratio for PD versus HD based on the scaled Schoenfeld residuals [31] was estimated. We used this method by Grambsch & Therneau (which originally was proposed to check for proportional hazards) to visualize the time-dependency of the hazard ratio. The curves are generated based on Schoenfeld residuals from the (multivariate/adjusted) Cox models separately for each cohort and subgroup. The curves employ a simple Lowess smoother with bandwidth .8.

Subgroup analyses for the last analysis were performed for 1. DM diagnosis (yes), 2. age >= 65 years, 3. patients older than 65 years and with diabetic nephropathy and 4. patients with an early & routine initiation.

A supplementary analysis was performed for those patients who were still on dialysis after 90 days, where the study period started 90 days after ESRD, and the patients were classified according to their dialysis modality on that date. Type of ESRD initiation was not considered in this analysis.

The proportional hazard assumption is violated for modality in the first model, but this is not a major problem. The first model estimates the average hazard ratio over time (since the estimated hazard ratio based on a Cox model is shown to be fairly close to the exact calculation of the average hazard ratio over time). Thus, the true underlying proportional hazard ratio is not measured, just the overall/average effect. The next step was to fit piecewise

Table 4. Patient mortality according to modality, age and diabetic status.

			Two-year Mortality (%)				Four-year Mortality (%)			
Modality	**Diagnosis**	**Age (yrs)**	**90-94**	**95-99**	**00-04**	**05-10**	**90-94**	**95-99**	**00-04**	**05-10**
PD	NonDM	<65	18	16	10	11	47	30	23	23
		>=65	41	40	37	33	69	67	63	60
	DM	<65	34	22	19	21	71	53	48	46
		>=65	74	39	36	39	100	79	74	74
HD	NonDM	<65	24	25	25	23	44	42	41	36
		>=65	55	49	48	44	76	73	70	68
	DM	<65	43	42	31	31	64	64	56	57
		>=65	51	60	59	49	89	84	83	74

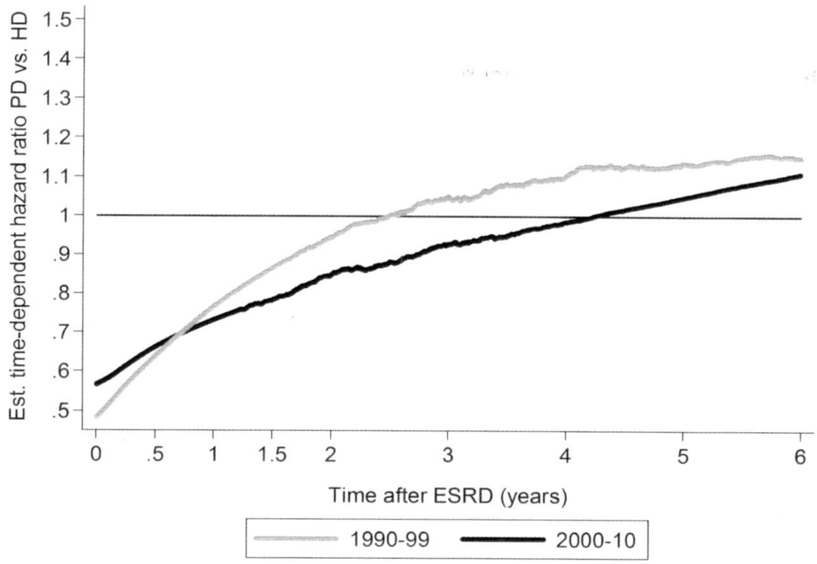

Figure 3. Relationship of relative mortality risk PD/HD to dialysis duration. 1990–99 versus 2000–10.

models, and the last was to show time-dependent hazard ratios. This last method was originally proposed as a model check (violation of proportional hazards) but can conveniently be applied to visualize time-dependency.

Since there was a tendency over cohorts for "increased superiority", a cohort x modality effect analysis was performed to investigate whether there were any significant effects.

Reported *p*-values are based on Wald tests. All analyses were done using Stata (StataCorp 2011. Stata Statistical Software: Release 12. College Station TX: StataCorp LP).

Results

The patient characteristics are shown in Table 1. Patients treated with PD were generally younger, with a lower Comorbidity and a more planned ESRD initiation. Type 1 diabetic nephropathy was more prevalent in PD patients and Type 2 less. Average age increased significantly by 10.6 years for HD patients and 5.3 years for PD patients. Over cohorts, mean age ±SD increased from 55.0±15.8 in the cohort 1990–94 (HD: 55.3±16.5; PD: 54.4.±16.6) to 64.0±15.8 in the cohort 2005–10 (HD: 65.9±14.8; PD: 59.7±16.9). Mean CCI rose from

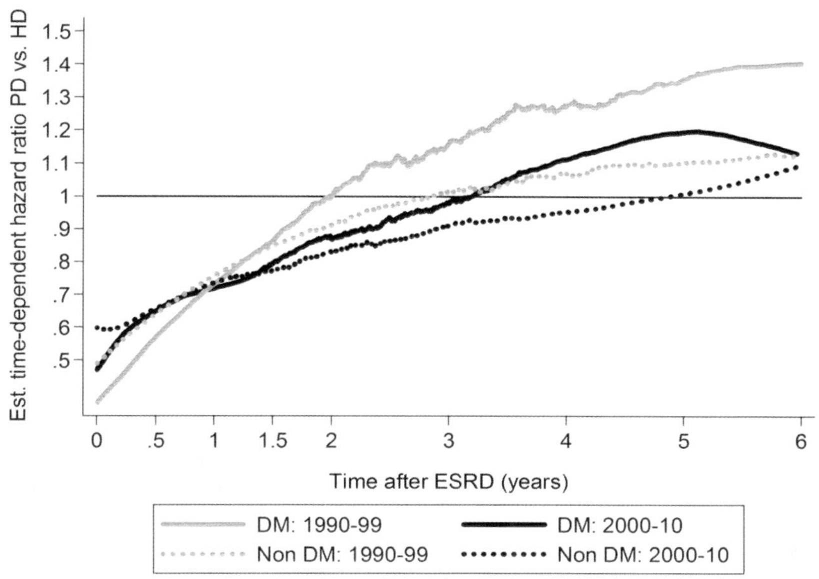

Figure 4. Relationship of relative mortality risk PD/HD to dialysis duration. DM versus Non-DM.

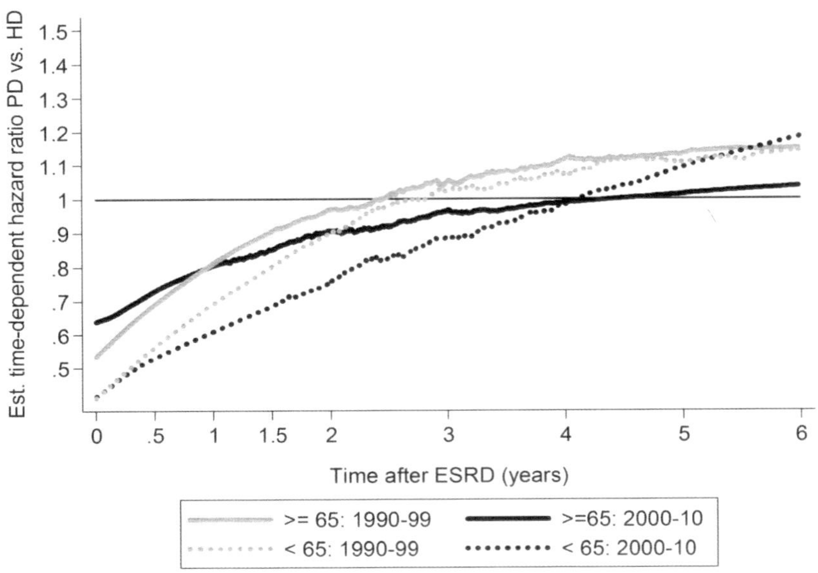

Figure 5. Relationship of relative mortality risk PD/HD to dialysis duration. <65 years versus >=65 years.

0.9±1.4 in 1990–94 to 1.6±1.8 in 2005–2010. This was not just due to increasing age. The CCI for patients aged 60–69-years rose from 1.3±1.5 to 1.8±1.9, 70–79 years from 1.2±1.6 to 2.1±1.9 and 80+ years from 0.7±1.2 to 2.1±1.7.

Improvements in referral pattern were seen during the period of observation. L&A initiations fell from 37 to 16% and E&R rose from 10 to 43%.

The hazard ratios for the factors analyzed are shown in Table 1. All factors except for (female) sex had a highly significant influence on mortality in model 2. The unadjusted prognosis according to cohort and initial dialysis modality is shown in Table 2, and the adjusted in Table 3. Overall, there was a significant improvement in patient prognosis during the period of observation (HR for cohort, Table 1). Adjusted mortality fell overall by 34%. Estimated relative mortality of PD versus HD improved from .95 in 1990–94 to .8 in 2005–10 (Table 3, based on model 2 with an additional interaction term between cohort and dialysis modality).

For HD patients improvement consisted of largely unchanged mortality despite rapidly increasing age and morbidity (Figs. 1 & 2), while for PD patients non-DM median survival increased by 10

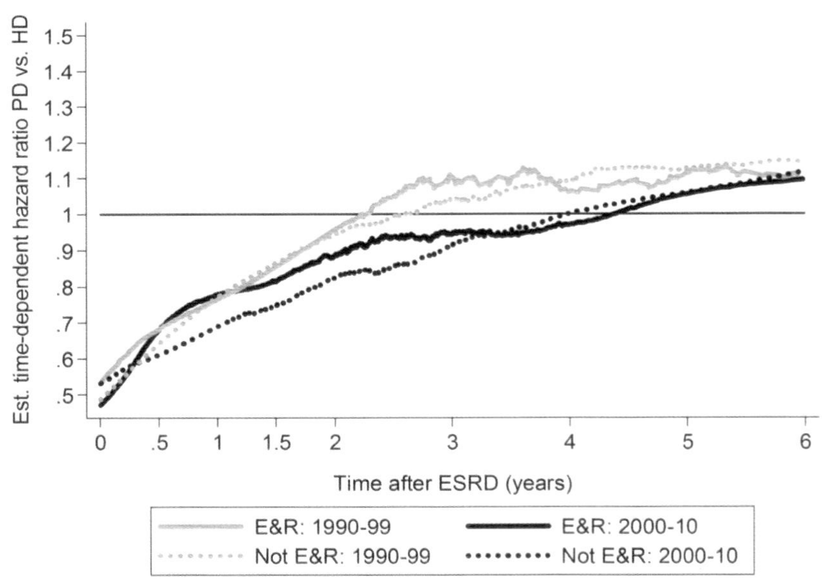

Figure 6. Relationship of relative mortality risk PD/HD to dialysis duration. Early & routine versus not E&R referral pattern.

months from 1990–99 to 2000–10, while DM survival increased by 8 months, despite a seven-year increase in average age. For some subgroups, the PD improvement was dramatic: 4-year mortality for young, non-DM patients fell from 47% to 23%, and two-year mortality for elderly diabetics from 74% to 39% (Table 4).

PD was associated with a significant initial survival advantage, both overall and for all subgroups (Table 5, Figs. 3, 4, 5, & 6). Late prognosis was generally poorer for PD patients, but less so for the later cohort. Relative PD prognosis improved for all subgroups from 1990–99 to 2000–10. The "crossover point" from better to poorer PD prognosis increased from about 30 months to 52 months, and for no subgroup was less than 24 months. PD results were mostly better for non-DM patients than DM, and younger (<65 years) than older. Improvements in referral pattern were seen during the period of observation. Relative PD prognosis was better for patients with E&R initiation in the later cohort for the initial 36 months. There were no significant differences in age or CCI index between the E&R group and other patients.

Results for the 90-day analysis were broadly similar and are therefore not shown.

Discussion

Substantial improvements in prognosis were seen for both HD and PD during the period of observation. This is in accordance with USRDS and DOPPS data [32,33]. This is particularly remarkable, since the period has been characterized by an absence of major randomized controlled trials with a positive therapeutic result. Possible factors contributing to this general improvement include defined standards for adequate dialysis, increased attention to calcium, phosphate and PTH control, better anemia control, better preparation of dialysis initiation, and a tendency towards earlier dialysis initiation. Furthemore, advances in non-nephrological areas, such as reduced tobacco consumption, improved treatment of cardiovascular disease will also have contributed. It is possible that some of the improved prognosis is a statistical artifact, due to increased registration of comorbidity over time.

A trend to improvement in the relative prognosis of PD patients compared to HD patients were also seen, despite employing a conservative intention-to-treat analysis (ITT) strategy where the "true" group differences tend to be under- rather than overestimated. This is in accordance with previous studies [15,19,23,25]. Substantial changes in the practice of PD occurred during the period. The observation of an increased mortality of patients with fast peritoneal transport [34] and the observation that automated PD (APD) seems to solve the problem [35–37] suggests that a major cause of PD mortality during the nineties was due to inadequate ultrafiltration secondary to rapid dissipation of the glucose osmotic gradient in fast transporters, with consequent overhydration, hypertension, pulmonary edema and death. Better fluid control using icodextrin and APD seems to have solved the problem of fast transport [36,38]. Icodextrin became available in Denmark from 1999 and the use of APD rose rapidly from 3% in 1990 to 30% in 2000 and 66% in 2008 [39]. Biocompatible PD fluids became available in 2000, and have recently been demonstrated to preserve residual renal function (RRF), peritoneal membrane function and reduce the incidence of peritonitis and possibly other infections [40,41]. The possible contribution of a reduction in peritonitis frequency in this study is unknown. Peritonitis frequency registration was first introduced in 2000, and has since showed a moderate improvement from 1/25 patient months to 1/31 [39]. HD-specific improvements have also occurred during the period. The introduction of biocompatible

Table 5. Relationship between relative mortality PD/HD and dialysis duration.

	All		DM		>=65 yrs		DM and >=65 yrs		Early & Routine	
Duration (months)	**1990-99**	**2000-10**	**1990-99**	**2000-10**	**1990-99**	**2000-10**	**1990-99**	**2000-10**	**1990-99**	**2000-10**
0-6	.45 (.36-.57)**	.54 (.44-.66)**	.34 (.2-.56)**	.48 (.32-.73)*	.51 (.38-.68)**	.60 (.48-.76)**	.19 (.07-.53)*	.33 (.17-.63)*	.52 (.25-1.1)	.50 (.35-.72)**
6-12	.79 (.63-1.00)	.69 (.56-.86)*	.78 (.49-1.25)	.76 (.52-1.11)	.84 (.61-1.15)	.78 (.60-1.01)	1.36 (.65-2.86)	.81 (.49-1.32)	.64 (.32-1.28)	.87 (.61-1.24)
12-18	.96 (.75-1.22)	.79 (.64-.99)*	1.01 (.66-1.55)	.73 (.49-1.08)	0.97 (.7-1.36)	.83 (.64-1.09)	1.25 (.59-2.65)	.66 (.37-1.16)	1.15 (.62-2.14)	1.12 (.8-1.57)
18-24	.97 (.74-1.26)	.84 (.65-1.08)	.65 (.39-1.07)	.81 (.51-1.29)	1.06 (.74-1.52)	.97 (.71-1.33)	.84 (.33-2.15)	1.04 (.54-2.01)	.73 (.39-1.38)	.66 (.43-1)
24-36	1.17 (.97-1.42)	.88 (.74-1.06)	1.43 (.98-2.08)	.9 (.65-1.24)	1.2 (.92-1.56)	.93 (.74-1.16)	1.65 (.87-3.13)	1.03 (.62-1.69)	1.22 (.78-1.89)	.81 (.6-1.1)
36-48	1.1 (.87-1.38)	1.03 (.83-1.28)	1.28 (.8-2.04)	1.32 (.91-1.9)	.94 (.67-1.32)	1.08 (.83-1.41)	1.01 (.36-2.84)	1.32 (.78-2.24)	1.18 (.65-2.14)	1.28 (.9-1.81)
>48	1.15 (1-1.31)*	1.12 (.96-1.32)	1.52 (1.08-2.12)*	1.11 (.81-1.53)	1.17 (.96-1.43)	1.04 (.83-1.31)	3.09 (1.38-6.90)*	1.62 (.93-2.83)	1.05 (.76-1.47)	1.05 (.8-1.38)
Overall	.94 (.87-1.01)	.83 (.77-.89)**	.97 (.84-1.12)	.85 (.75-.97)*	.94 (.85-1.04)	.86 (.78-.94)*	1 (.77-1.29)	.85 (.71-1.01)	.97 (.81-1.17)	.88 (.78-.99)*

membranes and the use of "floating dry weight" (whereby fluid balance is controlled by fluid restriction rather than ultrafiltration in nonoliguric HD patients) may help to preserve RRF [42,43]. The beneficial effects on mortality of high flux dialysis and hemodiafiltration remain however unproved [44,45]. In conclusion, the improvement in PD prognosis has been greater than HD, and therefore cohorts from the nineties can no longer be used for comparing treatment results. Furthermore, randomized, controlled trials comparing HD and PD should offer patients the full range of PD products, including biocompatible fluids, icodextrin and APD.

As mentioned in the introduction, PD is characterized by a better initial prognosis, and an equal or worse late prognosis. One possible cause is better preservation of RRF in PD [46], perhaps due to intradialytic renal dehydration and ischemia during HD [47]. Preservation of RRF is a major determinant of dialysis survival [48]. One important exception to the general pattern is the ANZA study, which showed a poorer prognosis for PD patients, albeit with considerable improvement in the latest cohort [19]. Closer perusal of these results however [49] show that the good HD prognosis was mainly related to the high home HD prevalence in this population. If these patients are excluded from the analysis, the traditional pattern reappears, with an initial PD advantage disappearing after two years. The present study also showed a better initial prognosis, and an insignificantly worse late prognosis, again, despite a conservative ITT approach. The overall prognosis since 2000 was significantly better for PD for each of the four major subgroups.

Regardless of the overall result, most studies show a better relative effect of PD in younger [1–3,5,8,9,11,12,14–16,19–21,25], non-diabetic [1–3,5–11,14–16,18,20,21,23,25] patients, and patients without comorbidity [8–12,16,19–21,23,24]. The present study also showed a relatively better prognosis for younger and non-diabetic patients, but for no subgroup was PD worse than HD. After 2000, there was no difference between relative diabetic and non-diabetic prognosis. It has been suggested [22] that the better initial prognosis is due to differences in dialysis planning, in that PD patients are more likely to have been referred earlier and started ESRD therapy as out-patients. The present study has the advantage that ESRD planning, which was found to have a major impact on prognosis, was included in the statistical analysis. In a separate analysis of patients with early, out-patient ESRD initiation, the initial PD advantage remained. Thus, differences in ESRD planning do not explain the initial PD survival advantage in this study. This conclusion is substantially different from the Quinn study [22]. It is possible that differences in patient population, protocol design and hospital practice may explain some of the differences.

All patients in the E&R group were out-patient at the time of initiation, and had been referred early to a nephrologist. This does not, of course exclude the possibility that they were acutely sick at the time of dialysis start, just that they did not need hospital admission. Furthermore, the vast majority of these patients will have been started using an AV fistula or graft, since a central catheter always requires hospital admission in Denmark. The initial PD advantage holds for all subgroups analysed, and may therefore be a universal phenomenon. Possible causes include early loss of residual function after HD initiation [47,50] and the detrimental effects of myocardial stunning after HD initiation.

The practical consequences of this study remain controversial. Questions may be made as to the validity of the CCI and patient referral pattern. Discharge diagnosis registration may vary between centers and over time, particularly if quality measures or reimbursement rules are based on the CCI. This is not however the case in Denmark. The CCI measures only discharge diagnoses, and will thus underestimate the true comorbidity; this underestimation is not necessarily uniform between the groups studied. Despite these reservations, both CCI and referral patient were indeed very significant markers of death. As it is an epidemiological study, no causal conclusions can be drawn. The initial PD results may be due to better preservation of RRF, or to hitherto unidentified comorbid factors. The present consensus is that dialysis patients should continue to choose modality on the basis of personal preference. Patients, in particular younger, non-diabetic patients, should be informed of the possible advantage of PD. If survival is the primary motivating factor, this group of patients should however consider home HD as an alternative. It offers better phosphate, PTH, anemia and blood pressure control, fewer dietary restrictions, and removes the dangers of the long weekend [51]. Probably as a direct consequence, patient survival is greater than conventional PD and HD [49] and on a par with cadaver renal transplantation [52].

Author Contributions

Conceived and designed the experiments: JGH. Performed the experiments: JGH. Analyzed the data: SW. Contributed reagents/materials/analysis tools: SW. Wrote the paper: JGH. Performed statistical analysis: SW.

References

1. Fenton SS, Schaubel DE, Desmeules M, Morrison HI, Mao Y, et al. (1997) Hemodialysis versus peritoneal dialysis: a comparison of adjusted mortality rates. Am J Kidney Dis 30: 334–342. S0272638697001686 [pii].
2. Schaubel DE, Morrison HI, Fenton SS (1998) Comparing mortality rates on CAPD/CCPD and hemodialysis. The Canadian experience: fact or fiction? Perit Dial Int 18: 478–484.
3. Vonesh EF, Moran J (1999) Mortality in end-stage renal disease: a reassessment of differences between patients treated with hemodialysis and peritoneal dialysis. J Am Soc Nephrol 10: 354–365.
4. Locatelli F, Marcelli D, Conte F, D'Amico M, Del VL, et al. (2001) Survival and development of cardiovascular disease by modality of treatment in patients with end-stage renal disease. J Am Soc Nephrol 12: 2411–2417.
5. Heaf JG, Lokkegaard H, Madsen M (2002) Initial survival advantage of peritoneal dialysis relative to haemodialysis. Nephrol Dial Transplant 17: 112–117.
6. Winkelmayer WC, Glynn RJ, Mittleman MA, Levin R, Pliskin JS, et al. (2002) Comparing mortality of elderly patients on hemodialysis versus peritoneal dialysis: a propensity score approach. J Am Soc Nephrol 13: 2353–2362.
7. Collins AJ, Weinhandl E, Snyder JJ, Chen SC, Gilbertson D (2002) Comparison and survival of hemodialysis and peritoneal dialysis in the elderly. Semin Dial 15: 98–102. 0032 [pii].
8. Termorshuizen F, Korevaar JC, Dekker FW, Van Manen JG, Boeschoten EW, et al. (2003) Hemodialysis and peritoneal dialysis: comparison of adjusted mortality rates according to the duration of dialysis: analysis of The Netherlands Cooperative Study on the Adequacy of Dialysis 2. J Am Soc Nephrol 14: 2851–2860.
9. Ganesh SK, Hulbert-Shearon T, Port FK, Eagle K, Stack AG (2003) Mortality differences by dialysis modality among incident ESRD patients with and without coronary artery disease. J Am Soc Nephrol 14: 415–424.
10. Stack AG, Molony DA, Rahman NS, Dosekun A, Murthy B (2003) Impact of dialysis modality on survival of new ESRD patients with congestive heart failure in the United States. Kidney Int 64: 1071–1079. kid165 [pii];10.1046/j.1523-1755.2003.00165.x [doi].
11. Vonesh EF, Snyder JJ, Foley RN, Collins AJ (2004) The differential impact of risk factors on mortality in hemodialysis and peritoneal dialysis. Kidney Int 66: 2389–2401. KID66028 [pii];10.1111/j.1523-1755.2004.66028.x [doi].
12. Jaar BG, Coresh J, Plantinga LC, Fink NE, Klag MJ, et al. (2005) Comparing the risk for death with peritoneal dialysis and hemodialysis in a national cohort of patients with chronic kidney disease. Ann Intern Med 143: 174–183. 143/3/174 [pii].
13. Frimat L, Durand PY, Loos-Ayav C, Villar E, Panescu V, et al. (2006) Impact of first dialysis modality on outcome of patients contraindicated for kidney transplant. Perit Dial Int 26: 231–239.

14. Mircescu G, Garneata L, Florea L, Cepoi V, Capsa D, et al. (2006) The success story of peritoneal dialysis in Romania: analysis of differences in mortality by dialysis modality and influence of risk factors in a national cohort. Perit Dial Int 26: 266–275.
15. Liem YS, Wong JB, Hunink MG, de Charro FT, Winkelmayer WC (2007) Comparison of hemodialysis and peritoneal dialysis survival in The Netherlands. Kidney Int 71: 153–158. 5002014 [pii];10.1038/sj.ki.5002014 [doi].
16. Huang CC, Cheng KF, Wu HD (2008) Survival analysis: comparing peritoneal dialysis and hemodialysis in Taiwan. Perit Dial Int 28 Suppl 3: S15–S20. 28/Supplement_3/S15 [pii].
17. Sanabria M, Munoz J, Trillos C, Hernandez G, Latorre C, et al. (2008) Dialysis outcomes in Colombia (DOC) study: a comparison of patient survival on peritoneal dialysis vs hemodialysis in Colombia. Kidney Int Suppl S165–S172. 5002619 [pii];10.1038/sj.ki.5002619 [doi].
18. Lee CC, Sun CY, Wu MS (2009) Long-term modality-related mortality analysis in incident dialysis patients. Perit Dial Int 29: 182–190. 29/2/182 [pii].
19. McDonald SP, Marshall MR, Johnson DW, Polkinghorne KR (2009) Relationship between dialysis modality and mortality. J Am Soc Nephrol 20: 155–163. ASN.2007111188 [pii];10.1681/ASN.2007111188 [doi].
20. Weinhandl ED, Foley RN, Gilbertson DT, Arneson TJ, Snyder J, et al. (2010) Propensity-matched mortality comparison of incident hemodialysis and peritoneal dialysis patients. J Am Soc Nephrol 21: 499–506. ASN.2009060635 [pii];10.1681/ASN.2009060635 [doi].
21. van de Luijtgaarden MW, Noordzij M, Stel VS, Ravani P, Jarraya F, et al. (2011) Effects of comorbid and demographic factors on dialysis modality choice and related patient survival in Europe. Nephrol Dial Transplant 26: 2940–2947. gfq845 [pii];10.1093/ndt/gfq845 [doi].
22. Quinn RR, Hux JE, Oliver MJ, Austin PC, Tonelli M, et al. (2011) Selection bias explains apparent differential mortality between dialysis modalities. J Am Soc Nephrol 22: 1534–1542. ASN.2010121232 [pii];10.1681/ASN.2010121232 [doi].
23. Mehrotra R, Chiu YW, Kalantar-Zadeh K, Bargman J, Vonesh E (2011) Similar outcomes with hemodialysis and peritoneal dialysis in patients with end-stage renal disease. Arch Intern Med 171: 110–118. archinternmed.2010.352 [pii];10.1001/archinternmed.2010.352 [doi].
24. Sens F, Schott-Pethelaz AM, Labeeuw M, Colin C, Villar E (2011) Survival advantage of hemodialysis relative to peritoneal dialysis in patients with end-stage renal disease and congestive heart failure. Kidney Int 80: 970–977. ki2011233 [pii];10.1038/ki.2011.233 [doi].
25. Yeates K, Zhu N, Vonesh E, Trpeski L, Blake P, et al. (2012) Hemodialysis and peritoneal dialysis are associated with similar outcomes for end-stage renal disease treatment in Canada. Nephrol Dial Transplant 27: 3568–3575. gfr674 [pii];10.1093/ndt/gfr674 [doi].
26. Wehberg S (2010) Datagrundlag og analysemetode. Danish Nephrology Registry Annual Report 2009. Available: www.nephrology.dk: 14–21. Accessed 2014 Feb 8.
27. Charlson ME, Pompei P, Ales KL, MacKenzie CR (1987) A new method of classifying prognostic comorbidity in longitudinal studies: development and validation. J Chronic Dis 40: 373–383.
28. Lynge E, Sandegaard JL, Rebolj M (2011) The Danish National Patient Register. Scand J Public Health 39: 30–33. 39/7_suppl/30 [pii];10.1177/1403494811401482 [doi].
29. Pedersen CB, Gotzsche H, Moller JO, Mortensen PB (2006) The Danish Civil Registration System. A cohort of eight million persons. Dan Med Bull 53: 441–449. DMB3816 [pii].
30. Andersen TF, Madsen M, Jorgensen J, Mellemkjoer L, Olsen JH (1999) The Danish National Hospital Register. A valuable source of data for modern health sciences. Dan Med Bull 46: 263–268.
31. Grambsch PM, Therneau TM (2010) Proportional hazards tests and diagnostics based on weighted residuals. Biometrika 81: 515–526.
32. Collins AJ, Foley RN, Chavers B, Gilbertson D, Herzog C, et al. (2012) 'United States Renal Data System 2011 Annual Data Report: Atlas of chronic kidney disease & end-stage renal disease in the United States. Am J Kidney Dis 59: A7, e1–A7,420. S0272-6386(11)01571-X [pii];10.1053/j.ajkd.2011.11.015 [doi].
33. Port FK, Pisoni RL, Bommer J, Locatelli F, Jadoul M, et al. (2006) Improving outcomes for dialysis patients in the international Dialysis Outcomes and Practice Patterns Study. Clin J Am Soc Nephrol 1: 246–255. CJN.01050905 [pii];10.2215/CJN.01050905 [doi].
34. Churchill DN, Thorpe KE, Nolph KD, Keshaviah PR, Oreopoulos DG, et al. (1998) Increased peritoneal membrane transport is associated with decreased patient and technique survival for continuous peritoneal dialysis patients. The Canada-USA (CANUSA) Peritoneal Dialysis Study Group. J Am Soc Nephrol 9: 1285–1292.
35. Brimble KS, Walker M, Margetts PJ, Kundhal KK, Rabbat CG (2006) Meta-analysis: peritoneal membrane transport, mortality, and technique failure in peritoneal dialysis. J Am Soc Nephrol 17: 2591–2598. ASN.2006030194 [pii];10.1681/ASN.2006030194 [doi].
36. Yang X, Fang W, Bargman JM, Oreopoulos DG (2008) High peritoneal permeability is not associated with higher mortality or technique failure in patients on automated peritoneal dialysis. Perit Dial Int 28: 82–92. 28/1/82 [pii].
37. Johnson DW, Hawley CM, McDonald SP, Brown FG, Rosman JB, et al. (2010) Superior survival of high transporters treated with automated versus continuous ambulatory peritoneal dialysis. Nephrol Dial Transplant 25: 1973–1979. gfp780 [pii];10.1093/ndt/gfp780 [doi].
38. Davies SJ (2006) Mitigating peritoneal membrane characteristics in modern peritoneal dialysis therapy. Kidney Int Suppl S76–S83. 5001920 [pii];10.1038/sj.ki.5001920 [doi].
39. Heaf JG (2011) Danish Nephrology Registry Annual Report. Available: www.nephrology.dk: 1–109. Accessed 2014 Feb 8
40. Johnson DW, Brown FG, Clarke M, Boudville N, Elias TJ, et al. (2012) Effects of biocompatible versus standard fluid on peritoneal dialysis outcomes. J Am Soc Nephrol 23: 1097–1107. ASN.2011121201 [pii];10.1681/ASN.2011121201 [doi].
41. Johnson DW, Brown FG, Clarke M, Boudville N, Elias TJ, et al. (2012) The effect of low glucose degradation product, neutral pH versus standard peritoneal dialysis solutions on peritoneal membrane function: the balANZ trial. Nephrol Dial Transplant 27: 4445–4453. gfs314 [pii];10.1093/ndt/gfs314 [doi].
42. Lang SM, Bergner A, Topfer M, Schiffl H (2001) Preservation of residual renal function in dialysis patients: effects of dialysis-technique-related factors. Perit Dial Int 21: 52–57.
43. Vilar E, Wellsted D, Chandna SM, Greenwood RN, Farrington K (2009) Residual renal function improves outcome in incremental haemodialysis despite reduced dialysis dose. Nephrol Dial Transplant 24: 2502–2510. gfp071 [pii];10.1093/ndt/gfp071 [doi].
44. Eknoyan G, Beck GJ, Cheung AK, Daugirdas JT, Greene T, et al. (2002) Effect of dialysis dose and membrane flux in maintenance hemodialysis. N Engl J Med 347: 2010–2019. 10.1056/NEJMoa021583 [doi];347/25/2010 [pii].
45. Grooteman MP, van den Dorpel MA, Bots ML, Penne EL, van der Weerd NC, et al. (2012) Effect of online hemodiafiltration on all-cause mortality and cardiovascular outcomes. J Am Soc Nephrol 23: 1087–1096. ASN.2011121140 [pii];10.1681/ASN.2011121140 [doi].
46. Moist LM, Port FK, Orzol SM, Young EW, Ostbye T, et al. (2000) Predictors of loss of residual renal function among new dialysis patients. J Am Soc Nephrol 11: 556–564.
47. Jansen MA, Hart AA, Korevaar JC, Dekker FW, Boeschoten EW, et al. (2002) Predictors of the rate of decline of residual renal function in incident dialysis patients. Kidney Int 62: 1046–1053. kid505 [pii];10.1046/j.1523-1755.2002.00505.x [doi].
48. Paniagua R, Amato D, Vonesh E, Correa-Rotter R, Ramos A, et al. (2002) Effects of increased peritoneal clearances on mortality rates in peritoneal dialysis: ADEMEX, a prospective, randomized, controlled trial. J Am Soc Nephrol 13: 1307–1320.
49. Marshall MR, Hawley CM, Kerr PG, Polkinghorne KR, Marshall RJ, et al. (2011) Home hemodialysis and mortality risk in Australian and New Zealand populations. Am J Kidney Dis 58: 782–793. S0272-6386(11)00942-5 [pii];10.1053/j.ajkd.2011.04.027 [doi].
50. Burton JO, Jefferies HJ, Selby NM, McIntyre CW (2009) Hemodialysis-induced cardiac injury: determinants and associated outcomes. Clin J Am Soc Nephrol 4: 914–920. CJN.03900808 [pii];10.2215/CJN.03900808 [doi].
51. Foley RN, Gilbertson DT, Murray T, Collins AJ (2011) Long interdialytic interval and mortality among patients receiving hemodialysis. N Engl J Med 365: 1099–1107. 10.1056/NEJMoa1103313 [doi].
52. Pauly RP, Gill JS, Rose CL, Asad RA, Chery A, et al. (2009) Survival among nocturnal home haemodialysis patients compared to kidney transplant recipients. Nephrol Dial Transplant 24: 2915–2919. gfp295 [pii];10.1093/ndt/gfp295 [doi].

6

Left Ventricular Myocardial Function in Hemodialysis and Nondialysis Uremia Patients: A Three-Dimensional Speckle-Tracking Echocardiography Study

Ran Chen[1], Xia Wu[2], Li-Jun Shen[3], Bei Wang[1], Ming-Ming Ma[1], Yuan Yang[1], Bo-Wen Zhao[1]*

1 Department of Diagnostic Ultrasound and Echocardiography, Sir Run Run Shaw Hospital, Zhejiang University College of Medicine and Sir Run Run Shaw Institute of Clinical Medicine of Zhejiang University, Hangzhou, China, **2** Department of Radiology, Sir Run Run Shaw Hospital, Zhejiang University College of Medicine and Sir Run Run Shaw Institute of Clinical Medicine of Zhejiang University, Hangzhou, China, **3** Department of Ultrasound, The First People's Hospital, Hangzhou Xiao Shan District, Hangzhou, China

Abstract

Background: Several studies have demonstrated that uremic patients who have preserved left ventricular ejection fraction (LVEF) could still have the potential for systolic dysfunction. The aim of this study was to assess the differences between the left ventricular (LV) myocardial function in hemodialysis and nondialysis uremic patients based on three-dimensional speckle-tracking echocardiography.

Methods: The study population consisted of 35 maintenance hemodialysis patients (the hemodialysis group), 30 uremic patients who were hospitalized for the creation of a primary arteriovenous fistula (the nondialysis group), and 32 healthy volunteers. All of the patients had normal left ventricular ejection fractions (i.e., 55% or greater). Three-dimensional speckle tracking echocardiography was performed to assess the left ventricle's global three-dimensional strain, regional longitudinal strain, circumferential strain, and radial strain.

Results: The left ventricular regional longitudinal strain, radial strain, circumferential strain, and global three-dimensional strain were significantly decreased in the nondialysis patients compared with the other two groups (all, $P<0.001$). However, the three-dimensional strain and the regional longitudinal strain were lower in the hemodialysis patients than in the controls ($P<0.01$). In the hemodialysis patients and the control group, the longitudinal strain, circumferential strain, and radial strain were higher at the apical level than they were at the basal level and midlevels. A multivariate linear regression analysis showed that the blood urea nitrogen and creatinine levels were independently associated with the values of the global three-dimensional strain ($\beta=-0.217$, $P=0.000$; $\beta=-0.243$, $P=0.011$, respectively) and the longitudinal strain ($\beta=-0.154$, $P=0.032$; $\beta=-0.188$, $P=0.029$, respectively).

Conclusions: Three-dimensional speckle-tracking echocardiography may detect myocardial dysfunction in patients with uremia who have preserved LVEF. The global three-dimensional strain and the regional longitudinal strain appear to be superior in hemodialysis patients compared with nondialysis patients.

Editor: Xiongwen Chen, Temple University, United States of America

Funding: The research is supported by Specialized Research Fund for the Doctoral Program of Higher Education (20110101120136). The funders had no role in study design, data collection and analysis, decision to publish, or preparation of the manuscript.

Competing Interests: The authors have declared that no competing interests exist.

* Email: zbwcjp@163.com

Introduction

Uremia is associated with an increased risk of cardiovascular diseases, including coronary artery disease, myocardial infarction, and heart failure. Mortality is increased by 10- to 20-fold in dialysis patients compared with healthy individuals [1]. Most studies have used the conventional echocardiographic parameters of cardiac function, such as ejection fraction and fraction shortening, which are frequently normal in uremic patients [2,3]. A previous study showed that the ejection fraction and fraction shortening do not adequately describe the regional systolic function and the loading conditions affecting these parameters [4]. Attention has recently been focused on using Doppler tissue imaging to assess LV regional systolic function through the measurement of tissue velocities, displacement, strain, and strain rate. However, tissue Doppler imaging is limited by Doppler angle dependence, which can identify only the myocardial motion and deformation occurring in the direction of the ultrasound beam [5]. Therefore, it has been used primarily to assess longitudinal strain. However, longitudinal strain is only 1 of the 3 principle components of the regional systolic function [6]. Two-dimensional speckle-tracking echocardiography was also recently adopted to detect the subtle impairment of the LV systolic function in uremic patients who have normal LVEF [7,8]. However, a major limitation of two-dimensional speckle-tracking echocardiography (2D STE) is that it is unable to quantify one of the three components of the local displacement vector because of the three-dimensional (3D) anatomy of the LV and the complex 3D patterns of the wall motion [9].

Three-dimensional speckle-tracking echocardiography (3D STE) is a new and emerging technique. It relies on 3D echocardiographic datasets and tracks the motion of speckles within a scanned volume, irrespective of direction. Yu et al. demonstrated that the 3D strain (3DS), which is best described as the "principle tangential strain," may display the resulting direction's muscle fiber contractions, which are aligned either parallel to or tangential to the myocardial surface [10]. The combination of the three components, 3D optical flow and 3D phase correlation, as well as the 3D intensity correlation, allows the calculation of the 3D motion vector field of the subendocardium. Kleijn et al. confirmed the accuracy of 3D STE for the quantitative assessment of global LV function by using cardiac magnetic resonance imaging as a reference method [11], suggesting that 3D STE has the potential to overcome the limitations of Doppler tissue imaging and 2D STE [12,13]. Therefore, the aim of this study was use 3D STE to investigate the LV global and regional myocardial function in hemodialysis and nondialysis uremic patients who have normal LVEF.

Materials and Methods

Study Participants

Between August 2012 and June 2013, 75 uremic patients with a LVEF of 55% or greater were consecutively enrolled from the nephrology clinic. The cases excluded from the study were 2 patients with arrhythmias, 2 patients with severe valvular disease, 3 patients with uncontrolled hypertension (i.e., systolic blood pressure greater than 140 mmHg and/or diastolic blood pressure greater than 90 mmHg), and 3 patients for whom the 3D STE image quality was inadequate. Finally, 65 patients with uremia were analyzed in this study. The uremia patients included 35 patients on maintenance hemodialysis (the hemodialysis group; 4-hour sessions, 3 times weekly for 3 months or more) who were prescribed a standard dose of dialysis targeting an equilibrated dose (Kt/V of urea) of 1.2 or more and 30 patients who were hospitalized for the creation of a primary arteriovenous fistula (the nondialysis group). We recruited 32 age-matched control volunteers from among individuals who received routine checkups at our hospital who had normal results on electrocardiography, transthoracic echocardiography, multi-slice spiral computed tomography (CT), and coronary angiography and had normal blood pressure. The biochemical indexes of all of the study participants were evaluated at the hospital laboratory. The indexes included total cholesterol, glyceride, hemoglobin, creatinine, and urea nitrogen levels in the blood. Written and informed consent was obtained from all of the study participants. The study was approved by the local ethics committee of the Sir Run Run Shaw Hospital (Hangzhou, China).

Echocardiography Measurements

All of the echocardiographic studies were performed using a commercial scanner (iE33; Philips Medical System, N.A., Bothell, WA, USA). Real-time 3D echocardiographic imaging was performed from the cardiac apex by a fully sampled matrix-array transducer. The full-volume acquisition (which included 6 wedge-shaped volumes) was recorded with 6 consecutive cardiac cycles during a single breath-hold. Moreover, the temporal and spatial resolutions of the images were optimized by decreasing the depth and adjusting the sector width to ensure that the entire LV cavity was included within the pyramidal volume. An experienced echocardiographer obtained all of the echocardiographic images using a standard protocol, and another echocardiographer who was blinded to the clinical data of the study participants analyzed the images. An offline analysis of the data was performed using Tom-Tec 4.0 analysis software (Tom Tec Imaging Systems Gmbh, Unterschleissheim, Bayern, Germany). For the tracing of the endocardium and epicardium, the following five views were displayed: (1) the apical four-chamber view; (2) the apical two-chamber view and the three short-axis views; (3) the apex of the LV; (4) the midlevel of the LV; and (5) the basal level of the LV.

Table 1. Clinical Characteristics of the Uremia and Control Groups.

Parameters	Control (n = 32)	Hemodialysis (n = 35)	Nondialysis (n = 30)
Age (year)	53.05±6.83	52.78±7.65	53.16±5.69
Male/female	20/20	19/21	17/23
Course of disease (year)	--------	5.5±3.3	6.2±2.8
Heart rate (bpm)	75±11	73±10	74±12
Systolic BP (mmHg)	120±15	125±13	128±12
Diastolic BP (mmHg)	75±8	80±9	83±8
Body surface area (m^2)	1.5±0.4	1.6 ±0.3	1.6±0.5
Total cholesterol (mmol/;L)	3.3±0.8	6.8±0.9*	8.0±1.2*
Glyceride (mmol/L)	1.2±0.8	4.8±1.2*	6.3±1.3*
Hb (g/dL)	12.4±0.9	11.3±0.8	8.5±0.6*†
CRE (umol/L)	100.5±26.3	580.5±53.3**	897.8±186.9** ††
BUN (mmol/L)	6.8±1.3	20.6±6.4**	48.6±7.0**††
KT/V	NA	1.3±0.2	NA

BP = blood pressure; BUN = blood urea nitrogen; CRE = creatinine; Hb = hemoglobin; Kt/V = dose of dialysis.
$P<0.01$, compared with the control group.
**$P<0.001$, compared with the control group.
†$P<0.01$, compared with the hemodialysis patient group.
††$P<0.001$, compared with the hemodialysis patient group.

Table 2. Echocardiographic Characteristics of the Uremia and Control Groups.

	Control (n = 32)	Hemodialysis (n = 35)	Nondialysis (n = 30)
LVEDV(mL)	78.9±5.1	95.8±8.1*	109.4±7.2*
LVSDV(mL)	3 5.1±3.5	45.4±2.5*	54.3±2.9*
LVEDD(mm)	49.4±3.5	58.6±3.2*	60.2±2.8*
LVESD(mm)	30.5±4.3	41.3±2.6*	43.5±3.0*
LVEF(%)	62.9±2.4	57.8±1.9	56.7±2.0
IVST(mm)	9.2±0.4	13.8±0.5**	14.5±0.3**
LVPWT(mm)	8.8±0.3	12.8±0.2**	13.3±0.3**
E	85.3± 22.1	83.6±17.8	72.3±10.4*
A	78.61±2.5	85.3±20.1	93.9±19.4*
E/A	1.1±0.5	0.83±0.2	0.8±0.3*
E'	8.3±1.6	7.0±1.0	6.2±0.8*
A'	6.8±1.5	8.0±2.1	9.0±2.2*
E'/A'	1.12±0.3	0.92±0.2	0.71±0.1*
E/E'	10.3±2.7	14.3±2.5**	15.8±3.2**

A = transmitral peak velocity of late-diastole; E = transmitral peak velocity of early-diastole; A', velocity of late diastole of the mitral annulus; E' = velocity of early diastole of the mitral annulus; E/A = the ratio of velocity of early and late diastole; E'/A' = ratio of velocity of early and late diastole of mitral annulus; IVST = interventricular septum thickness; LVEDV, left ventricular end-diastolic volume; LVEDD, left ventricular end-diastolic diameter; LVEF = left ventricular ejection fraction; LVESD, left ventricular end- systolic diameter; LVESV, left ventricular end-systolic volume; LVPWT = left ventricular posterior wall thickness.
*$P<0.01$, compared to the control group.
**$P<0.001$, compared to the control group.

The LV epicardium and endocardium were traced automatically, and the tracings were refined with further adjustment. Thus, in a cardiac cycle, the software was able to perform both global and segmental strain analyses, including the global 3D strain (3DS), regional longitudinal strain (LS), radial strain (RS), and circumferential strain (CS). Meanwhile, the end-systolic and end-diastolic LV volumes and ejection fractions were observed automatically. On the parasternal long-axis view, the thickness of the interventricular septum and LV posterior wall were measured at the end-diastole of the LV. The LV diameters were measured at the end-systole and end-diastole phases. The early (E) and late (A) diastolic peak velocities of the mitral inflow and the early (E') and late (A') diastolic peak velocities of the septal mitral annulus were measured by pulse wave Doppler and Doppler tissue imaging. Subsequently, the E/A ratio, E'/A' ratio, and E/E' ratio were calculated to evaluate the diastolic function of the LV.

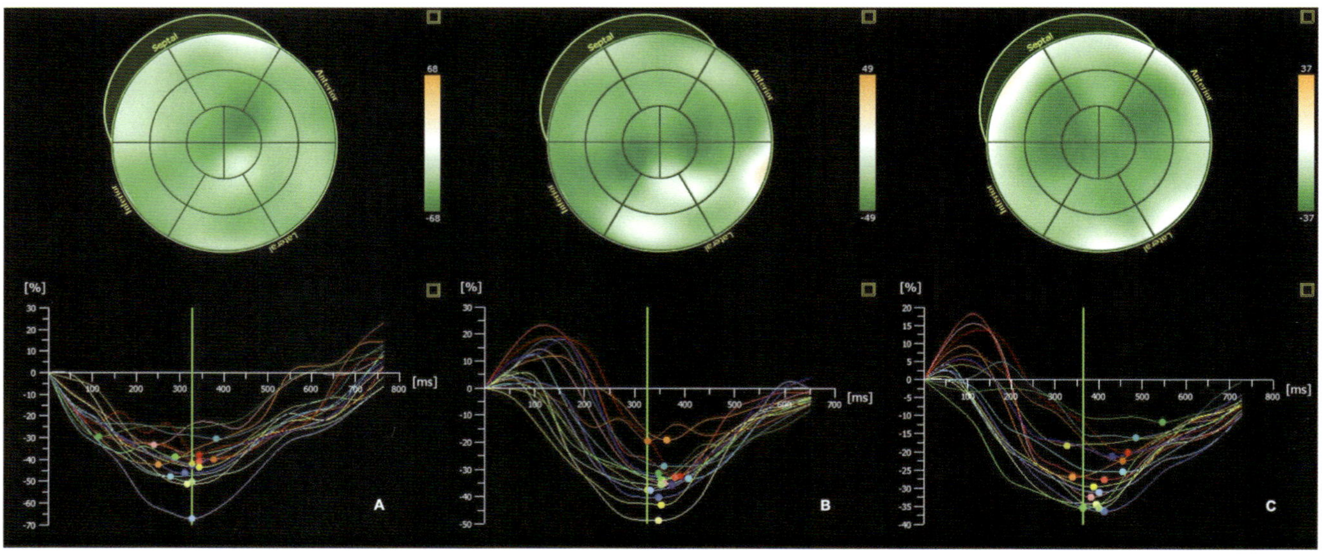

Figure 1. The three-dimensional strain curves of the 16 segments of LV in (A) the controls, (B) the patients in the hemodialysis group, and (C) the nondialysis patients. The color-coded curves indicate the different myocardial segments of the LV. The peak strain values of the different myocardial regions are more decreased in the uremic patients than in the controls. The peak strain is lowest in the nondialysis group.

Table 3. 3D-STE parameters of the Uremia and Control Groups.

		Control (n = 29)	Hemodialysis (n = 30)	Nondialysis (n = 28)
Global	3DS(%)	−38.58±4.25	−25.52±6.81*	−17.75±5.87*,†
Basal	LS	−21.09±3.45	−16.98±2.35*	−10.78±3.08*,†
	CS	−40.63±2.96	−41.69±3.69	−28.58±5.10*,†
	RS	78.08±18.06	77.36±13.37	60.58±12.95*,†
Mid	LS	−22.96±2.65	−15.45±5.23*	−10.39±2.89*,†
	CS	−44.48±5.32	−42.39±4.56	−30.28±2.64*,†
	RS	92.37±8.69	90.78±6.31	64.58±5.87**,††
Apex	LS	−32.43±4.51§,‖	−23.87±3.41*,§,‖	−12.27±2.14*,†
	CS	−50.25±5.68§,‖	−49.24±3.59§,‖	−30.23±3.14**,††
	RS	100.58±10.21§,‖	101.58±16.31§,‖	62.89±7.19**,††

3DS = three-dimensional strain; CS = circumferential strain; LS = longitudinal strain; RS = radial strain; STE = speckle-tracking echocardiography.
*$P<0.01$, compared with the control group.
**$P<0.001$, compared with the control group.
†$P<0.01$, compared with the hemodialysis patient group.
††$P<0.001$, compared with the hemodialysis patient group $P<0.01$, compared with the hemodialysis patient group.
§$P<0.01$, compared with the values at the basal level.
‖$P<0.01$, compared with the values at the midlevel.

Intraobserver Reproducibility and Interobserver Reliability

For the intraobserver reproducibility, 10 subjects were analyzed twice within 4 weeks by one investigator, and the mean values of 16 segments at three levels of LV for RS, CS, LS and 3DS were calculated. The interobserver reliability assessment was performed by analyzing 10 subjects who were chosen randomly by 2 independent investigators. Both observers were blinded to the previous measurements.

Statistical Analysis

All statistical analyses were performed using SPSS version 16.0 software (SPSS, Inc., Chicago, IL, USA). All data were presented as the mean ± the standard deviation (SD). The duration of uremia and hypertension were presented as median values. Differences in the continuous data and categorical data between the patients and the controls were compared using a one-way analysis of variance and χ^2 tests. Independent determinations of subclinical myocardial systolic dysfunction in patients with uremia were examined using multivariate linear regression. The intraclass correlation coefficients (ICCs) method was used to assess the intraobserver reproducibility and the interobserver reliability for the values of the 3D global strain and regional strain. The ICCs were expressed as percentages. The clinical significance was categorized as follows: "excellent," if the ICC was 0.80 or greater; "good," if the ICC was between 0.61 and 0.79; "moderate," if the ICC was between 0.41 and 0.60; and "poor," if the ICC was 0.4 or less [14].

Results

Clinical Parameters

The general clinical indexes and the blood indexes of the hemodialysis group, the nondialysis group, and the control group are summarized in Table 1. Among the three groups, there were no significant differences in sex, age, heart rate, and blood pressure (all, $P>0.05$). However, the total cholesterol and glyceride levels were greater in the hemodialysis and nondialysis groups than in the control group (6.8±0.9 mmol/L and 8.0±1.2 mmol/L vs. 3.3±0.8 mmol/L; 4.8±1.2 mmol/L and 6.3±1.3 mmol/L vs. 1.2±0.8 mmol/L, respectively; $P<0.01$). The total cholesterol and glyceride levels were not significantly different between the hemodialysis and the nondialysis groups. The hemoglobin level was lower in the nondialysis group than in the hemodialysis group and the control group (8.5±0.6 g/dL vs. 11.3±0.8 g/dL and 8.5±0.6 g/dL vs. 12.4±0.9 g/dL, respectively; $P<0.01$). No difference was observed between the hemodialysis group and control group. The creatinine (CRE) and blood urea nitrogen (BUN) levels were significantly greater in the hemodialysis and nondialysis groups than in the control group (580.5±53.3 μmol/L and 897.8±186.9 umol/L vs. 100.5±26.3 umol/L; 20.6±6.4 mmol/L and 48.6±7.0 mmol/L vs. 6.8±1.3 mmol/L, respectively; $P<0.001$). These two levels were significantly decreased in the hemodialysis group compared with the nondialysis group (580.5±53.3 umol/L vs. 897.8±186.9 umol/L and 20.6±6.4 mmol/L vs. 48.6±7.0 mmol/L, respectively; $P<0.001$).

Echocardiographic Characteristics

The echocardiographic parameters of the study groups are shown in Table 2. Compared with the control group, both the nondialysis group and the hemodialysis group demonstrated higher left ventricular end-diastolic volume, left ventricular end-diastolic volume, left ventricular end-diastolic diameter, left ventricular end-systolic diameter, left ventricular septum thickness, left ventricular posterior wall thickness, and E/E′ ratio (all, $P<0.01$). However, there were no significant differences in these factors between the hemodialysis and nondialysis groups. The LVEF was similar in the three groups. Furthermore, the E, A, E/A ratio, E′, A′, and E′/A′ ratio (all, $P<0.01$) were decreased significantly only in the nondialysis group compared with the hemodialysis group and the control group. However, no difference was found between the hemodialysis group and the control group.

Speckle-Tracking Echocardiography Analysis

One hundred and sixty (10%) of 1552 segments were excluded from the 3D STE analysis because of drop-out. The 3D STE analyses of the three groups are shown in Table 3. The LS, CS,

Table 4. Independent factors associated with the systolic functional parameters.

	3DS		LS		RS		CS	
	β	*P*	*β*	*P*	*β*	*P*	*β*	*P*
Duration of Uremia	0.074	.463	0.056	.379	0.021	.089	0.013	.089
Systolic BP	−0.125	.142	−0.074	.284	−0.058	.315	−0.252	.074
LVST	0.062	.326.	0.087	.365	0.021	.064	0.700	.125
E/E'	0.004	.245	0.025	.157	0.085	.310	0.018	.584
Total cholesterol	−0.035	.638	−0.042	.793	−0.038	.157	−0.098	.243
Glyceride	−0.041	.548	−0.058	.547	−0.024	.857	−0.035	.142
Hb	0.025	.336	0.102	.970	0.054	.634	0.047	.639
CRE	−0.243	.011	−0.188	.029	−0.116	.213	−0.137	.105
BUN	−0.217	.000	−0.154	.032	−0.128	.122	−0.092	.174

3DS = three-dimensional strain; CS = circumferential strain; LS = longitudinal strain; RS = radial strain; BP = blood pressure; IVST = interventricular septum thickness; E/E' = the ratio of transmitral peak velocity of early-diastole and velocity of early diastole of the mitral annulu; Hb = hemoglobin; BUN = blood urea nitrogen; CRE = creatinine; *β = Beta coeffident*

and RS at the three levels of LV and 3DS were decreased in the nondialysis group compared with both the control group and the hemodialysis group (all, $P<0.01$) (Figure 1). In addition, the 3DS and LS at the three levels of LV were lower in the hemodialysis group than in the control group (all, $P<0.01$). In the CS and RS, there was no significant difference between the hemodialysis and the control group. The LS, CS, and RS were higher at the apical level than they were at the basal level and the midlevel in the hemodialysis patients and the control patients. However, these values were not significantly changed in the nondialysis group. Based on the multivariate linear regression analysis, the duration of the uremia, systolic blood pressure, LVST, E/E' ratio, and the levels of the total cholesterol, glyceride, Hb, CRE, and BUN were associated with the 3DS, LS, RS and CS, which were used to examine the risk factors for preclinical myocardial systolic dysfunction. The levels of CRE and BUN were independently associated with the 3DS value ($\beta = -0.217$, $P = 0.000$; $\beta = -0.243$, $P = 0.011$) and the LS value ($\beta = -0.154$, $P = 0.032$; $\beta = -0.188$, $P = 0.029$) (Table 4).

Interobserver and Intraobserver Reproducibility

The ICCs are shown in Table 5. The ICCs were all above 0.8. The mean absolute percentage error of all of the measurements did not exceed 0.1. The intraobserver and interobserver reproducibility for the mean measurements of the LS, CS, and RS in the sixteen segments of the three levels of LV and 3DS were acceptable.

Discussion

Cardiac function is still incompletely characterized in uremia patients. This is the first study to compare the differences in the global and regional myocardial functions in hemodialysis and nondialysis patients based on 3D STE. The primary findings of this study are as follows: (1) the global LV systolic function (EF) was normal in the uremic group; however, the global 3DS and the regional LS, RS, and CS were decreased in the nondialysis group, indicating that the LV regional long-axis, short-axis, and global functions were already impaired; (2) the 3DS and LS were higher in the hemodialysis group than in the nondialysis group, indicating that the LV global and regional long-axis functions were superior in the hemodialysis patients; and (3) the decreased CS and RS were observed only in the nondialysis patients and not in the hemodialysis patients. These results demonstrate that, in myocardial dysfunction, the global LV dysfunction and LV regional long-axis systolic dysfunction appear to be more vulnerable to change compared with the short-axis function.

The LVEF reflects the sum of all of the regional shortening in the left ventricle, and regional wall motion impairment may not reduce the LVEF unless several segments are involved.

In our study, the LVEF was normal in the uremia group; however, the LV regional long-axis, short-axis and global functions were already impaired in the uremia patients as assessed by 3D STE, regardless of whether they were undergoing hemodialysis. The underlying mechanisms of the decreased LV function in uremia patients are complex and not thoroughly understood. We speculated that hypertension, LV hypertrophy, LV remodeling, coronary artery disease, myocardial fibrosis, and apoptosis may contribute to LV dysfunction in uremia patients with preserved LVEF. In addition, we found that the LV global function and regional long-axis function were superior in the hemodialysis patients, as shown by the higher 3DS and LS in the hemodialysis group than in the nondialysis group. We believe that the improvement in the LV function in the hemodialysis patients

Table 5. Reproducibility of interobserver and intraobserver by 3D STE.

		Interobserver		Intraobserver	
		ICC	MAPE	ICC	MAPE
Global	3DS(%)	0.84	0.04	0.85	0.03
Basal	LS	0.85	0.05	0.81	0.05
	CS	0.87	0.07	0.91	0.08
	RS	0.85	0.05	0.89	0.07
Mid	LS	0.83	0.08	0.82	0.04
	CS	0.90	0.04	0.86	0.09
	RS	0.87	0.06	0.85	0.05
Apex	LS	0.81	0.08	0.87	0.07
	CS	0.84	0.07	0.90	0.06
	RS	0.82	0.06	0.84	0.05

3DS = three-dimensional strain; CS = circumferential strain; ICC = intraclass correlation coefficient; LS = longitudinal strain; MAPE = mean absolute percentage error; RS = radial strain.

may have resulted from factors such as improvements in their anemia, malnutrition, calcium-phosphorus metabolism disorder and acid-base balance, etc. These factors may decrease the volume load of the LV and thereby improve the anoxic condition of the tissues and organs. The increase in the myocardial oxygen and blood flow as well as the improvement in the LV remodeling may also promote LV systolic function. Therefore, the results from the current study indicate that the 3DS and LS may be sensitive predictors of preclinical LV dysfunction in patients with uremia, particularly in hemodialysis patients. The detection of subclinical myocardial dysfunction may assist clinical doctors in treating uremia patients earlier (even if the LVEF is normal), and thereby reduce the incidence of cardiovascular disease while improving long-term outcomes.

Yan et al. also demonstrated that the CS and RS decreased only in the nondialysis patients based on the 2D STE [3]. This is similar to the results of our study, showing that the impairment in the short-axis function occurred later than the impairment in the regional long-axis function based on the 3D STE. The possible reasons for this result are (1) the augmented LV wall thickness and cross-fiber shortening, which exert their effects as the interaction between a contraction and a systolic increase in the cross-sectional area of all differently aligned myocardial layers; and (2) the curvature radius of the circumferentially oriented myocardial fibers is smaller than that of the longitudinal fibers, which may entail lower stress and consequently delay the appearance of functional abnormalities [15–17].

In addition, myocardial deformation occurs in three dimensions and can be characterized in the longitudinal direction, as well as in the circumferential and radial directions. Subepicardial fibers play a major role in both the RS and LS [18], and subendocardial fibers are important components in CS [19]. The subepicardium is more susceptible to myocardial ischemia and stiffness than the subendocardium. Maizel et al. reported that myocardial stiffness in the uremic mouse may represent an autonomic nervous dysfunction, cellular calcium, or an energy metabolism disorder, for example [20]. Our study showed that the CS and RS were observed in the nondialysis patients but not in the hemodialysis patients. Therefore, myocardial stiffness may be one factor that causes changes in the LV long-axis function earlier than in the short-axis function in uremia patients.

The LV's contractions travel from the apex to the basal region. Our study also found that the LS, CS, and RS were higher at the apical level than at the basal level and the midlevels in the control and hemodialysis groups. However, this phenomenon did not appear in the nondialysis group. A previous study has shown that myocardial contractility reflects the influence of preload [21]. We postulated that the improvement in water-sodium retention and the removal of fluid decrease the preload in hemodialysis patients compared with the nondialysis patients.

A decreased myocardial strain in uremia patients reportedly results from LV hypertrophy rather than from uremic toxicity [22]. In fact, in this study, the myocardial strain was superior in the hemodialysis patients, and the prevalence of hypertrophy was similar in the hemodialysis and nondialysis groups. Moreover, the multiple linear regression showed that the CRE and BUN levels were independent predictors of the global LV systolic function. The CRE and BUN levels were lower in the hemodialysis group than in the nondialysis group. We therefore assumed that the superior LV systolic function in the hemodialysis patients may result from the removal of uremic toxins. A previous study demonstrated that the injury of the myocardial cell membrane structure could cause cardiac dysfunction in uremic patients that was possibly related to the accumulation of uremic toxins [23]. Mark demonstrated that CRE could inhibit the activity of succinate dehydrogenase (SDH) in myocardial cells, which could lead both to obstacles in ATP production and mitochondrial swelling and fragmentation, and thus imbalance and damage to the nutrition and function of the myocardial cells [24]. Moreover, in some studies, BUN is a powerful predictor of increased mortality in patients hospitalized for heart failure. In older patients hospitalized for heart failure [25], a positive linear relationship was found between the BUN and the occurrence of 1-year mortality. According to our study, both the BUN and the CRE possibly contributed to myocardial dysfunction to a certain degree. In addition, indoxyl sulfate (IS), a uremic toxin, can induce TGF-$\beta$and phospho-NFkB p65 protein expression, and the reactive oxygen species-NF-kB-TGF-β_1 pathway may play a role in cardiac fibrosis. Lekawanvijit et al. showed that cardiac fibrosis is reversible by reducing the serum IS level in uremic rats [26]. Therefore, the reduction in uremic toxins possibly alleviates the injury to the myocardial function in hemodialysis patients.

Study Limitations

The temporal and spatial resolutions are relatively lower in the 3D STE than in the 2D STE. Therefore, several patients had to be excluded because the image quality in 1 or more segments was insufficient for the STE analysis. Moreover, our study included a relatively small number of patients. In addition, the long-term cardiovascular event rates or survival assessment in the patients on maintenance hemodialysis was not presented in this study.

Conclusions

Three-dimensional STE analysis offers a useful tool for predicting the myocardial function of the LV in uremic patients. The global LV systolic function and the short-axis and long-axis regional LV myocardial function may be impaired in nondialysis patients who have preserved ejection fraction. However, the global LV function and regional LV systolic function appeared to be superior in the hemodialysis patients over those in the nondialysis patients. 3DS and LS may be sensitive predictors of LV global and regional systolic dysfunction.

Acknowledgments

The authors wish to thank the study subjects for their participation.

Author Contributions

Conceived and designed the experiments: RC BWZ LJS. Performed the experiments: XW BW MMM. Analyzed the data: RC MMM YY. Wrote the paper: RC XW.

References

1. Foley RN, Parfrey PS, Sarnak MJ (1998) Epidemiology of cardiovascular disease in chronic renal disease. J Am Soc Nephrol 9: S16–23.
2. Hayashi SY, Brodin LA, Alvestrand A, Lind B, Stenvinkel P, et al. (2004) Improvement of cardiac function after haemodialysis. Quantitative evaluation by colour tissue velocity imaging. Nephrol Dial Transplant 19: 1497–1506.
3. Yan P, Li H, Hao C, Shi H, Gu Y, et al. (2011) 2D-speckle tracking echocardiography contributes to early identification of impaired left ventricular myocardial function in patients with chronic kidney disease. Nephron Clin Pract 118: c232–240.
4. Semple D, Smith K, Bhandari S, Seymour AM (2011) Uremic cardiomyopathy and insulin resistance: a critical role for akt? J Am Soc Nephrol 22: 207–215.
5. Aurigemma GP, Gaasch WH, Villegas B, Meyer TE (1995) Noninvasive assessment of left ventricular mass, chamber volume, and contractile function. Curr Probl Cardiol 20: 361–440.
6. Mendes L, Ribeiras R, Adragao T, Lima S, Horta E, et al. (2008) Load-independent parameters of diastolic and systolic function by speckle tracking and tissue doppler in hemodialysis patients. Rev Port Cardiol 27: 1011–1025.
7. Kim HK, Sohn DW, Lee SE, Choi SY, Park JS, et al. (2007) Assessment of left ventricular rotation and torsion with two-dimensional speckle tracking echocardiography. J Am Soc Echocardiogr 20: 45–53.
8. Liu YW, Su CT, Huang YY, Yang CS, Huang JW, et al. (2011) Left ventricular systolic strain in chronic kidney disease and hemodialysis patients. Am J Nephrol 33: 84–90.
9. Saito K, Okura H, Watanabe N, Hayashida A, Obase K, et al. (2009) Comprehensive evaluation of left ventricular strain using speckle tracking echocardiography in normal adults: comparison of three-dimensional and two-dimensional approaches. J Am Soc Echocardiogr 22: 1025–1030.
10. Kang Y, Sun MM, Cui J, Chen HY, Su YG, et al. (2012) Three-dimensional speckle tracking echocardiography for the assessment of left ventricular function and mechanical dyssynchrony. Acta Cardiol 67: 423–430.
11. Kleijn SA, Brouwer WP, Aly MF, Russel IK, de Roest GJ, et al. (2012) Comparison between three-dimensional speckle-tracking echocardiography and cardiac magnetic resonance imaging for quantification of left ventricular volumes and function. Eur Heart J Cardiovasc Imaging 13: 834–839.
12. Perk G, Tunick PA, Kronzon I (2007) Non-Doppler two-dimensional strain imaging by echocardiography—from technical considerations to clinical applications. J Am Soc Echocardiogr 20: 234–243.
13. Ng AC, Tran da T, Newman M, Allman C, Vidaic J, et al. (2008) Comparison of myocardial tissue velocities measured by two-dimensional speckle tracking and tissue Doppler imaging. Am J Cardiol 102: 784–789.
14. Fleiss JL (1986) The design and analysis of clinical experiments. New York: Wiley. xiv, 432 p. p..
15. Rakhit DJ, Zhang XH, Leano R, Armstrong KA, Isbel NM, et al. (2007) Prognostic role of subclinical left ventricular abnormalities and impact of transplantation in chronic kidney disease. Am Heart J 153: 656–664.
16. Fagugli RM, Reboldi G, Quintaliani G, Pasini P, Ciao G, et al. (2001) Short daily hemodialysis: blood pressure control and left ventricular mass reduction in hypertensive hemodialysis patients. Am J Kidney Dis 38: 371–376.
17. Serri K, Reant P, Lafitte M, Berhouet M, Le Bouffos V, et al. (2006) Global and regional myocardial function quantification by two-dimensional strain: application in hypertrophic cardiomyopathy. J Am Coll Cardiol 47: 1175–1181.
18. Buckberg GD, Coghlan HC, Hoffman JI, Torrent-Guasp F (2001) The structure and function of the helical heart and its buttress wrapping. VII. Critical importance of septum for right ventricular function. Semin Thorac Cardiovasc Surg 13: 402–416.
19. Gotte MJ, Germans T, Russel IK, Zwanenburg JJ, Marcus JT, et al. (2006) Myocardial strain and torsion quantified by cardiovascular magnetic resonance tissue tagging: studies in normal and impaired left ventricular function. J Am Coll Cardiol 48: 2002–2011.
20. Maizel J, Six I, Slama M, Tribouilloy C, Sevestre H, et al. (2009) Mechanisms of aortic and cardiac dysfunction in uremic mice with aortic calcification. Circulation 119: 306–313.
21. Bogaert J, Rademakers FE (2001) Regional nonuniformity of normal adult human left ventricle. Am J Physiol Heart Circ Physiol 280: H610–620.
22. Popovic ZB, Kwon DH, Mishra M, Buakhamsri A, Greenberg NL, et al. (2008) Association between regional ventricular function and myocardial fibrosis in hypertrophic cardiomyopathy assessed by speckle tracking echocardiography and delayed hyperenhancement magnetic resonance imaging. J Am Soc Echocardiogr 21: 1299–1305.
23. Sarnak MJ, Levey AS, Schoolwerth AC, Coresh J, Culleton B, et al. (2003) Kidney disease as a risk factor for development of cardiovascular disease: a statement from the American Heart Association Councils on Kidney in Cardiovascular Disease, High Blood Pressure Research, Clinical Cardiology, and Epidemiology and Prevention. Circulation 108: 2154–2169.
24. Marks AR (1997) Intracellular calcium-release channels: regulators of cell life and death. Am J Physiol 272: H597–605.
25. Smith GL, Shlipak MG, Havranek EP, Foody JM, Masoudi FA, et al. (2006) Serum urea nitrogen, creatinine, and estimators of renal function: mortality in older patients with cardiovascular disease. Arch Intern Med 166: 1134–1142.
26. Lekawanvijit S, Kompa AR, Manabe M, Wang BH, Langham RG, et al. (2012) Chronic kidney disease-induced cardiac fibrosis is ameliorated by reducing circulating levels of a non-dialysable uremic toxin, indoxyl sulfate. PLoS One 7: e41281.

7

Statins for the Prevention of Stroke

Wen Wang, Bo Zhang*

Department of Neurosurgery, First Affiliated Hospital of Dalian Medical University, Dalian, PR China

Abstract

Background: Stroke is a frequently encountered clinical event that has a detrimental impact on the quality of life. Evidence has increasingly shown that statins can substantially reduce the risk of coronary heart disease. However, it remains to be determined whether statins are definitively effective in preventing stroke.

Methods: We systematically searched the PubMed, Embase, and Central databases for studies that compared the effects of statins and placebo in patients at high risk for stroke. The outcome measures were overall incidence of stroke, incidence of fatal stroke, and incidence of hemorrhagic stroke.

Results: Eighteen randomized controlled trials satisfied all the inclusion criteria for the meta-analysis. The analysis revealed that statins reduced the overall incidence of stroke than placebo (odds ratio [OR]: 0.80; 95% confidence interval [CI]: 0.74–0.87; P<0.00001). In particular, statins showed efficacy in reducing the incidence of fatal stroke (OR: 0.90; 95% CI: 0.67–1.21; P = 0.47) and hemorrhagic stroke (OR: 0.87; 95% CI: 0.60–1.25; P = 0.45). On the contrary, they were found to increase the overall incidence of stroke (OR: 1.12; 95% CI: 0.89–1.41; P = 0.32) and fatal stroke (OR: 1.37; 95% CI: 0.93–2.03; P = 0.11) in renal transplant recipients and patients undergoing regular hemodialysis.

Conclusion: The results of this analysis suggest that statins may be beneficial in reducing the overall incidence of stroke and they may decrease the risk of fatal stroke and hemorrhagic stroke. However, statins should be used with caution in patients with a history of renal transplantation, regular hemodialysis, transient ischemic attack, or stroke. Further analyses should focus on multicentre, double-blind, placebo-controlled randomized trials with data stratification according to the nature of primary diseases and dose–effect relationship, to clarify the benefits of statins in protection against stroke.

Editor: Michael Fehlings, University of Toronto, Canada

Funding: The authors have no support or funding to report.

Competing Interests: The authors have declared that no competing interests exist.

* E-mail: zhangbodl@126.com

Introduction

Stroke leads to disturbances in the blood supply to the brain, which can lead to the rapid deterioration of brain function. On the basis of etiology, stroke can be broadly classified into two types: ischemic and hemorrhagic; it is a heterogeneous condition that involves several causative factors in high-risk populations [1], such as patients with coronary heart disease (CHD), diabetes mellitus, and hypertension. A salient feature of stroke is that the type of stroke is not correlated with the prognosis of the patient [2].

Many studies have indicated that inhibitors of 3-hydroxy-3-methylglutaryl coenzyme A reductase (statins) reduce cardiovascular mortality by bringing about a reduction in the serum low-density lipoprotein (LDL) levels; this reduction has been shown to substantially lower the risk of CHD [3–6]. Further, several large-scale clinical trials have been conducted to evaluate the efficiency of statins in the primary and secondary prevention of atherosclerosis and stroke [7–9]. While some of these trials have shown the beneficial effect of statins in stroke prevention, others have not. This discrepancy in the currently available evidences leads to uncertainty regarding the effect of statins on the prevention of stroke in general and fatal stroke and hemorrhagic stroke in particular.

In the light of the prevalent confusion regarding the efficacy of statins in various high-risk populations, we sought to conduct a meta-analysis of randomized clinical trials (RCTs) evaluating the efficacy of statins in the primary and secondary prevention of stroke in high-risk populations.

Methods

Search strategy

In this meta-analysis, we conducted a thorough search of the PubMed, Embase, and Central databases for the reports of all the RCTs conducted up to October 2012 on the comparison of statins with placebo in the prevention of stroke, without any language restriction. The following search terms were used in various combinations: "stroke," "pravastatin," "lovastatin," "atorvastatin," "simvastatin," "fluvastatin," "cerivastatin," "rosuvastatin," "pitavastatin," "HMG-CoA reductase inhibitor," and "statins." To account for both published and unpublished studies, we performed a cited references search by using Web of Science, checked the reference lists of the identified relevant trials, and contacted the authors of the respective papers and investigators. The primary endpoint of the analysis was the overall incidence of

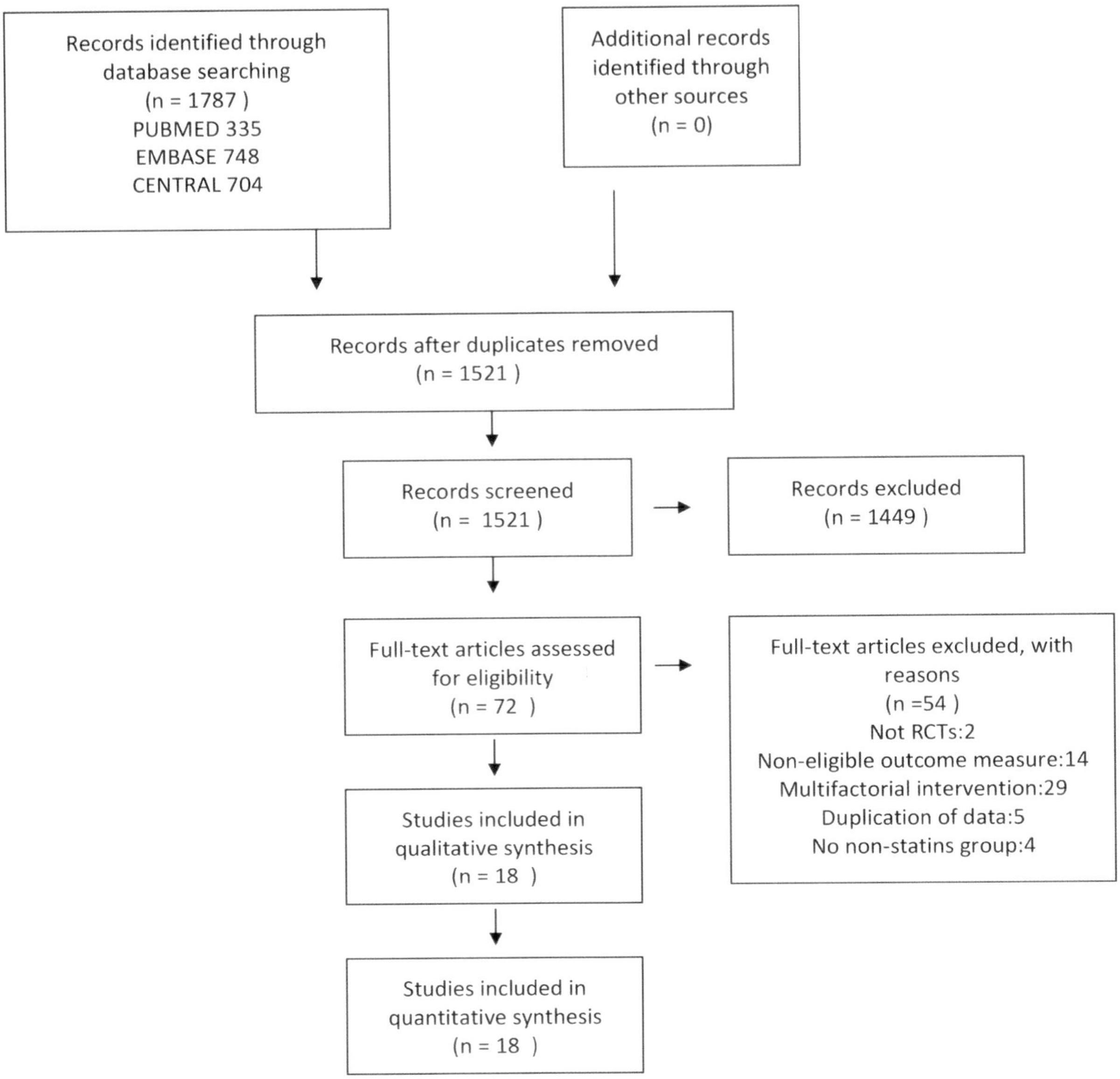

Figure 1. Flow chart indicating the selection process for this meta-analysis.

stroke, incidence of fatal stroke, and incidence of hemorrhagic stroke. The data extraction was independently performed by WW and BZ, and differences in opinion were resolved through discussion.

Inclusion criteria

Studies were included in the meta-analysis if they fulfilled the following criteria: (1) enrolled subjects had high risk of stroke due to prevalent conditions (CHD, diabetes mellitus, hypertension, myocardial ischemia, and hypercholesterolemia) and were of mean age≥50 y; (2) the studies were RCTs conducted on humans; (3) the dosage of statin therapy was specified; (4) the details regarding the type of stroke, including fatal stroke and hemorrhagic stroke, were reported; and (5) the incidence of stroke in the study population was specified or could be calculated.

Subgroup analysis

In order to specifically evaluate the efficacy of statins in patients with end-stage renal disease, a subgroup analysis was performed on trials that included only renal transplant recipients or patients undergoing regular hemodialysis.

Quality assessment

The risk of bias in each study was evaluated by using the Cochrane Collaboration's tool following the instructions given in the Cochrane Handbook for Systematic Reviews. The assessment was made across six domains: sequence generation, allocation concealment, blinding, incomplete data outcomes, selective outcome reporting, and other causes of bias. We studied the influence of the methodological quality of the trials on their results by reviewing the reported randomization protocol and follow-up procedures adopted in each trial.

Table 1. Baseline characteristics of included studies.

STUDY ID	AGE	FEMALE %	TREATMENT	Follow-up year	N(I/C)	Overall Stroke(OS)	Fatal Stroke(FS)	Hemorrhagic Stroke(HS)
Athyros VG et al. 2002 [10]	59 y	22%	Atorvastatin 10–80	3 y	800/800	9/17	ND	ND
Koren MJ et al. 2004 [11]	61 y	17%	Simvastatin 10–80	4.3 y	1217/1225	35/39	ND	ND
Knopp RH et al. 2006 [12]	61 y	34%	Simvastatin 10	4 y	1211/1199	34/38	ND	ND
Sever PS et al. 2007 [13]	63 y	19%	Atorvastatin 10	3.3 y	5168/5163	110/139	ND	ND
White HD et al. 2000 [14]	62 y	17%	Pravastatin 40	6 y	4512/4502	169/204	ND	9/18
Nakamura H et al. 2006 [15]	58 y	69%	Simvastatin 10–20	5.3 y	3866/3966	50/62	ND	16/14
ALLHAT 2002 [16]	66 y	49%	Pravastatin 40	4.8 y	5170/5185	209/231	53/56	ND
Shepherd J et al. 2002 [17]	75 y	52%	Pravastatin 40	3.2 y	2891/2913	135/131	22/14	ND
Hitman GA et al. 2007 [18]	62 y	32%	Atorvastatin 10	3.9 y	1428/1410	21/39	1/7	ND
Amarenco P et al. 2006 [19]	63 y	40%	Simvastatin 80	4.9 y	2365/2366	265/311	24/41	55/33
Plehn JF et al. 1999 [20]	59 y	14%	Pravastatin 40	5 y	2081/2078	52/76	5/1	2/6
HPSI 2003 [21]	65 y	25%	Simvastatin 40	5 y	10269/10267	444/585	96/119	51/53
Waters DD et al. 2002 [22]	65 y	35%	Atorvastatin 80	0.3 y	1538/1548	13/25	3/2	0/3
Kjekshus J et al. 2007 [23]	73 y	24%	Simvastatin 10	2.7 y	2514/2497	103/115	14/11	15/9
Everett BM et al. 2010 [24]	66 y	38%	Rosuvastatin 20	1.9 y	8901/8901	33/64	3/6	6/9
Wanner C et al. 2005 [25]	66 y	46%	Simvastatin 20	4 y	619/636	60/45	27/13	3/5
Fellstrom BC et al. 2009 [26]	64 y	38%	Simvastatin 10	3.2 y	1389/1384	93/81	40/36	25/21
Abedini S et al. 2009 [27]	50 y	34%	Fluvastatin 80	6.7 y	1050/1052	77/83	21/17	10/17

ND: No Data; I/C: Intervention/Control.

Table 2. GRADE profile evidence of the included studies.

Quality assessment							No of patients		Effect		Quality	Importance
No of studies	**Design**	**Risk of bias**	**Inconsistency**	**Indirectness**	**Imprecision**	**Other considerations**	**Statins**	**Control**	**Relative (95% CI)**	**Absolute**		
Overall Stroke (follow-up mean 4 years)												
18	Randomized trials	No serious risk of bias	No serious inconsistency	No serious indirectness	No serious imprecision	Reporting bias	1912/56989 (3.4%)	2285/57092 (4%); 4.1%	OR 0.84 (0.76 to 0.92)	6 fewer per 1000 (from 3 fewer to 9 fewer); 6 fewer per 1000 (from 3 fewer to 10 fewer)	MODERATE	IMPORTANT
Fatal Stroke (follow-up mean 3.8 years)												
12	Randomized trials	No serious risk of bias	No serious inconsistency	No serious indirectness	No serious imprecision	Reporting bias	309/40215 (0.8%)	323/40237 (0.8%); 0.8%	OR 1.03 (0.79 to 1.35)	0 more per 1000 (from 2 fewer to 3 more); 0 more per 1000 (from 2 fewer to 3 more)	MODERATE	CRITICAL
Hemorrhagic Stroke (follow-up mean 4 years)												
10	Randomized trials	No serious risk of bias	No serious inconsistency	No serious indirectness	No serious imprecision	Reporting bias	137/36739 (0.4%)	155/36831 (0.4%); 0.4%	OR 0.88 (0.67 to 1.15)	1 fewer per 1000 (from 1 fewer to 1 more); 0 fewer per 1000 (from 1 fewer to 1 more)	MODERATE	CRITICAL

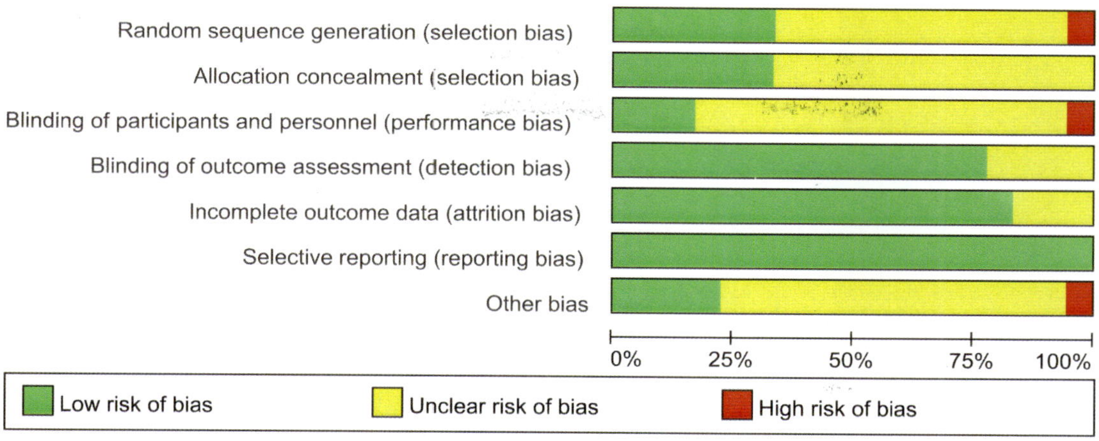

Figure 2. Risk of bias graph.

The quality of evidence was rated using the Grade of Recommendation, Assessment, Development, and Evaluation (GRADE) approach by using the GRADEpro software (version 3.6). As per the GRADE approach, the evidences were graded into the following levels of quality according to the likelihood of change in the estimate of the effect in the light of further research: (1) high quality, if the estimate was extremely unlikely to change; (2) moderate quality, if the estimate was moderately likely to change; (3) low quality, if the estimate effect was highly likely to change; (4) very low quality, if the estimate appeared to be extremely uncertain.

Statistical analysis

The overall incidence of stroke was expressed in dichotomous variables, and the results were expressed as odds ratio (OR) with 95% confidence interval (CI). Data on the incidence of fatal stroke and hemorrhagic stroke were available in 12 and 11 trials, respectively. The pooled estimate of efficacy was calculated using the Mantel-Haenszel method, and the random-effects model was used because various types and strengths of statins were used in the analyzed studies. Significant heterogeneity was defined at $P<0.05$. Heterogeneity was assessed using the I^2 statistic: when I^2 was< 25%, heterogeneity was considered absent; when I^2 was 25–50%, heterogeneity was considered low; when I^2 was 50–75%, heterogeneity was considered moderate; and when I^2 was>75%, heterogeneity was considered high. All statistical analyses were performed using Review Manager 5.2 (version 5.2.4; http://ims.cochrane.org/revman).

Results

Literature search

The initial database search retrieved 1787 studies (335 from PubMed, 748 from Embase, 704 from Central) that were limited to humans, RCTs, and published before October 2012. After eliminating duplicate entries, the number of entries was reduced to 1521. Finally, after applying all the inclusion criteria, 18 RCTs, conducted on 114,081 subjects in all, were selected for the analysis (Figure 1).

Study characteristics

The salient features of the 18 selected studies [10–27] are summarized in Table 1. The studies were published between 1999 and 2010, included 1255 to 20536 subjects each, and had a mean follow-up duration of 4 y. Various statins were investigated in these trials: rosuvastatin, fluvastatin, atorvastatin, pravastatin, and simvastatin. The mean serum level of LDL recorded in the studies was 136 mg/dl.

All the studies were conducted on populations at high risk of stroke, including those with CHD, diabetes mellitus, hypertension and myocardial ischemia. Additionally, one RCT [27] included renal transplant recipients, and two RCTs [25,26] included patients undergoing regular hemodialysis. A subgroup analysis was conducted with these three RCTs. In addition, patients in one of the RCTs [19] had history of stroke or transient ischemic attack (TIA) within the past one to six months, and statins were used in this population for the secondary prevention of stroke.

GRADE evidence profile

All the included RCTs had the same endpoints, which were overall incidence of stroke, incidence of fatal stroke, and incidence of hemorrhagic stroke. The GRADE evidence profiles for upgrading or downgrading each outcome level are shown in Table 2.

Risk of bias

The risk of bias in the included studies is summarized through a graph (Figure 2) and summary (Figure 3). The 18 trials were conducted across eight different countries, namely, USA, UK, Norway, Sweden, Greece, Japan, Germany, and New Zealand, and were mostly based in hospitals or clinics. Only four of the included trials [16,17,23,25] had adequate allocation concealment. All the included trials were considered to have adequate sequence generation because they were essentially randomized in nature. The reports of 12 trials did not describe the method used for generating the allocation sequence. One trial [10] report indicated that patients were randomly allocated to the intervention or placebo group at the out-patient clinic, and therefore, the risk of bias for random sequence generation was considered to be high. While most trials reported blinding of outcome assessment, that of participants, personnel, and outcome assessment was reported only in the case of three [10,19,25] trials. One study [16] was a nonblinded trial, and the risk of bias due to inadequate blinding of participants and personnel was considered high in this case. In most of the selected RCTs, participant flow and important outcomes were reported; therefore, we assessed the incomplete outcome data bias and considered all trials to be of low risk of

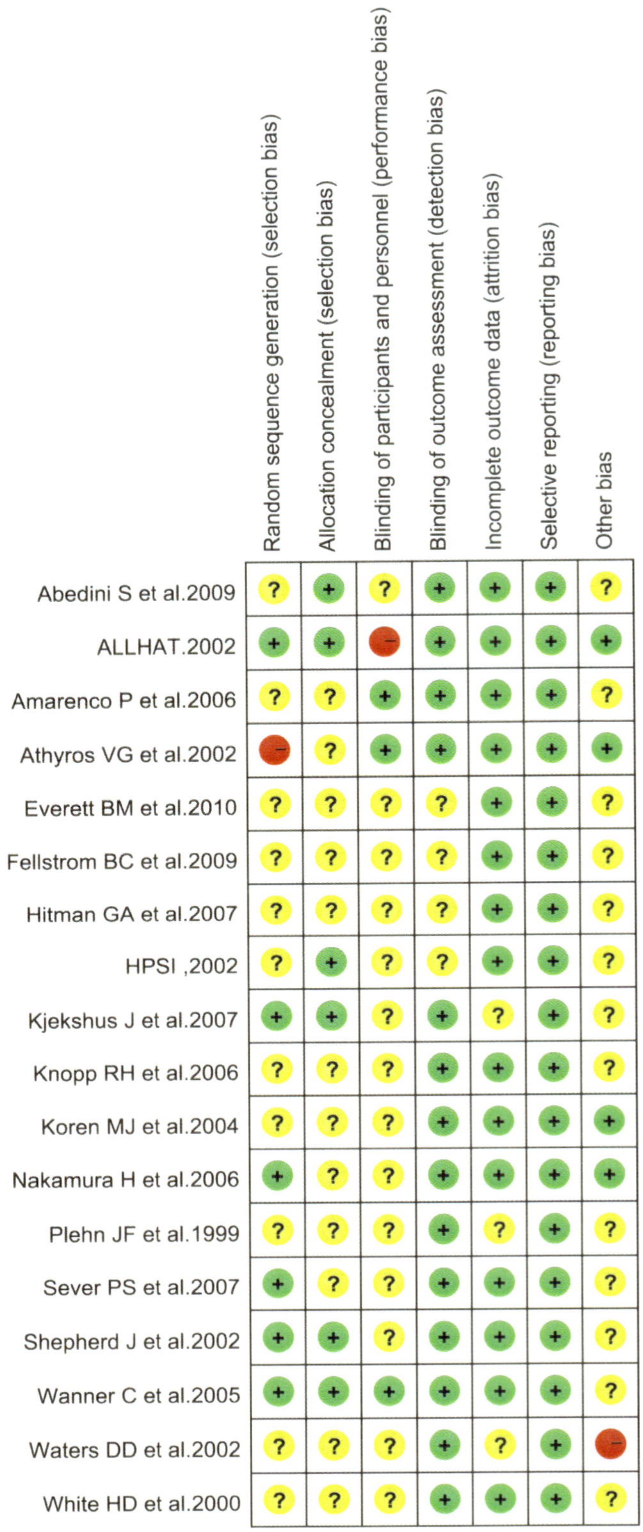

Figure 3. Risk of bias summary.

selective reporting. In one trial [22], the duration of follow up was only 0.3 y, which made the long-term effect of statins on stroke incidence unclear; therefore, the risk of bias due to other causes was considered to be high for that trial.

Overall stroke incidence

The overall incidence of stroke was indicated in all the trial reports. The pooled percentages in the intervention and placebo groups were 3.36% and 4%, respectively. The result of the meta-analysis of all the included studies showed a significant reduction in the incidence of overall stroke in patients treated with statins (OR: 0.80; 95% CI: 0.74–0.87; $P<0.00001$; Figure 4).

The trial by Amarenco et al. [19] included patients with history of stroke or TIA. Pooled results obtained after excluding this study did not differ significantly from those obtained after its inclusion (OR: 0.80; 95% CI: 0.72–0.87; $P<0.00001$), and neither did the heterogeneity ($I^2 = 28\%$, heterogeneity, $P = 0.15$).

Fatal stroke incidence

Nine trial reports provided data on the incidence of fatal stroke [16–24] among 74,322 patients (Table 1). Meta-analysis using the random-effects model showed that statin treatment induced no significant reduction in the incidence of fatal stroke (OR: 0.90; 95% CI: 0.67–1.21; $P = 0.47$; Figure 5) and that heterogeneity among the trials was low ($I^2 = 40\%$; heterogeneity, $P = 0.10$).

Hemorrhagic stroke incidence

Data regarding the efficiency of statins in the prevention of hemorrhagic stroke were available for 11 RCTs. Pooled analysis of data from 7 [14,15,20–24] of these studies, using the random-effects model, revealed that statins did not significantly reduce the incidence of hemorrhagic stroke (OR: 0.87; 95% CI: 0.60–1.25; $P = 0.45$; Figure 6) and had low statistical heterogeneity ($I^2 = 26\%$; heterogeneity, $P = 0.23$). Analysis including the study performed by Amarenco et al. [19] showed a different result (OR: 0.98; 95% CI: 0.67–1.43; $P = 0.91$), with low heterogeneity ($I^2 = 49\%$; heterogeneity, $P = 0.06$).

Subgroup analysis

Subgroup analysis was performed on the three trials [25–27] conducted on renal transplant recipients or patients undergoing regular hemodialysis, by using the random-effects model. The analysis revealed the following: statins reduced the overall incidence of stroke, although this reduction had low statistical significance (OR: 1.12; 95% CI: 0.89–1.41; $P = 0.32$; Figure 4); statins may, in fact, increase the incidence of fatal stroke (OR: 1.37; 95% CI: 0.93–2.03; $P = 0.11$; Figure 5); and statins had a beneficial effect on the incidence of hemorrhagic stroke (OR: 0.87; 95% CI: 0.53–1.42; $P = 0.58$; Figure 6), but with low statistical significance.

Publication bias

Publication bias was assessed using the funnel plot, and the results indicated that the risk of significant bias was low (Figure 7).

Discussion

Current evidences indicate that statins can reduce the incidence of cardiovascular disease via various mechanisms, which include reduced lipid and platelet aggregation, improved endothelial function, anti-inflammation activity, and neuroprotective action [28–31]. Through this meta-analysis, we sought to determine whether statins can indeed prevent stroke, especially fatal stroke and hemorrhagic stroke.

Our analysis of 18 RCTs revealed that statins did, in fact, significantly reduce the overall incidence of stroke. Further, statins

Study or Subgroup	Intervention Events	Intervention Total	Control Events	Control Total	Weight	Odds Ratio M-H, Random, 95% CI
2.1.1 Overall						
ALLHAT.2002	209	5170	231	5185	9.1%	0.90 [0.75, 1.09]
Amarenco P et al.2006	265	2365	311	2366	9.7%	0.83 [0.70, 0.99]
Athyros VG et al.2002	9	800	17	800	1.2%	0.52 [0.23, 1.18]
Everett BM et al.2010	33	8901	64	8901	3.7%	0.51 [0.34, 0.78]
Hitman GA et al.2007	21	1428	39	1410	2.6%	0.52 [0.31, 0.90]
HPSI ,2002	444	10269	585	10267	11.6%	0.75 [0.66, 0.85]
Kjekshus J et al.2007	103	2514	115	2497	6.6%	0.88 [0.67, 1.16]
Knopp RH et al.2006	34	1211	38	1199	3.2%	0.88 [0.55, 1.41]
Koren MJ et al.2004	35	1217	39	1225	3.2%	0.90 [0.57, 1.43]
Nakamura H et al.2006	50	3866	62	3966	4.4%	0.83 [0.57, 1.20]
Plehn JF et al.1999	52	2081	76	2078	4.7%	0.68 [0.47, 0.97]
Sever PS et al.2007	110	5168	139	5163	7.1%	0.79 [0.61, 1.01]
Shepherd J et al.2002	135	2891	131	2913	7.3%	1.04 [0.81, 1.33]
Waters DD et al.2002	13	1538	25	1548	1.7%	0.52 [0.26, 1.02]
White HD et al.2000	169	4512	204	4502	8.5%	0.82 [0.67, 1.01]
Subtotal (95% CI)		**53931**		**54020**	**84.9%**	**0.80 [0.74, 0.87]**
Total events	1682		2076			
Heterogeneity: Tau² = 0.01; Chi² = 18.38, df = 14 (P = 0.19); I² = 24%						
Test for overall effect: Z = 5.20 (P < 0.00001)						
2.1.2 Renal						
Abedini S et al.2009	77	1050	83	1052	5.4%	0.92 [0.67, 1.28]
Fellstrom BC et al.2009	93	1389	81	1384	5.7%	1.15 [0.85, 1.57]
Wanner C et al.2005	60	619	45	636	4.0%	1.41 [0.94, 2.11]
Subtotal (95% CI)		**3058**		**3072**	**15.1%**	**1.12 [0.89, 1.41]**
Total events	230		209			
Heterogeneity: Tau² = 0.01; Chi² = 2.65, df = 2 (P = 0.27); I² = 25%						
Test for overall effect: Z = 0.99 (P = 0.32)						
Total (95% CI)		**56989**		**57092**	**100.0%**	**0.84 [0.76, 0.92]**
Total events	1912		2285			
Heterogeneity: Tau² = 0.02; Chi² = 30.81, df = 17 (P = 0.02); I² = 45%						
Test for overall effect: Z = 3.68 (P = 0.0002)						
Test for subgroup differences: Chi² = 7.43, df = 1 (P = 0.006), I² = 86.5%						

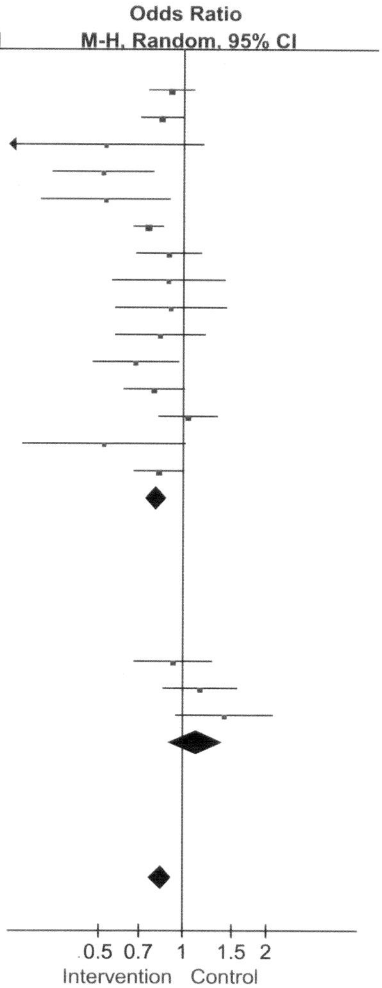

Figure 4. Forest plot for overall stroke incidence.

were found to be effective in the prevention of fatal stroke, although this effect was not statistically significant. On the contrary, three RCTs [25–27] showed that statins may potentially increase the incidence of overall stroke and fatal stroke in patients with a history of renal transplantation, regular hemodialysis, TIA, or stroke, but not significantly. Since this finding was not statistically significant, further investigations are warranted to confirm this. Nevertheless, statins have been previously shown to protect against kidney disease through various immunomodulatory mechanisms [7–9,32]. Therefore, when treating kidney transplant recipients or patients undergoing regular hemodialysis, clinicians should carefully assess the requirement and the dosage of statins administered in relation to the patient's renal function.

This meta-analysis revealed that the use of statins may decrease the incidence of hemorrhagic stroke, although not in a statistically significant manner. This finding is consistent with previous reports indicating the safety of statins in the prevention of hemorrhagic stroke [33,34]. A study by Amarenco et al. [19] on the secondary prevention of stroke revealed that patients treated with statins had a significantly greater frequency of hemorrhagic stroke (55 events) than those treated with placebo (33 events), thereby indicating that the incidence of hemorrhagic stroke in the intervention group was 67% (95% CI: 1.09–2.60). Subsequent analysis revealed that the incidence of hemorrhagic stroke was particularly high in older male patients who had a history of hypertension or stroke [35]. This may be explained by the fact that statins are reported to cause vascular dilatation with rising levels of nitric oxide in the vascular endothelium, which has been implicated in the pathogenesis of hemorrhagic stroke. This may render statins unsuitable for the secondary prevention of stroke.

With regard to the quality of evidence, evaluation using the GRADE system indicated that the data from the included studies were of moderate quality. Since all the 18 included RCTs yielded important outcomes, all trials were to be at low risk of selective reporting.

Our findings should be interpreted in the light of a few limitations. This meta-analysis included only three RCTs comprising renal transplant recipients or patients undergoing regular hemodialysis and only one trial comprising patients with a history of TIA or stroke. This could have led to an underestimation or overestimation of the true incidence of stroke among the analyzed population. Further, we could not account for the impact of the type of coexisting primary diseases (e.g., CHD, diabetes mellitus, hypertension etc.), because the evaluated reports did not contain separate records for the various conditions. Another drawback is that from the current evidences, we were unable to analyze the

Study or Subgroup	Intervention Events	Intervention Total	Control Events	Control Total	Weight	Odds Ratio M-H, Random, 95% CI
1.2.1 Fatal						
ALLHAT.2002	53	5170	56	5185	14.9%	0.95 [0.65, 1.38]
Amarenco P et al.2006	24	2365	41	2366	12.0%	0.58 [0.35, 0.97]
Everett BM et al.2010	3	8901	6	8901	3.1%	0.50 [0.12, 2.00]
Hitman GA et al.2007	1	1428	7	1410	1.5%	0.14 [0.02, 1.14]
HPSI ,2002	96	10269	119	10267	17.4%	0.80 [0.61, 1.05]
Kjekshus J et al.2007	14	2514	11	2497	7.3%	1.27 [0.57, 2.79]
Plehn JF et al.1999	5	2081	1	2078	1.4%	5.00 [0.58, 42.85]
Shepherd J et al.2002	22	2891	14	2913	9.0%	1.59 [0.81, 3.11]
Waters DD et al.2002	3	1538	2	1548	2.0%	1.51 [0.25, 9.05]
Subtotal (95% CI)		**37157**		**37165**	**68.6%**	**0.90 [0.67, 1.21]**
Total events	221		257			
Heterogeneity: Tau² = 0.07; Chi² = 13.32, df = 8 (P = 0.10); I² = 40%						
Test for overall effect: Z = 0.72 (P = 0.47)						
1.2.2 Renal						
Abedini S et al.2009	21	1050	17	1052	9.4%	1.24 [0.65, 2.37]
Fellstrom BC et al.2009	40	1389	36	1384	13.0%	1.11 [0.70, 1.75]
Wanner C et al.2005	27	619	13	636	9.0%	2.19 [1.12, 4.28]
Subtotal (95% CI)		**3058**		**3072**	**31.4%**	**1.37 [0.93, 2.03]**
Total events	88		66			
Heterogeneity: Tau² = 0.03; Chi² = 2.75, df = 2 (P = 0.25); I² = 27%						
Test for overall effect: Z = 1.58 (P = 0.11)						
Total (95% CI)		**40215**		**40237**	**100.0%**	**1.03 [0.79, 1.35]**
Total events	309		323			
Heterogeneity: Tau² = 0.09; Chi² = 21.39, df = 11 (P = 0.03); I² = 49%						
Test for overall effect: Z = 0.24 (P = 0.81)						
Test for subgroup differences: Chi² = 2.86, df = 1 (P = 0.09), I² = 65.0%						

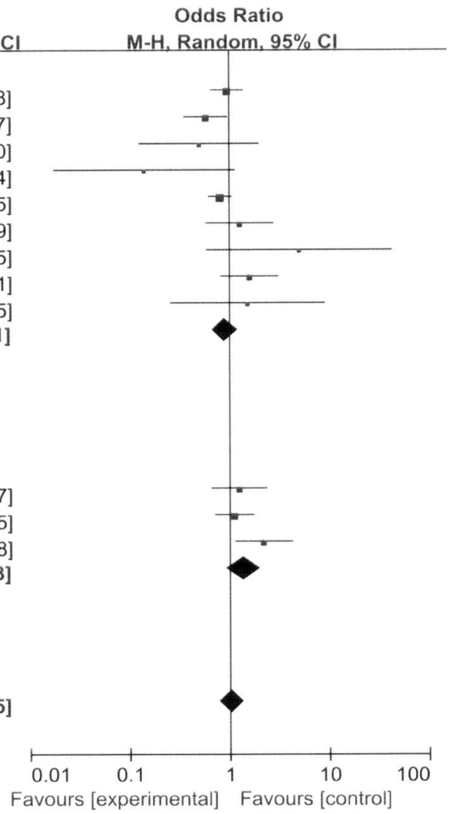

Figure 5. Forest plot for fatal stroke incidence.

Study or Subgroup	Intervention Events	Intervention Total	Control Events	Control Total	Weight	Odds Ratio M-H, Random, 95% CI
1.3.1 Hemorrhagic						
Everett BM et al.2010	6	8901	9	8901	6.2%	0.67 [0.24, 1.87]
HPSI ,2002	51	10269	53	10267	29.4%	0.96 [0.65, 1.41]
Kjekshus J et al.2007	15	2514	9	2497	9.3%	1.66 [0.72, 3.80]
Nakamura H et al.2006	16	3866	14	3966	11.8%	1.17 [0.57, 2.41]
Plehn JF et al.1999	2	2081	6	2078	2.7%	0.33 [0.07, 1.65]
Waters DD et al.2002	0	1538	3	1548	0.8%	0.14 [0.01, 2.78]
White HD et al.2000	9	4512	18	4502	9.8%	0.50 [0.22, 1.11]
Subtotal (95% CI)		**33681**		**33759**	**70.0%**	**0.87 [0.60, 1.25]**
Total events	99		112			
Heterogeneity: Tau² = 0.06; Chi² = 8.13, df = 6 (P = 0.23); I² = 26%						
Test for overall effect: Z = 0.76 (P = 0.45)						
1.3.2 Renal						
Abedini S et al.2009	10	1050	17	1052	10.1%	0.59 [0.27, 1.28]
Fellstrom BC et al.2009	25	1389	21	1384	16.5%	1.19 [0.66, 2.14]
Wanner C et al.2005	3	619	5	636	3.4%	0.61 [0.15, 2.58]
Subtotal (95% CI)		**3058**		**3072**	**30.0%**	**0.87 [0.53, 1.42]**
Total events	38		43			
Heterogeneity: Tau² = 0.03; Chi² = 2.29, df = 2 (P = 0.32); I² = 13%						
Test for overall effect: Z = 0.56 (P = 0.58)						
Total (95% CI)		**36739**		**36831**	**100.0%**	**0.88 [0.67, 1.15]**
Total events	137		155			
Heterogeneity: Tau² = 0.03; Chi² = 10.43, df = 9 (P = 0.32); I² = 14%						
Test for overall effect: Z = 0.93 (P = 0.35)						
Test for subgroup differences: Chi² = 0.00, df = 1 (P = 1.00), I² = 0%						

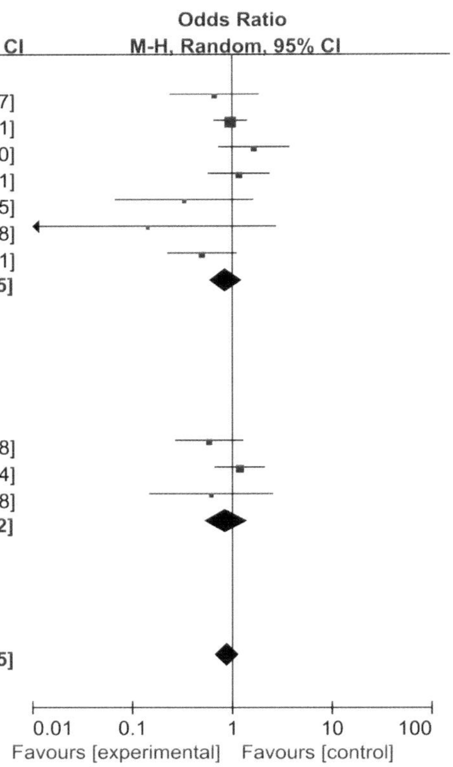

Figure 6. Forest plot for hemorrhagic stroke incidence.

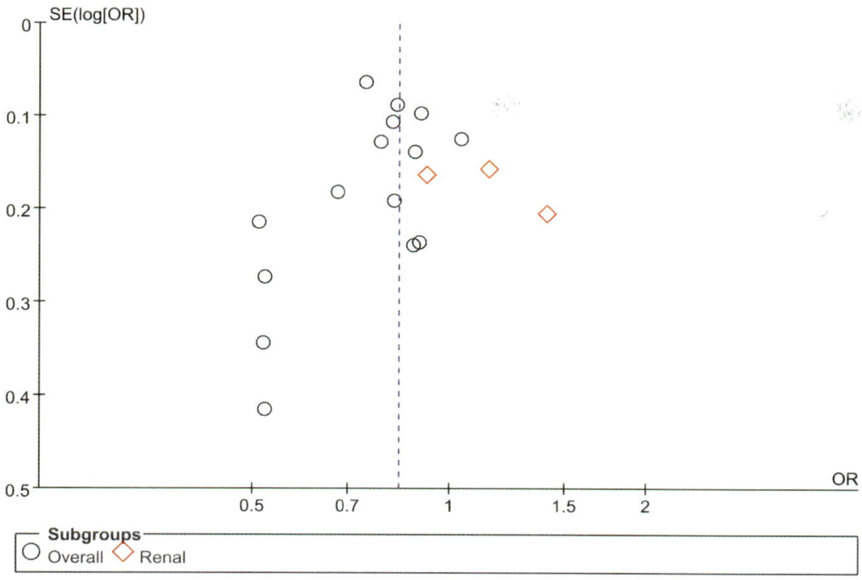

Figure 7. Funnel plot for 18 randomized controlled trials.

possible dose–effect relationship for different types of statins. This highlights the need for more multicentre, double-blind, placebo-controlled randomized trials focusing on the nature of the coexisting primary disease and dose–effect relationship.

Conclusion

The findings of this meta-analysis indicate that statins may be beneficial in preventing the occurrence of stroke in general. In particular, it may potentially reduce the incidence of fatal stroke and hemorrhagic stroke. However, caution must be exercised when using statins in patients with a history of renal transplantation, regular hemodialysis, TIA, or stroke. Further analyses based on data collected in multicentre, double-blind, placebo-controlled, randomized trials and stratified by primary diseases and dose–effect relationship are warranted to substantiate the findings of this meta-analysis.

Author Contributions

Conceived and designed the experiments: BZ WW. Performed the experiments: BZ WW. Analyzed the data: BZ WW. Contributed reagents/materials/analysis tools: BZ WW. Wrote the paper: WW.

References

1. Mohr JP, Albers GW, Amarenco P, Babikian VL, Biller J, et al. (1997) American Heart Association Prevention Conference. IV. Prevention and Rehabilitation of Stroke. Etiology of stroke. Stroke 28: 1501–1506.
2. Kent DM (2006) Stroke—an equal opportunity for the initiation of statin therapy. N Engl J Med 355: 613–615.
3. Robinson JG, Smith B, Maheshwari N, Schrott H (2005) Pleiotropic effects of statins: benefit beyond cholesterol reduction? A meta-regression analysis. J Am Coll Cardiol 46: 1855–1862.
4. Calabro P, Yeh ET (2005) The pleiotropic effects of statins. Curr Opin Cardiol 20: 541–546.
5. Chen J, Zhang ZG, Li Y, Wang Y, Wang L, et al. (2003) Statins induce angiogenesis, neurogenesis, and synaptogenesis after stroke. Ann Neurol 53: 743–751.
6. Grundy SM (1997) Cholesterol and coronary heart disease. The 21st century. Arch Intern Med 157: 1177–1184.
7. (1994) Randomised trial of cholesterol lowering in 4444 patients with coronary heart disease: the Scandinavian Simvastatin Survival Study (4S). Lancet 344: 1383–1389.
8. (1998) Prevention of cardiovascular events and death with pravastatin in patients with coronary heart disease and a broad range of initial cholesterol levels. The Long-Term Intervention with Pravastatin in Ischaemic Disease (LIPID) Study Group. N Engl J Med 339: 1349–1357.
9. Heart Protection Study Collaborative G (2002) MRC/BHF Heart Protection Study of cholesterol lowering with simvastatin in 20,536 high-risk individuals: a randomised placebo-controlled trial. Lancet 360: 7–22.
10. Athyros VG, Papageorgiou AA, Mercouris BR, Athyrou VV, Symeonidis AN, et al. (2002) Treatment with atorvastatin to the National Cholesterol Educational Program goal versus 'usual' care in secondary coronary heart disease prevention. The GREek Atorvastatin and Coronary-heart-disease Evaluation (GREACE) study. Curr Med Res Opin 18: 220–228.
11. Koren MJ, Hunninghake DB, Investigators A (2004) Clinical outcomes in managed-care patients with coronary heart disease treated aggressively in lipid-lowering disease management clinics: the alliance study. J Am Coll Cardiol 44: 1772–1779.
12. Knopp RH, d'Emden M, Smilde JG, Pocock SJ (2006) Efficacy and safety of atorvastatin in the prevention of cardiovascular end points in subjects with type 2 diabetes: the Atorvastatin Study for Prevention of Coronary Heart Disease Endpoints in non-insulin-dependent diabetes mellitus (ASPEN). Diabetes Care 29: 1478–1485.
13. Sever PS, Poulter NR, Dahlof B, Wedel H, Beevers G, et al. (2008) The Anglo-Scandinavian Cardiac Outcomes Trial lipid lowering arm: extended observations 2 years after trial closure. Eur Heart J 29: 499–508.
14. White HD, Simes RJ, Anderson NE, Hankey GJ, Watson JD, et al. (2000) Pravastatin therapy and the risk of stroke. N Engl J Med 343: 317–326.
15. Nakamura H, Arakawa K, Itakura H, Kitabatake A, Goto Y, et al. (2006) Primary prevention of cardiovascular disease with pravastatin in Japan (MEGA Study): a prospective randomised controlled trial. Lancet 368: 1155–1163.
16. Officers A, Coordinators for the ACRGTA, Lipid-Lowering Treatment to Prevent Heart Attack T (2002) Major outcomes in moderately hypercholesterolemic, hypertensive patients randomized to pravastatin vs usual care: The

Antihypertensive and Lipid-Lowering Treatment to Prevent Heart Attack Trial (ALLHAT-LLT). JAMA 288: 2998–3007.
17. Shepherd J, Blauw GJ, Murphy MB, Bollen EL, Buckley BM, et al. (2002) Pravastatin in elderly individuals at risk of vascular disease (PROSPER): a randomised controlled trial. Lancet 360: 1623–1630.
18. Hitman GA, Colhoun H, Newman C, Szarek M, Betteridge DJ, et al. (2007) Stroke prediction and stroke prevention with atorvastatin in the Collaborative Atorvastatin Diabetes Study (CARDS). Diabet Med 24: 1313–1321.
19. Amarenco P, Bogousslavsky J, Callahan A, 3rd, Goldstein LB, Hennerici M, et al. (2006) High-dose atorvastatin after stroke or transient ischemic attack. N Engl J Med 355: 549–559.
20. Plehn JF, Davis BR, Sacks FM, Rouleau JL, Pfeffer MA, et al. (1999) Reduction of stroke incidence after myocardial infarction with pravastatin: the Cholesterol and Recurrent Events (CARE) study. The Care Investigators. Circulation 99: 216–223.
21. Heart Protection Study Collaborative G (2002) MRC/BHF Heart Protection Study of cholesterol lowering with simvastatin in 20,536 high-risk individuals: a randomised placebo-controlled trial. Lancet 360: 7–22.
22. Waters DD, Schwartz GG, Olsson AG, Zeiher A, Oliver MF, et al. (2002) Effects of atorvastatin on stroke in patients with unstable angina or non-Q-wave myocardial infarction: a Myocardial Ischemia Reduction with Aggressive Cholesterol Lowering (MIRACL) substudy. Circulation 106: 1690–1695.
23. Kjekshus J, Apetrei E, Barrios V, Bohm M, Cleland JG, et al. (2007) Rosuvastatin in older patients with systolic heart failure. N Engl J Med 357: 2248–2261.
24. Everett BM, Glynn RJ, MacFadyen JG, Ridker PM (2010) Rosuvastatin in the prevention of stroke among men and women with elevated levels of C-reactive protein: justification for the Use of Statins in Prevention: an Intervention Trial Evaluating Rosuvastatin (JUPITER). Circulation 121: 143–150.
25. Wanner C, Krane V, Marz W, Olschewski M, Mann JF, et al. (2005) Atorvastatin in patients with type 2 diabetes mellitus undergoing hemodialysis. N Engl J Med 353: 238–248.
26. Fellstrom BC, Jardine AG, Schmieder RE, Holdaas H, Bannister K, et al. (2009) Rosuvastatin and cardiovascular events in patients undergoing hemodialysis. N Engl J Med 360: 1395–1407.
27. Abedini S, Holme I, Fellstrom B, Jardine A, Cole E, et al. (2009) Cerebrovascular events in renal transplant recipients. Transplantation 87: 112–117.
28. Vaughan CJ, Delanty N (1999) Neuroprotective properties of statins in cerebral ischemia and stroke. Stroke 30: 1969–1973.
29. Moonis M, Kane K, Schwiderski U, Sandage BW, Fisher M (2005) HMG-CoA reductase inhibitors improve acute ischemic stroke outcome. Stroke 36: 1298–1300.
30. Amarenco P, Lavallee P, Touboul PJ (2004) Stroke prevention, blood cholesterol, and statins. Lancet Neurol 3: 271–278.
31. Willey JZ, Elkind MS (2010) 3-Hydroxy-3-methylglutaryl-coenzyme A reductase inhibitors in the treatment of central nervous system diseases. Arch Neurol 67: 1062–1067.
32. Rysz J, Aronow WS, Stolarek RS, Hannam S, Mikhailidis DP, et al. (2009) Nephroprotective and clinical potential of statins in dialyzed patients. Expert Opin Ther Targets 13: 541–550.
33. Baigent C, Keech A, Kearney PM, Blackwell L, Buck G, et al. (2005) Efficacy and safety of cholesterol-lowering treatment: prospective meta-analysis of data from 90,056 participants in 14 randomised trials of statins. Lancet 366: 1267–1278.
34. Lakhan SE, Bagchi S, Hofer M (2010) Statins and clinical outcome of acute ischemic stroke: a systematic review. Int Arch Med 3: 22.
35. Goldstein LB, Amarenco P, Szarek M, Callahan A, 3rd, Hennerici M, et al. (2008) Hemorrhagic stroke in the Stroke Prevention by Aggressive Reduction in Cholesterol Levels study. Neurology 70: 2364–2370.

Predicting Mortality in Patients with Diabetes Starting Dialysis

Merel van Diepen[1]☯, Marielle A. Schroijen[1,2]*☯, Olaf M. Dekkers[1,2], Joris I. Rotmans[3], Raymond T. Krediet[4], Elisabeth W. Boeschoten[5], Friedo W. Dekker[1]

1 Department of Clinical Epidemiology, Leiden University Medical Center, Leiden, the Netherlands, **2** Department of Endocrinology and Metabolic Diseases, Leiden University Medical Center, Leiden, the Netherlands, **3** Department of Nephrology, Leiden University Medical Center, Leiden, the Netherlands, **4** Department of Nephrology, Academic Medical Center, Amsterdam, the Netherlands, **5** Hans Mak Institute, Naarden, the Netherlands

Abstract

Background: While some prediction models have been developed for diabetic populations, prediction rules for mortality in diabetic dialysis patients are still lacking. Therefore, the objective of this study was to identify predictors for 1-year mortality in diabetic dialysis patients and use these results to develop a prediction model.

Methods: Data were used from the Netherlands Cooperative Study on the Adequacy of Dialysis (NECOSAD), a multicenter, prospective cohort study in which incident patients with end stage renal disease (ESRD) were monitored until transplantation or death. For the present analysis, patients with DM at baseline were included. A prediction algorithm for 1-year all-cause mortality was developed through multivariate logistic regression. Candidate predictors were selected based on literature and clinical expertise. The final model was constructed through backward selection. The model's predictive performance, measured by calibration and discrimination, was assessed and internally validated through bootstrapping.

Results: A total of 394 patients were available for statistical analysis; 82 (21%) patients died within one year after baseline (3 months after starting dialysis therapy). The final prediction model contained seven predictors; age, smoking, history of macrovascular complications, duration of diabetes mellitus, Karnofsky scale, serum albumin and hemoglobin level. Predictive performance was good, as shown by the c-statistic of 0.810. Internal validation showed a slightly lower, but still adequate performance. Sensitivity analyses showed stability of results.

Conclusions: A prediction model containing seven predictors has been identified in order to predict 1-year mortality for diabetic incident dialysis patients. Predictive performance of the model was good. Before implementing the model in clinical practice, for example for counseling patients regarding their prognosis, external validation is necessary.

Editor: Rosa Maria Affonso Moysés, Universidade de São Paulo, Brazil

Funding: This research was performed within the framework of CTMM, the Center for Translational Molecular Medicine (www.ctmm.nl), project PREDICCt (grant 01C-104), and supported by the Dutch Heart Foundation, Dutch Diabetes Research Foundation and Dutch Kidney Foundation. This study was supported by grants from the Dutch Kidney Foundation (E.018) and the Dutch National Health Insurance Board (OG97/005). The funders had no role in study design, data collection and analysis, decision to publish, or preparation of the manuscript.

Competing Interests: Olaf Dekkers is a PLOS ONE Editorial Board member. This does not alter the authors' adherence to all the PLOS ONE policies on sharing data and materials.

* E-mail: m.a.schroijen@lumc.nl

☯ These authors contributed equally to this work.

Introduction

Diabetic patients have a high risk of developing micro- and macrovascular complications such as retinopathy, (cardio)vascular disease and renal disease. According to data in the ERA-EDTA Registry, 23% of the incident end-stage renal disease (ESRD) patients had diabetes as primary renal disease [1]. Survival of diabetic dialysis patients appears inferior compared to ESRD patients without diabetes [2,3], mainly due to cardiovascular disease [4]. Mortality in the diabetic dialysis population is high but varies significantly among patients [5,6].

A prediction model for mortality in diabetic dialysis patients could be a helpful tool in clinical decision-making. For example, it could inform patients about their mortality risk and guide doctors and patients in their decisions on treatment. Furthermore, a prediction model that could accurately stratify patients according to their mortality risk would be useful to evaluate the composition of patients treated in a given center and provide the opportunity to compare baseline risks in comparative studies [7]. Finally, it could aid in designing a clinical trial and selecting subjects for inclusion [8]. Although some prediction models have been developed in patients with diabetes and diabetic nephropathy to predict ESRD [9–13], no prediction model exists in diabetic dialysis patients to predict mortality.

The primary aim of this study was to construct a prediction model to predict 1-year mortality in diabetic dialysis patients. We aimed to include easily obtainable patient characteristics, comorbid conditions and basic laboratory variables, for the model to be convenient for clinical practice.

Materials and Methods

Study population

Data were collected from the Netherlands Cooperative Study on the Adequacy of Dialysis (NECOSAD), a multicenter, prospective cohort study in which 38 dialysis centers throughout the Netherlands participated. Incident adult patients were included at the start of dialysis treatment, between 1997 and 2007. Follow-up data on death were available until 2011. In the present analysis, all patients with diabetes mellitus (patients with diabetic nephropathy and patients with non- diabetic origin of ESRD but diabetes as co-morbid condition) at 3 months after the start of dialysis, which was considered the baseline of the study, were included. We chose 3 months as the start of the study for several reasons: First, at 3 months renal replacement therapy is likely to be a chronic therapy and the choice of treatment modality, hemodialysis or peritoneal dialysis, would be more definitive [14]. Furthermore, patients who recovered or died from acute renal failure within 3 months were excluded from the analysis in this way, creating a more robust model. Finally, at 3 months the clinical condition of patients is more likely to have stabilized and prognostic questions may arise at this point in time. Patients were monitored until renal transplantation or death. Informed consent was obtained before inclusion, and the Medical Ethics Committees of all participating centers approved the study (Maasstad Hospital Rotterdam, Deventer Hospital Deventer, Sint Lucas Andreas Hospital Amsterdam, Academic Medical Center Amsterdam, Maxima Medical Center Veldhoven, Catharina Hospital Eindhoven, Medical Center Haaglanden Den Haag, University Medical Center Groningen, Kennemer Gasthuis Haarlem, Atrium Medical Center Heerlen, Medical Center Leeuwarden, Leiden University Medical Center Leiden, Elisabeth Hospital Tilburg, University Medical Center Utrecht, Antonius Ziekenhuis Nieuwegein, Hospital Gelderse Vallei Ede, Haga Hospital Leyenburg Den Haag, Academic Hospital Maastricht, Jeroen Bosch Hospital Den Bosch, Medisch Spectrum Twente Enschede, Albert Schweitzer Hospital Dordrecht, Alysis Zorg-groep Rijnstate Hospital Arnhem, Dianet Dialysis Center Lunetten Utrecht, Canisius Wilhelmina Hospital Nijmegen, Vie Curi Medical Center Venlo, Leveste Scheper Hospital Emmen, Dianet Dialysis Center Holendrecht Amsterdam, Haga Hospital Rode Kruis Den Haag, Rijnland Hospital Leiderdorp, Admiraal de Ruyter ziekenhuis Goes, Medical Center Alkmaar, Laurentius Ziekenhuis Roermond, Dialysis Center 't Gooi Hilversum, Groene Hart Hospital Gouda, Westfries Gasthuis Hoorn, TergooiHospitals Hilversum, Martini Ziekenhuis Groningen, Zaans Medical Center Zaandam).

Outcome and candidate predictors

The outcome of interest was all-cause mortality within one year after inclusion (3 months). To minimize the risk of overfitting which would harm generalizability of the model and lead to poor performance in new datasets, the number of candidate predictors considered in the analysis should be limited [15,16]. Also, decisions regarding the list of candidate predictors should be made independently of the data at hand [17]. Therefore, we composed a limited candidate predictor list a priori, that is prior to the statistical modelling process. To this end, we first made a selection of promising prognostic factors for one year mortality among incident dialysis patients with diabetes mellitus from the available variables based on a literature review. Next, we reduced this list by combining the rankings of these prognostic factors by both nephrologists and endocrinologists, resulting in the candidate predictors as described below.

Age, sex, smoking status and data on comorbidity were collected at the start of dialysis therapy. Currently smoking or smoking cessation in the three months preceding dialysis initiation was considered smoking. Comorbidity data included a history of cerebral vascular accident, myocardial infarction and peripheral vascular disease with or without amputation. At three months, laboratory values and other clinical parameters were collected. For each patient, data on diabetes mellitus were collected. To indicate the severity of diabetes mellitus, insulin-dependency, a history of diabetic retinopathy for which laser therapy was performed and patient-reported duration of diabetes mellitus were considered for the analysis. Body mass index, blood pressure and levels of hemoglobin, phosphate and serum albumin were included in the analysis. In addition, residual renal function was expressed as the residual glomerular filtration rate (rGFR), which was calculated as the mean of 24-hour creatinine and urea clearance corrected for body surface area (ml/min/1.73 m2). Finally, dialysis treatment modality (HD/PD) and the Karnofsky scale, which is a clinician-assessed scale of functional status, were included. The Karnofsky scale consists of ten levels, ranging from 10 (moribund) to 100 (normal, without limitations).

Next, the list of candidate predictors was further reduced as follows. Instead of including all selected comorbidities separately, history of cerebral vascular accident (CVA), myocardial infarction (MI) and peripheral vascular disease with amputation were combined into one predictor to indicate whether a patient had suffered from macrovascular complications. Systolic blood pressure was chosen to represent blood pressure, as this has been shown to be most predictive of mortality in dialysis patients [18]. Next, although the Karnofsky scale was registered as a categorical variable, it is of an ordinal nature and it was therefore included as a continuous variable [17]. Finally, although data on measured residual GFR (rGFR) based on 24-hour urine collection were available in NECOSAD, rGFR was not included in the main analysis since rGFR is not measured everywhere in this way as a standard procedure. Including rGFR in a prediction rule would therefore make it less practical for use in clinical practice and generalizability would be questionable. Indeed, also in the NECOSAD database a large part (18.8%) of this variable was missing. This would mean no prediction could be made for one out of every five patients. However, as most researchers and clinicians would agree rGFR could potentially be an important predictor for mortality in kidney patients and should not be overlooked a priori, we did perform an additional analysis where rGFR was included in the candidate variable list (see below). In total, these procedures resulted in a list of 14 candidate predictors for the main analysis.

Statistical analyses

Baseline characteristics were summarized as means with standard deviations for continuous variables and as numbers with valid percentages for categorical variables, unless stated otherwise. Missing data were handled by multiple imputation methods using the fully conditional specification [19–21]. All predictors were imputed through linear or logistic regression as appropriate, with two exceptions: the square root of duration of DM was imputed because of non-normality, and the Karnofsky scale was imputed continuously. All candidate predictor variables were entered in a multivariate logistic regression analysis, with one-year mortality as dependent variable. Backward selection with the Akaike Information Criterion (AIC) stopping rule [17,22] was used to identify the

Table 1. Baseline characteristics of the study population.

Baseline characteristics (n = 394)	
Sex (% male)	55
Age at start dialysis (median, years)	65.3 (54.4–72.4)
BMI (kg/m^2)	26.6 (5.0)
Smoking status (current or recently quit) (%)	21
BP (mmHg)	
Systolic	149 (21)
Diastolic	78 (10)
Comorbidities (%)	
Cerebrovascular accident	13
Myocardial infarction	18
Peripheral vascular disease with amputation	5
Macrovascular complications	32
Severity of DM	
Insulin-dependency (%)	64
Duration of DM (median, years)	14 (7–22)
Retinopathy (lasercoagulation) (%)	47
Treatment modality (% HD)	69
Karnofsky scale (%)	
0–40	4
50–70	47
80–100	49
Laboratory values	
Hemoglobin (g/dl)	11.1 (1.6)
Phosphate (mmol/l)	1.8 (0.5)
Serum albumin (g/l)	34.9 (5.0)
rGFR (ml/min per 1.73 m^2)	4.1 (2.9)

Age and duration of DM are presented as median (interquartile range). Other continuous predictors are presented as means (SD); categorical variables are presented as %.
Abbreviations: BMI, body mass index; BP, blood pressure; DM, diabetes mellitus; HD, hemodialysis; rGFR, residual glomerular filtration rate.

most significant independent predictors. In logistic regression analysis, the AIC stopping rule corresponds to a p-value<0.157 for predictor variables with one degree of freedom. Subsequently, forward selection was applied to check stability of the results. Results were pooled over imputed datasets according to Rubin's rules [23,24].

The model's predictive performance was assessed by estimating calibration and discrimination of the model. Calibration indicates how well the model's predictions agree with the observed outcomes and was represented by the calibration slope (which is the regression coefficient of the logistic regression model with the prognostic index as the only predictor) [17,25]. Discrimination indicates how well the model can distinguish between individuals with and without the outcome and was represented by Harrell's c-statistic (which is equal to the area under the receiver operator curve (AUC) for logistic regression analysis) [15,17]. The apparent predictive performance, meaning the performance in the data that were used to develop the model, generally overestimates the predictive performance in new patients. Therefore, validation of the model's predictive performance is necessary to control for this potential overfitting, and internal validation was established through bootstrapping [26,27]. The bootstrapped calibration slope was used as a shrinkage factor to adjust the model for potential overfitting and adjusted coefficients were computed [17].

To assess the robustness of the model a number of sensitivity analyses were performed by (1) checking for non-linearity of continuous variables, (2) excluding all patients with competing endpoints that were treated as alive in the original analysis, (3) including rGFR in the candidate list after imputation of missing values, (4) extending the outcome to 3-year mortality and (5) relaxing the backward selection removal criterion. Bootstrap analysis was performed using the Design package in R [28,29] All other statistical analyses were performed using SPSS (version 20.0; SPSS Inc, Chicago, IL).

Results

Baseline characteristics

Baseline characteristics of the study population of diabetic incident dialysis patients (n = 394 out of a total of 2051 incident dialysis patients in NECOSAD) are shown in *Table 1*. Patients had a median age of 65 years (interquartile range 54–72) and were on average overweight (mean BMI 26.6 (5.0)). In 69% of patients the initial treatment modality was hemodialysis. Thirty-two percent of patients had macrovascular complications and 47% of patients had clinically relevant microvascular complications (retinopathy for which laser coagulation was performed). Eighty-two patients (21%) died within one year after inclusion.

Predictive variables for 1-year mortality

Fourteen candidate predictors (age, sex, BMI, smoking status, systolic blood pressure, macrovascular complications, insulin dependency, duration of diabetes, retinopathy, treatment modality, Karnofsky scale, hemoglobin level, serum phosphate and serum albumin) were included in this analysis. Percentage of missing data was on average 1.9% with a maximum of 8.9% for duration of diabetes mellitus. Five imputed datasets were created. Backward selection with the Akaike information criterion (AIC) stopping rule resulted in the final model with seven predictors; age, smoking status, Karnofsky scale, history of macrovascular complications, duration of DM, serum albumin and hemoglobin level. The pooled estimation results are presented in *Table 2*. Forward selection led to the same results, indicating stability of results.

All predictor variables in the final model had estimated coefficients in the expected directions. For example, smoking status had a positive coefficient, so a smoking patient has a higher

Table 2. Predictive variables for 1-year mortality based on multivariate regression analysis.

Predictor	**B**	**S.E.**	**P-value**	**B_adj**
Age (years)	0.047	0.014	0.001	0.042
Smoking	0.631	0.364	0.083	0.570
Macrovascular complications	1.195	0.291	<0.001	1.078
Duration of DM (years)	0.026	0.013	0.047	0.023
Karnofsky scale	−0.043	0.010	<0.001	−0.039
Hemoglobin level (g/dl)	−0.186	0.097	0.056	−0.168
Albumin level (g/l)	−0.060	0.029	0.042	−0.054

Abbreviations: B, estimated coefficient; S.E., standard error of estimate; B_adj, estimated coefficient adjusted for overfitting.
The intercept of the model, which is necessary for computing predicted mortality risks, was 1.692 (1.610), and 1.427 when adjusted for overfitting.

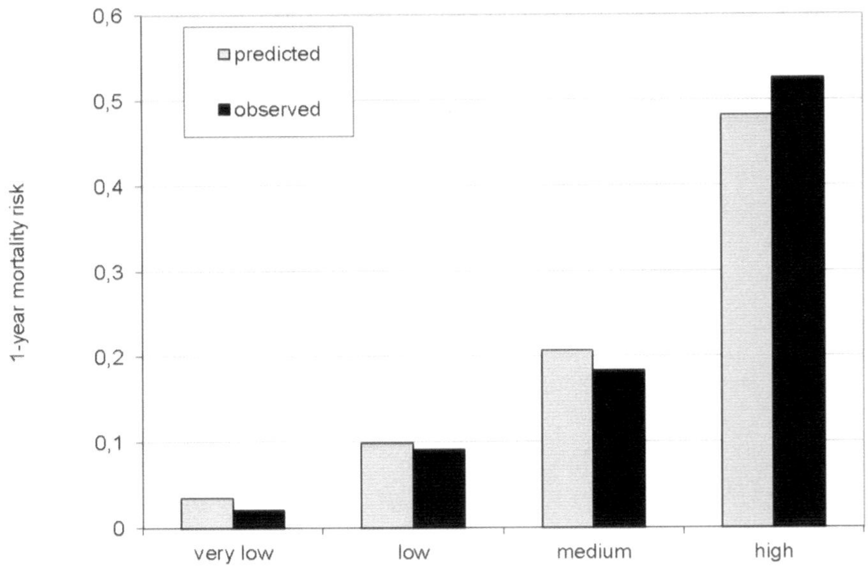

Figure 1. One-year mortality according to risk quartiles. Grey bars represent predicted 1-year mortality risk and black bars represent observed 1-year mortality risk.

probability of dying within a year. On the other hand, Karnofsky scale had a negative coefficient, so the higher the Karnofsky scale of a patient, the lower the probability of dying within a year.

To illustrate the predictions of the model, consider a non-smoking diabetic dialysis patient of 60 years old, with a previous history of myocardial infarction and a duration of diabetes mellitus of 14 years. His Karnofsky scale was 70, his Hb level was 10.5 g/dl and his albumin level was 35 g/l. This resulted in a 1-year mortality risk of 27% (95%-CI: 18%–37%). The same patient, but 10 years older and with a Karnofsky scale of only 40, would have a 1-year mortality risk of 68% (95%-CI: 51%–81%). See Table A.1 in Appendix S1 for computational details and Appendix S2 for a risk calculator.

Validation of the model

To illustrate the calibration of the model, the model was used to predict the risk of one-year mortality for every patient in each imputed dataset used to develop the model and pooled over imputations. Then predicted mortality risk was divided into quartiles from very low to high risk, where the very low risk category represented an average risk of less than 5%, while the average predicted risk in the high risk category was about 50%. Calibration of the model was investigated by comparing observed to predicted risk across the four risk strata and is shown in *Figure 1*.

Discrimination was assessed by calculating the c-statistic using the receiver operator curve (ROC) for each imputed dataset and pooling results. *Figure 2* shows the ROC of the logistic regression model. The c-statistic of the model was 0.810 [0.759–0.860], indicating good discriminative ability. That is, in 81% of the cases the model will assign the highest mortality risk to a patient that dies within a year compared to a random patient that is still alive after a year.

Our model was subsequently internally validated by bootstrapping in each imputed dataset after which results were pooled. *Table 3* compares the apparent performance of the full model (before backward selection), the apparent performance of the final model, and the bootstrapped performance of the final model. The bootstrapped performance is an indication of the external performance, so how the model will perform in a new set of patients.

The c-statistic of the final model was 0.810, which is only slightly lower than that of the full model (0.816). Hence, the final seven predictors were able to discriminate almost as well as the total set of fourteen predictors, justifying the backward selection procedure. By definition, the calibration slope equalled 1 in the original data. After bootstrapping the calibration slope was 0.903, indicating that some overfitting was present. However, it did not

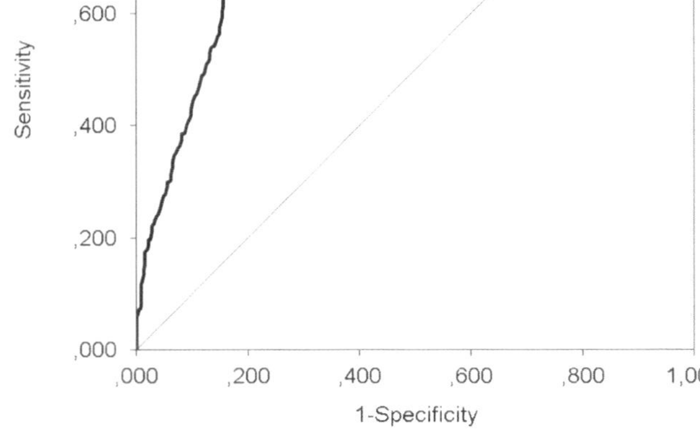

Figure 2. Receiver operating characteristic curve for the logistic regression model. The c-statistic was 0.810.

Table 3. Internal validation: apparent & optimism-corrected performance.

Performance measure	full model	final model	bootstrap
Calibration: slope	1.000	1.000	0.903
Discrimination: c-statistic	0.816	0.810	0.790

substantially affect discrimination, as the c-statistic was still 0.790. For clinical purposes, the bootstrapped calibration slope estimate can be used as a shrinkage factor to compute more reliable parameter estimates, which are presented in the final column of *Table 2*.

Next, several sensitivity analyses were performed to check stability of results. First, to test for non-linearities, quadratic terms of the continuous predictors in the final model were added one by one. None of them were found significant and discrimination did not improve substantially, with a maximum c-statistic of 0.812. Second, patients with competing endpoints such as transplantation or refusal to participate within one year were treated as alive, although their actual status at one year was unknown. Excluding these patients (n = 33) from the analysis did not alter results; the same seven predictors constituted the final model with similar coefficients and model performance. Third, residual GFR was added to the candidate predictor list. In 18.8% of the cases rGFR was missing. Because of non-normality, rGFR was imputed as a square root. It was not significant on top of the seven original predictors in the final model (point estimate of −0.068 with p = 0.275), nor did it substantially improve discrimination (improvement of 0.005 in c-statistic). In an additional analysis with only patients with available rGFR, adding rGFR did not substantially improve predictive performance of the model either (improvement of 0.007 in c-statistic). As a more concise model would be preferred in clinical practice and a recent rGFR may not be available for all patients, rGFR was hence not included in the final model. Fourth, the prediction procedure was repeated for 3-year mortality. Of the 394 patients, 174 (44%) died within three years. Backward selection resulted in predominantly the same final predictor list, where smoking status and hemoglobin level in the model were replaced by sex and therapy modality. Thus, even with a broader timeframe for the outcome, the model is quite stable. The predictive performance was slightly lower, as indicated by a c-statistic of 0.784. Finally, the backwards selection removal criterion was relaxed to p-value = 0.25, which did not change the final model. Further backwards selection removal criterion to p-value = 0.50, resulted in three extra predictors in the final model (sex, BMI and insulin-dependence), but only slightly improved discrimination (c-statistic = 0.815). Since a smaller model is more convenient in practice, the final model with seven predictors was retained.

Discussion

In this cohort study we aimed to identify predictors for 1-year all-cause mortality in diabetic patients on dialysis treatment and used the results to develop a prediction model for this population. Three hundred and ninety four incident diabetic patients were included in this analysis and 82 patients (21%) died within one year after inclusion. Candidate predictors were selected a priori based on existing literature and clinical expertise. The final prediction model contained seven predictors; age, smoking, history of macrovascular complications, duration of diabetes mellitus, Karnofsky scale, serum albumin and hemoglobin level.

Several prediction models have been developed to predict mortality in dialysis patients. Wagner et al. developed a prediction model for 3-year mortality in incident dialysis patients and found that basic patient characteristics, co-morbid conditions and laboratory values can predict 3-year mortality with a c-statistic of 0.75 [13]. Mortality in this study was somewhat lower (30%) than our 3-year mortality (44%). Holme et al. made a prediction model for total 3-year mortality in patients on hemodialysis with a c-statistic of 0.73 [30]. Mortality in this study (47%) was in line with our 3-year mortality. These prediction models included diabetes mellitus as a comorbid condition.

The current prediction model adds to existing models because it is a special model for diabetic incident dialysis patients, which includes specific diabetes-related patient characteristics and co-morbid conditions. Therefore, it is probably more accurate than existing prediction models [13,30] in predicting mortality in this diabetic patient group, as indicated by the c-statistic of 0.810. This model will provide the opportunity to individualize treatment options. Furthermore it allows identifying and informing patients with the highest risk of death within one year. Also, as (novel) biomarkers for outcomes in this patient population are currently being developed [31,32], an adequate basic prediction model is a requisite for assessing the additional predictive value of these biomarkers. Note that our model is not developed as a decision-tool in a pre-dialysis setting, as for such a tool, one would need both different data and different methods. Instead, our model was developed for risk stratification, i.e., to make risk predictions for new chronic dialysis patients after the clinical situation has stabilized.

There are some potential limitations in the present study. First, although the percentage of patients with diabetes in our cohort was similar to that in other European studies [5], the number of diabetic patients was relatively small for developing a prediction model. However, we controlled for potential overfitting by limiting the number of candidate predictors and bootstrapping performance measures. Second, other risk factors - such as if dialysis was started as an elective or urgent treatment, if access for dialysis was already available and social and educational variables - have been found or hypothesized to be related to mortality in diabetic or dialysis patients but have not been included in our analysis because of data restrictions. Specific examples of promising predictors lacking in the NECOSAD data are neuropathy, HbA1c level and diabetes type. Regarding neuropathy, however, adding severity of co-morbid conditions did not seem to increase their predictive power for survival in a study comparing several commonly used co-morbidity indices [33]. As for glycaemic control, we cannot exclude that difference in HbA1c level might translate into different mortality risk [34] and could improve the predictive performance of our model. Regarding diabetes type, as information on this predictor was lacking we included insulin use in our candidate predictor list, which may have been a weaker predictor. However, even without these variables, our prediction model performs well. In contrast to an etiologic study, the value of a prediction model is not judged on individual variables, but on the quality and validity of the predictions that can be made with the variables available. Predicting outcomes is different from explaining their cause [35]. All variables potentially associated with the outcome, not necessarily causally, can be considered in a prognostic study and confounding does not play a role [36,37]. Thus, the lack of potentially important covariates in a prognostic study means there may be room for improvement of the predictive performance, but does not invalidate the current results. Because of data restrictions we could not take all mentioned risk factors into account, but it would be an interesting future research avenue to investigate whether these also contribute prognostically, and improve the predictive performance of the current model. As a third limitation, some may argue that it might be warranted to develop separate prediction models for hemodialysis and peritoneal dialysis patients. Indeed, this may result in even better predictive performance, as it could be that predictor effects differ for PD and HD patients. However, our sample size does not suffice for developing separate models or including interaction terms with therapy modality and we therefore leave this exercise to future research. And fourth, this prediction model has not been evaluated in an external data set yet, which is a necessary condition before introducing the model in clinical practice, by means of an easy to use clinical application.

Despite these limitations this prediction model is the first model that predicts mortality in diabetic incident dialysis patients with good discriminative ability, indicated by the c-statistic of 0.810. To minimize the risk of overfitting we considered a ratio of five endpoints to one candidate predictor acceptable. As larger ratios have been suggested, we additionally controlled for overfitting with internal validation through bootstrapping. Also several sensitivity analyses were performed to check robustness of the model, which showed stability of the results. For example, even a broader time frame of the predicted outcome resulted in predominantly the same final predictor list. Furthermore, the simplicity of the model with parameters that are easily to obtain makes this prediction model potentially useful for clinical practice, for example for counseling patients regarding their prognosis, and guiding doctors and patients in their decisions on future treatment.

In conclusion; a prediction algorithm for 1-year all-cause mortality has been developed for incident diabetic dialysis patients. The performance of this model is good as indicated by good outcomes for discrimination and calibration. For future research our study results need to be evaluated in an external data set. Preferentially this prediction model would be evaluated in other international and larger cohort studies before implementing in clinical practice.

Acknowledgments

The nursing staffs of the participating dialysis centers are gratefully acknowledged for collecting most of the clinical data. The authors also wish to thank the staff of the NECOSAD trial office for their assistance in the logistics of this study.

Author Contributions

Analyzed the data: MD MAS OMD FWD. Contributed reagents/materials/analysis tools: MD MAS OMD FWD. Wrote the paper: MD MAS OMD JIR RTK EWB FWD.

References

1. Stel VS, van de Luijtgaarden MW, Wanner C, Jager KJ (2011) The 2008 ERA-EDTA Registry Annual Report-a precis. NDT Plus 4: 1–13.
2. Liem YS, Wong JB, Hunink MG, de Charro FT, Winkelmayer WC (2007) Comparison of hemodialysis and peritoneal dialysis survival in The Netherlands. Kidney Int 71: 153–158.
3. Vonesh EF, Snyder JJ, Foley RN, Collins AJ (2004) The differential impact of risk factors on mortality in hemodialysis and peritoneal dialysis. Kidney Int 66: 2389–2401.
4. Sarnak MJ (2003) Cardiovascular complications in chronic kidney disease. Am J Kidney Dis 41: 11–17.
5. van Dijk PC, Jager KJ, Stengel B, Gronhagen-Riska C, Feest TG, et al (2005) Renal replacement therapy for diabetic end-stage renal disease: data from 10 registries in Europe (1991–2000). Kidney Int 67: 1489–1499.
6. Villar E, Chang SH, McDonald SP (2007) Incidences, treatments, outcomes, and sex effect on survival in patients with end-stage renal disease by diabetes status in Australia and New Zealand (1991–2005). Diabetes Care 30: 3070–3076.
7. Goodkin DA, Young EW, Kurokawa K, Prutz KG, Levin NW (2004) Mortality among hemodialysis patients in Europe, Japan, and the United States: case-mix effects. Am J Kidney Dis 44: 16–21.
8. Moons KG, Royston P, Vergouwe Y, Grobbee DE, Altman DG (2009) Prognosis and prognostic research: what, why, and how? BMJ 338: b375.
9. Berhane AM, Weil EJ, Knowler WC, Nelson RG, Hanson RL (2011) Albuminuria and estimated glomerular filtration rate as predictors of diabetic end-stage renal disease and death. Clin J Am Soc Nephrol 6: 2444–2451.
10. Forsblom C, Harjutsalo V, Thorn LM, Waden J, Tolonen N, et al (2011) Competing-risk analysis of ESRD and death among patients with type 1 diabetes and macroalbuminuria. J Am Soc Nephrol 22: 537–544.
11. Keane WF, Zhang Z, Lyle PA, Cooper ME, de Zeeuw D, et al (2006) Risk scores for predicting outcomes in patients with type 2 diabetes and nephropathy: the RENAAL study. Clin J Am Soc Nephrol 1: 761–767.
12. Vupputuri S, Nichols GA, Lau H, Joski P, Thorp ML (2011) Risk of progression of nephropathy in a population-based sample with type 2 diabetes. Diabetes Res Clin Pract 91: 246–252.
13. Wagner M, Ansell D, Kent DM, Griffith JL, Naimark D, et al (2011) Predicting mortality in incident dialysis patients: an analysis of the United Kingdom Renal Registry. Am J Kidney Dis 57: 894–902.
14. Termorshuizen F, Korevaar JC, Dekker FW, van Manen JG, Boeschoten EW, et al (2003) Hemodialysis and peritoneal dialysis: comparison of adjusted mortality rates according to the duration of dialysis: analysis of The Netherlands Cooperative Study on the Adequacy of Dialysis 2. J Am Soc Nephrol 14: 2851–2860.
15. Harrell FE Jr., Lee KL, Mark DB (1996) Multivariable prognostic models: issues in developing models, evaluating assumptions and adequacy, and measuring and reducing errors. Stat Med 15: 361–387.
16. Royston P, Moons KG, Altman DG, Vergouwe Y (2009) Prognosis and prognostic research: Developing a prognostic model. BMJ 338: b604.
17. Steyerberg EW (2012) Clinical Prediction Models: A Practical Approach to Development, Validation, and Updating. New York: Springer; 2009.
18. Bos WJ, van Manen JG, Noordzij M, Boeschoten EW, Krediet RT, et al (2010) Is the inverse relation between blood pressure and mortality normalized in 'low-risk' dialysis patients? J Hypertens 28: 439–445.
19. Schafer JL (1999) Multiple imputation: a primer. Stat Methods Med Res 8: 3–15.
20. van Buuren S (2007) Multiple imputation of discrete and continuous data by fully conditional specification. Stat Methods Med Res 16: 219–242.
21. de Goeij MC, van Diepen M, Jager KJ, Tripepi G, Zoccali C, et al (2013) Multiple imputation: dealing with missing data. Nephrol Dial Transplant 28: 2415–2420.
22. Akaike H (1973) Information Theory and an Extension of the Maximum Likelihood Principle. In: Pretov BN, Csaki F, editors. Second International Symposium on Information Theory. Budapest: Akademiai Kaido. pp. 267–281.
23. Kenward MG, Carpenter J (2007) Multiple imputation: current perspectives. Stat Methods Med Res 16: 199–218.
24. Rubin DB (1987) Multiple Imputation for Nonresponse in Surveys.
25. Cox DR (2012) Two further applications of a model for binary regression. Biometrika 1958. 45:562–565.
26. Efron B, Tibshirani RJ (1994) An Introduction to the Bootstrap.
27. Steyerberg EW, Harrell FE Jr., Borsboom GJ, Eijkemans MJ, Vergouwe Y, et al (2001) Internal validation of predictive models: efficiency of some procedures for logistic regression analysis. J Clin Epidemiol 54: 774–781.
28. Harrell FE (2009). Design Package. R package version 2.3-0.
29. R Development Core Team (2009). R: A language and environment for statistical computing. R Foundation for Statistical Computing, Vienna, Austria. ISBN 3-900051-07-0, http://www.R-project.org.
30. Holme I, Fellstrom BC, Jardin AG, Schmieder RE, Zannad F, et al (2012) Prognostic model for total mortality in patients with haemodialysis from the Assessments of Survival and Cardiovascular Events (AURORA) study. J Intern Med 271: 463–471.
31. Bazeley J, Bieber B, Li Y, Morgenstern H, de Sequera P, et al (2011) C-reactive protein and prediction of 1-year mortality in prevalent hemodialysis patients. Clin J Am Soc Nephrol 6: 2452–2461.

32. Desai AS, Toto R, Jarolim P, Uno H, Eckardt KU, et al (2011) Association between cardiac biomarkers and the development of ESRD in patients with type 2 diabetes mellitus, anemia, and CKD. Am J Kidney Dis 58: 717–728.
33. van Manen JG, Korevaar JC, Dekker FW, Boeschoten EW, Bossuyt PM, et al (2002) How to adjust for comorbidity in survival studies in ESRD patients: a comparison of different indices. Am J Kidney Dis 40: 82–89.
34. Hill CJ, Maxwell AP, Cardwell CR, Freedman BI, Tonelli M, et al (2014) Glycated Hemoglobin and Risk of Death in Diabetic Patients Treated With Hemodialysis: A Meta-analysis. Am J Kidney Dis 63(1):84–94.
35. Brotman DJ, Walker E, Lauer MS, O'Brien RG (2005) In search of fewer independent risk factors. Arch Intern Med 165: 138–145.
36. Moons KG, Altman DG, Vergouwe Y, Royston P (2009) Prognosis and prognostic research: application and impact of prognostic models in clinical practice. BMJ 338: b606.
37. Tripepi G, Jager KJ, Dekker FW, Zoccali C (2008) Testing for causality and prognosis: etiological and prognostic models. Kidney Int 74: 1512–1515.

Estimated Glomerular Filtration Rate Decline Is a Better Risk Factor for Outcomes of Systemic Disease-Related Nephropathy than for Outcomes of Primary Renal Diseases

Shuo-Chun Weng[1,2,3]¶, Der-Cherng Tarng[3,4,5]¶, Chyong-Mei Chen[6], Chi-Hung Cheng[2,7], Ming-Ju Wu[2,3,8,9], Cheng-Hsu Chen[2,9], Tung-Min Yu[2], Kuo-Hsiung Shu[2,8]* on behalf of the CKDBHPDH investigators

1 Center for Geriatrics and Gerontology, Taichung Veterans General Hospital, Taichung, Taiwan, **2** Division of Nephrology, Department of Internal Medicine, Taichung Veterans General Hospital, Taichung, Taiwan, **3** Institute of Clinical Medicine, National Yang-Ming University, Taipei, Taiwan, **4** Department and Institute of Physiology, National Yang-Ming University, Taipei, Taiwan, **5** Division of Nephrology, Department of Medicine and Immunology Research Center, Taipei Veterans General Hospital, Taipei, Taiwan, **6** Department of Statistics and Informatics Science, Providence University, Taichung, Taiwan, **7** Department of Biotechnology, HungKuang University, Taichung, Taiwan, **8** School of Medicine, Chung Shan Medical University, Taichung, Taiwan, **9** School of Medicine, College of Medicine, China Medical University, Taichung, Taiwan

Abstract

Background: Currently, the contribution of kidney function decline in renal and patient outcomes is unclear. There are few data on the associations of different etiologies of estimated glomerular filtration rate (eGFR) decline with outcomes in multidisciplinary care. The purpose of this investigation was to establish whether eGFR decline in patients with disease is an important risk factor for developing end-stage renal disease (ESRD) and death.

Methods: From December 1, 2001 to December 31, 2011, 5097 adults with chronic kidney disease (CKD) received biochemical tests, physical examinations, a pathological examination, and a comprehensive questionnaire. We used linear regression models and multivariate Cox proportional hazards model to examine the outcome of eGFR decline in renal diseases with different etiologies.

Results: Mean age was 68.1±16.1 (standard deviation, SD) years, and 63.3% patients were male. In the studied cohort, 58.2% of the patients had systemic disease-related nephropathy (SDRN), 29.4% had primary renal diseases (PRDs), and 12.4% had other etiologies. The eGFR decline in SDRN had a significant association with dialysis in the Cox proportional hazards model [crude hazard ratio (HR) = 1.07, 95% confidence interval (CI), 1.04 to 1.10; adjusted HR 1.05, 95% CI, 1.02 to 1.08]. Diabetic nephropathy (DN) had the most severe eGFR decline in CKD stages 3, 4, and 5, and all contributed to the initiation of dialysis and death regardless of whether DN with or without eGFR decline was considered to be the cause. Although hypertensive nephropathy (HN) was related to significant acceleration of eGFR decline, it did not lead to poor outcome. There were still discrepancies between eGFR decline and outcomes in PRDs, hypertensive nephropathy, and lupus nephritis.

Conclusions: eGFR decline and CKD staging provide an informative guide for physicians to make proper clinical judgments in the treatment of CKD, especially SDRN. Poor control of the underlying systemic disease will thus lead to more rapid progression of SDRN.

Editor: Valquiria Bueno, UNIFESP Federal University of São Paulo, Brazil

Funding: The authors are very grateful for the study grants provided by TCVGH, Taiwan, R.O.C. (TCVGH-1003606A, TCVGH-1013602A, TCVGH-1023601A, CGG-TCVGH1020101-4.4), and Taipei Veterans General Hospital (V97S5-004, V98S5-002, V99S5-002, V100E4-003, V101E4-001), and the Ministry of Education, Taiwan, Aim for the Top University Plan. The funders had no role in study design, data collection and analysis, decision to publish, or preparation of the manuscript.

Competing Interests: The authors have declared that no competing interests exist.

* E-mail: khshu@vghtc.gov.tw

¶ These authors contributed equally to this work.

Introduction

The prediction of need for dialysis and risk of death in chronic kidney disease (CKD) patients has been shown to underestimate the importance of the rate of decline in renal function [1–4]. Although global guidelines have been proposed for estimating the need for preventive services for dialysis, in practice, they might not have been used for those purposes. Renal function is affected by both intrinsic mechanisms of renal disease (e.g., impaired autoregulation [5–6], renal micro-inflammation [7–8], or limited renal functional reserve [9]) and extrinsic factors, such as hemodynamic changes, diabetes mellitus, hypertension, cardiovascular diseases

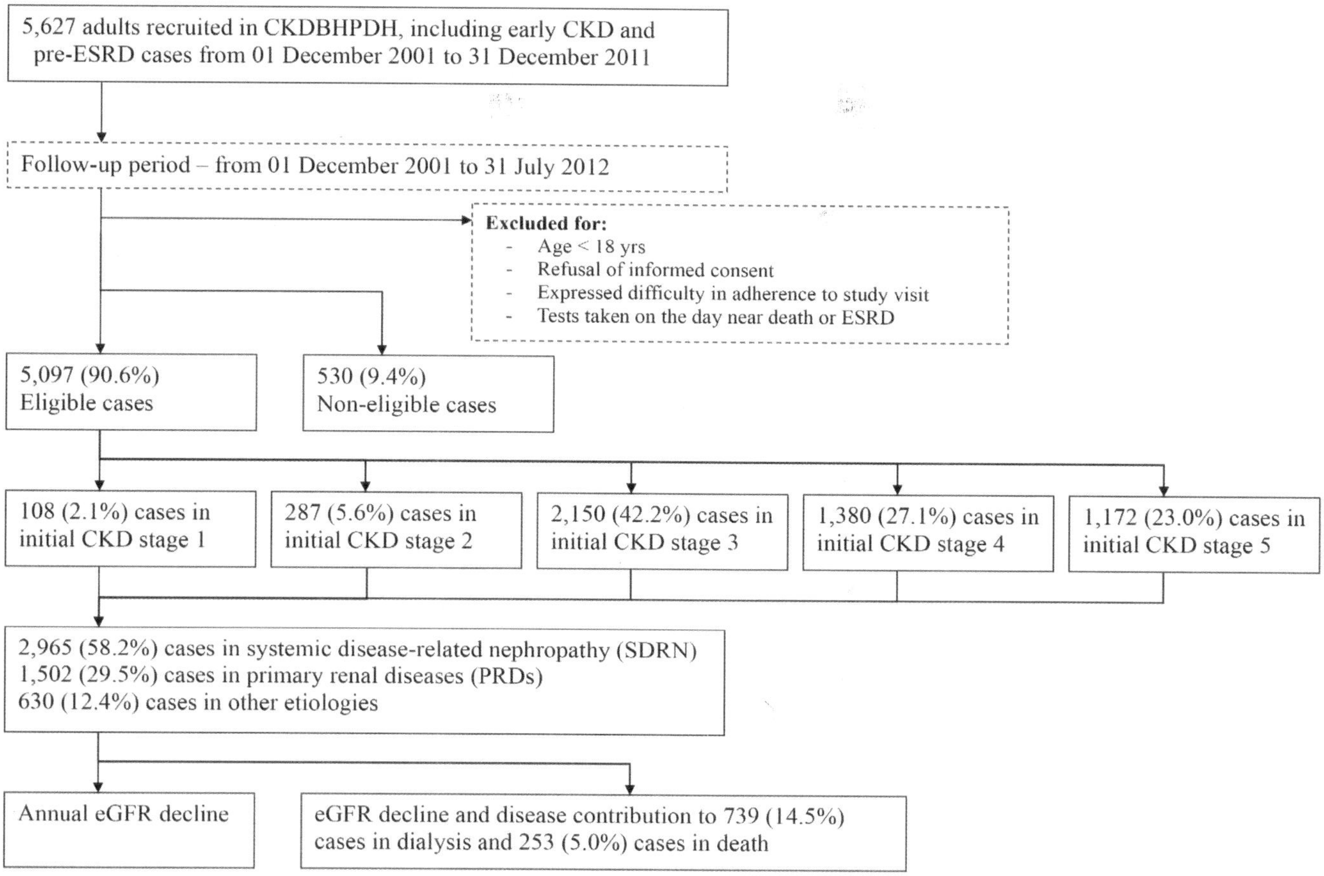

CKDBHPDH – case management care system of Chronic Kidney Disease Division of the Bureau of Health Promotion, Department of Health, R.O.C.

Figure 1. Study diagram of study cohort.

or medication [6]. Physiological decline in kidney occurs due to the aging process, with approximately 10% of eGFR and 10% of renal plasma flow lost per decade after age 40 [10].

Systemic disease-related nephropathy (SDRN) more specifically refers to renal manifestations of systemic disease. A huge variety of systemic conditions can affect the function of the kidneys, from acute illnesses (including, for example, prolonged hypotension) to drugs and more insidious illnesses [2,11,12]. The highest prevalence of secondary glomerular diseases was diabetic nephropathy (44.3%) in the United States and systemic lupus erythematous (54.3%) in China [11]. Primary renal diseases include most common forms of glomerulonephritis, tubulointerstitial diseases, and microvascular or infectious etiologies without diabetic nephropathy, hypertensive nephropathy, lupus nephritis, congestive heart failure, human immunodeficiency virus (HIV) infection, liver disease, and dysproteinemias [11,13,17,18]. It has been shown that extreme eGFR variation may occur in blacks with established CKD (from 1st percentile, -23.6 mL/min/1.73 m^2 per year to 99th percentile, 18.5 mL/min/1.73 m^2 per year), but annual change in eGFR was similar in all race groups with CKD (-3.7% to -4.3% per year) [3]. Biopsy-proved normo- and micro-albuminuric diabetic nephropathy ($-4.9 \sim -2.3$ ml/min/1.73 m^2 per year) [14], and overt diabetic nephropathy (-3.8 ± 3.7 ml/min per 1.73 m^2 per year) were reported in an observational retrospective study [15]. Renal function rates in lupus nephritis (LN) stratified by average urine protein excretion over time, i.e., 0–1, 1–2, and >2 g/day, respectively, were -1.15 ± 5.37, 0.32 ± 8.98, and -6.68 ± 14.6 ml/min per 1.73 m^2 per year [16]. For PRDs, the focal and segmental glomerulosclerosis (FSGS) displayed the highest incidence of ESRD (25.8%) and the fastest decline of eGFR (-4.6 ± 17.6 ml/min per 1.73 m^2 per year) [17]. The prognoses of SDRN and PRDs can be complicated by various modifiable risk factors, racial differences, glomerular hyperfiltration, interstitial fibrosis, tubular atrophy, and primitive etiologies [19]. However, relatively few studies have been conducted to establish whether the effects of different rates of eGFR decline, due to ordinary renal disease etiologies, on outcomes in the same cohort are dependent on SDRN and PRDs [14–20]. Therefore, in the present study, we investigated whether eGFR decline or diseases themselves have different pathological effects superimposed on physiological decline in the overall outcomes. Annual eGFR decline based on the coefficient of variation of the regression line is the most widely used method for estimation, and is used to show correlations with distinct histopathology and clinical diagnosis of CKD [1–6].

In this study, we investigated the effect of eGFR decline on the outcomes of different disease etiologies by conducting a prospective cohort study. The subjects were mostly middle-aged. We hypothesized that eGFR decline in patients with disease is an important risk factor for developing ESRD and death in cause-specific groups.

Materials and Methods

Study Population

Using administrative data from the Chronic Kidney Disease division of the Bureau of Health Promotion, Department of Health, R.O.C. (CKDBHPDH), we identified records of men and women aged older than 18 years with CKD from five counties and cities in central Taiwan from 2001 to 2011. Study participants were recruited and followed up in three major hospitals under the Veterans Affairs Commission, Taiwan, namely, Taichung Veterans General Hospital (VGHTC; main institute), VGHTC Puli branch, and VGHTC Chiayi Branch. The referral centers included more than 4 million residents and the in-charge area was 10,660 square kilometers. The cohort database enrolled early CKD and pre-ESRD patients who were followed-up for longer than 6 months, from December 1, 2001, to July 31, 2012 (Figure 1). Reasons for disenrollment included initiation of dialysis, transfer to another hospital, all-cause mortality, and loss of contact. This study was approved by the institutional review board of Taichung Veterans General Hospital (No.CE12252). Although informed consent was required, the multidisciplinary care did not interfere with clinical decisions related to patient care. Whether written informed consent was given by participants (or next of kin/caregiver in the case of children) for their clinical records to be used in this study, every consent was obtained before the patient records/information was anonymized and de-identified prior to analysis.

Study Design

Patients who had electronic medical records (visits for emergency department, outpatient clinic or hospitalization) in three hospitals were screened for potential recruitment. Screening for recruitment identified in previous units, the acute change in serum creatinine may have been affected by other factors during hospitalizations/emergency department presentations. We recruited the CKD cases under a relatively stable condition which may necessarily reflect their true eGFR change. To examine this question, we assembled a cohort with initial and subsequent eGFR using the 4-variable composite index (serum creatinine, age, race, and gender) – Modification of Diet in Renal Disease (MDRD) equation [1,21]. The enrolled participants were allocated to five CKD groups, from stage 1 to stage 5. The eGFR decline (ml/min/1.73 m^2 per year) with respect to time in different etiologies was analyzed by linear regression models. The coefficient of variation of the eGFR regression line accounts for the eGFR slope in repeated measurements [1–6]. This study considered three separate time intervals, 0–20, 20–40, and 40–60 months because the chosen cut-off points provided adequate statistical power for performing various subgroup analyses during the follow-up period. The cases with representative values of eGFR decline in each time interval excluded the cases that were censored when a value occurred outside the range of a measuring instrument. Such a situation can occur if an individual withdraws from the follow-up study, or if the individual is currently alive and on dialysis at the observational age.

A checklist providing information on socio-demographic characteristics, initial registration day, symptoms and signs of CKD, pre-existing comorbidity, current medication, and laboratory data requested from the Taiwan Society of Nephrology (TSN) for each patient, was completed by research nurses. Demographic information including age, sex, current smoking status, alcohol status, and malignancy were recorded. Diabetes mellitus, hypertension, and current medications were self-reported by the patients or retrieved from electronic records. Presence of cardiovascular diseases, i.e., coronary artery disease, stroke, congestive heart failure, arrhythmia, and peripheral arterial disease, was defined when identified in medical records. Body mass index (BMI) was calculated from the recorded height and weight. Serum creatinine was measured by the Jaffe method using a Beckman Synchron CX5 analyzer (USA) calibrated in accordance with the standards of the Chinese National Laboratory Accreditation program. Measurements of serum uric acid were obtained using the uricase method. Serum albumin was measured using bromocresol green (BCG) assay. Serum glycosylated hemoglobin A1c (HbA1c) was assessed by high-performance liquid chromatography (HPLC), and urine protein to creatinine ratio was measured by strip test. All biochemical laboratory tests were conducted by the Pathology and Laboratory Medicine Department of VGHTC. The time interval between the two eGFR tests or laboratory tests was required to be at least 3 months. Furthermore, we reviewed the medical records of clinical or pathological diagnoses of SDRN and PRDs partly with the assistance of our Clinical Informatics Research and Development Center. The primary outcome measures were incident ESRD warranting renal replacement therapy initiation and mortality due to eGFR decline based on etiological differences.

Statistical Analyses

Our primary goal was to investigate the contribution of eGFR decline to the outcome of CKD patients with SDRN or PRDs after adjusting for age, sex, traditional risk factors (proteinuria, angiotensin-converting-enzyme inhibitor, ACEI/angiotensin receptor blocker, ARB, diabetes mellitus, and hypertension), and antilipemic agents in different stages of CKD [6,19,22–30]. For continuous variables, descriptive results were summarized by mean ± standard deviation and differences were tested by one-way ANOVA if the normality assumption was satisfied, or by Kruskall-Wallis test when the normal assumption was violated. For categorical variables, analyses were conducted using the Pearson χ^2 test. Moreover, the *P*-value for trends was calculated using the Pearson correlation test when a variable was normal and using the Spearman's rank test for continuous non-normal variables. Normality of continuous variables was tested with the Kolmogorov-Smirnov method. If the overall test for homogeneity was rejected, we further conducted pairwise comparison for post-hoc analysis to determine significant differences in risk factors among the five CKD groups.

For each patient, the eGFR decline rate (ml/min/1.73 m^2) with respect to time in different etiologies was estimated by linear regression analysis for all outpatient measures of eGFR during different time intervals. If a patient had at least two outpatient eGFR measures in a specified interval, the eGFR decline for the corresponding etiology would be used.

We performed survival analysis to analyze the duration prior to events. Cox proportional hazards regression was used to determine the associations of eGFR decline in different CKD stages, except CKD stage 1 and 2, with initiation of chronic dialysis and all-cause mortality. Since early eGFR decline has less effect on the later outcome of CKD, this study investigated the contribution of eGFR decline in the last year of follow-up. Unadjusted rates were also reported because these represent actual etiological differences and the full burden of the diseases. Multivariate Cox proportional hazards model was conducted to assess the association of different eGFR decline rates as well as SDRN and PRDs with the primary endpoints, dialysis and death. A two-tailed P value <0.05 was considered statistically significant. Statistical analyses were implemented using **R** statistical software, version 2.15.3.

Table 1. Participants' characteristics by different initial CKD stages.

	Stage 1	Stage 2	Stage 3	Stage 4	Stage 5	*P* value[a]
No. of participants	108	287	2,150	1,380	1,172	
Age (years)	38.6±16.7	52.2±17.7	67.5±14.9	67.2±14.8	63.5±14.6	<0.001[b]
Male gender (%)	46.3	57.1	74.8	59.9	48.9	<0.001[c]
Smoking history (%)	17.6	23.7	40.7	35.0	26.9	0.001[c]
Alcohol history (%)	53.7	42.9	25.2	40.1	51.1	<0.001[c]
Diabetes mellitus (%)	13.9	18.5	34.1	42.3	34.0	<0.001[c]
Hypertension (%)	25.9	47.4	71.4	70.5	65.7	<0.001[c]
Cardiovascular disease (%)	2.8	1.7	8.4	9.5	6.2	0.337[c]
Malignancy (%)	0.0	2.1	6.0	7.4	5.1	0.080[c]
BMI (kg/m2)[†]						
Male, abnormal (%)	71.2	61.7	65.4	61.8	61.4	0.094[c]
Female, abnormal (%)	55.4	59.8	71.6	70.3	59.5	0.085[c]
Average initial eGFR, MDRD (ml/min, median [IQR])	104.5 (95.3–113.0)	71.6 (65.3–79.2)	39.9 (35.1–44.4)	23.1 (19.1–26.6)	9.2 (6.5–12.0)	<0.001[d]
Average initial eGFR, CKD-EPI (ml/min, median [IQR]) [††]	106.3 (100.2–117.0)	73.1 (66.3–81.7)	37.5 (32.9–42.6)	21.3 (17.6–21.2)	8.3 (5.8–10.8)	<0.001[d]
Urine PCR (mg/mmol, median [IQR])	2.9 (1.2–6.5)	1.5 (0.8–3.2)	0.5 (0.1–1.4)	1.0 (0.3–2.5)	1.5 (0.7–2.9)	<0.001[d]
Serum albumin <3.5g/dL, (%)	52.8	33.1	10.2	16.4	23.3	0.718[c]
Serum uric acid ≥7.2mg/dL, (%)	37.0	42.9	58.6	67.8	71.5	<0.001[c]
HbA1C						<0.001[c]
≥6.5 (%)	10.2	13.6	22.8	26.4	14.2	
<6.5 (%)	9.3	7.0	16.4	17.7	18.6	
NA (%)	80.5	79.4	60.8	55.9	67.2	
ACEI & ARB (%)	44.4	54.3	57	58.2	32.4	<0.001[c]
Insulin (%)	3.7	2.1	9.3	18.0	13.6	<0.001[c]
OAD (%)	13.0	16.0	31.3	38.0	24.7	0.105[c]
Antilipemic agents (%)	54.6	36.6	37.2	40.1	18.6	<0.001[c]
ESA (%)	0.9	0.7	2.2	12.9	47.9	<0.001[c]
Final status – Dialysis (%)	0.9	1.0	2.0	10.6	46.7	<0.001[c]
Final status – Death (%)	0.9	4.5	4.6	6.2	4.7	0.158[c]
Median follow-up in months (IQR)	20.3 (12.0–31.5)	27.5 (15.5–40.6)	27.7 (15.8–41.1)	25.7 (14.3–41.6)	16.0 (9.4–27.5)	<0.001[d]

Note: Data for categorical variables are given as percentage; data for continuous variables are given as mean ± standard deviation or median (interquartile range).
[†]The normal BMI value: male is 19.2–23.7 kg/m^2 and female is 18.3–22.7 kg/m^2 (Department of Health, Executive Yuan, Taiwan, R.O.C.). [Spindle 2009 health education advocacy plan survey summary report - The definition of body mass index in adults in Taiwan. February 2009 36(1) 23–26].
[a]For trend; [b]By one-way ANOVA test; [c]By Chi-square test; [d]By Kruskal-Wallis test.
Abbreviations: BMI, body mass index; MDRD, Modification of Diet in Renal Disease equation; CKD-EPI, Chronic Kidney Disease Epidemiology Collaboration formula; PCR, urine protein to urine creatinine ratio; eGFR, estimated glomerular filtration rate; NA, non-available; ACEI & ARB, angiotensin-converting enzyme inhibitors & angiotensin II receptor blockers; OAD, oral antidiabetics; ESA, erythropoiesis-stimulating agent.
[††]CKD-EPI formula, references:
1. Delanaye, P, Mariat, C. (2013) The applicability of eGFR equations to different populations. Nat. Rev. Nephrol 9: 513–522.
2. Levey AS, Stevens LA, Schmid CH, Zhang YL, Castro AF 3rd, et al. (2009) A new equation to estimate glomerular filtration rate. Ann Intern Med 150: 604–612.
3. Matsushita K, Mahmoodi BK, Woodward M, Emberson JR, Jafar TH, et al. (2012) Comparison of risk prediction using the CKD-EPI equation and the MDRD study equation for estimated glomerular filtration rate. JAMA. 307: 1941–1951.

Results

Baseline Demographics

Participants' characteristics were stratified by initial eGFR (Table 1). We also simulated the CKD cohort with the Chronic Kidney Disease Epidemiology Collaboration (CKD-EPI) formula which included variables such as age, sex, and serum creatinine, and concordance was found with a positive correlation between MDRD and CKD-EPI (Figure S1, Figure S2, Figure S3). Of the 5,097 patients included in the cohort, the mean age was 68.1±16.1 years. Patients with late-stage (stage 3, 4, 5) CKD were slightly older, more likely to have diabetes (CKD stage 3, 34.1%; stage 4, 42.3%; stage 5, 34.0%, *P* for trend <0.001), hypertension (CKD stage 3, 71.4%; stage 4, 70.5%; stage 5, 65.7%, *P* for trend <0.001), and hyperuricemia (CKD stage 3, 58.6%; stage 4, 67.8%; stage 5, 71.5%, *P* for trend <0.001). There was a high rate of prescription of patients on insulin (CKD stage 3, 9.3%; stage 4, 18.0%; stage 5, 13.6%, *P* for trend <0.001) and using an erythropoiesis-stimulating agent (ESA) in late-stage CKD patients (CKD stage 3, 2.2%; stage 4, 12.9%; stage 5, 47.9%, *P* for trend <0.001). Those with early-stage (stage 1 and 2) CKD were younger and smoking was less prevalent, but were more likely to have significant proteinuria. There were no differences in the distributions of cardiovascular disease, malignancy, abnormal

Table 2. Diagnosed etiologies by different initial CKD stages.

	Stage 1	Stage 2	Stage 3	Stage 4	Stage 5	*P value*[a]
No. of participants	108	287	2,150	1,380	1,172	
Systemic disease-related nephropathy (n = 2,965, 58.2%)						
Diabetic nephropathy (%)	9.3	16.0	29.0	38.1	32.1	<0.001
Hypertensive nephropathy (%)	4.6	10.1	23.9	19.2	22.4	0.011
Lupus nephrophritis (%)	4.6	3.1	0.6	1.0	2.2	0.641
Others (%)[††]	0.0	2.8	5.6	5.4	3.4	0.034
Primary renal diseases (n = 1,502, 29.4%)						
IgA nephropathy (%)	14.8	11.5	3.1	3.4	1.6	<0.001
Membranous nephropathy (%)	16.7	11.5	1.5	0.8	0.6	<0.001
Focal segmental glomerulosclerosis (%)	3.7	3.8	1.8	1.8	1.3	0.012
Minimal change disease (%)	10.2	3.5	0.4	0.1	0.1	<0.001
Membranoproliferative glomerulonephritis (%)	0.0	0.7	0.2	0.4	0.1	0.524
Crescentic GN, RPGN (%)	0.0	0.0	0.1	0.2	0.6	0.002
Other renal parenchyma disease (%)*	33.3	26.5	21.6	18.0	20.7	0.001
Other etiology (n = 630, 12.4%)**						<0.001
	2.8	10.5	12.2	11.6	14.9	

[a]By Chi-square test.
[††]Other systemic disease-related nephropathy included amyloidosis, scleroderma, multiple myeloma, gouty nephropathy, liver cirrhosis, heart failure, eclampsia, metabolic diseases causing renal failure, and other systemic disease causing renal failure.
*Other renal parenchyma disease of the primary renal diseases including chronic pyelonephritis, unrecovered acute renal failure, chronic glomerulonephritis, post-infectious glomerulonephritis, chronic interstitial nephritis, rejection of kidney allograft.
**Other etiology included obstructive nephropathy, urinary tract diseases, renal vascular diseases, hereditary diseases, other causes of renal failure, and renal failure with unknown causes.

body mass index (BMI) by gender, serum albumin, oral antidiabetics (OADs), and final death status among the five groups.

After using pairwise comparison for post-hoc analysis, males were distributed equally in all CKD stages, except for 1,608 cases (74.8%) in CKD stage 3. With regard to lifestyle behaviors, never-smoking patients were more prevalent in early-stage CKD and the highest proportions of never-alcohol patients were observed in CKD stages 3 and 4. During follow-up, patients with CKD stages 4 or 5 were more likely to have dialysis (10.6% and 46.7%). But for the other rigorous outcome, all-cause mortality, there were no differences among the five groups. Furthermore, patients with CKD stage 5 had a shorter median follow-up in months (Table 1).

Systemic Disease-related Nephropathy (SDRN) and Primary Renal Disease (PRD) Based on Initial Clinical or Pathological Diagnosis

Most SDRN was diagnosed by clinical judgment (96.1%). SDRN was diagnosed by pathological report in 3.9% of cases, but almost all cases of lupus nephritis were diagnosed by pathology. For entry eGFRs, diabetic nephropathy (DN) and hypertensive nephropathy (HN) were largely found in patients with relatively late-stage CKD (DN, stage 3, 29.0%; stage 4, 38.1%; stage 5, 32.1%, *P* for trend <0.001; HN, stage 3, 23.9%; stage 4, 19.2%; stage 5, 22.4%, *P* for trend 0.011, Table 2). Patients with diagnosis of PRDs included 32.8% cases diagnosed by renal-biopsy report and 67.2% cases that were identified in a search of index hospitals in Taiwan's National Health Insurance Research Database (NHIRD). Several subgroups in PRDs had early-stage CKD, such as IgA nephropathy (IgAN) (stage 1, 14.8% and stage 2, 11.5% *vs.* other stages, *P* for trend <0.001), membranous nephropathy (MN) (stage 1, 16.7% and stage 2, 11.5% *vs.* other stages, *P* for trend <0.001), FSGS (stage 1, 3.7% and stage 2, 3.8% *vs.* other stages, *P* for trend = 0.012), and minimal change disease (MCD) (stage 1, 10.2% and stage 2, 3.5% *vs.* other stages, *P* for trend <0.001). Crescentic glomerulonephritis (GN) and rapidly progressive glomerulonephritis (RPGN) were found to be more prevalent in late-stage CKD (3, 4, 5). For other renal parenchymal diseases, most patients with chronic interstitial nephritis or rejection of kidney allograft had CKD stage 1, 2, or 3. Other etiologies, including obstructive nephropathy, urinary tract diseases, renal vascular diseases, hereditary diseases, and unknown causes were less prevalent in CKD stage 1 (Table 2).

Different eGFR Decline Rates in Systemic or Primary Renal Etiology among Different Time Intervals

The data revealed the more skewed the linear regression line in disease etiology, the higher the variation in primitive eGFR. The importance of eGFR variation and decline can be seen in figure 2, which shows the serial eGFR changes in early-stage CKD (1 and 2) in SDRN during different time intervals was quite diverse. Rapid and significant eGFR decline was obvious in late-stage diabetic nephropathy (stage 3: −1.792 mL/min/1.73 m^2 per year during 0–20th month, $P<0.001$; stage 4: −1.29 mL/min/1.73 m^2 per year during 0–20th month, $P<0.001$, −0.867 mL/min/1.73 m^2 per year during 20–40th month, $P = 0.033$, and −1.982 mL/min/1.73 m^2 per year during 40–60th month, $P = 0.023$; stage 5: −1.208 mL/min/1.73 m^2 per year during 0–20th month, $P = 0.008$ and −1.741 mL/min/1.73 m^2 per year during 20–40th month, $P<0.001$, Figure 2A). There were also significantly faster rates of eGFR decline in the later stages of hypertensive nephropathy (stage 4: −1.197 mL/min/1.73 m^2 per year during 20th–40th month, $P = 0.006$, −2.601 mL/min/1.73 m^2 per year during 40th–60th month, $P = 0.003$; stage 5:

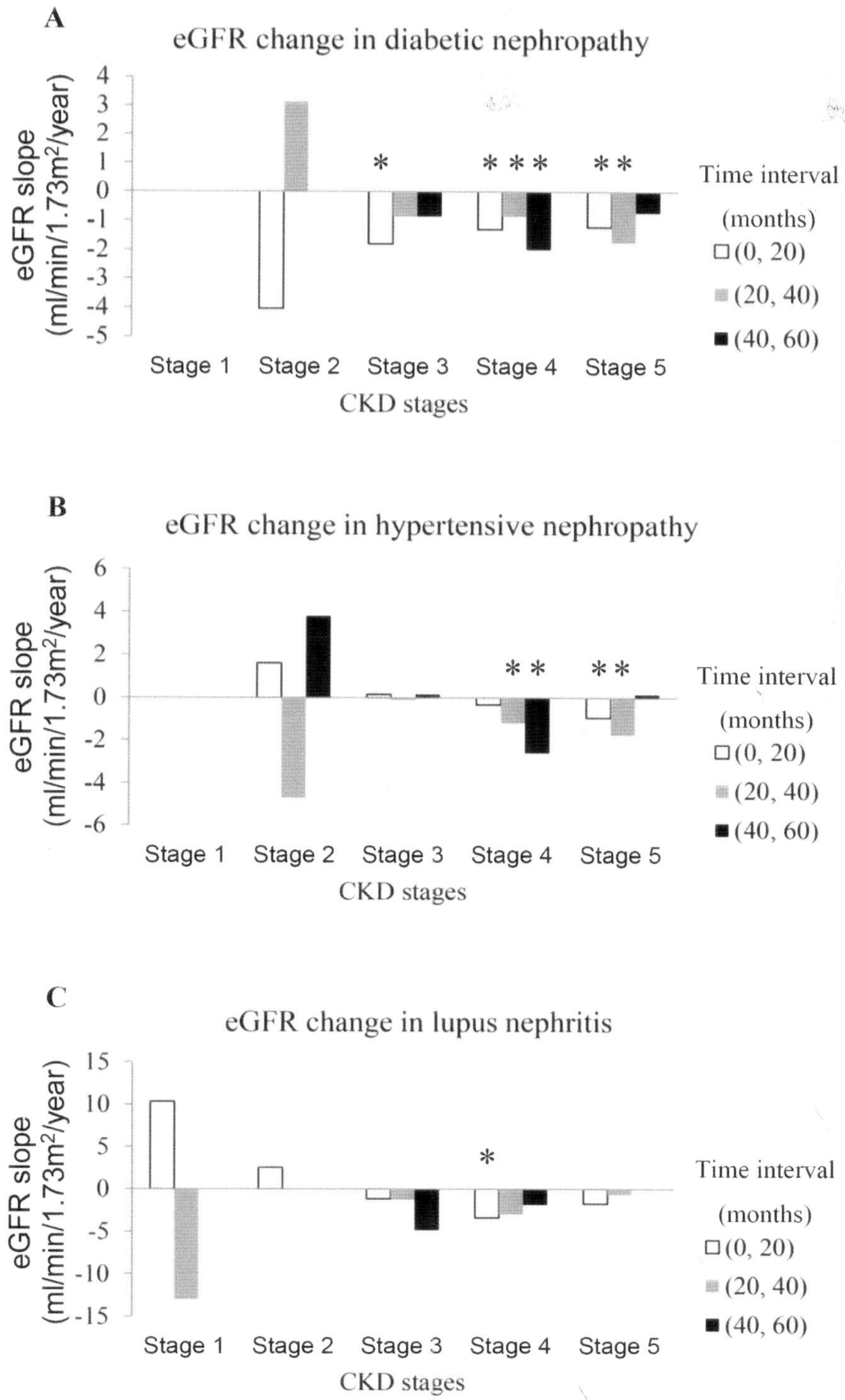

Figure 2. eGFR decline in systemic disease-related nephropathy (Significant codes: *, <0.05 means the eGFR decline is a significant value during this time interval under lineal regression model).

−0.942 mL/min/1.73 m^2 per year during 0–20th, $P<0.001$, −1.761 mL/min/1.73 m^2 per year during 0–20th, $P<0.001$, Figure 2B). Lupus nephritis was not significantly associated with eGFR decline, except in CKD stage 4, with −3.384 mL/min/1.73 m^2 per year during 0–20th, $P=0.027$ (Figure 2C).

For PRDs, membranous nephropathy (MN) was associated with rapid eGFR decline in the early follow-up period (−4.210 mL/min/1.73 m^2 per year during 0–20th month). Minimal change disease was correlated with significantly elevated eGFR in the early follow-up period (7.551 mL/min/1.73 m^2 per year during 0–20th month). Focal segmental glomerulosclerosis (FSGS) was

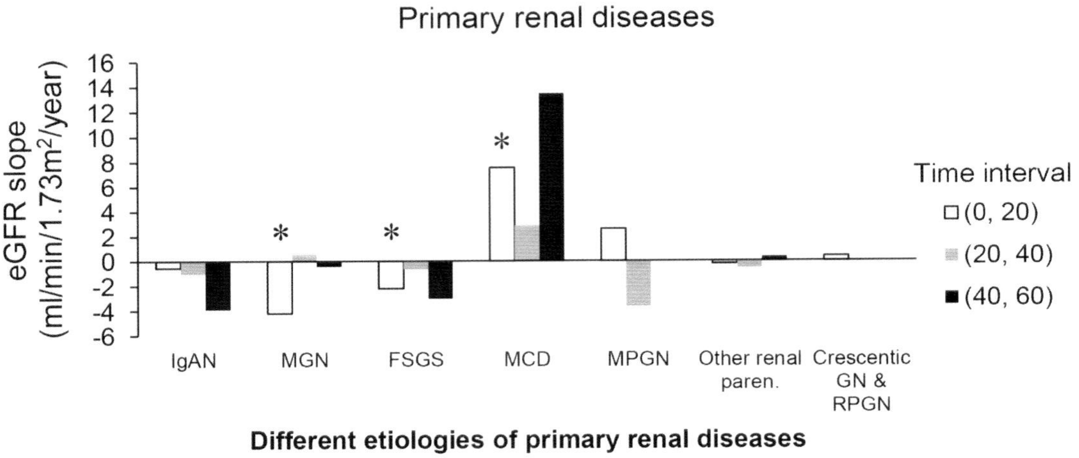

Figure 3. eGFR decline in primary renal diseases; IgAN, IgA nephropathy; MGN, membranous glomerulonephritis; FSGS, focal and segmental glomerulosclerosis; MCD, minimal change disease; MPGN, membranoproliferative glomerulonephritis; Other renal paren., other renal parenchymal disease; Crescentic GN& RPGN, crescentic glomerulonephritis and rapidly progressive glomerulonephritis (Significant codes: *, <0.05 means the eGFR decline is a significant value during this time interval under lineal regression model).

related to rapid eGFR decline in the early follow-up period (-2.203 mL/min/1.73 m^2 per year during 0–20th month) (Figure 3).

eGFR Decline Independently Predicted Poor Outcomes, Especially for SDRN in Maintenance of Dialysis

With regard to the primary endpoint, (434/2,723) 15.9% dialysis cases were stage 1–5 SDRN patients compared with (56/432) 13.0% dialysis cases who were stage 1–5 PRD ($P = 0.113$) (Table 3). The crude eGFR decline and adjusted (age, gender, eGFR decline, proteinuria, ACEI/ARB, and antilipemic agents) risk of dialysis and all-cause mortality in those with SDRN and PRDs are listed in Table 3. Several disease types categorized as SDRN (e.g., multiple myeloma) that could potentially be successfully treated were excluded. In addition, PRDs (e.g., Crescentic GN or RPGN, obstructive nephropathy, acute rejection in kidney transplant recipients, and pyelonephritis) with extreme values were excluded in the preliminary analysis.

SDRN individuals with eGFR decline (per 1 ml/min/1.73 m^2 per month) had a greater risk of initiating dialysis than that of PRDs (crude HR = 1.07, 95% CI = 1.04–1.10 and multivariate analysis, adjusted HR = 1.05, 95% CI = 1.02–1.08). That is to say, each unit of eGFR decline in SDRN increased the risk for dialysis by 5% after multivariate analysis. For the other outcome, (164/2,723) the mortality rate was 6.0% in stage 1–5 SDRN patients compared with (4/432) 0.9% in stage 1–5 PRDs ($P < 0.001$), which was significantly different. However, there was no significant difference in the HR of eGFR decline to death between SDRN and PRD stages 1–5 in the analysis.

Table 4 presents an overall view of the average effects on outcomes (dialysis and all-cause mortality based on the most impactful CKD stages 3–5. eGFR declined independently and

Table 3. Association of eGFR decline with outcomes during study period by different disease etiologies.

	HR and 95% C.I. for dialysis	HR and 95% C.I. for death
	CKD stage 1–5	**CKD stage 1–5**
Systemic disease-related nephropathy, eGFR decline		
Number of events/Total numbers	434/2,723	164/2,723
Model 1	1.07 (1.04–1.10)***	0.95 (0.88–1.02)
Model 2	1.05 (1.02–1.08)***	0.99 (0.91–1.07)
Primary renal disease, eGFR decline		
Number of events/Total numbers	56/432	4/432
Model 1	1.01 (0.93–1.09)	1.02 (0.91–1.14)
Model 2	0.99 (0.92–1.08)	1.03 (0.75–1.43)

Model 1 is crude. Model 2 is adjusted for age, gender, eGFR decline, proteinuria, ACEI/ARB, and antilipemic agents.
Several disease types categorized as SDRN (e.g., multiple myeloma) that could potentially be successfully treated were excluded. In addition, PRDs (e.g., Crescentic GN or RPGN, obstructive nephropathy, acute rejection in kidney transplant recipients, and pyelonephritis) with extreme values were excluded in the preliminary analysis.
HR, hazard ratio; C.I., confidence interval.
Significant codes: *, <0.05; **, <0.01; ***, <0.001.

Table 4. Association of eGFR decline with dialysis and death in CKD stages 3~5 cohort using univariate and multivariate cox proportional hazards analysis.

	HR and 95% C.I. for dialysis			HR and 95% C.I. for death		
CKD	**Stage 3**	**Stage 4**	**Stage 5**	**Stage 3**	**Stage 4**	**Stage 5**
Average eGFR decline (ml/min)	−0.115	−0.143	−0.272	−0.115	−0.143	−0.272
Number of events/Total numbers	42/2,150	146/1,380	547/1,172	98/2,150	86/1,380	55/1,172
Model 1	1.40 (1.24–1.58)***	1.79 (1.52–2.12)***	1.61 (1.44–1.80)***	0.87 (0.77–0.98)*	1.39 (1.01–1.89)*	1.61 (0.70–3.71)
Model 2	1.50 (1.30–1.73)***	1.60 (1.37–1.88)***	1.69 (1.49–1.92)***	0.91 (0.79–1.04)	1.69 (1.23–2.33)**	1.82 (0.62–5.32)

Model 1 is crude. Model 2 is further adjusted for age, gender, proteinuria, ACEI/ARB, antilipemic agents, diseases with a relatively large subgroup of patients (diabetic nephropathy, hypertensive nephropathy, IgA nephropathy, and membranous nephropathy).
HR, hazard ratio; C.I., confidence interval
Significant codes: *, <0.05; **, <0.01; ***, <0.001.

significantly increased the risk of poor outcome of dialysis in patients with CKD stages 3, 4, and 5 (Table 3B). However, only in CKD stage 4 did eGFR decline have a positive association with death after univariate and multivariate analysis. The effect of eGFR decline on death in patients with CKD stage 3 was observed to be inversely correlated with risk of death (HR = 0.87, 95% C.I. = 0.77–0.98, Table 4).

Table 5 shows the associations of disease etiologies and eGFR decline with dialysis and all-cause mortality in the cohort with CKD stages 3, 4, and 5 using multivariate Cox proportional hazards analysis. Regarding SDRN, diabetic nephropathy (DN) had the greatest effect on initiation of dialysis (model 1: CKD stage 3: HR = 3.04, 95% C.I. = 1.66–5.58; CKD stage 5: HR = 1.29, 95% C.I. = 1.08–1.55). DN also had the greatest contribution to initiation of dialysis after adjustment for traditional risk factors (model 2: CKD stage 3: HR = 5.06, 95% C.I. = 2.63–9.71; CKD stage 4: HR = 2.02, 95% C.I. = 1.42–2.87; CKD stage 5: HR = 1.51, 95% C.I. = 1.26–1.82). Furthermore, when additive eGFR decline was added to the model, there was a strong association between CKD stages of DN and dialysis. We also found a correlation of DN with additive eGFR decline to all-cause mortality among CKD stages 3,4, and 5 with the application of the same statistical analysis. A small increase in the percentage of dialysis in patients with hypertensive nephropathy (HN) was found after adjusting for conventional risk factors with additive eGFR decline. However, in CKD stage 5 in the HN group, there was a lower mortality rate (model 1: CKD stage 5: HR = 0.62, 95% C.I. = 0.33–1.26; model 2: CKD stage 5: HR = 0.47, 95% C.I. = 0.23–0.97; model 3: CKD stage 5: HR = 0.47, 95% C.I. = 0.23–0.97) after adjusting for eGFR decline and traditional risk factors. Multiple post hoc comparisons showed a greater prevalence of ACEI/ARB usage in patients with stage 5 CKD in the HN group compared with usage rates in the other groups.

For PRDs, IgA nephropathy had a greater effect on initiation of dialysis (model 1: CKD stage 3: HR = 2.94, 95% C.I. = 1.14–7.42; CKD stage 5: HR = 1.81, 95% C.I. = 1.07–3.08). However, no worse effects for CKD progression were observed after adjusting for conventional risk factors as well as the additive eGFR decline factors. Those non-available data were small sample size (Table 4); 95% confidence interval of hazard ratio is wide, which is the reasons for the data being inadequate for appropriate analysis. There was a large diversity of other renal parenchymal diseases and thus the data were difficult to interpret.

Discussion

In this study, we found that eGFR decline independently predicted poor outcomes, especially the initiation of dialysis in systemic disease-related nephropathy (SDRN). For DN, each unit of eGFR decline had 5.20 times more risk for dialysis than that for other etiologies in CKD stage 3, 1.91 times more risk for dialysis than that for other etiologies in CKD stage 4, and 1.48 times more risk for dialysis than that for other etiologies in CKD stage 5 after multivariate analysis. The eGFR decline in primary renal diseases only makes a small contribution to the renal outcome and patients' outcome in a unified and integrated health care system. This risk was independent of traditional risk factors (age, diabetes mellitus, proteinuria, baseline eGFR, and hypertension), and was recently shown to be a non-traditional risk factor reflecting both intrinsic and extrinsic factors in the kidney [2,6,19]. In this multi-center study we attempted to better understand the association of eGFR decline with the renal outcome and all-cause mortality. We found eGFR decline had a major effect on risk of dialysis and all-cause mortality after univariate and multi-variate analysis with specific primary renal disease etiologies (Table 3 and 4). This study demonstrated that eGFR decline rate, defined as ml/min per 1.73 m^2 per year decrease, was associated with an increased risk for initiation of dialysis in SDRN, especially DN. Even after adjustment for age, the overall effect of eGFR decline beyond the normal aging process may be due to multiple co-morbidities, metabolic syndrome, and insulin resistance, which are risk factors for progression of CKD, and the rapid decline in renal function in the elderly [1].

One of the strengths of this study is that it is a long-term follow-up study spanning 10 years. In addition, a large sample size was analyzed which provided important information on the major etiologies of renal diseases. This study comprehensively examined long-term changes of eGFR in different renal diseases and showed associations of long-term outcomes with CKD. We explored the changes in eGFR over different time intervals in order to establish the relationships between longitudinal behavior of renal function and renal etiologies. Importantly, we investigated the contribution of eGFR decline (non-traditional risk factors) [2,6,19] in the final year of follow-up to the outcomes of CKD stages 3–5. Slopes were not calculated based on ordinary least squares as the renal outcome is technically problematic due to autocorrelation and heteroskedasticity. We did not adjust for baseline eGFR in slope models in order to avoid the so-called "horse-racing effect" [31].

Most predictors for ESRD and all-cause mortality found in ethnic Chinese cohorts showed similar findings in previous studies

Table 5. Associations of Disease Etiologies eGFR Decline with Dialysis and Death in CKD Stages 3~5 Cohort Using Multivariate Cox Proportional Hazards Analysis.

	HR and 95% C.I. for dialysis			HR and 95% C.I. for death		
CKD	**Stage 3**	**Stage 4**	**Stage 5**	**Stage 3**	**Stage 4**	**Stage 5**
Systemic disease-related nephropathy						
DM nephropathy						
Model 1	3.04 (1.66–5.58)***	1.37 (0.99–1.90)	1.29 (1.08–1.55)**	1.58 (1.05–2.39)*	1.35 (0.88 – 2.07)	2.42 (1.42 – 4.12)**
Model 2	5.06 (2.63–9.71)***	2.02 (1.42–2.87)***	1.51 (1.26–1.82)***	1.77 (1.17 – 2.69)**	1.62 (1.05 – 2.50)*	2.93 (1.70 – 5.03)***
Model 3	5.20 (2.72– 9.96)***	1.91 (1.34–2.70)***	1.48 (1.23–1.78)***	1.74 (1.15–2.65)**	1.59 (1.03–2.46)*	2.87 (1.66–4.95)***
Hypertensive nephropathy						
Model 1	0.24 (0.07–0.77)*	0.99 (0.66–1.50)	0.91 (0.74–1.12)	1.23 (0.80 – 1.91)	1.04 (0.61 – 1.77)	0.62 (0.33 – 1.26)
Model 2	0.32 (0.10–1.07)	1.14 (0.75–1.74)	0.98 (0.80–1.20)	0.92 (0.59 – 1.43)	0.68 (0.39 – 1.16)	0.47 (0.23 – 0.97)*
Model 3	0.36 (0.11–1.18)	1.18 (0.77–1.80)	0.97 (0.79–1.20)	0.90 (0.57–1.41)	0.68 (0.40–1.18)	0.47 (0.23–0.97)*
Lupus nephritis						
Model 1	–	2.78 (0.88–8.73)	1.49 (0.86–2.59)	–	–	–
Model 2	–	1.47 (0.46–4.72)	1.32 (0.75–2.31)	–	–	–
Model 3	–	1.60(0.50–5.16)	1.31(0.75–2.31)	–	–	–
Primary renal diseases						
IgA nephropathy						
Model 1	2.91 (1.14–7.42)*	1.68 (0.85–3.29)	1.81 (1.07–3.08)*	–	–	–
Model 2	1.48 (0.55–3.93)	0.93 (0.46–1.89)	1.25 (0.73–2.14)	–	–	–
Model 3	1.43 (0.54–3.82)	0.89 (0.44–1.82)	0.90 (0.52–1.57)	–	–	–
MGN						
Model 1	2.39 (0.58–9.92)	0.74 (0.10–5.31)	1.43 (0.53–3.82)	1.1 (0.27 – 4.47)	–	–
Model 2	2.74 (0.65–11.56)	1.13 (0.16–8.12)	1.25 (0.47–3.36)	2.42 (0.58 – 10.09)	–	–
Model 3	2.28 (0.54–9.67)	1.22 (0.17–8.82)	1.34 (0.50–3.61)	2.54 (0.61–10.65)	–	–
FSGS						
Model 1	–	1.66 (0.68–4.06)	1.29 (0.64–2.59)	0.40 (0.06 – 2.88)	–	–
Model 2	–	0.95 (0.38–2.38)	0.99 (0.49–2.01)	–	–	–
Model 3	–	0.82 (0.33–2.08)	0.98 (0.48–1.98)	–	–	–
MCD						
Models 1 & 2 & 3	–	–	–	–	–	–
MPGN						
Model 1	–	2.63 (0.65 – 10.65)	–	–	–	–
Model 2	–	1.80 (0.44 – 7.36)	–	–	–	–
Model 3	–	1.81 (0.44 – 7.40)	–	–	–	–
Crescentic GN & RPGN						
Model 1	–	–	1.34 (0.50–3.57)	–	–	–
Model 2	–	–	1.17 (0.44–3.14)	–	–	0.96 (0.51 – 1.81)
Model 3	–	–	1.21 (0.45–3.25)	–	–	–
Other renal parenchymal diseases						
Model 1	0.80 (0.37–1.73)	0.86 (0.56–1.32)	0.82 (0.66–1.00)	0.89 (0.54 – 1.45)	0.78 (0.44 – 1.38)	0.94 (0.50 – 1.76)
Model 2	0.57 (0.26–1.25)	0.73 (0.48–1.12)	0.75 (0.61–0.92)*	0.96 (0.58 – 1.58)	0.85 (0.48 – 1.50)	–
Model 3	0.55 (0.25 – 1.22)	0.73 (0.48–1.13)	0.78 (0.63–0.96)*	0.99 (0.60–1.64)	0.88 (0.49–1.55)	0.95 (0.50–1.79)

Model 1 is crude for disease itself. Model 2 is further adjusted for age, gender, proteinuria, ACEI/ARB, antilipemic agents. Model 3 is further adjusted for all the items in model 2+ eGFR decline.
Significant codes: *, <0.05; **, <0.01; ***, <0.001.

[32–36]. Taiwan is the only country to have achieved a hugely significant reduction in the incidence of ESRD in recent years, partly due to the inclusion of early CKD and pre-end-stage renal disease (ESRD) management programs in the National Health Insurance scheme [17,32]. Despite the successful reduction of CKD, it must be remembered that there is a growing burden of CKD. In part this is due to the growth of other non-communicable diseases (NCDs), most notably diabetes. However, the emergence of new epidemics of CKD in the developing world, some of which appear to have environmental causes, has also contributed to the overall burden. Rapid decline of eGFR is a clinical concern for physicians and patients. GFR decline with aging is a sign of normal senescence, not disease [10]. However, among patients with similar levels of eGFR, clinical outcomes vary substantially by age. The well-known reasons for risk of rapid GFR decline are aging, racial difference (young blacks), albuminuria, hypertension, diabetes, and variable primary renal diseases [19]. However, the discrepancy between eGFR decline and clinical outcomes in long-term observational studies has yet to be fully elucidated.

To the best of our knowledge, the present study is the first to investigate the importance of eGFR decline and its differing contributions to rigorous clinical endpoints. However, several equivocal findings could be partly explained by different behaviors of medical practice. In clinical practice, eGFR decline in DN was kept under control in stage 2–4 CKD, but the improvements in stage 4 CKD of DN were lost after 40 months of follow-up. The decline of eGFR could be seen in stage 5 CKD in DN, and the decreased eGFR decline in the last period (40–60 months) was due to the ceiling effect of the lowest value of the eGFR (Figure 2A). Efforts to retard eGFR decline in stage 1–3 CKD in HN were effective, but no benefit was found after stage 4–5 CKD (Figure 2B). For PRDs, IgA nephropathy, FSGS, and memrano-proliferative glomerulonephritis (MPGN) the decline rates were difficult to control (Figure 3). MN required more time to observe due to its chronic disease status and changes in eGFR were not obvious (Figure 3). In the episodic 12-month follow-up of eGFR decline, it was shown that multidisciplinary predialysis education (MPE) can be efficacious in motivated systemic-disease patients, especially for prolonging survival. Questions remain about its effectiveness (i.e., whether it works in everyday life) as it may be very hard to convince "non-compliant" patients. Skilled non-medical educators are often better than physicians at conveying information to patients, as they tend to have a more solid pedagogic and methodological background. There is no need for strong experimental, multidisciplinary care and non-randomized observational trials [36]. However, long-term follow-up studies are still worthwhile as they are capable of identifying potential risk factors.

In conclusion, eGFR decline was demonstrated to be superior to absolute GFR value as an indicator of kidney disease progression by the overall changes in kidney function over time. Diverse eGFR variations had better predictive values in systemic disease-related nephropathy than those in primary renal diseases. Diabetic nephropathy and hypertensive nephropathy were correlated with significantly greater eGFR decline in CKD stages 3, 4, and 5 compared with that of other disease etiologies. eGFR decline has a predictive value for dialysis and death in CKD stages 3, 4, and 5 in SDRN patients, especially DN. There were still discrepancies between eGFR decline and clinical outcomes in PRDs, hypertensive nephropathy, and lupus nephritis.

Supporting Information

Figure S1 Concordance was found with a positive correlation between MDRD and CKD-EPI.

Figure S2 The similar distribution of estimated GFR and eGFR-risk relationship were found between the CKD-EPI equation (red) and the MDRD Study equation (black) in our CKD cohort.

Figure S3 The positive correlation and distribution of eGFR between MDRD and CKD-EPI were shown by age categories (< and ≥65 years) in the CKD cohorts (female).

Acknowledgments

The authors thank the Clinical Informatics Research and Development Center and the Biostatistics Task Force of Taichung Veterans General Hospital (TCVGH), Taichung, Taiwan, R.O.C., for their help with the statistical analysis. This study was also conducted on behalf of the GREEnS Project, Tunghai University, Taiwan, and the CKDBHPDH investigators (Division of Nephrology, RN. Chia-Fang Hung, RN. Chia-Ying Tung, RN. Su-Chi Hung, RN. Tzu-Mei Lin, email: tmlin@vghtc.gov.tw), Taichung Veterans General Hospital, Taiwan, R.O.C.

Author Contributions

Conceived and designed the experiments: S-CW D-CT. Performed the experiments: K-HS C-H. Cheng C-H. Chen T-MY M-JW. Analyzed the data: S-CW C-MC. Wrote the paper: S-CW D-CT.

References

1. Cheng HT, Huang JW, Chiang CK, Yen CJ, Hung KY, et al. (2012) Metabolic syndrome and insulin resistance as risk factors for development of chronic kidney disease and rapid decline in renal function in elderly. J Clin Endocrinol Metab 97: 1268–1276.
2. Al-Aly Z, Balasubramanian S, McDonald JR, Scherrer JF, O'Hare AM (2012) Greater variability in kidney function is associated with an increased risk of death. Kidney Int 82: 1208–1214.
3. Derose SF, Rutkowski MP, Crooks PW, Shi JM, Wang JG, et al. (2013) Racial differences in estimated GFR decline, ESRD, and mortality in an integrated health system. Am J Kidney Dis 62: 236–244.
4. Peralta CA, Vittinghoff E, Bansal N, Jacobs D Jr, Muntner P, et al. (2013) Trajectories of kidney function decline in young black and white adults with preserved GFR: results from the Coronary Artery Risk Development in Young Adults (CARDIA) study. Am J Kidney Dis 62: 261–266.
5. Hansen HP, Hovind P, Jensen BR, Parving HH (2002) Diurnal variations of glomerular filtration rate and albuminuria in diabetic nephropathy. Kidney Int 61: 163–168.
6. Perkins RM, Tang X, Bengier AC, Kirchner HL, Bucaloiu ID (2012) Variability in estimated glomerular filtration rate is an independent risk factor for death among patients with stage 3 chronic kidney disease. Kidney Int 82: 1332–1338.
7. Kajitani N, Shikata K, Nakamura A, Nakatou T, Hiramatsu M, et al. (2010) Microinflammation is a common risk factor for progression of nephropathy and atherosclerosis in Japanese patients with type 2 diabetes. Diabetes Res Clin Pract 88: 171–176.
8. Shikata K Makino H (2013) Microinflammation in the pathogenesis of diabetic nephropathy. J Diabetes Investig 4: 142–149.
9. Hinchliffe SA, Lynch MR, Sargent PH, Howard CV, Van Velzen D (1992) The effect of intrauterine growth retardation on the development of renal nephrons. Br J Obstet Gynaecol 99: 296–301.
10. Jocelyn W, Sanjeevkumar RP (2009) Changes in Kidney Function. Hazzard's geriatric medicine and gerontology. 6th ed. Seattle, USA: McGraw-Hill; p.1009–1015.
11. Li LS, Liu ZH (2004) Epidemiologic data of renal diseases from a single unit in China: analysis based on 13,519 renal biopsies. Kidney Int 66: 920–923.
12. Sowers JR, Epstein M (1995) Diabetes mellitus and associated hypertension, vascular disease, and nephropathy. An update. Hypertension 26: 869–879.
13. Crook ED, Flack JM, Salem M, Salahudeen AK, Hall J (2002) Primary renal disease as a cardiovascular risk factor. Am J Med Sci 324: 138–145.
14. Moriya T, Tsuchiya A, Okizaki S, Hayashi A, Tanaka K, et al. (2012) Glomerular hyperfiltration and increased glomerular filtration surface are associated with renal function decline in normo- and microalbuminuric type 2 diabetes. Kidney Int 81: 486–493.
15. Mulec H, Blohmé G, Grände B, Björck S (1998) The effect of metabolic control on rate of decline in renal function in insulin-dependent diabetes mellitus with overt diabetic nephropathy. Nephrol Dial Transplant 13: 651–655.
16. Reich HN, Gladman DD, Urowitz MB, Bargman JM, Hladunewich MA, et al. (2011) Persistent proteinuria and dyslipidemia increase the risk of progressive chronic kidney disease in lupus erythematosus. Kidney Int 79: 914–920.

17. Chou YH, Lien YC, Hu FC, Lin WC, Kao CC, et al. (2012) Clinical outcomes and predictors for ESRD and mortality in primary GN. Clin J Am Soc Nephrol 7: 1401–1408.
18. Andreoli SP (1998) Renal manifestations of systemic diseases. Semin Nephrol 18: 270–279.
19. Al-Aly Z (2013) Prediction of renal endpoints in chronic kidney disease. Kidney Int 83: 189–191.
20. Mahajan A, Simoni J, Sheather SJ, Broglio KR, Rajab MH, et al. (2010) Daily oral sodium bicarbonate preserves glomerular filtration rate by slowing its decline in early hypertensive nephropathy. Kidney Int 78: 303–309.
21. Estimation of GFR. KDOQI Clinical Practice Guidelines for Chronic Kidney Disease: Evaluation, Classification, and Stratification (Guideline 4). National Kidney Foundation, Inc. http://www.kidney.org/professionals/kdoqi/guidelines_ckd/p5_lab_g4.htm. Accessed 2002.
22. Chang TI, Li S, Chen SC, Peralta CA, Shlipak MG, et al. (2013) Risk factors for ESRD in individuals with preserved estimated GFR with and without albuminuria: results from the Kidney Early Evaluation Program (KEEP) Am J Kidney Dis 61(4 Suppl 2): S4–S11.
23. Kuo HW, Tsai SS, Tiao MM, Yang CY (2007) Epidemiological features of CKD in Taiwan. Am J Kidney Dis 49: 46–55.
24. Chadban SJ, Briganti EM, Kerr PG, Dunstan DW, Welborn TA, et al. (2003) Prevalence of kidney damage in Australian adults: The AusDiab kidney study. J Am Soc Nephrol 14(7 Suppl 2): S131–138.
25. Hallan SI, Matsushita K, Sang Y, Mahmoodi BK, Black C, et al. (2012) Age and association of kidney measures with mortality and end-stage renal disease. JAMA 308: 2349–2360.
26. Gansevoort RT, Correa-Rotter R, Hemmelgarn BR, Jafar TH, Heerspink HJ, et al. (2013) Chronic kidney disease and cardiovascular risk: epidemiology, mechanisms, and prevention. Lancet 382: 339–352.
27. Mahmoodi BK, Matsushita K, Woodward M, Blankestijn PJ, Cirillo M, et al. (2012) Associations of kidney disease measures with mortality and end-stage renal disease in individuals with and without hypertension: a meta-analysis. Lancet 380: 1649–1661.
28. Nitsch D, Grams M, Sang Y, Black C, Cirillo M, et al. (2013) Associations of estimated glomerular filtration rate and albuminuria with mortality and renal failure by sex: a meta-analysis. BMJ 346: f324.
29. Hsu TW, Liu JS, Hung SC, Kuo KL, Chang YK, et al. (2013) Renoprotective Effect of Renin-Angiotensin-Aldosterone System Blockade in Patients With Predialysis Advanced Chronic Kidney Disease, Hypertension, and Anemia. JAMA Intern Med Dec 16. doi: 10.1001/jamainternmed.2013.12700 [Epub ahead of print].
30. Wen CP, David Cheng TY, Chan HT, Tsai MK, Chung WS, et al. (2010) Is high serum uric acid a risk marker or a target for treatment? Examination of its independent effect in a large cohort with low cardiovascular risk. Am J Kidney Dis 56: 273–288.
31. Glymour MM, Weuve J, Berkman LF, Kawachi I, Robins JM (2005) When is baseline adjustment useful in analyses of change? An example with education and cognitive change. Am J Epidemiol 162: 267–278.
32. Yang WC, Hwang SJ, Taiwan Society of Nephrology (2008) Incidence, prevalence and mortality trends of dialysis end-stage renal disease in Taiwan from 1990 to 2001: the impact of national health insurance. Nephrol Dial Transplant 23: 3977–3982.
33. Chiu YL, Chien KL, Lin SL, Chen YM, Tsai TJ, et al. (2008) Outcomes of stage 3–5 chronic kidney disease before end-stage renal disease at a single center in Taiwan. Nephron Clin Pract 109: c109–118.
34. Wu IW, Wang SY, Hsu KH, Lee CC, Sun CY, et al. (2009) Multidisciplinary predialysis education decreases the incidence of dialysis and reduces mortality–a controlled cohort study based on the NKF/DOQI guidelines. Nephrol Dial Transplant 24: 3426–3433.
35. Chen YR, Yang Y, Wang SC, Chiu PF, Chou WY, et al. (2013) Effectiveness of multidisciplinary care for chronic kidney disease in Taiwan: a 3-year prospective cohort study. Nephrol Dial Transplant 28: 671–682.
36. Van Biesen W, Verbeke F, Vanholder R (2009) We don't need no education .... (Pink Floyd, The Wall) Multidisciplinary predialysis education programmes: pass or fail? Nephrol Dial Transplant 24: 3277–3279.

Non-Adherence in Patients on Peritoneal Dialysis

Konstadina Griva[1,4]*, Alden Yuanhong Lai[1], Haikel Asyraf Lim[1], Zhenli Yu[2], Marjorie Wai Yin Foo[3], Stanton P. Newman[4,5]

1 Department of Psychology, National University of Singapore, Singapore, **2** Department of Renal Medicine, Khoo Teck Puat Hospital, Singapore, **3** Department of Nephrology, Peritoneal Dialysis Centre, Singapore General Hospital, Singapore, **4** Unit of Behavioural Medicine, University College London, London, United Kingdom, **5** Health Services Research Group, City University London, London, United Kingdom

Abstract

Background: It has been increasingly recognized that non-adherence is an important factor that determines the outcome of peritoneal dialysis (PD) therapy. There is therefore a need to establish the levels of non-adherence to different aspects of the PD regimen (dialysis procedures, medications, and dietary/fluid restrictions).

Methods: A systematic review of peer-reviewed literature was performed in PubMed, PsycINFO and CINAHL databases using PRISMA guidelines in May 2013. Publications on non-adherence in PD were selected by two reviewers independently according to predefined inclusion and exclusion criteria. Relevant data on patient characteristics, measures, rates and factors associated with non-adherence were extracted. The quality of studies was also evaluated independently by two reviewers according to a revised version of the Effective Public Health Practice Project assessment tool.

Results: The search retrieved 204 studies, of which a total of 25 studies met inclusion criteria. Reported rates of non-adherence varied across studies: 2.6–53% for dialysis exchanges, 3.9–85% for medication, and 14.4–67% for diet/fluid restrictions. Methodological differences in measurement and definition of non-adherence underlie the observed variation. Factors associated with non-adherence that showed a degree of consistency were mostly socio-demographical, such as age, employment status, ethnicity, sex, and time period on PD treatment.

Conclusion: Non-adherence to different dimensions of the dialysis regimen appears to be prevalent in PD patients. There is a need for further, high-quality research to explore these factors in more detail, with the aim of informing intervention designs to facilitate adherence in this patient population.

Editor: D. William Cameron, University of Ottawa, Canada

Funding: The authors have no support or funding to report.

Competing Interests: The authors have declared that no competing interests exist.

* E-mail: psygk@nus.edu.sg

Background

While the majority of End-Stage Renal Disease (ESRD) patients undergo in-center maintenance hemodialysis (HD) in most settings, chronic peritoneal dialysis (PD) is the dominant home dialysis therapy utilized by 11% of the dialysis population worldwide [1]. PD offers patients the convenience of home-based care and continuous clearance, but requires a daily commitment and a high level of involvement by patient and/or carer with scrupulous attention to hygiene so as to avoid infection of the peritoneum.

With increasing numbers of ESRD patients in need of Renal Replacement Therapy (RRT) and the need to expand dialysis delivery in home settings away from overburdened hospital and tertiary care settings, there is renewed interest in outcomes in patients who are established on PD regimes. Adherence to treatment is of paramount importance as non-adherence has been shown to have major consequences including an increased risk of mortality and hospitalization in patients on HD (see [2] for a review) and in PD [3,4], which in turn lead to increased costs and expenditure for patient care [5,6,7]. However, in contrast to research on adherence in HD patients [2,8,9,10,11,12] and other patient populations, little is known about adherence to PD regimes.

Researchers often use the terms compliance and adherence interchangeably, although they have slightly different implications. Compliance, principally used extensively in older literature, has drawn criticism for its emphasis on medical authority and an implication for patients as passive recipients of care. In response, the term adherence was introduced to recognize patients' right to choose whether or not to follow advice, calling attention to the importance of patients' active participation in their treatment regimes. It is also important and increasingly recognized that a distinction needs to made between intentional and unintentional non-adherence [13]. Non-adherence is unintentional when it is not deliberate through patients' lack of understanding, forgetfulness or miscommunication with health care professionals [14]. Intentional non-adherence, on the other hand, is when patients actively choose not to follow treatment recommendations, such as when they choose to delay, alter or skip dosages of prescribed medication, or to forego dietary or fluid intake recommendations. In this review the term adherence will be adopted, defined as the extent to which a person's behavior (taking medication, following a diet and/or executing lifestyle changes) corresponds with agreed recommendations from a healthcare provider [15]. Where available, intentional and unintentional non-adherence behaviors will be explored.

Overall, adherence among patients with chronic conditions is disappointingly low with rates estimated at 24.8% [16]. Evidence in HD patients shows a similar problem with non-adherence being common [17], occurring in 22–74% of dialysis patients depending on the definition of adherence and the type of treatment [10]. A review has documented up to 74% of HD patients as non-adherent to fluid restrictions, 81.4% for diet restrictions, and 73% for medication non-adherence [2]. The PD regimen is no less complicated and time-consuming than HD. PD patients are required to adhere to a demanding dialysis regime that involves regular manual exchanges at least thrice daily (in the case of continuous ambulatory peritoneal dialysis; CAPD), or long overnight dialysis exchange (in the case of automated peritoneal dialysis; APD), as well as lifelong changes in lifestyle related to diet, intake of multiple medications, and safety and preventive measures. None of the existing systematic reviews on adherence in dialysis to date has distinguished between adherence in HD and PD. PD patients tend to be younger, have fewer comorbidities, and be newer to RRT across varying populations [18,19,20,21]. As the profile of the HD and PD populations differs, the value of a review focused on adherence in PD is therefore accentuated. Individual studies on the other hand have produced mixed results, with some reported higher levels of adherence in PD vs. HD, while others indicated lowered rates of adherence in PD [22] or no differences between the two dialysis modalities [23].

Because of this lack of evidence specific to PD patients in previous reviews, we have undertaken and report here a systematic literature review in which we aimed to:

1. Summarize and synthesize the frequency of (non-) adherence to dialysis exchanges, medication and diet/fluid intake in the PD population;
2. Compare rates of (non-) adherence to dialysis exchanges, medication and diet/fluid intake between patients on different PD modalities, i.e. APD and CAPD;
3. Examine socio-demographic, clinical, and psychological factors associated with adherence to dialysis exchanges, medication and diet/fluid intake.

Methods

This systematic review follows the Preferred Reporting Items for Systematic Reviews and Meta-analyses (PRISMA) guidelines [24].

Search strategy

Articles were identified through PubMed, PsychInfo, and CINAHL electronic databases using combinations of Medical Subject Heading (MeSH; where appropriate) terms and keywords: peritoneal dialysis; adheren*; complian*; medication*; diet*; fluid*; regimen*; session*; schedule*. Search results were downloaded and imported directly into EndNote X6, after which their bibliographic reference lists were scanned to identify additional relevant studies. The search was carried out in May 2013. Refer to Table 1 for an example of the search strategy for PubMed.

Table 1. Example Search Strategy (PubMed on 20/05/2013).

ID	Search
#1	Peritoneal Dialysis [MeSH Terms]
#2	Peritoneal Dialysis, Continuous Ambulatory [MeSH Terms]
#3	#1 OR #2
#4	Medication Adherence [MeSH Terms]
#5	Patient Compliance [MeSH Terms]
#6	#4 OR #5
#7	Medication*
#8	Diet
#9	Diets
#10	Dietary
#11	#8 OR #9 OR #10
#12	Fluid*
#13	#7 OR #11 OR #12
#14	Regimen*
#15	Session*
#16	Schedule*
#17	Exchange*
#18	#14 OR #15 OR #16 OR #17
#19	#13 OR #18
#20	#3 AND #6 AND #19

Note: Search string for PsycINFO and CINAHL was "(peritoneal AND dialysis) AND ((((((adheren*) OR nonadheren*) OR non-adheren*) OR complian*) OR noncomplian*) OR non-complian*) AND (((((((medication*) OR diet*) OR fluid*) OR regimen*) OR session*) OR schedule*) OR exchange*)".

Study selection

We used a three-step process to select the studies. First, using EndNote, duplicate articles were eliminated. Second, to discard irrelevant studies, two authors (HL and KG) screened all titles and abstracts of the papers. Disagreements between the authors were resolved by a consensus. The full paper was obtained where there was insufficient information in the abstract or title to determine eligibility. Third, to select studies that met our inclusion criteria, one analyst (HL) read the full papers identified at abstract screen. If the results of a study were reported in more than one publication, only the publication with the most complete results was retained. Only if publications on the same study focused on different outcomes (i.e. adherence to different aspects of treatment) or different populations were they included in this review.

Publications were included in this review only if full papers met the following criteria:

a. written in English.
b. published in peer-reviewed journals.
c. included measure(s) of (non)-adherence outcome in either dialysis exchanges, medication, diet/fluid restrictions or exercise.
d. explicated criteria/methods or cut offs to calculate and define (non-) adherence.

The papers were required to include details of the methods used to determine non-adherence in any one of the treatment aspects (i.e. dialysis exchanges, medication, diet/fluid restrictions, or exercise) and some numeric results on rates of non-adherence. As there is no gold standard adherence measure, all measures were considered (e.g., self-report, physician/nurse estimate, tablet count, and prescription refill, electronic monitoring, inventory checks/delivery records, built-in software or electronic monitoring systems) as long as the criteria for definition of non-adherence based on these measures and data on frequencies were reported. All definitions of (non-) adherence, such as the percentage of doses taken/exchanges performed over a given time period and percentage of patients achieving a specified adherence level or clinical target, were considered. Where multiple measures were reported, the percentage of patients achieving a specified adherence level was used in this review as this was common to the majority of studies.

Cohort studies, both prospective and retrospective, and cross-sectional designs were all included. For intervention studies, they were only considered if baseline rates were reported. Dissertations, systematic reviews, meta-analyses, case series, editorials, opinion papers, and interventions without any baseline rates on non-adherence were excluded. Studies were also excluded if they did not examine (non-) adherence on either performance of dialysis exchanges, medication, diet/fluid or exercise; did not report on methods to measure or define (non-) adherence; or did not present numerical data on (non-) adherence for PD patients separately to HD. Studies reporting on performance of different steps of PD protocol procedures such as preparation of materials, sterilization, connection/disconnection, or disposal of dialysate bags rather than performance of dialysis exchanges per se were also excluded. These were deemed more related to quality of performance of the recommended procedures among patients who perform PD exchanges rather than (non-) adherence to dialysis exchanges.

Data extraction

Data from the studies were extracted by one analyst (HL) and second analyst (KG) verified all extractions against the original studies. Information extracted included: authors, year of publication, country, study design, PD modality, age, gender, adherence assessment method, definition of non-adherence, non-adherence rates, and factors associated with adherence/non-adherence. Where information on mean age and proportion of male vs. female study participants were unavailable, estimates were calculated based on available data.

We grouped non-adherence into three categories: non-adherence to dialysis exchanges (e.g., missing, shortening or altering schedules), medications (which include not only prescribed phosphate binders but also other medications, e.g., erythropoietin), and dietary/fluid restrictions. When studies did not distinguish between non-adherence rates of their modality sub-population (APD/CAPD), we extracted the available data for the overall study sample.

Quality assessment

The methodological quality of the studies was assessed using a shortened version of the Effective Public Health Practice Project (EPHPP) Quality Assessment Tool for Quantitative Studies [25] employing only the sections pertaining to selection bias, data collection and withdrawals/dropouts. Other sections were not used as they were tailored towards interventional, comparative study designs and were not deemed relevant to many of the studies included in this review. Two researchers (KG and AYL) assessed the quality of the studies independently. Discrepancies were resolved by discussion until consensus was reached.

Results

Search results and study characteristics

Figure 1 shows the flow of literature into this systematic review. We obtained a total of 204 articles from electronic databases and additional searches, of which 147 were excluded at the title/abstract screen stage. Full papers and references lists were reviewed for the remaining 57 studies. A final total of 25 (out of the identified 204) studies were judged to meet the criteria for inclusion in the review (see Table 2). The main reasons for exclusion at both the abstract and full paper screens were that studies: did not clearly define or report the numerical rates of non-adherence, were not written in English, assessed the effects of biochemical markers on clinical outcomes such as survival, were intervention studies aimed at improving adherence without baseline rates reported, or did not distinguish between adherence rates in HD and PD patients among the mixed sample pools.

Study locations and settings

As seen in Table 2, approximately half (N = 12) of the included adherence-related studies were conducted in North America [3,4,23,26,27,28,29,30,31,32,33,34], six were conducted in Europe [35,36,37,38,39,40], and six studies were conducted in Asia [41,42,43,44,45,46]. One study was conducted in South America [47].

Patient populations and sample sizes

All of studies included patients on PD yet exact PD modality (i.e. CAPD, APD/Continuous Cycle Peritoneal Dialysis; CCPD) was not always clearly stated (N = 12). Of those where modality was specified, N = 4 studies included CAPD only [29,32,41,44], N = 4 included APD only [28,31,38,39] and N = 5 included both CAPD and APD/CCPD patients [3,23,26,37,46]. More often than not adherence rates were reported for the pooled PD sample and not separately for the different PD modalities with the exception of adherence to dialysis prescription, where rates for APD and CAPD were separately provided [3,26,37,46].

Sample sizes varied greatly from N = 19 in [38] to N = 2001 in [30]; only 20% (N = 5) of the studies had sample sizes of more than 100 participants [27,30,37,40,44] (Table 2).

More than half (N = 15) of the included studies were cross-sectional [3,4,23,26,27,33,34,35,36,37,41,43,44,46,47], with another seven as longitudinal [30,31,32,39,40,42,45]. Two were retrospective investigations [28,38]. One study reported presented a mixture of cross sectional/retrospective data with some overlap in their sample [29].

While there was no limit to the dates of identification of studies and the earliest was published in 1994 [33], the majority (N = 19) were conducted and published in or after 2000.

Study quality

Overall, the studies were judged as being of moderate quality, as measured using the Effective Public Health Practice Project tool. The most common reasons for being of moderate quality were that non-validated tools were used to assess adherence and that the study recruited small numbers of volunteers, or the selection procedures were not outlined so representativeness could not be inferred.

Definition and measurement of non-adherence

Although some studies report studying adherence and others report non-adherence the studies are implicitly studying both adherence and non-adherence as the one is the converse of the other. Most studies used the same, conceptual definition for non-

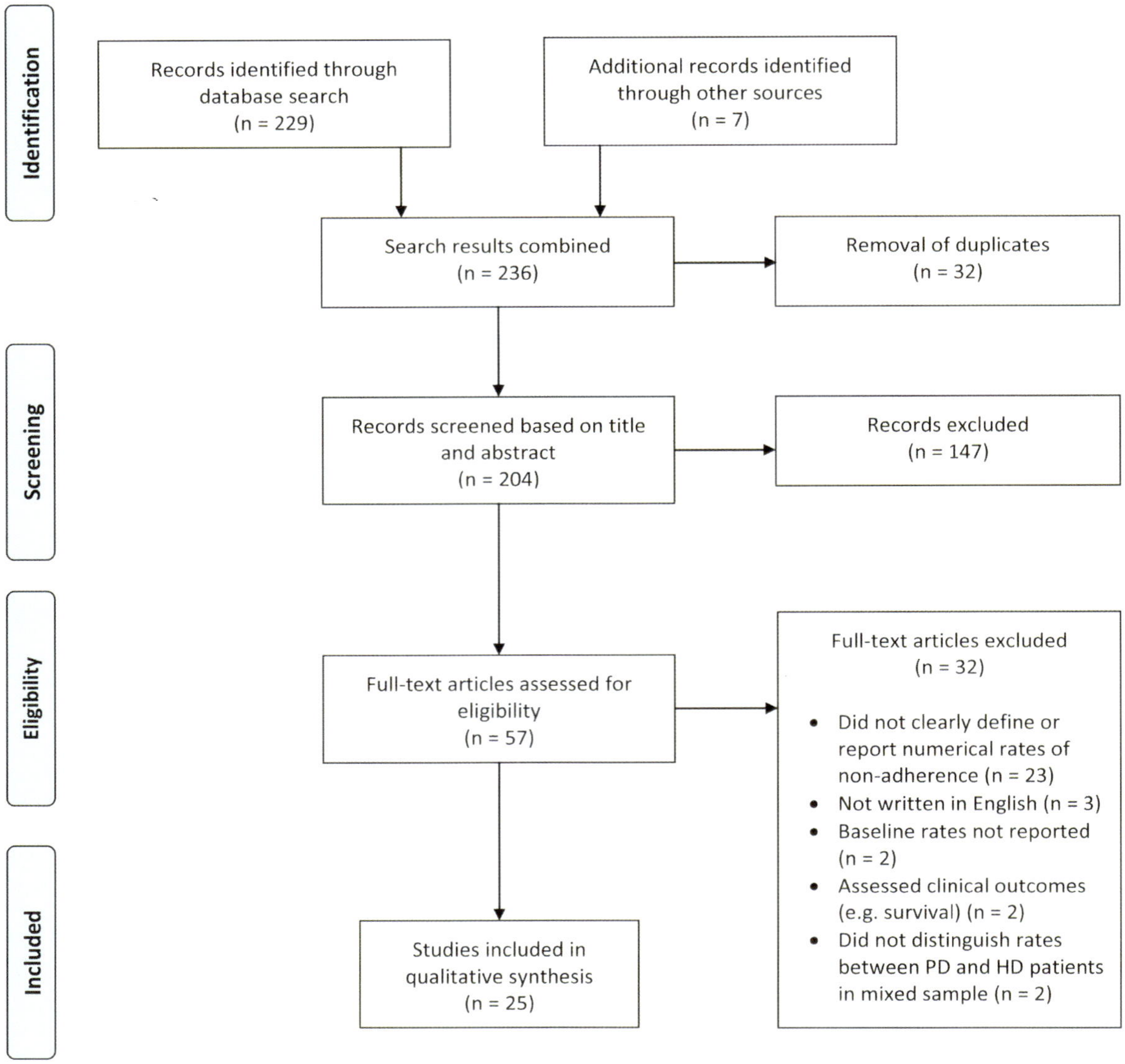

Figure 1. Flowchart of Study Selection.

adherence, namely 'not following doctor's instructions'. This was operationalized in 20 studies as 'performing less than prescribed dialysis or deviating from instructions' and in one study as not meeting clinical targets, while four studies used both definitions. Notably, one study [37] chose to avoid the use of term "non-adherence/non compliance" in favor of the term "any modification on PD regime". Although all studies included some form of definition of non-adherence, the timeframes of measuring non-adherence were not stated in all studies.

The majority of the studies (80%; N = 20) examined adherence with regards to only one aspect of treatment regimen – either dialysis procedures [3,4,26,27,28,29,30,31,32,33,35,37,38,39,47], medication [34,36,43] or diet/fluid restrictions [42,45]. Two studies considered at least two of these aspects [23,40] and another three studies considered all three aspects of treatment (dialysis, medication and diet) [41,44,46].

There was a greater degree of research that focused on adherence to dialysis and medication as opposed to dietary recommendations. Adherence to dialysis exchanges was the most commonly assessed treatment aspect (80%; N = 20) [3,4,23,26,27,28,29,30,31,32,33,35,37,38,39,40,41,44,46,47], eight studies assessed adherence to medication [23,34,36,40,41,43,44,46] and five studies assessed adherence to diet/fluid restrictions [41,42,44,45,46]. None of the studies assessed adherence to physical activity despite the fact that it is widely recommended for patients on dialysis and has been found to improve clinical and psychological outcomes.

The methods used to assess non-adherence fell into three categories: (1) subjective measures based on patient self-report, or reporting by nurses/physicians (2) objective/direct measures based on inventory checks/delivery records, built-in software or electronic monitoring systems (e.g. Baxter Home-Choice Pro Card or Baxter PD Link software) and (3) physiological and biochemical indicators that included micronutrients (e.g. serum phosphate, serum potassium), and interdialytic weight gain to evaluate respectively adherence to diet and to fluid intake. Serum creatinine levels were used to quantify adherence to dialysis prescription.

Table 2. Non-Adherence Rates Documented in PD Patients.

Author, Pub. Year	Area	Sample		Design	Method	Definition of NA	NA Rates		
		Modality	Mean Age (% Female)[a]				Dialysis	Medication	Diet
Amici et al., 1996	Italy	50 PD	65.9(–)	Cross-sectional	Self report	Not always observing dialysis prescription (time frame not stated)	18%	–	–
					PD Adequest Software	The % of patients below 95% CI of mean difference between measured and estimated weekly CrCl derived as per software in the patients reported no deviations	22%		
Bernardini et al., 1997	USA	15 CAPD; 5CCPD	46.8 (45)	Cross-sectional	Inventory check	Performing less than 90% of prescribed exchanges over interval period of 4–8 weeks	40%	–	–
Bernardini et al., 1998	USA	35 CAPD; 15 CCPD	48.7 (50)	Cross-sectional	Inventory check	Performing less than 90% of prescribed exchanges over interval period of 1–3 months	35%	–	–
Bernardini et al., 2000	USA	92 PD	52.8 (22)	Cross-sectional	Inventory check	Performing less than 90% of prescribed exchanges over interval period of 6 months, or until transplantation for 4 years	30%	–	–
Blake et al., 2000	USA	656 PD	56.0 (52)	Cross-sectional	Self-report	Missing ≥1 exchange per week, or ≥2 exchanges per month	15%	–	–
Chan et al., 2009[b]	Hong Kong	76 CAPD	66.1 (60.5)	Cross-sectional	Self-report (DDFQ)	Mild, moderate, severe, or very severe deviation from therapeutic regimen (i.e., >0)	2.6%	3.9%	Diet/Fluid: 34.2/55.9%
		77 CAPD	53.1 (31.2)				39%	37.7%	14.4%/33.8%
Chen et al., 2006	China	35 PD	57.6 (57)	Prospective	Laboratory data	Excessive dietary protein intake (DPI) beyond the range 0.8–1.2 g/kg/d	–	–	67%
Chua et al., 2011	USA	51 APD	11.8 (43)	Retrospective	Baxter Home-Choice PRO Card	Following a prescription variable (number of sessions/duration of cycles/number of cycles/dialysate volume) by ≤95% of the time	18%/4%/8%/22%	–	–
						Following a prescription variable (number of sessions/duration of cycles/number of cycles/dialysate volume) by <90% of the time	12%/6%/2%/2%		
Figueiredo et al., 2005	Brazil	30 PD	52.8 (63)	Cross-sectional	Self-report	Performing less than 90% of prescribed exchanges over interval period of 1–2 months for 4 months	30%	–	–
Fine, 1997[b]	Canada	67 CAPD	–	Cross sectional	Records of dialysate delivery and pick-up visit)	Using less than 90% of prescribed dialysate based on data (over a mean of 18 months)	3%	–	–
		77 CAPD		Retrospective	Records of dialysate delivery and pick-up visit)	Using less than 90% of prescribed dialysate based on data (over a mean of 18 months in retrospective)	5%		
		26 CAPD		Prospective	Inventory check (nurse)	Using less than 90% for an interval period of 4–6 weeks	12%		
García-Llana et al., 2013	Spain	31 PD	47.9 (19)	Cross-sectional	Self-report (Morisky-Green-Levine Test)	At least one positive (non-adherent) response on the Green-Levine Test	–	82.8% (antihypertensives); 85.2% (phosphate binders)	–

Table 2. Cont.

Author, Pub. Year	Area	Sample		Design	Method	Definition of NA	NA Rates		
		Modality	Mean Age (% Female)[a]				Dialysis	Medication	Diet
Hall et al., 2004	USA	2001 PD	53.7 (49)	Prospective	Nurse evaluation	At least 3 of the following: not attending clinics, ordering enough supplies, avoiding expedited delivery, bringing adequacy samples	10%	–	–
Hollis et al., 2006	Belgium, Italy, UK	149 APD 227 CAPD	60.0 (45)	Cross-sectional	Self-report	Any modification of treatment regimen in the past month	20%	–	–
Hung et al., 2013	Taiwan	76 PD	43.6 (62)	Cross-sectional	Interview	Not meeting all of: taking full prescribed dose, taking dose regularly with meals, and taking dose using correct method	–	43% total	–
Juergensen et al., 2004	USA	42 APD	58.0 (43)	Prospective	Baxter Home-Choice PRO Card	(Delivered dialysis volume/prescribed dialysis volume)*100<90%	17%	–	–
Kutner et al., 2002	USA	21 APD; 30 CAPD	49.2 (51)	Cross-sectional	Self-report/Laboratory data (Medication)	*APD*: Missed/shortened at least 1 session during past 2 weeks	30% (missed);10% (shortened APD)	10%	–
						CAPD: Missed at least 1 session during past 7 days			
						Medication: Serum phosphate >7.5 mg/dl over 3 months			
Lam et al., 2010	Hong Kong	173 CAPD	Median =60 (49)	Cross-sectional	Self-report (DDFQ)	Mild, moderate, severe, or very severe deviation from therapeutic regimen (i.e., >0)	7%	17%	Diet/Fluid: 62%/36%
Neri et al., 2002	Italy	19 APD	67.9 (21)	Retrospective	Baxter PD Link software	Missing PD sessions in 90 days	53%	–	–
Quan et al., 2006	China	30 PD (diabetic)	65.4 (53)	Prospective	3-day Dietary diary and fluid intake history	Deviating from dietician's instructions	–	–	19.5%
Rivetti et al., 2002	Italy	23 APD	68.0 (25)	Prospective	Baxter Home-Choice PRO Card	Number of missed sessions in 30 days	4.3%	–	–
Russo et al., 2006	Italy	191 PD	61.0 (41)	Prospective	Nurse evaluation (home visit and completion of nurse scoring card)	*Dialysis*: deviation from exchange protocol procedures/excessive of inadequate quantity of supplies present	23%/10%	25%	–
						Medication: incongruence between drugs at home and prescribed in the clinical file			
Sevick et al., 1999	USA	20 CAPD	56.2 (42)	Prospective	Self report (2 week log); APREX Medication Event Monitoring System	Missed exchanges (self report/ MEMS)	2.5%/22.7%	–	–
						Missing ≥10% of exchanges	36.8%		
						Missing >50% of exchanges	26%		
Warren et al., 1994	USA	64 PD	53.0 (–)	Cross-sectional	Self report (patient)	Non compliance to prescribed exchanges (time frame not stated)	14%	–	–
					Laboratory data	The % of patients with 24% difference between measured and estimated creatinine (cut-off based on (99% CI of the patients reported either compliance of non-compliance in the history taking)	26%		

Table 2. Cont.

Author, Pub. Year	Area	Sample		Design	Method	Definition of NA	NA Rates		
		Modality	Mean Age (% Female)[a]				Dialysis	Medication	Diet
Wazny et al., 2002	Canada	54 PD	55.9 (56)	Cross-sectional	Pharmacy record review; Self-report	Using less than 90% of prescribed dose in EPO treatment as per records or reporting missing EOP injections	–	35%	–
Yu et al., 2012	Singapore	15 APD; 5 CAPD	64.4 (40)	Cross-sectional	Self-report; Laboratory data	*Dialysis:* Skipping or shortening exchanges at least 1 exchange during past 4 weeks	15% total (5% APD /10% CAPD)	15%/30%/16%	26%/26%/16%
						Medication: Skipping/forgetting doses/Serum phosphate >1.78 mmol/L			
						Diet: intentional/unintentional dietary plan deviations / Serum potassium <3.5 mmol/L			

Note: PD = Peritoneal Dialysis. HD = Haemodialysis. CAPD = Continuous Ambulatory PD. APD = Automated PD. CCPD = Continuous Cycling PD. NA = Non-adherence. DDFQ = Dialysis Diet and Fluid Questionnaire. EPO = Erythropoietin. [a]Age and gender characteristics are presented only if reported in (or able to be calculated from) the study. [b]Articles that included more than one patient sub-group, hence sample size was separated to accurately reflect adherence rates reported in these studies.

By far, the most frequently used method to assess (non-) adherence across all treatment aspects was self-report either by the patient or healthcare provider (nurse or physician) [3,4,23,26,27,32,33,34,35,36,37,40,41,43,44,45,46,47,48]. Specific methodologies varied across studies. A total of 17 studies used a self-report by interview or an ad hoc (non-validated) patient questionnaire to measure adherence whereas three studies used self-report with a validated questionnaire (Morisky-Green-Levine Test; Dialysis Diet and Fluid Non-adherence Questionnaire) to measure adherence [36,41,44].

Biochemical measures/markers were used to quantify adherence to medication (e.g., serum phosphate for phosphate binders [23,46]) or diet (e.g., protein intake and serum potassium [42,46]). Only one study used creatinine levels as a marker of adherence to dialysis [33].

Seven out of the 25 reviewed studies used two or more adherence instruments [23,29,32,33,34,35,46], and one [34] combined the different instruments in their analyses to estimate non-adherence rates.

Occurrence of non-adherence

Overall, non-adherence rates ranged from 2.6% to 85.2%. The lowest non-adherence rates were those that measured adherence with built-in software/dialysis delivery records and the highest non-adherence rates measured adherence by either patient self-report or laboratory data. The rates differed across treatment aspects and various definitions for non-adherence. Estimates were typically higher when non-adherence was defined as any deviation from prescribed or recommended activity, and were lower when more specific criteria were applied (e.g. clinical targets for serum biochemistry or duration or numbers of cycles for APD). These issues are presented below.

Non-adherence to dialysis procedures

Non adherence to dialysis was measured in 20 of the 25 studies, and was typically defined as missing exchange(s) [27,28,32,38,39,41,46]; shortening sessions [28,46] (relevant only to APD/CCPD), or using less than the prescribed amount of dialysate, typically verified by delivery records or built-in software in PD cyclers [3,4,23,26,28,29,31,32,47] (e.g. Baxter HomeChoice PRO Card or Baxter PD Link Software) (see Table 2). In the study with the largest sample size, non adherence to dialysis encompassed a range of distinct behaviors and was defined as doing at least three of the following: not attending clinics, not ordering enough supplies, avoiding expedited delivery, or not bringing adequate samples to scheduled outpatient PD appointments [30].

Criteria and the window of observations varied. For 40% of the studies (N = 8/20) that investigated adherence to dialysis, performing less than 90% of prescribed exchanges typically over a period of 1 to 6 months was considered as indicative of non-adherence [3,4,26,28,29,30,31,47]. The remaining studies had varied criteria to identify non-adherence. Four studies (20%; N = 4/20) adopted more inclusive criteria, i.e. any deviation from regime or procedures [37,40,41,44], or at least one missed exchange during either the past one, two or four weeks [23,27,46] while others opted for a more rigid approach in which non adherence was signified by missing 50% of more of the exchanges [32]. Indirect methods based on physiological data (biochemistry or dialysis adequacy data) were also employed mainly in earlier studies [33,35].

Appreciating the heterogeneity of methods, the observed rates of non-adherence to dialysis procedures ranged from 2.6–53%. In general, rates of non-adherence to dialysis exchanges based on self-report ranged from 2.6–39%, while rates based on objective/direct measures such as inventory/delivery records or built-in software in PD cyclers ranged from 3–53% [28,29,31,32,35,38,39].

Missing PD exchanges/sessions was reported to be in range of 2.5–53% [28,32,38,39,46], shortening (as in reducing duration of cycles or number of cycles) by 4–15% of patients [23,28,46] and performing less than 90% of prescribed exchanges (as per dialysate volume) was evident in 2–40% of patients. Indirect biochemical/physiological measures (e.g. creatinine levels and/or analysis urine/dialysate data and peritoneal equilibration tests) indicate non-adherence rates at 22–26% [33,35].

Over half of the studies (65%; N = 13/20) reported the rates of non-adherence to dialysis procedures to be higher than 20% [3,4,23,26,28,32,33,35,37,38,40,41,47] suggesting that non-adherence to dialysis prescription estimates are closer to upper bounds estimates reaching 25–30% of patients on PD regimes. In the largest study to date (N = 2001) that employed composite indices, a total 10% of PD patients were found to be non-adherent to dialysis exchanges based on the definition of doing at least three of the following: not attending clinics, ordering enough supplies, avoiding expedited delivery, or bringing in their adequacy samples at scheduled outpatient PD appointments [30].

It is important to note that there is no clear consensus on definitions regarding non-adherence to dialysis sessions, which is likely to have attributed to the high degree of variability in reported non-adherence rates. Missing was defined as absence of one or more session per week, or two or more sessions per month [27]. Definitions were also different between CAPD and APD; non-adherence to the former was conceptualized as missing at least one session during the past week, while for the latter as missing at least one session during the past two weeks [23].

Non-adherence to medication

Non-adherence behaviors to medication included: not completing the full course of a prescribed medication (non-persistence), or incorrectly taking or missing doses of medication.

The range of non-adherence to medication was 3.9–85% (see Table 2 for details). Further investigation revealed that this large spread was due primarily to one outlier, which used more inclusive criteria for non-adherence: i.e., at least one instance of a non-adherent response on the eight-item Morisky-Green-Levine Test (self-report) for anti-hypertensive medication [36]. Removing this paper indicated a range of non-adherence to medication of 3.9–43% for the remaining seven papers.

Both renal specific medications (e.g. phosphate binders, erythropoietin) [23,34,36,43], and other generic/non-renal medications (e.g. medication for extra-renal morbidity such as hypertension) [36] were studied. Several studies assessed non-adherence to medication in general but not to a specific prescribed medication(s) (e.g. [44]). Non adherence rates to generic/non-renal medications ranged from 3.9–37.7% for self-report [41,44,46], compared to non-adherence rates of 25% by pill count [40].

Despite the importance of phosphate control in dialysis [49,50], only three of the studies focused on use of phosphate binders in PD, with self-reported non-adherence rates ranging from 15–85.2% [36,46] and estimates based on (serum phosphate levels) being more conservative at 10–16% [23,46].

Non-adherence to diet/fluid restrictions

Out of all identified studies, only a fraction (20%; N = 5/25) investigated dietary non-adherence in PD patients, with 14.4–67% of patients found to be non-adherent to their dietary guidelines. Of these five, two examined fluid adherence presenting the rate of self-reported non-adherence to fluid restrictions as 33.8–55.9% [41,44]. Studies that used self report showed non-adherence to diet ranging from 14.4–62% [44,45]. Unintentional and intentional dietary non-adherence behaviors were equally common at 26% [46]. Biochemical indicators of non-adherence produced divergent findings, with rates of dietary non adherence at 16% based on potassium levels [46] while a total of 67% of patients had excessive dietary protein intake in another study [42].

Factors associated with non-adherence

To explore factors associated with non-adherence in the primary studies we have adopted a narrative synthesis approach. The focus was on directionality of associations rather than the magnitude as the variation on type of statistical analyses and inconsistent reporting did not allow a more effective synthesis of results. This involved tabulating factors examined in the included studies, their reported relationship with non-adherence outcomes, defined in terms of significance and direction (negative, positive, or no relationship), and tallying studies falling into each respective grouping with the majority of studies falling into any specific category being considered to indicate a likely relationship.

Nine studies (36%; N = 9/25) [23,27,28,34,36,37,41,44,46] identified in this review evaluated factors associated with non-adherence in PD. The focus was mainly on socio-demographic parameters (i.e. age, employment status, education level, sex, race, household income and smoking status), followed by medical/treatment-related factors (duration of renal replacement therapy, presence of carer, number of comorbidities, contact with healthcare professionals) [23,27,28,34,37,41,44,46]. Psychosocial resources variables (i.e. self-efficacy, perceived burden/control, Quality of Life, satisfaction) have not been examined by more than one study per parameter [23,36]. Five of the studies that explored factors associated with non-adherence relied on univariate and correlations analyses [28,36,37,44,46], with four using more rigorous multivariate methods [23,27,34,41].

Although some variables were identified to influence non-adherence, overall there was little agreement between the studies on observed associations to allow identification of high risk sub-groups or determinants in terms of predisposing or maintaining factors. Out of the parameters that have been examined by more than one study, consistent associations with non-adherence were identified for five factors: younger age [23,34,37,41,44], being employed [27,37,41,44,46], being male [28,41,44], being on treatment for a longer period of time [34,37,44], and non-white ethnicity [23,27,28]. The correlation between education and adherence levels produced mixed results – lower education was shown to be associated with non-adherence in one study [44], but an opposite trend was observed in three other studies [27,34,41].

There is limited evidence for psychosocial factors as each of the various parameters were not examined by more than one of the studies included in this review. The patterns of associations however suggest that non-adherence is associated with low self-efficacy [46], high depression and low quality of life [23] or poor satisfaction with treatment [37]. The presence of a caregiver was found in two studies to be associated with lower rates of non-adherence to dialysis [27,46].

The association of PD modality with adherence outcomes received very little attention. We are unable to provide clear evidence for the role of PD modality as this issue has not been explored in most studies that have recruited both CAPD and APD patients or studies merged patients on PD modalities and reported overall PD non-adherence rates. Based on the limited number of studies to report rates separately for CAPD and APD patients

[3,26,37,46], non-adherence to APD procedures range from 5–20%, in comparison to 10–47% in CAPD. Although no systematic comparisons have been conducted, a trend of higher non-adherence rates in CAPD compared to APD patients is evident.

Discussion

This is the first systematic review to summarize data on (non-)adherence rates in PD and to identify factors influencing adherence in this patient group. Overall, 25 studies fulfilled the inclusion criteria with the majority focused solely on adherence to dialysis procedures/exchanges or medication, and only five on adherence to diet/fluid. As noted in previous reviews of the adherence literature across a range of patient populations, heterogeneity in methods used is more the rule than the exception. Data source and quality, sample size, and definitions of non-adherence and methods used in the included studies varied widely, thus limiting comparability and summation of results. Methodological variation is expected as there is no 'gold standard' to measure adherence [51] nor any clinical 'benchmark' on levels of adherence required for clinical benefits in PD. In the studies reported here, cut-offs of performing less than 50%, 90% or 95% of dialysis exchanges were employed as definitions of non-adherence.

Nevertheless, despite disparate operationalizations of non-adherence, evidence indicated that a substantial proportion of patients on PD regimes reported or were found to deviate from prescribed dialytic, medication regimens or dietary recommendations. The overall rates were 2.6% to 85%, with most studies reporting non-adherence rates over 30%. Most notably, regardless of methods used to operationalize non-adherence (i.e., self-report, software, delivery records) non-adherence rates were closer to upper bound estimates than lower bound rates. Non-adherence across the different treatment aspects ranged up to 53% for dialysis procedures, 43% for medication (85% when over-inclusive definition was employed) and 67% for dietary guidelines, confirming that adherence to all key aspects of PD regime is generally poor. In general, although non-adherence rates were somewhat higher for medication and diet compared to dialysis procedures, the rates of missing dialysis exchanges/sessions were far from negligible. In most studies, more than 20% of PD patients performed less than 90% of prescribed exchanges. Given the potential repercussions of non-adherence such as technique failure, peritonitis, and hospitalization [3,4], these rates are alarming.

Comparing these data in PD to those in HD [2,10], non-adherence rates to dialysis ranged from 4–53% for PD, as compared to 35% in HD, indicating higher non-adherence in PD patients. Non-adherence to medication and diet on the other hand appears to be lower in PD (3.9–43% and 14.4–67% respectively) relative to those reported in HD, where non-adherence to medication has been reported to range from 3–80.4% [52,53] and non-adherence to diet between 24–81.4% [54,55,56,57]. The intermittent nature of HD necessitates more rigid dietary requirements relative to PD, which may account for the divergent findings. It is notable however that diet or medication intake (especially related to particular types of medications) have largely been overlooked in the adherence literature in PD, hence making it difficult to assess the true extent of the problem in this population. For instance, only eight studies were identified in our review that looked at adherence to phosphate binders and dietary behaviors in PD. The small sample sizes do cast doubts on the precision of the estimates and their generalizability in PD population, yet the findings from these small studies suggest that a problem of non-adherence does exist in this area. Likewise there have been no studies that examine exercise or other important self-management/self-care behaviors in PD, such as prevention, recognition and help-seeking behaviors in response to signs of infection. Practices and skills related to connect/disconnect, hygiene or sterilization procedures are also important [58]. A study on CAPD patients indicated poor performance of the CAPD steps (most notably not using face mask) for 16.5% patients [59]. Clearly, more research is warranted to explore these behaviours and practices in both CAPD and APD as they may be linked to clinical outcomes such as technique or patient survival.

Based on four studies that compared rates of non-adherence to dialysis prescriptions in APD and CAPD populations in the same study, CAPD patients exhibited higher non-adherence to exchanges (10–47%) than APD (5–20%) patients [3,26,37,46]. This might be related to the procedural differences between the two techniques. CAPD requires multiple manual exchanges administered by the patient/care-giver, whereas APD requires only one overnight session. Higher non-adherence might occur in CAPD given the higher frequency of exchanges leading to greater opportunity to detect non-adherence.

Only one of the included studies explored rates of intentional and unintentional non-adherence [46]. In line with work with other patient populations, unintentional non-adherence was found to occur more frequently. More research will need to be undertaken in this area as these two types of non-adherence lead to very different interventions to improve adherence.

The second goal of this review was to identify factors that are associated with non-adherence in PD. Nine studies identified in this review have investigated potential determinants or correlates with adherence. Considering the lack of adequate statistical power due to small sample size and the suboptimal quality of analyses we would call for caution in the interpretation of associations, and emphasize the need for further work. However, being younger in age, male, employed, of non-white ethnicity or on PD treatment for longer was found to have consistent associations with non-adherence in PD. Patients' self care ability and/or presence of a caregiver may moderate the effect of age [46,60] as older patients assisted by a caregiver were found to be less likely to miss exchanges than an older patient who is conducting the exchanges him/herself [61].

The role of psychosocial factors of adherence received little attention despite evidence from reviews in other patient populations and HD [10,62]. Two studies have assessed some factors but none has explicitly used a theoretical framework to understand what facilitates and what inhibits adherence. There is some limited evidence that low Quality of Life, low satisfaction, low self-efficacy and depression are associated with non-adherence but replication is necessary as none of these factors was identified in more than one study. It is only once these associations are conclusively known that evidence-based interventions to increase adherence can be developed and tested.

A first step to improving adherence is being able to define, assess and recognize it. Arriving at a consensual definition for non-adherence in the context of PD and developing reliable methods of assessment so as to establish accurate frequencies of non-adherence are essential to determine the extent of the problem and provide basis for prevention, support and intervention that can improve care and outcomes for PD patients. Although methods are not yet available for routine use, renal health care professionals should regularly enquire of patients as to how they manage their treatment requirements so that difficulties can be identified early and action or support can be rendered.

To our knowledge, this is the first comprehensive systematic review to focus on adherence in PD, and it has been conducted according to PRISMA guidelines. Despite the rigorous methodology used to search, select and extract data, the study has several limitations, most of which are inherent to the studies included. First, evidence gathered is based largely on cross-sectional data. We found that recruited study samples were very small, thus limiting the generalizability of findings. Only five studies had sample sizes above 100 and the majority of studies opted to merge between APD and CAPD groups due to small sample sizes. Longitudinal data are needed to evaluate course of adherence over time in the PD population. Second, there was very little consistency in methodologies and the description and rigor of self-reported measures of adherence were generally poor.

We had also hoped to compare non-adherence across PD modalities but only four studies reported adherence separately for modality subgroups, hence limiting any analysis. Other possible limitations of this study is the potential publication bias introduced by excluding non-English studies and not conducting a search for grey literature via contacting relevant experts for unpublished manuscripts due to limited resources and rapid time frame for the review. Finally our approach to rely on directionality and statistical significance when exploring factors associated with non-adherence, albeit deemed necessary to overcome caveats in the reporting of relevant statistical data failed to consider the magnitude of reported effects and may therefore have resulted in taking a conservative stance in interpreting the evidence.

In conclusion, the results of this review suggest that non-adherence is a persistent concern in PD and needs to be given serious consideration in order to improve outcomes. Additional high quality, adequately powered studies are required to investigate adherence to all aspects of treatment particularly with respect to diet, types of medication, lifestyle recommendations and other self-care behaviors that are critical to PD success. The use of multiple measurement methods would be recommended as a triangulation of methods can help gain better understanding and more reliable estimates of rates or magnitude of non-adherence. Due consideration should be given to identifying factors that influence non-adherence as these remain inadequately addressed. The role of PD modality, psychosocial and interpersonal factors guided by relevant theoretical frameworks can advance understandings of non-adherence and inform interventions for this patient group.

Author Contributions

Conceived and designed the experiments: KG MWYF SPN. Performed the experiments: KG AYL HAL ZY. Analyzed the data: KG AYL HAL ZY MWYF SPN. Contributed reagents/materials/analysis tools: KG AYL HAL ZY MWYF SPN. Wrote the paper: KG AYL HAL SPN.

References

1. Jain AK, Blake P, Cordy P, Garg AX (2012) Global trends in rates of peritoneal dialysis. J Am Soc Nephrol 23: 533–544.
2. Denhaerynck K, Manhaeve D, Dobbels F, Garzoni D, Nolte C, et al. (2007) Prevalence and consequences of nonadherence to hemodialysis regimens. Am J Crit Care 16: 222–235.
3. Bernardini J, Piraino B (1998) Compliance in CAPD and CCPD patients as measured by supply inventories during home visits. Am J Kidney Dis 31: 101–107.
4. Bernardini J, Nagy M, Piraino B (2000) Pattern of noncompliance with dialysis exchanges in peritoneal dialysis patients. Am J Kidney Dis 35: 1104–1110.
5. Bender B, Rand C (2004) Medication non-adherence and asthma treatment cost. Current Opinion in Allergy & Clinical Immunology 4: 191–195.
6. Sokol MC, McGuigan KA, Verbrugge RR, Epstein RS (2005) Impact of medication adherence on hospitalization risk and healthcare cost. Medical care 43: 521–530.
7. Sunanda K, Fadia S (2008) Medication non-adherence is associate with increased medical health care costs. Digestive diseases and sciences 53: 1020–1024.
8. Denhaerynck K, Dobbels F, Cleemput I, Desmyttere A, Schafer-Keller P, et al. (2005) Prevalence, consequences and determinants of nonadherence in adults renal transplant patients: A literature review. Transpl Int 18: 1121–1133.
9. Denhaerynck K, Burkhalter F, Schäfer-Keller P, Steiger J, Bock A, et al. (2009) Clinical consequences of non adherence to immunosuppresive medication in kidney transplant patients. Transpl Int 22: 441–446.
10. Karamanidou C, Clatworthy J, Weinman J, Horne R (2008) A systematic review of the prevalence and determinants of nonadherence to phosphate binrding medication in patients with end-stage renal disease. BMC Nephol 9.
11. Khalil AA, Frazier SK (2010) Depressive symptoms and dietary nonadherence in patients with end-stage renal disease receiving hemodialysis: a review of quantitative evidence. Issues Ment Health Nurs 31: 324–330.
12. Schmid H, Hartmann B, Schiffl H (2009) Adherence to prescribed oral medication in adult patients undergoing chronic hemodialysis: a critical review of the literature. Eur J Med Res 14: 185–190.
13. Lehane E, McCarthy G (2007) Intentional and unintentional medication non-adherence: a comprehensive framework for clinical research and practice? A discussion paper. Int J Nurs Stud 44.
14. Bland RJ, Cottrell RR, Guyler LR (2008) Medicaton compliance of hemodialysis patients and factors contributing to non-compliance. Dial Transpl 37: 174–178.
15. Sabate E (2003) Adherence to Long-Term Therapies: Evidence for Action. Geneva: World Health Organization.
16. DiMatteo MR (2004) Variations in patients' adherence to medical recommendations: a quantitative review of 50 years of research. Med Care 42: 200–209.
17. Hailey BJ, Moss SB (2000) Compliance behaviour in patients undergoing haemodialysis: A review of the literature. Psychol Health Med 5: 395–406.
18. Lulowsky L, Mehrotra R, Kheifets L, Arah OA, Nissenson AR, et al. (2013) Comparing mortality of peritoneal and hemodialysis patients in the first 2 years of dialysis therapy: a marginal structural model analysis. Clin J Am Soc Nephrol 8.
19. Pruthi R, Steenkamp R, Feest TG (2013) UK Renal Registry 16th Annual Report: Chapter 8 Survival and cause of death of UK adult patients on renal replacement therapy in 2012: national and centre-specific analyses. Bristol: The Renal Association.
20. Termorshuizen F, Korevaar JC, Dekker FW, Van Manen JG, Boeschoten EW, et al. (2003) Hemodialysis and peritoneal dialysis: comparison of adjusted mortality rates according to the duration of dialysis: analysis of the Netherlands Cooperative Study on the Adequacy of Dialysis 2. J Am Soc Nephrol 14: 2851–2860.
21. Vonesh E, Snyder JJ, Foley R, Collins A (2004) The differential impact of risk factors on mortality in hemodialysis and peritoneal dialysis. Kidney Int 66.
22. Wright M, Woodrow G, O'Brien S, King N, Dye L, et al. (2004) Polydipsia: a feature of peritoneal dialysis. Nephrol Dial Transpl 19: 1581–1586.
23. Kutner NG, Zhang R, McClellan WM, Cole SA (2002) Psychosocial predictors of non-compliance in haemodialysis and peritoneal dialysis patients. Nephrol Dial Transpl 17: 93v99.
24. Liberati A, Altman DG, Tetzlaff J, Mulrow C, Gotzsche PC, et al. (2009) The PRISMA statement for reporting for systematic reviews and meta-analyses of studies that evaluate health care interventions: explanation and elaboration. Ann Intern Med 151: W65–94.
25. Effective Public Health Practice Project (1998) Quality Assessment Tool for Quantitative Studies. In: Project EPHP, editor.
26. Bernardini J, Piraino B (1997) Measuring compliance with prescribed exchanges in CAPD and CCPD patients. Perit Dial Dial 17: 338v342.
27. Blake PG, Korbet SM, Blake R, Bargman JM, Burkart JM, et al. (2000) A multicenter study of noncompliance with continuous ambulatory peritoneal dialysis exchanges in US and Canadian patients. Am J Kidney Dis 35: 506–514.
28. Chua AN, Warady BA (2011) Adherence of pediatric patients to automated peritoneal dialysis. Pediatr Nephrol 26: 789–793.
29. Fine A (1997) Compliance with CAPD prescription is good. Perit Dial Dial 17: 343–346.
30. Hall G, Bogan A, Dreis S, Duffy A, Greene A, et al. (2004) New directions in peritoneal dialysis patient training. Nephrol Nurs J 31: 149–154, 159–163.
31. Juergensen PH, Gorban-Brennan N, Finkelstein FO (2004) Compliance with the dialysis regimen in chronic peritoneal dialysis patients: Utility of the pro card and impact of patient education. Adv Perit Dial 20: 90–92.
32. Sevick MA, Levine D, Burkart JM, Rocco M, Keith J, et al. (1999) Measurement of continuous ambulatory peritoneal dialysis prescription adherence using a novel approach. Perit Dial Dial 19: 23–30.
33. Warren PJ, Brandes JC (1994) Compliance with the peritoneal dialysis prescription is poor. J Am Soc Nephrol 4: 1627–1629.

34. Wazny LD, Stojimirovic BB, Heidenheim P, Blake PG (2002) Factors influencing erythropoietin compliance in peritoneal dialysis patients. Am J Kidney Dis 40: 623–628.
35. Amici G, Viglino G, Virga G, Gandolfo G, Ra Rin G, et al. (1996) Compliance study in peritoneal dialysis using PD Adequent software. Perit Dial Dial 16: S176–178.
36. García-Llana H, Remor E, Selgar R (2013) Adherence to treatment, emotional state and quality of life in patients with end-stage renal disease undergoing dialysis. Psicothema 25: 79–86.
37. Hollis J, Harman W, Goovearts T, Paris V, Chivers G, et al. (2006) Managing peritoneal dialysis (PD) —factors that influence patients' modification of their recommended dialysis regimen. A European study of 376 patients. J Ren Care 32: 202–207.
38. Neri L, Viglino G, Cappelletti A, Gandolfo G, Barbieri S (2002) Compliance in automated peritoneal dialysis. Adv Perit Dial 18.
39. Rivetti M, Battú S, Barrile P, Benotto S, Berruto L, et al. (2002) Compliance with automated peritoneal dialysis. EDTNA ERCA J 28: 40–43, 55.
40. Russo R, Manili L, Tiraboschi G, Amar K, De Luca M, et al. (2006) Patient re-training in peritoneal dialysis: why and when it is needed. Kidney Int Suppl 70: S127–132.
41. Chan MF, Wong FKY, Chow SKY (2009) Investigating the health profile of patients with end-stage renal failure receiving peritoneal dialysis: a cluster analysis. J Clin Nurs 19: 649–657.
42. Chen W, Lu X, Wang T (2006) Menu suggestion: An effective way to improve dietary compliance in peritoneal dialysis patients. J Renal Nutr 16: 132–136.
43. Hung KY, Liao SC, Chen TH, Chao MC, Chen JB (2013) Adherence to phosphate binder therapy is the primary determinant of hyperphosphatemia incidence in patients receiving peritoneal dialysis. Ther Apher Dial 17: 72–77.
44. Lam LW, Twinn SF, Chan SWC (2010) Self-reported adherence to a therapeutic regimen among patients undergoing continuous ambulatory peritoneal dialysis. J Adv Nurs 66: 763–773.
45. Quan L, Xu Y, Luo SP, Wang L, LeBlanc D, et al. (2006) Negotiated care improves fluid status in diabetic peritoneal dialysis patients. Perit Dial Dial 26: 95–100.
46. Yu ZL, Yeoh LY, Seow YY, Luo XC, Griva K (2012) Evaluation of adherence and depression among patients on peritoneal dialysis. Singapore Med J 53: 474–480.
47. Figueiredo AE, Santos KS, Creutzberg M (2005) Compliance in peritoneal dialysis measured by supply inventories. Adv Perit Dial 21: 77–79.
48. Fine A (1997) Compliance with CAPD prescription is good. Perit Dial Dial 17: 343–346.
49. Weed-Collins M, Hogan R (1989) Knowledge and health beliefs regarding phosphate-binding medication in predicting compliance. ANNA J 16: 278–282.
50. National Kidney Foundation (2012) Dialysis.
51. Morris LS, Schulz RM (1992) Patient compliance: an overview. J Clin Pharm Ther 17: 183–195.
52. Hirth RA, Greer SL, Albert JM, Young EW, John D (2008) Out-of-pocket spending and medication adherence among dialysis patients in twelve countries. Health affairs 27: 89–102.
53. Lindberg M, Lindberg P, Wikstrom B (2007) Medication discrepancy: A concordance problem between dialysis patients and caregivers. Scandinavian journal of urology and nephrology 41: 546–552.
54. Kara B, Caglar K, Kilic S (2007) Nonadherence with diet and fluid restrictions and perceived social support in patients receiving hemodialysis. J Nurs Scholarship 39: 243–248.
55. Kugler C, Maeding I, Russell CL (2011) Non-adherence in patients on chronic hemodialysis: an international comparison study. J Nephrol 24: 366–375.
56. Lin CC, Liang CC (1997) The relationship between health locus of control and compliance of hemodialysis patients. Kaohsiung J Med Sci 13: 243–254.
57. Vlaminck H, Maes B, Jacobs A, Reyntjens S, Evers G (2001) The dialysis diet and fluid non-adherence questionnaire: validity testing of a self-report instrument for clinical practice. J Clin Nurs 10: 707–715.
58. Bender FH, Bernardini J, Piraino B (2006) Prevention of infectious complications in peritoneal dialysis: best demonstrated practices. Kidney Int 70: S44–54.
59. Mawar S, Gupta S, Mahajan S (2012) Non-compliance to he continuous ambulatory peritoneal dialysis procedure increases the risk of peritonitis. Int Urol Nephrol 44: 1243–1249.
60. Blake PG (1999) Individualized prescription of peritoneal dialysis therapy? Perit Dial Dial 19: S495–498.
61. Ricka R, Vanrenterghem Y, Evers GCM (2002) Adequate self-care of dialysed patients: a review of the literature. Int J Nurs Stud 39: 329–339.
62. Bane C, Hughes CM, McElnay JC (2006) The impact of depressive symptoms and psychosocial factors on medication adherence in cardiovascular disease. Patient Educ Couns 60: 187–193.

Structural and Functional Brain Alterations in End Stage Renal Disease Patients on Routine Hemodialysis: A Voxel-Based Morphometry and Resting State Functional Connectivity Study

Yingwei Qiu[1,2]*, Xiaofei Lv[3], Huanhuan Su[1], Guihua Jiang[1], Cheng Li[4], Junzhang Tian[1]

1 Department of Medical Imaging, Guangdong No. 2 Provincial People's Hospital, Guangzhou, PR China, **2** Department of Medical Imaging, The First Affiliated Hospital of Gannan Medical University, Ganzhou, PR China, **3** Departments of Medical Imaging and Interventional Radiology, Cancer Center, Sun Yat-Sen University, Guangzhou, PR China, **4** Department of Renal Transplantation, Guangdong No. 2 Provincial People's Hospital, Guangzhou, PR China

Abstract

Background and Purpose: Cognitive impairment is a well-described phenomenon in end-stage renal disease (ESRD) patients. However, its pathogenesis remains poorly understood. The primary focus of this study was to examine structural and functional brain deficits in ESRD patients.

Materials and Methods: Thirty ESRD patients on hemodialysis (without clinical neurological disease) and 30 age- and gender-matched control individuals (without renal or neurological problems) were recruited in a prospective, single-center study. High-resolution structural magnetic resonance imaging (MRI) and resting state functional MRI were performed on both groups to detect the subtle cerebral deficits in ESRD patients. Voxel-based morphometry was used to characterize gray matter deficits in ESRD patients. The impact of abnormal morphometry on the cerebral functional integrity was investigated by evaluating the alterations in resting state functional connectivity when brain regions with gray matter volume reduction were used as seed areas.

Results: A significant decrease in gray matter volume was observed in ESRD patients in the bilateral medial orbito-prefrontal cortices, bilateral dorsal lateral prefrontal cortices, and the left middle temporal cortex. When brain regions with gray matter volume reduction were used as seed areas, the integration was found to be significantly decreased in ESRD patients in the fronto-cerebellum circuits and within prefrontal circuits. In addition, significantly enhanced functional connectivity was found between the prefrontal cortex and the left temporal cortex and within the prefrontal circuits.

Conclusions: Our study revealed that both the structural and functional cerebral cortices were impaired in ESRD patients on routine hemodialysis.

Editor: Satoru Hayasaka, Wake Forest School of Medicine, United States of America

Funding: This work was supported by the grants from the Natural Scientific Foundation of China [Grant No. 81201084 for YQ], and the Planned Science and Technology Project of Guangdong Province, China [Grant No. 2011B031800044 for GJ]. The funders had no role in study design, data collection and analysis, decision to publish, or preparation of the manuscript.

Competing Interests: The authors have declared that no competing interests exist.

* E-mail: qiuyw1201@gmail.com

These authors contributed equally to this work.

Introduction

End stage renal disease (ESRD) is the last stage (stage 5) of chronic kidney disease (CKD), and corresponds to complete or almost complete loss of kidney function. Cognitive impairment is highly prevalent in ESRD patients [1,2]. Deficits involve a range of cognitive domains, including concentration, memory and planning, which may be associated with increased staff time in caring for the patients, greater utilization of healthcare resources, more frequent hospitalizations and an increased number of days spent in the hospital [3,4]. Recognizing the cerebral deficits of ESRD could help us understand the underlying neuronal mechanisms and lead to earlier interventions that might reduce morbidity.

Imaging plays an important role in detecting structural and functional abnormalities of the brain in ESRD patients. Conventional MR and computed tomography (CT) imaging studies with visual assessment and manual measurements of structures of interest have demonstrated that patients with ESRD have reduced brain volumes, reduced deep white matter volumes, a high prevalence of subcortical white matter lesions, and a high incidence rate for stroke [5–8]. MR spectroscopy (MRS) studies have demonstrated that CKD patients (stage 4–5) without clinical signs of uremic encephalopathy showed metabolic disturbances in multiple brain regions, including the parieto-occipital white matter, the occipital grey matter, the basal ganglia and the pons [8–10]. Positron emission tomography (PET) studies have displayed that hemispheric oxygen [11] and glucose metabolism [12], especially for bilateral pre-frontal cortices (PFC), are depressed in patients with ESRD. However, due to the methodological limitations, insensitivity to the early and small lesions (conventional MRI and CT with visual assessment and manual measurements of structures of interest) [13], need for a predetermined region of interest, time-consuming manual measurements or subjective visual assessments (conventional MRI and CT with visual assessment and manual measurements of structures of interest and single-voxel MRS) [13,14], and radiation exposure and low spatial resolution (PET) [15], their applications are restricted in a large cohort.

Resting state functional MRI (rs-fMRI) has the ability to record spontaneous brain activity fluctuations when subjects lie still in the scanner. Low-frequency (0.01–0.8 Hz) fluctuations of the blood-oxygen-level-dependent (BOLD) signal in the resting state are considered to be physiologically meaningful and related to spontaneous neural activity [16]. Recently, using rs-fMRI and the regional homogeneity analysis method, Liang et al. found that patients with ESRD showed decreased regional homogeneity in multiple areas of the bilateral frontal, parietal and temporal lobes. Moreover, they found the progressively decreased regional homogeneity in the default mode network (DMN), indicating that frontal and parietal lobes might be trait-related in ESRD patients with minimal nephro-encephalopathy [17]. Voxel-based morphometry (VBM) is a spatially specific and unbiased method of analyzing MR images reflecting the regional gray matter volume at a voxel scale [18]. This technique has already been successfully applied to normal aging [18], schizophrenia [19], dementia [20], mild cognitive impairment (MCI) [21], drug addicts [22] and hepatic encephalopathy [23]. In ESRD patients, Zhang and colleagues found diffusely decreased gray matter volume that was further decreased in the presence of encephalopathy [24]; while Prohovnik and coworkers found significant cerebral atrophy, most notably bilaterally in the caudate nuclei in ESRD patients [25]. These morphometric deficits may also relate to the functional integrity alterations in the ESRD patients. However, no studies have investigated the effects of the observed gray matter impairment on functional integrity. Studies combining VBM with rs-fMRI can explore the structural and functional cerebral deficits simultaneously [26,27]. This method can be an ideal way to explore the neurobiological mechanisms of ESRD patients.

The purposes of the present study were to 1) identify brain regions with gray matter volume deficits, using voxel-based morphometry, and 2) investigate the brain network effect of these anatomic deficits in ESRD patients using the observed structural deficits as seed regions in functional connectivity analysis.

Materials and Methods

Participants

This prospective study was approved by the Research Ethics Review Board of the Institute of Mental Health at the Guangdong No. 2 Provincial People's Hospital. Written informed consent was obtained from all subjects. Sixty subjects, including 30 control subjects and 30 ESRD patients participated in this study. The ESRD patients were recruited from the Renal and Hemodialysis Clinics and Department of Renal Transplantation at Guangdong No. 2 Provincial People's Hospital. Demographic characteristics and chronic health conditions of each ESRD patient were obtained from the patient's electronic medical records. Laboratory values from ESRD patients included serum calcium, serum phosphorus, serum uric acid and creatinine. As part of the routine clinical care, these laboratory tests were drawn monthly on dialysis days prior to the treatment. Values for serum calcium, serum phosphorus, serum uric acid and serum urea were calculated by averaging the monthly laboratory tests for 3 consecutive months prior to MR imaging. All tests were performed at a single central laboratory using standard methods. Measured blood pressure was determined by averaging the 3 office blood pressure readings prior to MR imaging. The control group was recruited from the local community.

Exclusion criteria for both groups were as follows: a history of stroke or dementia either reported or documented in the medical chart, a history of Parkinson's or neurodegenerative disease, diabetes, alcoholism, drug abuse, psychiatric disorder, or major neurologic disorders (severe head injury, stroke, epilepsy, or visible lesions), liver function enzymes (AST and ALT) more than twice the upper limit of normal, or a hemoglobin level <10 g. In all of the ESRD patients MRI was performed on non-dialysis days to limit the effect of the potential temporal relationship between brain changes and time since last dialysis.

MR imaging

MR data were obtained on a Philips Achieva 1.5 T Nova dual MR scanner using a 16-channel Neuro-Vascular (NV) coil. None of the subjects were taking any medications at the time of the scans. Tight but comfortable foam padding was used to minimize head motion, and earplugs were used to reduce scanner noise. Sagittal structural images (160 sagittal slices, TR = 25 ms, TE = 4.1 ms, thickness = 1.0 mm, no gap, in-plane resolution = 231×232, FOV = 230×230 mm^2, flip angle = 30°) were acquired using a fast field echo (FFE) three-dimensional T1 weighted sequence. Resting-state functional MRI (fMRI) scans were performed by an echo planar imaging (EPI) sequence with scan parameters of TR = 3000 ms, TE = 50 ms, flip angle = 90°, matrix = 64×64, FOV = 230×230 mm^2, slice thickness = 4.5 mm and slice gap = 0 mm. Each brain volume comprised 33 axial slices and each functional run contained 160 volumes (8 minutes). During resting state fMRI scanning, subjects were instructed to close their eyes and keep as still as possible, and not to think of anything systematically or fall asleep.

After the scan, all the participants were asked the following questions to verify the degree of their cooperation: "what were you thinking during the scan?", "did you fall asleep just now?", "were your eyes closed during the scan?" and "did you feel uncomfortable during the scan?" Only when the participant answered "nothing", "no, I did not", "yes, I kept my eyes closed" and "no, I did not feel any uncomfortable", were their data used in the present study.

Voxel-Based Morphometry Analysis

Structural image processing was conducted using the Voxel-based morphometry toolbox (VBM8) (http://dbm.neuro.uni-jena.de/vbm/) implemented in Statistical Parametric Mapping-8 (SPM8) (http://www.fil.ion.ucl.ac.uk/spm, Welcome Department of Imaging Neuroscience, London). VBM8 in SPM8 combines tissue segmentation, bias correction, and spatial normalization into a unified model [27]. Hidden Markov Random Fields were applied to improve accuracy of tissue segmentation (medium HMRF 0.3). Otherwise, default parameters were used. Individual brains were normalized to tissue probability maps provided by International Consortium for Brain Mapping (ICBM). The optimally processed images were smoothed with an isotropic Gaussian kernel (full-width half maximum = 12 mm). At the second level, whole brain data were modeled across the groups using analysis of covariance (ANCOVA) with total gray matter volume and age as covariates. The effects of total gray matter volume were removed to allow inferences between regional differences in gray matter volume. An absolute threshold mask of .1 was used. The significance of group differences in each region was estimated by distributional approximations from the theory of random Gaussian fields, and significance levels were set at $p<0.05$ (corrected for multiple comparisons). To identify the association between structural abnormalities and clinical severity of kidney disease and times of hemodialysis, the average gray matter volume values for all voxels in the abnormal areas, revealed by voxel-based morphometry, were extracted and correlated with the duration of chronic kidney disease, duration of hemodialysis and the laboratory values (serum calcium level, serum phosphorus level, serum uric acid level and serum urea values) in individual ESRD patient.

Functional Connectivity Analysis

Preprocessing and statistical analysis of functional images were conducted using SPM8. For each subject, the first ten time points were discarded to avoid transient signal changes before magnetization reached steady-state and to allow subjects to get used to the fMRI scanning noise. Then echo-planar images were slice-time corrected and realigned to the first image in the first series and were subsequently unwarped to correct for susceptibility-by-movement interaction, subjects with head motion exceeding 1.0 mm of maximal translation (in any direction of x, y or z) or 1.0° of maximal rotation through the resting-state run were excluded from further analysis. All realigned images were spatially normalized to the Montreal Neurological Institute (MNI) echo-planar imaging template in SPM8, and each voxel was resampled to 3×3×3 mm^3. Functional connectivity was examined using a method based on a seed voxel correlation approach [27,28]. Since voxel-based morphometry analysis showed anatomic deficits in the bilateral medial PFC, the bilateral dorsal lateral PFC (dlPFC) and the left middle temporal gyrus, areas with gray matter volume reduction were defined as seeds for functional connectivity analysis. A reference time series for each seed was obtained by averaging the fMRI time series for all voxels within the region with anatomic deficits. Next, each time series was temporally bandpass filtered (0.01–0.08 Hz). Correlation analysis was conducted between the seed reference and the rest of the whole brain in a voxel-wise manner using the realigned images. To combine results across subjects and compute statistical significance, correlation coefficients were converted to a normal distribution by Fisher's z transform [29,30].

For each group, individual z value maps were analyzed with a random effect one-sample t test to identify voxels showing a significant positive or negative correlation to the seed time series, with correlations thresholded using a family-wise error correction at $p<0.05$. For between-group comparison, two-sample t tests were used to compare z value maps between ESRD patients and matched controls, with the significance threshold of group differences set at $p<0.05$ using AlphaSim correction in the REST software (http://www. restfmri.net), which applied Monte Carlo simulation to calculated the probability of false positive detection by taking both the individual voxel probability thresholding and cluster size into consideration [31]. To identify the association between functional connectivity and clinical severity of kidney disease in ESRD patients, the z value of the regions that showed aberrant functional connectivity with the anatomic abnormalities (revealed by group comparison) were extracted and correlated with the duration of chronic kidney disease, duration of hemodialysis and the laboratory values (serum calcium, serum phosphorus, serum uric acid and serum urea values) in individual ESRD patient.

A complementary analysis was carried out to investigate the link between the structural and functional results, i.e., we wanted to address whether the effects observed on functional connectivity in ESRD patients could be explained by the reduced gray matter volume observed in the seed areas. Therefor, we replicated the four between-groups comparisons of the functional connectivity maps in using the gray matter volume of the respective seed areas as covariates.

Results

Demographic Results

Table 1 demonstrates the basic characteristics of ESRD patients and controls. There were no significant differences in age ($p=0.737$), education ($p=0.506$), sex composition ($p=0.559$) between the ESRD and control groups. Table 2 demonstrates systolic blood pressure, diastolic blood pressure and hematocrit at the start and end of hemodialysis treatment session. In these patients, ESRD was secondary to glomerulonephritis.

Morphometry Analysis

Relative to controls, ESRD patients showed significantly decreased gray matter volume in bilateral medial orbito-prefrontal cortex (OFC, Brodmann's area 10, 11, 32, Talairach coordinates: 1.5, 43.5, −13.5; voxel size = 328 mm^3), left middle temporal gyrus (Brodmann's area 10, 11, 32, Talairach coordinates: −55.5, −9, −12; voxel size = 533 mm^3), left dorsal lateral prefrontal cortex (dlPFC, Brodmann's area 10, Talairach coordinates: −30, 51, 0; voxel size = 340 mm^3) and right dlPFC (Brodmann's area 11, Talairach coordinates: 27, 54, −9; voxel size = 182 mm^3) (Figure 1). No significant increases in gray matter volume were found in ESRD patients compared to controls. No significant negative/positive correlations were found between the abnormal gray matter volume and the duration of chronic kidney disease, duration of hemodialysis and laboratory values for serum calcium level, phosphorus, uric acid and urea levels in ESRD patients.

Functional Connectivity Analysis

The four seed areas, where reduced gray matter volume was detected among ESRD patients, were selected for functional connectivity analysis. When the seed was located in the bilateral medial OFC, the ESRD patients showed reduced functional connectivity in the bilateral posterior cerebellar lobes, right dlPFC, bilateral ACC, and enhanced FC in bilateral OFC, bilateral superior parietal lobe than controls (Table 3, Figure 2). When the seed was located in the left dlPFC, the ESRD patients demonstrated enhanced functional connectivity in the superior temporal gyrus compared to controls (Table 3, Figure 2). When the seed was located in the right dlPFC, the ESRD patients demonstrated reduced FC in bilateral posterior cerebellar lobes, the left inferior temporal gyrus, the right dlPFC, and enhanced FC in bilateral OFC, and the left posterior gyrus (Table 3, Figure 2). When the seed was located in the left middle temporal gyrus, enhanced FC was found in the right medial PFC in ESRD patients when compared to controls (Table 3, Figure 2).

The replication of the group comparisons for the four functional connectivity maps with the corresponding gray matter volume of the seeds as covariates resulted in similar results, except for the network corresponding to the seed of left dorsal lateral prefrontal cortex, which showed no significant differences between the two groups.

Table 1. Demographic and Clinical Characteristics for End Stage Renal Disease (ESRD) Patients and Controls.

Characteristic	*Group*				
	ESRD Patients (N = 30)		**Controls (N = 30)**		
	Mean	**SD**	**Mean**	**SD**	**P**
Age (years)	38.8	9.6	38.1	7.0	0.737
Education (years)	9.8	5.1	10.6	4.5	0.506
Laboratory tests					
S. uric acid (mg/dl)	5.98	1.20	N/A	N/A	-
S. urea (mmol/l)	19.2	5.4	N/A	N/A	-
S. calcium (mmol/l)	2.32	0.25	N/A	N/A	-
S. Phosphorus (mmol/l)	1.30	0.24	N/A	N/A	-
Illness duration (years)	12.5	4.8	N/A	N/A	-
Dialysis duration (mouths)	17.2	6.8	N/A	N/A	-
Mean hemodialysis duration (h/w)	14.5	3.5	N/A	N/A	-
	N	%	N	%	P
Gender					
Female	7	23.3	9	30	0.559
Male	23	76.7	21	70	0.559

There were no significant differences in age (p = 0.737), education (p = 0.506), sex composition (p = 0.559) between ESRD patients and controls.
Note. N/A = not applicable.

No significant positive or negative correlation was found between any of the Z values and the duration of chronic kidney disease, duration of hemodialysis and laboratory values for serum calcium, serum phosphorus, serum uric acid and serum serum urea values in ESRD patients.

Discussion

Our study revealed the following important findings. First, ESRD patients have several areas of decreased gray matter volume (including the bilateral medial OFC, the bilateral dlPFC and the left middle temporal gyrus) compared with healthy controls. Second, the decrease in gray matter volume in these regions was related to the functional network integrity deficits in ESRD patients. To the best of our knowledge, this is the first systemic investigation of anatomic and functional deficits in ESRD patients on routine hemodialysis with VBM and functional connectivity methods.

The loss of gray matter volumes includes the bilateral dlPFC, the bilateral medial OFC, and the left middle temporal gyrus. The reduced gray matter volume of the prefrontal cortex in ESRD patients observed in the present study is supported by a recent histological study by Migliori and coworkers [32]. These Authors compared normal rats, nephrectomized rats and nephrectomized rats treated with Fluoxetin, and found a significant decrease in brain derived neurotrophic factor (BDNF) at the level of the prefrontal cortex in the nephrectomized rats compared to normal rats. Moreover, they showed a partial recovery in the Nx-F rats [32]. The reduced BDNF had been widely related to atrophy and cellular death of glia and neurons in neurodegenerative disorder [32]. Previous PET studies also revealed abnormalities in these areas. In an F-18-fluorodeoxyglucose (FDG) PET study, Song et al. found several voxel clusters of significantly decreased cerebral glucose metabolism in pre-dialysis CKD patients, including the left prefrontal cortex (Brodmann's area 9), the right prefrontal cortex (Brodmann's area 10) and the right basolateral prefrontal cortex (Brodmann's area 46), the left anterior cingulate gyrus (Brodmann's area 32), the left premotor cortex (Brodmann's area 6), the left transverse temporal gyrus (Brodmann's area 41), the left superior temporal gyrus (Brodmann's area 42), the right basolateral prefrontal cortex (Brodmann's area 44), the right inferior parietal lobule (Brodmann's area 39), the left middle temporal gyrus (Brodmann's area 19), and the left angular gyrus (Brodmann's area 39). Moreover, they found a negative correlation between the cerebral glucose metabolism of the right orbitofrontal cortex and the Hamilton Depression Rating Scale (HDRS) in pre-dialysis CKD patients (Brodmann's area 11) [12]. Through measuring brain oxygen metabolism, Kanai et al.

Table 2. Blood pressure systolic, Blood pressure diastolic and Hematocrit of the ESRD patients at the start and end of hemodialysis treatment session.

variable	*Pre*	*Post*	*p*
Blood pressure systolic (mm Hg)	143±21	138±19	0.67
Blood pressure diastolic (mm Hg)	81±8	83±7	0.52
Hematocrit (vol%)	36.1±3.12	36.7±3.75	0.46

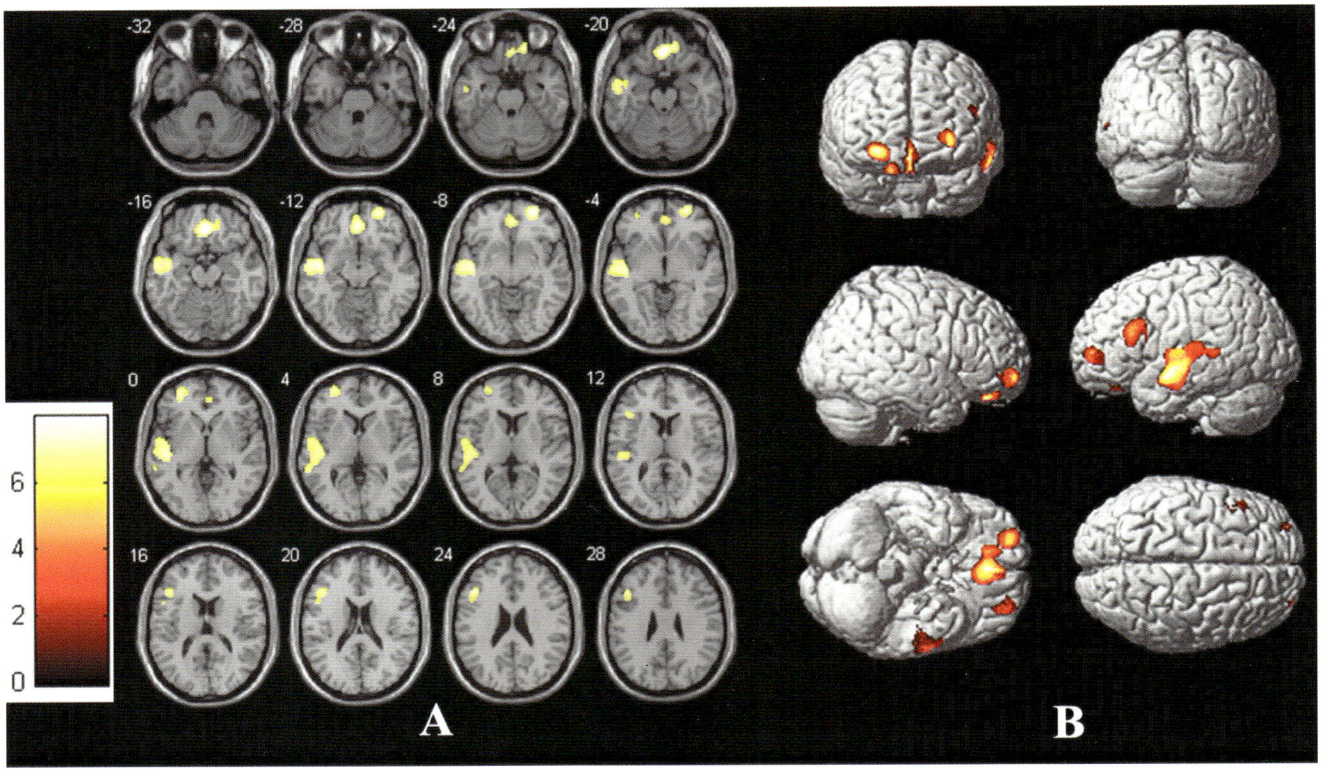

Figure 1. Statistical Parametric Images of Voxel-Based Morphometry Analysis for ESRD Patients and controls (Panels A: slices view, Panels B: whole brain rendering). Relative to controls, ERSD patients had significantly reduced gray matter volume in the bilateral medial orbitofrontal cortex, bilateral dorsal lateral prefrontal cortex and right middle temporal gyrus.

demonstrated significantly lower values of hemispheric and cerebral cortex oxygen metabolism in both hemodialysis and CKD patients compared with controls, and the frontal cortices tended to show the lowest values in patients with renal failure [11].

However, our VBM findings were somewhat different from previous VBM studies. Through comparing minimal nephro-encephalopathy (MNE) and Non-MNE, with controls, Zhang et al. reported diffusely decreased gray matter volumes in ESRD patients. In addition, they found that serum urea was negatively associated with changes in gray matter volume in many regions (bilateral occipital lobes, bilateral lingual lobes, bilateral calcarine, bilateral superior temporal gyri, bilateral temporal poles, bilateral uncus, posterior cingulate cortex/precuneus/cuneus, right fusiform, right parahippocampus, right amygdala, left hippocampus/parahippocampus) [24]. Thus, the differences in the laboratory tests (especially for the serum urea) might be one of the potential reasons. Another possible mechanism might be the hemodialysis differences in the ESRD patients between the two studies. In contrast to our present study, in which all the ESRD patients were undergoing hemodialysis, only 33 of 57 ESRD patients were on hemodialysis in their study [24]. Studies based on transcranial Doppler have indicated a decrease in the mean flow velocity (mfv) at the level of the middle cerebral artery (MCA) during hemodialysis, MCAmfv has been proposed as a reliable proxy for cerebral blood flow [33–35]. In addiction, lower cerebral blood flow has always been associated with lower brain gray matter volume and lower cortical thickness [36–38]. In a study by Prohovnik et al., 10 ESRD patients on hemodialysis and 6 controls were compared, and they found decreased gray volume only in bilateral caudate nuclei but not in other regions [25]. The most likely cause for the difference from our study may be the sample size.

The dorsal lateral prefrontal cortex serves as the highest cortical area responsible for motor planning, organization, and regulation [39]. OFC is involved in cognitive processing of decision-making [40]. Damage to either of these regions can result in the dysexecutive syndrome [41], which leads to problems with emotion, social judgment, executive memory, abstract thinking and intentionality. The decreased gray matter volume in these regions observed in the present study may imply executive function deficits in ESRD patients, which is supported by previous neuropsychological studies indicating that executive function deficits were the prominent feature of cognitive impairment among ESRD patients [42].

How the gray matter structural abnormalities in ESRD patients relate to cerebral functional integrity deficits is an interesting question. In the present study, regions with abnormal gray matter volume were used as seeds for functional connectivity analysis. We found a disconnect between the prefrontal cortex and the bilateral cerebellum (consist fronto-cerebellar circuits), and within the prefrontal cortex. We also found enhanced functional connectivity between the prefrontal cortex and left middle temporal gyrus as well as within the prefrontal cortex in ESRD patients when compared to the healthy controls (Figure 2, Table 3). Moreover, supplementary analysis showed that most of the results remained significant when local gray matter volumes (except the left dorsal lateral prefrontal cortex) were statistically controlled for. This suggests that local gray matter volumes partially influenced the functional results, but that the abnormalities we found regarding

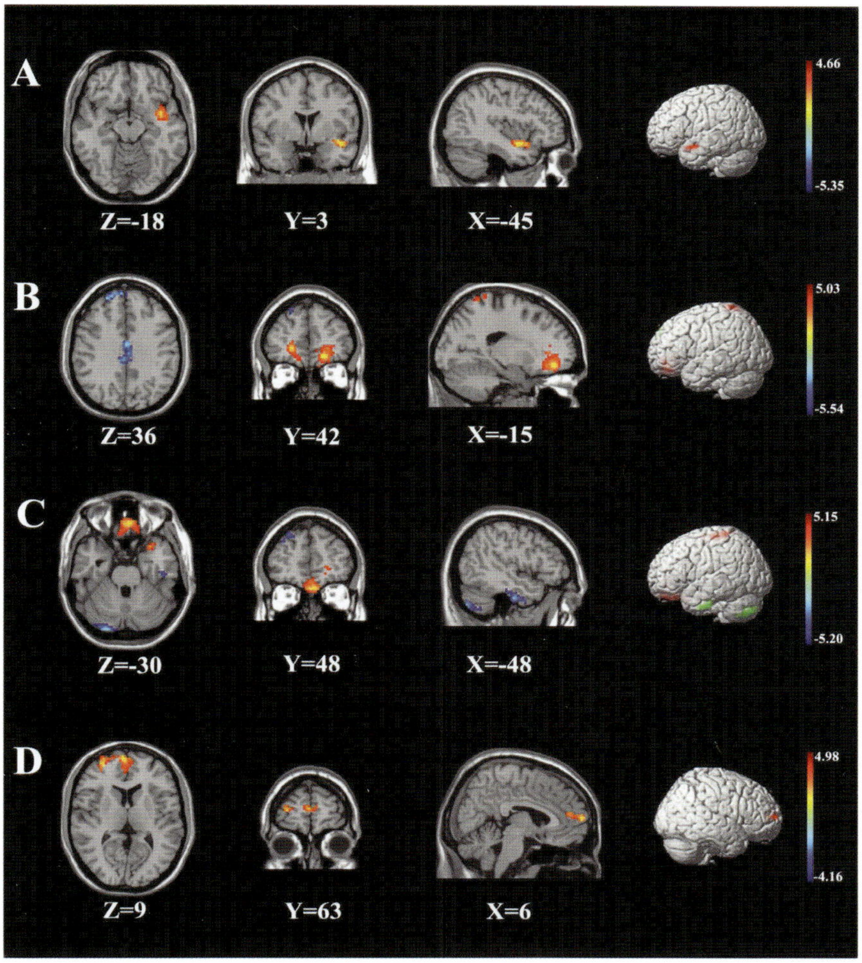

Figure 2. Statistical Parametric Images of Between-Group Functional Connectivity Analysis for ESRD Patients and Controls. Panels A demonstrated enhanced functional connectivity in superior temporal gyrus (Red) in ESRD patients when the seed areas were located in the left dorsal lateral prefrontal cortex ([Brodmann's area 10], panels B demonstrated reduced functional connectivity in bilateral cerebellum posterior lobe, left inferior temporal gyrus, right dlPFC (Blue), and enhanced functional connectivity in bilateral OFC, left posterior gyrus (Red) in ESRD patients when the seed areas were located in the right dorsal lateral prefrontal cortex ([Brodmann's area 11], panels C demonstrated reduced functional connectivity in bilateral cerebellum posterior lobe, right dlPFC, bilateral ACC (Blue), enhanced FC in bilateral OFC, bilateral superior parietal lobe (Red) when the seed areas were located in the medial orbito-frontal cortex ([Brodmann's area 10, 11, 32], and panels D demonstrated enhanced functional connectivity in right medial PFC (Red) in ESRD patients when the seed areas were located in the left middle temporal gyrus [Brodmann's area 10, 11, 32].

resting state functional connectivity in the ESRD group cannot entirely be explained by their lower gray matter volume.

Fronta-frontal circuits including the dorsolateral circuit, orbito-frontal circuit and anterior cingulate cortex circuit are thought to be involved in attention, cognition, action and emotion [43]. The separation performances of functional connectivity (enhance and reduce) within fronta-frontal circuits may represent different neural mechanisms, while reduced functional connectivity within the fronta-frontal circuits implies that the ESRD-related functional impairment, and enhanced functional connectivity may indicate compensatory mechanisms. Ideally, task-fMRI studies combined quantitative MRI imaging with neuropsychological testing should be planned to prove this hypothesis.

Fronto-cerebellar circuits include three distinct circuits that associate with the prefrontal cortex. These fronto-cerebellar circuits are thought to be involved in higher-order cognitive functioning. Studies have consistently demonstrated that the fronto-cerebellar circuits are associated with cognitive function [44,45]. Disconnection of the fronto-cerebellar connectivity observed in the present study may contribute to cognitive deficits in ESRD patients. This hypothesis can be partly supported by previous studies on alcoholism, which indicated that the disconnection between the fronto-cerebeller circuits related to the cognitive deficits in alcoholics and alcohol-naïve youth with a family history of alcoholism [44,45]. Further support to this hypothesis is also provided by a recent study performed in children with attention-deficit/hyperactivity disorder (ADHD), which found that the frontal and cerebellar circuits neural activity was enhanced in ADHD patients after cognitive training [46]. If this hypothesis holds, cognitive training can be used to enhance fronto-cerebellar connectivity of ESRD patients, which may improve the cognitive function in ESRD patients.

We also observed an enhanced FC between the left middle temporal gyrus and the medial PFC (Brodmann's area 10), while the fronto-temporal circuits function in language processing. The

Table 3. Significant differences between ESRD Patients and Controls in resting state functional connectivity for the four seed areas (showed different in group comparison) and the rest of the brain.

Seed area	*Cluster anatomical locations (Brodmann Area)*	*Cluster size (voxel)*	*Primary peak location*	*t-score*	*ESRD n = 30 Mean (zFC)*	*Controls n = 30 Mean (zFC)*
ESRD<Controls						
Bilateral medial OFC	Right cerebellum posterior lobe	388	36, −84, −33	−5.5361	−0.28	−0.04
	Left cerebellum posterior lobe	258	−36, −78, −45	−4.059	−0.28	−0.03
	right dlPFC (8,9,10)	139	24,51,36	−4.371	−0.13	0.08
	bilateral ACC(23,24,31)	234	18, −39,36	−4.6875	−0.10	0.08
Right DLPFC	Left Cerebellum Posterior Lobe	92	−48, −72, −48	−4.1573	−0.15	0.05
	Right Cerebellum Posterior Lobe	89	24, −93, −30	−5.196	−0.19	0.01
	Left Inferior Temporal Gyrus (20)	120	−48, −15, −36	−4.625	−0.14	0.07
	right dlPFC	110	42,33,42	−3.749	−0.11	0.10
ESRD>Controls						
Bilateral medial OFC	Left OFC (10, 11, 32)	276	−21,42, −15	5.0312	0.49	0.21
	Right OFC (10, 11)	153	21,45, −3	4.8567	0.56	0.25
	Left superior parietal lobe (4,5,7)	127	−12, −45,75	4.0437	0.14	−0.08
	Right superior parietal lobe (7)	108	24, −81,51	4.7056	0.11	−0.12
Left DLPFC	Left Superior Temporal Gyrus (38)	100	−45,3, −18	4.6605	0.09	−0.15
Right DLPFC	Bilateral OFC (10,11,25,38,47)	366	0,48, −30	4.5486	0.23	0.01
	Bilateral postcentral gyrus (1,2,3,4,5,6)	110	−36, −39,66	4.8554	0.13	−0.07
Left middle temporal gyurs	Right medial PFC (10,32)	129	6 63 9	4.2882	0.12	−0.09

All the coordinates are donated by Montreal Neurological Institute (MNI) space coordinates. t-score donates the statistic value of two sample t-test by contrasting ESRD patients to controls at $p<0.05$ AlphaSim corrected.

enhanced FC in this circuit may be compensatory for the GM volume reduction in the left temporal gyrus.

We did not find any correlation between the brain deficits (structural and functional) and clinical parameters in ESRD patients. Several factors might explain these findings. First, depression is the most common psychological disorder in ESRD patients with a prevalence as high as 20–25% by some contemporary estimates [47]. The reduced gray matter volume in the bilateral OFC, the left middle temporal gyrus and the bilateral dlPFC observed in present study is also found in patients with depression [48]. Thus, the brain deficits observed in the present study may result from the complication (depression) and not from the ESRD itself. A more rigorous experiment to exclude the effects of depression is needed in the future. Second, a relatively small sample size may lead to insufficient power. Although we did not find any significant correlation between the brain deficits and clinical parameters in ESRD patients, we found negative trends between the serum urea levels and the bilateral OFC, the left middle temporal gyrus and the right dlPFC gray matter volume. A larger sample size is needed in future studies.

Limitations

We acknowledge that our study has some limitations. The main limitation of the study is that all of the ESRD patients received regular hemodialysis at the time of the fMRI study. Whether and how hemodialysis itself can affect the brain is unknown; however, it can affect the patient's cognitive function [49,50]. Although we did not find any significant correlation between the abnormal gray matter volume, FC and times of hemodialysis, a more detailed experiment with chronic kidney disease (stage 4–5) without hemodialysis is required in the future study. Second, although we temporally bandpass filtered all fMRI data (0.01–0.08 Hz), and removed components with high correlation to cerebrospinal fluid or white matter or with low correlation to gray matter, we cannot completely rule out the influence of physiological noise on our findings due to its variation over time and across subjects. Simultaneous recording of heart rate and respiratory rate and depth during fMRI scanning might help further reduce physiological noise artifacts. Another limitation is that the current study did not include cognitive testing to allow the examination of any correlation with the structural brain abnormalities and functional connectivity. Such an investigation might potentially improve our understanding of the pathophysiological mechanisms of ESRD. In addition, this study is preliminary and our results are limited to a small sample size, which may affect the statistical analysis. Further studies with large-cohort are needed.

Conclusions

In conclusion, the present study applied morphometry analysis and resting-state functional connectivity to examine the structural and functional integrity changes in ESRD patients. Our findings document that patients with ESRD undergoing routine hemodialysis display clear-cut structural alterations in selected gray matter areas, Moreover, regions with gray matter volume reduction have significantly altered resting state functional connectivity with other brain regions. Our results provide support for future efforts to combine anatomical and functional data to explore the cognitive deficits of ESRD patients.

Acknowledgments

The authors express their appreciation to Zheng Guo at the University of Kentucky for her help on preparing this manuscript. Also, the authors are highly grateful to the anonymous reviewers for their significant and constructive comments and suggestions, which greatly improve the article.

Author Contributions

Conceived and designed the experiments: YQ HS XL. Performed the experiments: YQ GJ CL. Analyzed the data: YQ HS. Contributed reagents/materials/analysis tools: YQ JT. Wrote the paper: YQ.

References

1. Etgen T, Chonchol M, Förstl H, Sander D (2012) Chronic kidney disease and cognitive impairment: a systematic review and meta-analysis. Am J Nephrol 35(5):474–82.
2. Kurella M, Chertow GM, Luan J, Yaffe K (2004) Cognitive impairment in chronic kidney disease. J Am Geriatr Soc 52(11):1863–9.
3. Sehgal AR, Grey SF, DeOreo PB, Whitehouse PJ (1997) Prevalence, recognition and implications of mental impairment among hemodialysis patients. Am J Kidney Dis 30:41–49.
4. Bremer BA, Wert KM, Durica AL (1997) Neuropsychological, physical, and psychosocial functioning of individuals with end-stage renal disease. Ann Behav Med 19:348–352.
5. Fazekas G, Fazekas F, Schmidt R, Kapeller P, Offenbacher H, et al. (1995) Brain MRI findings and cognitive impairment in patients undergoing chronic hemodialysis treatment. J Neurol Sci 134:83–88.
6. Ikram MA, Vernooij MW, Hofman A, Niessen WJ, van der Lugt A, et al. (2008) Kidney function is related to cerebral small vessel disease. Stroke 39(1):55–61.
7. Kamata T, Hishida A, Takita T, Sawada K, Ikegaya N, et al. (2000) Morphologic abnormalities in the brain of chronically hemodialyzed patients without cerebrovascular disease. Am J Nephrol 20(1):27–31.
8. Savazzi GM, Cusmano F, Musini S (2001) Cerebral imaging changes in patients with chronic renal failure treated conservatively or in hemodialysis. Nephron 89(1):31–6.
9. Chiu ML, Li CW, Chang JM, Chiang IC, Ko CH, et al. (2010) Cerebral metabolic changes in neurologically presymptomatic patients undergoing haemodialysis: in vivo proton MR spectroscopic findings. Eur Radiol 20(6):1502–7.
10. Tryc AB, Alwan G, Bokemeyer M, Goldbecker A, Hecker H, et al. (2011) Cerebral metabolic alterations and cognitive dysfunction in chronic kidney disease. Nephrol Dial Transplant 26(8):2635–41.
11. Kanai H, Hirakata H, Nakane H, Fujii K, Hirakata E, et al. (2001) Depressed cerebral oxygen metabolism in patients with chronic renal failure: a positron emission tomography study. Am J Kidney Dis 38(4 Suppl 1):S129–33.
12. Song SH, Kim IJ, Kim SJ, Kwak IS, Kim YK (2008) Cerebral glucose metabolism abnormalities in patients with major depressive symptoms in pre-dialytic chronic kidney disease: statistical parametric mapping analysis of F-18-FDG PET, a preliminary study. Psychiatry Clin Neurosci 62(5):554–61.
13. Whitwell JL (2009) Voxel-based morphometry: an automated technique for assessing structural changes in the brain. J Neurosci 29(31):9661–4.
14. Maudsley AA, Domenig C, Ramsay RE, Bowen BC (2010) Application of volumetric MR spectroscopic imaging for localization of neocortical epilepsy. Epilepsy Res 88(2–3):127–38.
15. Kuperman S, Gaffney GR, Hamdan-Allen G, Preston DF, Venkatesh L (1990) Neuroimaging in child and adolescent psychiatry. J Am Acad Child Adolesc Psychiatry 29(2):159–72.
16. Rauch A, Rainer G, Logothetis NK (2008) The effect of a serotonin-induced dissociation between spiking and perisynaptic activity on BOLD functional MRI. Proc Natl Acad Sci U S A 105(18):6759–64.
17. Liang X, Wen J, Ni L, Zhong J, Qi R, et al. (2013) Altered Pattern of Spontaneous Brain Activity in the Patients with End-Stage Renal Disease: A Resting State Functional MRI Study with Regional Homogeneity Analysis. PLoS ONE 8(8): e71507.
18. Good CD, Johnsrude IS, Ashburner J, Henson RN, Friston KJ, et al. (2001) A voxel-based morphometric study of ageing in 465 normal adult human brains. Neuroimage 14:21–36.
19. Pomarol-Clotet E, Canales-Rodríguez EJ, Salvador R, Sarró S, Gomar JJ, et al. (2010) Medial prefrontal cortex pathology in schizophrenia as revealed by convergent findings from multimodal imaging. Mol Psychiatry 15(8):823–30.
20. Chételat G, Desgranges B, Landeau B, Mézenge F, Poline JB, et al. (2008) Direct voxel-based comparison between grey matter hypometabolism and atrophy in Alzheimer's disease. Brain 131(Pt 1):60–71.
21. Gili T, Cercignani M, Serra L, Perri R, Giove F, et al. (2011) Regional brain atrophy and functional disconnection across Alzheimer's disease evolution. J Neurol Neurosurg Psychiatry 82(1):58–66.
22. Qiu YW, Jiang GH, Su HH, Lv XF, Tian JZ, et al. (2013) The impulsivity behavior is correlated with prefrontal cortex gray matter volume reduction in heroin-dependent individuals. Neurosci Lett 538: 43–48.
23. Zhang LJ, Qi R, Zhong J, Xu Q, Zheng G, et al. (2012) The Effect of Hepatic Encephalopathy, Hepatic Failure, and Portosystemic Shunt on Brain Volume of Cirrhotic Patients: A Voxel-Based Morphometry Study. PLoS ONE 7(8): e42824.
24. Zhang LJ, Wen J, Ni L, Zhong J, Liang X, et al. (2013) Predominant gray matter volume loss in patients with end-stage renal disease: a voxel-based morphometry study. Metab Brain Dis 28(4):647–54.
25. Prohovnik I, Post J, Uribarri J, Lee H, Sandu O, et al. (2007) Cerebrovascular effects of hemodialysis in chronic kidney disease. J Cereb Blood Flow Metab 27(11):1861–1869.
26. Qiu YW, Lv XF, Jiang GH, Su HH, Yu T, et al. (2014) Reduced ventral medial prefrontal cortex (vmPFC) volume and impaired vmPFC-default mode network integration in codeine-containing cough syrups users. Drug Alcohol Depend 134:314–21.
27. Lui S, Deng W, Huang X, Jiang L, Ma X, et al. (2009) Association of cerebral deficits with clinical symptoms in antipsychotic-naive first-episode schizophrenia: an optimized voxel-based morphometry and resting state functional connectivity study. Am J Psychiatry 166: 196–205.
28. Horwitz B, Rumsey JM, Donohue BC (1998) Functional connectivity of the angular gyrus in normal reading and dyslexia. Proc Natl Acad Sci U S A 95:8939–8944.
29. Fox MD, Snyder AZ, Vincent JL, Corbetta M, Van Essen DC, et al. (2005) The human brain is intrinsically organized into dynamic, anticorrelated functional networks. Proc Natl Acad Sci U S A 102:9673–9678.
30. Jenkins GM, Watts DG (1968) Spectral Analysis and Its Applications. San Francisco
31. Yan CG, Zang YF (2010) DPARSF: A MATLAB Toolbox for "Pipeline" Data Analysis of Resting-State fMRI. Front Syst Neurosci 4:13.
32. Miglior M, Mannari C (2009) Role of brain derived neurotrophic factor (BDNF) in the development of neuropsychiatric disorders in chronic renal failure. Metabolic and other complications of ESRD – 1. abstract.
33. Regolisti G, Maggiore U, Cademartiri C, Cabassi A, Caiazza A, et al. (2013) Cerebral blood flow decreases during intermittent hemodialysis in patients with acute kidney injury, but not in patients with end-stage renal disease. Nephrol Dial Transplant 28(1):79–85.
34. Skinner H, Mackaness C, Bedforth N, Mahajan R (2005) Cerebral haemodynamics in patients with chronic renal failure: effects of haemodialysis. Br J Anaesth 94(2):203–5.
35. Stefanidis I, Bach R, Mertens PR, Liakopoulos V, Liapi G, et al. (2005) Influence of hemodialysis on the mean blood flow velocity in the middle cerebral artery. Clin Nephrol 64(2):129–37.
36. Denier N, Schmidt A, Gerber H, Schmid O, Riecher-Rössler A, et al. (2013) Association of frontal gray matter volume and cerebral perfusion in heroin addiction: a multimodal neuroimaging study. Front Psychiatry 4:135.
37. Alosco ML, Gunstad J, Jerskey BA, Xu X, Clark US, et al. (2013) The adverse effects of reduced cerebral perfusion on cognition and brain structure in older adults with cardiovascular disease. Brain Behav 3(6):626–36.
38. Drew DA, Bhadelia R, Tighiouart H, Novak V, Scott TM, et al. (2013) Anatomic brain disease in hemodialysis patients: a cross-sectional study. Am J Kidney Dis 61(2):271–8.
39. Zelazo PD, Müller U (2010) Executive Function in Typical and Atypical Development, in The Wiley-Blackwell Handbook of Childhood Cognitive Development, Second edition (ed U. Goswami), Wiley-Blackwell, Oxford, UK. doi: 10.1002/9781444325485.ch22.
40. Kringelbach ML (2005) The orbitofrontal cortex: linking reward to hedonic experience. Nature Reviews Neuroscience 6: 691–702.
41. John JP (2009) Fronto-temporal dysfunction in schizophrenia: A selective review. Indian J Psychiatry 51:180–90.
42. Kurella Tamura M, Yaffe K (2011) Dementia and cognitive impairment in ESRD: diagnostic and therapeutic strategies. Kidney Int 79(1):14–22.
43. Burruss JW, Hurley RA, Taber KH, Rauch RA, Norton RE, et al. (2000) Functional neuroanatomy of the frontal lobe circuits. Radiology 214(1):227–30.
44. Herting MM, Fair D, Nagel BJ (2011) Altered fronto-cerebellar connectivity in alcohol-naïve youth with a family history of alcoholism. Neuroimage 54(4):2582–9.
45. Rogers BP, Parks MH, Nickel MK, Katwal SB, Martin PR (2012) Reduced fronto-cerebellar functional connectivity in chronic alcoholic patients. Alcohol Clin Exp Res 36(2):294–301.
46. Hoekzema E, Carmona S, Tremols V, Gispert JD, Guitart M, et al. (2010) Enhanced neural activity in frontal and cerebellar circuits after cognitive training in children with attention-deficit/hyperactivity disorder. Hum Brain Mapp 31(12):1942–50.
47. Kimmel PL, Cukor D, Cohen SD, Peterson RA (2007) Depression in end-stage renal disease patients: a critical review. Adv Chronic Kidney Dis 14(4):328–34.
48. Grieve SM, Korgaonkar MS, Koslow SH, Gordon E, Williams LM (2013) Widespread reductions in gray matter volume in depression. Neuroimage Clin 3:332–9.
49. Nasser Mel T, Shawki S, El Shahawy Y, Sany D (2012) Assessment of cognitive dysfunction in kidney disease. Saudi J Kidney Dis Transpl 23(6):1208–14.
50. Kurella Tamura M, Unruh ML, Nissenson AR, Larive B, Eggers PW, et al. (2012) Effect of More Frequent Hemodialysis on Cognitive Function in the Frequent Hemodialysis Network Trials. Am J Kidney Dis 61(2):228–37.

12

Does Erythropoietin Cause Hemoglobin Variability- Is It 'Normal'?

Ashwani K Gupta*, Waseem David

Department of Nephrology, University of Florida-Jacksonville, Jacksonville, Florida, United States of America

Abstract

Hemoglobin variability (Hb-var) in patients with chronic kidney disease has been stipulated to be a result of exogenous treatment with erythropoiesis stimulating agents (ESA) and has been related to mortality in dialysis patients. We hypothesized the existence of Hb-var independent of ESA administration and compared it to that in healthy adults using data from the Scripps-Kaiser and NHANES III databases. We studied the Hb-var in 1571 peritoneal dialysis patients which included 116 patients not requiring treatment with erythropoietin. We systematically studied the differences between the groups that needed ESA therapy and those who did not. White race and male sex were significant predictors of need for erythropoietin therapy. We found peritoneal dialysis patients to exhibit significantly increased Hb-var independent of treatment with exogenous erythropoietin (0.99 gm/dL vs. 1.17 gm/dL, p-value$<$0.001). We found age to be a significant determinant of Hb-var in the ESA treated group. Hb-var in younger patients ($<$30 years) was increased by 50% compared to young healthy adults. The Hb-var in elderly ($>$60 years) peritoneal dialysis patients was similar to that seen in healthy elders, suggesting similarity with anemia of aging. We conclude that exogenous ESA administration does not explain Hb-var entirely but may enhance it. Intrinsic factors affecting erythropoiesis including age may be the major determinants of Hb-var.

Editor: Zoran Ivanovic, French Blood Institute, France

Funding: The authors have no support or funding to report.

Competing Interests: The authors have declared that no competing interests exist.

* E-mail: akgupta@ufl.edu

Introduction

The basal rate of Red Blood Cell (RBC) production is diminished in patients with chronic kidney disease (CKD). Usually, the anemia is proportional to the severity of renal dysfunction, caused due to a deficiency of erythropoietin (EPO) [1]. Supplementation with exogenous Erythropoiesis Stimulating Agents (ESA) partially corrects the EPO deficiency and is used for its treatment [2]. Treatment of anemia in this population has several benefits including improvement in exercise tolerance, functional and sexual capacity [3], along with reduction in left ventricular hypertrophy [4], and improved cardiovascular functioning. A large variability has been observed in the hemoglobin level of dialysis patients treated with ESAs [5]. The physiologic basis underlying hemoglobin variability (Hb-var) is poorly understood. It is thought that patient demographics, comorbidities, concurrent events (infections and hospitalizations) as well practice patterns of ESA and iron administration are related to Hb-var. Several investigations [6–11] have focused exclusively on the effects of ESA on Hb-var in hemodialysis patients. This phenomenon has been called Hb cycling [5,12] by clinical epidemiologists and has been related to mortality [13–16] and cardiovascular outcomes.

Data on Hb-var in peritoneal dialysis (PD) patients are limited to small reports from the Netherlands [17], the United Kingdom [18] and China [19]. Walker et al. [20] have reported the largest group of 558 PD patients receiving Erythropoietin and 528 PD patients receiving Darbepoetin from the Australian continent. They observed an Hb standard deviation of 1.5 gm/dL in the Darbepoetin group, as compared to 1.1 gm/dL in the erythropoietin treated group. No data have been reported from the United States or Canada. A large cohort of European dialysis patients [21] included data on 967 patients not receiving ESA, but the authors did not analyze this data separately. We hypothesize the existence of Hb-var in PD patients not receiving any ESA and that the Hb-var in PD patients would be comparable to or greater than healthy adults. This has not been reported in the literature previously. In this study, we examined Hb-var data on 1571 PD patients who received dialysis at various Dialysis Clinics Inc. (a large non-profit dialysis provider) facilities throughout the United States between January 2007 and December 2009. The study attempts to define "normal" Hb-var in CKD by comparing our results with population normal in healthy adults obtained from the Scripps-Kaiser and NHANESIII databases [22]. In order to determine the relationship of Hb variability to ESA administration, we compared the subset of PD patients not receiving any ESA to the group receiving ESAs. The study of the subset of CKD patients not receiving ESA is a natural first step in understanding the red blood cell dynamics in renal failure. We will attempt to describe how this subset of patients differs in characteristics from those who require ESA therapy. We will further attempt to investigate the factors that determine Hb variability in both subsets of patients.

Methods

Study Design

This was a retrospective observational study. The study protocol was approved by the University of Florida Institutional Review Board and adhered to the declaration of Helsinki. A limited data set consisting of de-identified data was provided by Dialysis Clinics Inc. through a data use agreement. It was not possible to identify individual patients directly or through identifiers linked to the patients. Therefore, it was exempted from requiring informed consent by the IRB. Prevalent peritoneal dialysis patients receiving services for 6 months or longer at any of the centers operated by Dialysis Clinic Inc., a large nonprofit dialysis provider in the United States between January 2007 and December 2009 were included in this study. Children less than 18 years of age were excluded from the study population. Demographic data including - age, sex, race, dialysis vintage were included in the data provided. Date of clinic visit, Hb measured per clinic protocol (monthly); ESA dose administered, types of ESA used were also recorded. Laboratory values obtained during routine clinical care including serum iron, ferritin, TIBC, percent saturation (usually every 3 months), serum Albumin, PTH, and Kt/V measured per clinic protocol were recorded.

Data Analysis

All data analysis was carried out using STATA v.9.0. Patients were stratified into those requiring any ESA therapy (n = 1455) and those not requiring ESA therapy (n = 116). Patients who were administered even a single dose of an ESA during the study period were stratified in the ESA group. ESA naïve patients did not receive any doses of an ESA during the entire follow-up period. Hb-var was calculated using a 1 month standard deviation (SD-Hb) and the coefficient of hemoglobin variation. The coefficient of hemoglobin variation is defined as the ratio of the SD-Hb to the mean Hb. Results are reported as mean ± standard deviation. Comparisons between groups were based on a two sided student's t-test of means. The patients were divided into deciles of age to compare Hb-var with the population means reported in the Scripps-Kaiser and NHANESIII databases [22]. A regression model was fit to SD-Hb in the ESA treated group to study the effect of various parameters on SD-Hb.

Results

Data was available for a total of 1571 patients followed over a mean 19 months (range 7–156 weeks). The data revealed that 7.4% (n = 116) of our sample did not require any ESA therapy over the entire follow-up period. The two groups did not differ with regards to mean patient age, dialysis vintage and follow up period in the study. The proportion of diabetics in either group was also similar. Table 1 shows the differences between the no-ESA vs. ESA group. As expected, the mean Hb in the no-ESA group was 13.0 explaining the lack of need for ESA therapy. The ESA group was treated to a mean Hb of 11.7. The standard deviation of hemoglobin in the ESA group was 1.17 gm/dL compared to 0.99 gm/dL in the no-ESA group (p-value$<$0.001).

The group not requiring ESA had a greater proportion of males (69%). The proportion of sexes was equally distributed in the ESA group (53% males vs. 47% females). Since females may have menstrual blood losses which can partly account for variability in their hemoglobin, males were analyzed separately as well. By limiting the analysis to males only, the results did not change. The male no-ESA group still had a standard deviation of 1.0 gm/dL compared to 1.15 gm/dL in males who received ESA.

Patients in the no-ESA group had significantly more residual renal function, perhaps explaining the lack of EPO requirement in this group. The no-ESA group had slightly higher serum albumin and lower ferritins and PTH. Other iron indices (TIBC, Transferrin and total iron) were lower in the ESA treated group. A racial difference was noted in EPO requirement. A greater proportion of whites than blacks (9.1% vs. 4.2%) did not need ESA therapy to maintain similar levels of Hb. Separate subgroup analysis of the no-ESA group by race did not find any significant differences in Hb levels, iron indices, ratio of sexes, dialysis vintage or Kt/V. The black patients had significantly higher PTH overall-an effect that was consistent across the ESA and no-ESA groups.

Figure 1a and 1b compare the SD-Hb seen in Peritoneal Dialysis not requiring any ESA therapy patients with population normals obtained from the Scripps-Kaiser database (Fig. 1a), and NHANESIII(Fig. 1b). Figure 2a and 2b compare the SD-Hb seen in ESA treated Peritoneal Dialysis patients with population normals obtained from the Scripps-Kaiser database (Fig. 2a), and NHANESIII (Fig. 2b). Hb-var in the ESA naïve group was similar in magnitude and trend as observed in the NHANESIII and Scripps-Kaiser populations (Fig. 3). In contrast the ESA treated group was distinctively different and the Hb-var was highest in younger patients. In older patients the Hb-var approached the population means and tended to decline in the patients with age more than 60 years. This was observed in both males and females as well as in Caucasians and African American patients.

Table 2 shows the results of a regression model with the p-values of significant predictors of SD-Hb in the ESA treated group. Age was again found to be a significant predictor of SD-Hb. SD-Hb declined by 0.05 gm/dL with each decile of age. Iron saturation and dialysis clearance (KT/V) were also found to be significant predictors of SD-Hb. Patient sex, race, vintage on dialysis, serum albumin, serum iron, transferrin and ferritin were not found to be significant predictors of SD-Hb. Using a stepwise regression model, in the ESA naïve group none of the factors studied were predictive of Hb-var.

Discussion

Hemoglobin Variability - Normal or Abnormal

In the absence of a disease condition RBC production is controlled by a negative feedback system. The rate of change of RBC concentration is the difference between their rates of production and destruction. Within the bone marrow there exists a population of committed lineage specific pluripotent stem cells, also called colony forming units (CFU). CFUs are capable of differentiating into mature RBC under the influence of hormone erythropoietin produced by the kidneys. Low density of circulating RBC signals EPO production, whereas an increase in the numbers of circulating RBCs provides negative feedback to EPO. The pluripotent cells in the bone marrow exist in either a resting state (G_0) or a proliferative state. In dialysis patients the effects of peripheral factors such as varying iron stores and circulating inflammatory mediators such as hepcidin [23] affecting bone marrow responsiveness to EPO have been studied extensively. It is not known, if these factors can also influence cell replication times within the marrow or change the rates of entry and exit of cells between the resting and proliferative states. Theoretically, hemoglobin variability in patients with CKD may originate from an altered rate of apoptosis of precursor cells within the proliferating compartment of the marrow(due to EPO deficiency), or it may occur due to an increased delay in cell maturation times within the marrow. Exogenous ESA administration may enhance

Table 1. Differences between ESA treated and ESA Naïve PD Patients.

	No-ESA			ESA			P-value
Variable	**Obs(n)**	**Mean**	**Std. Dev.**	**Obs(n)**	**Mean**	**Std. Dev.**	
Mean-Hb(gm/dL)	116	13.0	1.7	1455	11.7	0.9	<0.0001
SD-Hb*(gm/dL)	116	0.99	0.45	1455	1.17	0.43	<0.0001
CV-Hb#	116	7.70	3.60	1455	10.00	3.80	<0.0001
Age(years)	116	59.9	13.37	1455	59.9	14.25	0.9
Sex							
Male	80	69%		773	53%		0.004
Female	36	31%		682	47%		
Vintage(years)	114	6.3	2.8	1454	6.9	3.4	0.08
Race							
White	88	75%		883	60%		0.004
Black	20	17.20%		460	31.60%		
Other	8	7.80%		111	8.40%		
Follow-up	116	17.7	10.0	1455	19.5	10.0	0.06
Diabetes	29	25.0%		1455	32.3%		0.12
Albumin(gm/dL)	116	3.6	0.4	1455	3.4	0.4	<0.0001
Serum Ferritin(ng/dL)	116	442.3	87.8	1455	594.4	13.5	0.005
Serum Iron(μg/dL)	115	82.4	25.5	1442	73.9	23.7	0.0003
TSAT(%)	98	28.5	14.2	1279	27.3	9.6	0.29
TIBC(μg/dL)	98	312.7	61.1	1287	274.7	56.1	<0.0001
Transferrin(mg/dL)	113	218.4	40.6	1441	192.1	38.3	<0.0001
K/tV	113	2.47	0.74	1425	2.25	0.57	0.0002
Renal	113	0.99	0.86	1425	0.55	0.68	<0.0001
Peritoneal	114	1.43	0.48	1447	1.68	0.52	<0.0001
PTH	116	284.9	146.9	1453	322.6	192.1	0.0395

*Standard Deviation of Hemoglobin.
#Coefficient of Hemoglobin Variability.

(as is evident by a significantly greater Hb-var in the ESA treated group) or ameliorate this hemoglobin variability, but does not account for it entirely.

The existence of hemoglobin variability in the patients on dialysis not requiring ESA therapy provides useful insights into understanding RBC dynamics in CKD patients. Previous investigations have focused on the relationship between ESAs and Hb-var [6–11]; we think the Hb-var is inherent to the normal hematopoietic processes. In a review, Arneson et al. [24] have compared four different methodologies used to characterize hemoglobin variability. Using the mean, standard deviation or the absolute hemoglobin change [25], provides us with a summary measure that is easy to understand conceptually. A residual standard deviation methodology has been proposed by Feldman et al. It measures the deviation from a regression line and therefore controls for linear trends only in the data. Gilbertson et al. [8] have also used fluctuation across thresholds to characterize hemoglobin variability. These methods attempt to describe Hb-var but can be difficult to comprehend. They do not address the reasons for the hemoglobin variability and have not found clinical applications.

Peritoneal dialysis patients lack large volume shifts and do not have ongoing blood losses into dialysis tubings and dialyzers, which characterize hemodialysis which can affect Hb-var. Access related blood loss and use of hemodialysis catheters are also known to effect Hb-var [21] in hemodialysis patients but are not relevant to peritoneal dialysis patients. To test our hypothesis that Hb-var is present in chronic kidney disease independent of these factors, we chose to study patients on peritoneal dialysis. To exclude the effects of exogenous ESA on Hb-var, we studied patients who were not treated with any ESA. We found that patients on peritoneal dialysis with significantly preserved residual renal function still exhibited fluctuations in their Hb level. Hemoglobin variability (~1 gm/dL) was present in ESA naïve patients and was significantly increased to 1.17 gm/dL by ESA therapy. This indicates that variability in Hb is inherent to disturbed RBC dynamics in CKD, independent of exogenous ESA administration.

Determinants of Hemoglobin Variability

The inverse relationship between age and Hb-var in ESA treated hemodialysis patients has been observed previously [6,21], but no teleological argument has been made to explain it. In our study of peritoneal dialysis patients, we found that the youngest patients had the maximum degree of variation in their Hb and also the maximum deviation from the population means. It can be hypothesized that the inflammatory cytokines and uremic milieu characteristic of chronic kidney disease disrupts the hemostatic processes that maintain Hb in a narrow range in healthy adults. Aging has been associated with a pro-inflammatory state and higher levels of IL-6, a key regulator of hepcidin [26,27]. These

A

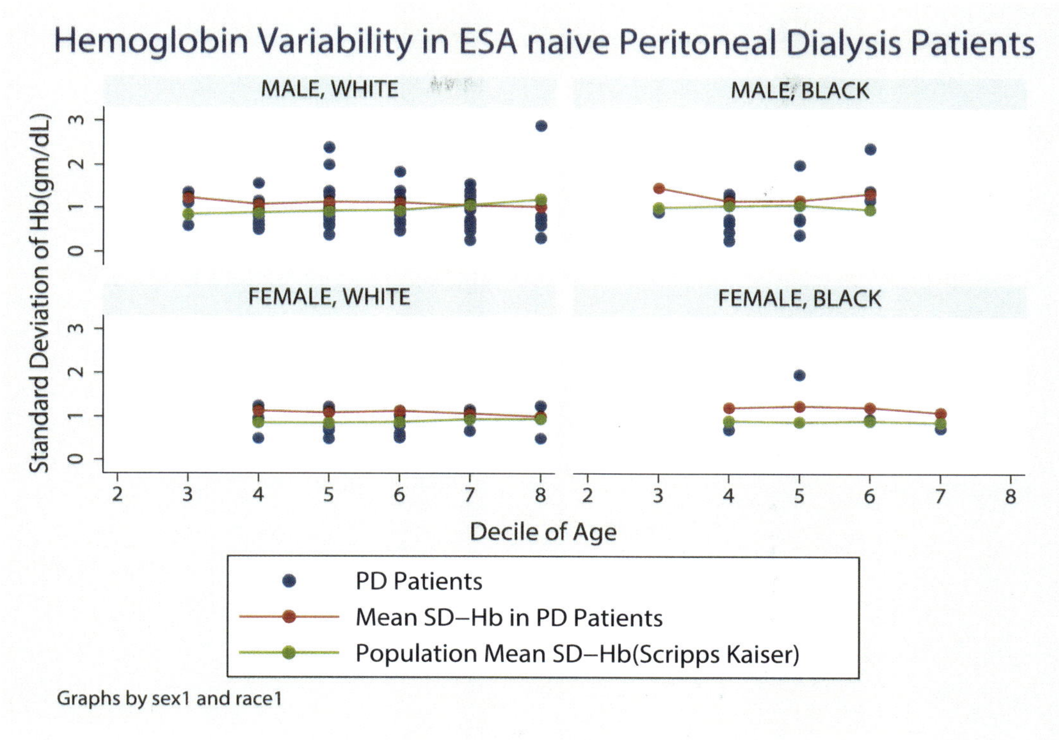

B

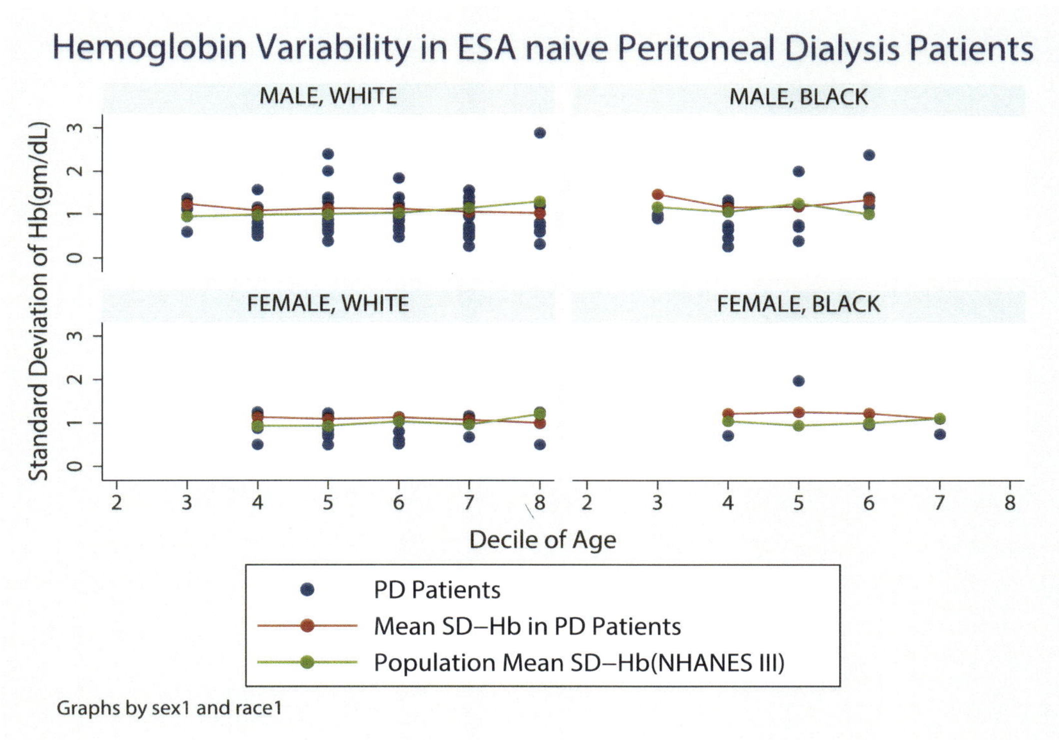

Figure 1. Hemoglobin Variability in ESA naïve Peritoneal Dialysis Patients.

A

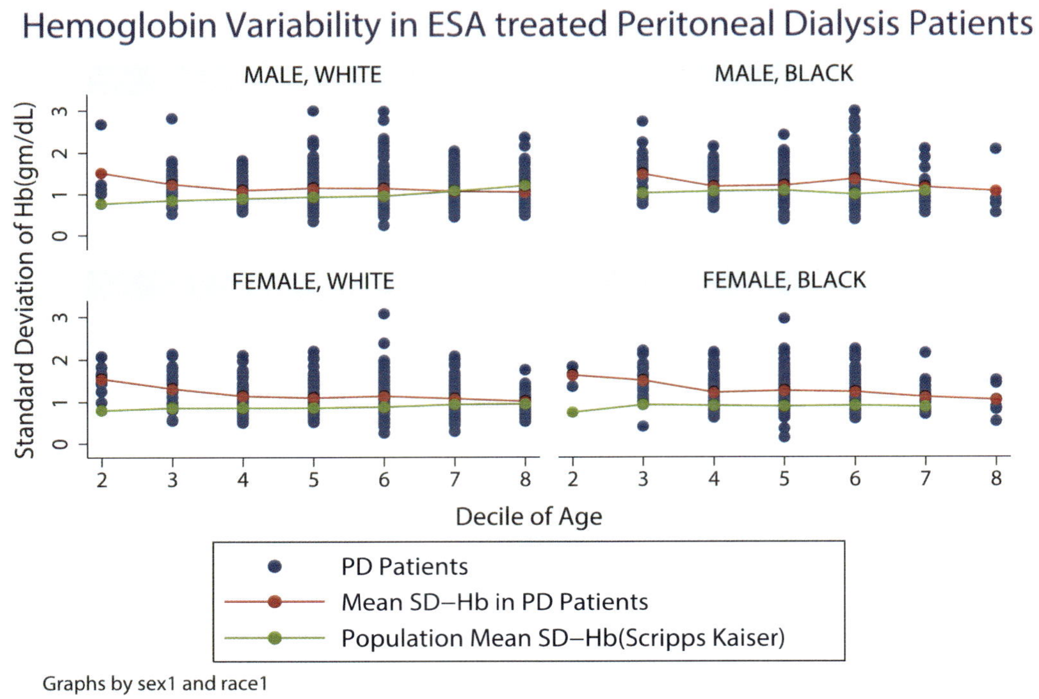

B

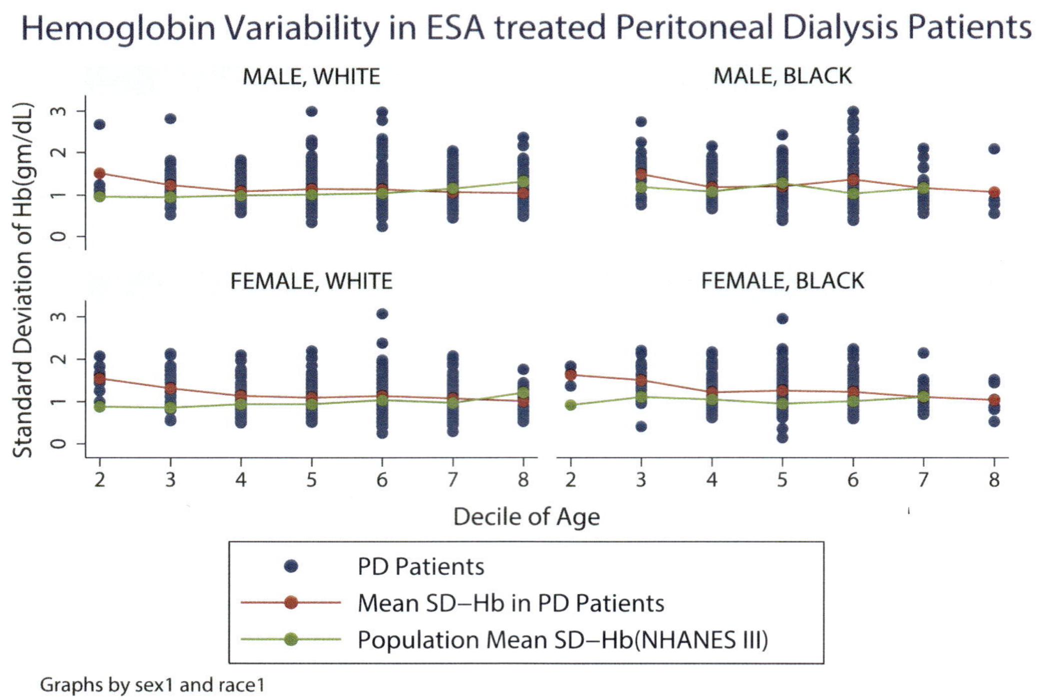

Figure 2. Hemoglobin Variability in ESA treated Peritoneal Dialysis Patients.

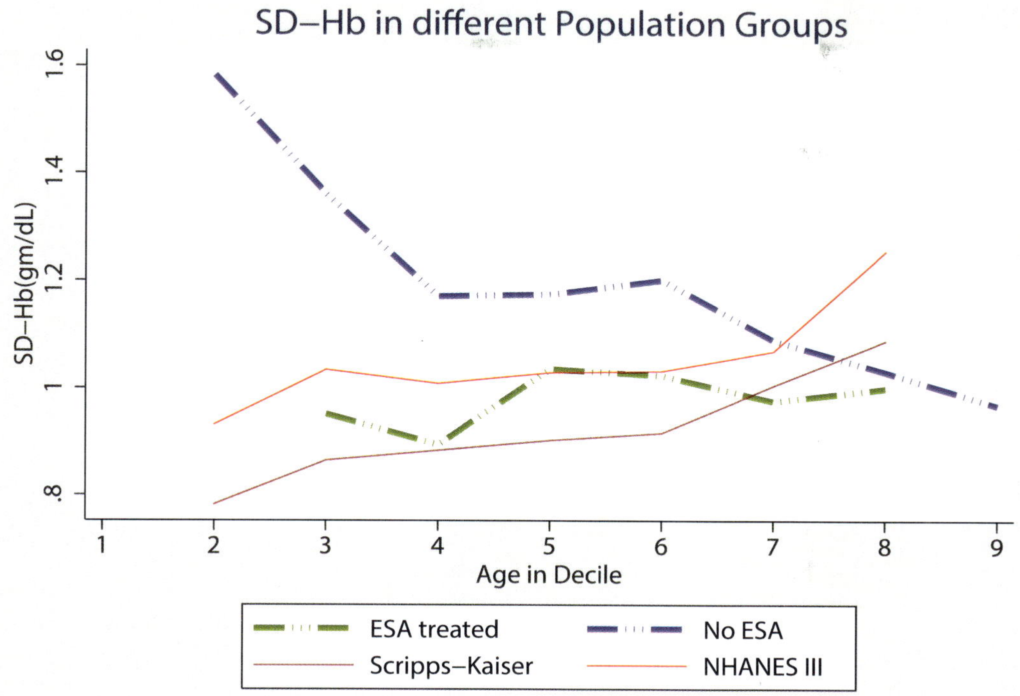

Figure 3. Hemoglobin Variability in different Population groups.

similarities with CKD may explain the closer degree of resemblance between elderly ESA treated peritoneal dialysis patients and the apparently healthy elders in the general population. Studying the factors that affect cell replication and control movement of cells between the resting and actively proliferating marrow pools may help us devise new treatments for anemia in CKD patients. Mathematical models of RBC dynamics can help us travel the path from normal physiology to disease pathophysiology and ultimately, allow us to devise more rational therapies. The factors affecting Hb-var in patients not treated with ESA have not been investigated before. In our regression models none of the clinical parameters being studied were significant predictors of Hb-var in this subgroup of patients. This may be a result of relatively small number of patients, to have enough power to detect a difference. Indeed however, this is the first time a systematic study of patients not needing ESA has been undertaken. Larger analysis will be needed to confirm this finding.

Table 2. Stepwise regression model of SD-Hb.

SD-Hb	Coef.	Std. Err.	t	P>t	[95% Conf.	Interval]
Kt/V	−0.05859	0.031955	−1.83	0.067	−0.12139	0.004215
T-Sat	0.011898	0.001898	6.27	0	0.008168	0.015629
Age	−0.0048	0.001315	−3.65	0	−0.00738	−0.00221
Followup	−0.00454	0.00177	−2.56	0.011	−0.00802	−0.00106
Regression Constant	1.322492	0.132143	10.01	0	1.062788	1.582196

Patient Sex, Race, Vintage on Diaysis, Serum Albumin, Iron, Transferrin and Ferretin were removed at a threshold level of $p = 0.1$.

Determinants of Need for ESA therapy

Higher EPO requirements have been observed in African American patients on dialysis in previous observational studies [28,29]. A race related genetic influence on hematopoiesis has been postulated earlier by Kauffman et al. [30]. Our finding that significantly more white patients did not need any ESA points to a stronger link to genetic factors effecting hematopoiesis. Similarly, greater proportion of males did not need ESA therapy. We did not have data related to hospitalizations, blood loss and infections which can also explain this apparent EPO hypo-responsiveness. The greater degree of residual renal function and total delivered dialysis dose (Kt/V) in the no-ESA group is not unexpected. The no-ESA group also had lower levels of various inflammatory markers including lower PTH, lower ferritin, and higher albumin level, once again pointing towards a role of inflammation in modulating erythropoiesis. Albumin levels have been found to be inversely correlated with inflammation in end stage renal disease patients [31–36]. Increased levels of cytokines INF-γ, TNF-α, IL-1 and IL-6 [37–39] have been implicated in producing ESA resistance and low hemoglobin levels. The low levels or absence of activation of these in patients not requiring ESA can be hypothesized but needs to be investigated. On the other hand ESA administration downregulates hepcidin [40,41] and may also suppress cytokine levels [42,43]. Lower levels hepcidin and pro-inflammatory cytokines may exert competing influence on erythropoiesis and can help explain the increased level of Hb-var in these patients. HFE gene mutations have been linked to lower ESA requirement [44], but their role in patients not needing ESA needs to be investigated. The prevalence of polymorphisms in genes for cytokine production can also provide useful insights. Compared to the study in hemodialysis patients [21] where inflammatory markers were significant predictors of Hb-var, serum albumin, PTH and ferritins were not found to be predictive of Hb-var in peritoneal dialysis patients. This is likely because peritoneal dialysis patients overall have lesser degree of inflammatory response compared to hemodialysis patients.

Conclusions

We conclude that Hb-var cannot be attributed to exogenous ESA administration alone. The physiologic bases of Hb-var are not completely understood. Deregulated homeostatic mechanisms in chronic kidney disease may enhance Hb-var. Hb-var in peritoneal dialysis patients younger than 50 years of age may be 50% greater than in healthy adults. The normal biology of aging may determine Hb-var. Effects of aging such as increased levels of inflammatory mediators and diminished capacity to secrete erythropoietin may mimic chronic kidney disease. The interaction and effects of exogenous ESA administration on these factors remains poorly understood and should be investigated. Identification of these mechanisms may help us identify unique targets for novel therapies. By choosing appropriate physiologic targets for therapy we may be able to improve patient outcomes and enhance our understanding of disease processes.

Acknowledgments

The authors would like to acknowledge James Leighton, MD and Charles W. Heilig, MD at the University of Florida-Jacksonville, for their support and help with reading the manuscript proofs and suggesting improvements. The authors would also like to thank Karen Majchrzak at Dialysis Clinics Inc. for administrative help with obtaining the database for analysis.

Author Contributions

Conceived and designed the experiments: AKG. Analyzed the data: AKG WD. Wrote the paper: AKG WD.

References

1. Eschbach JW, Adamson JW (1988) Modern aspects of the pathophysiology of renal anemia. Contrib Nephrol 66: 63–70.
2. Ahmad R, Hand M (1987) Recombinant erythropoietin for the anemia of chronic renal failure. N Engl J Med 317: 169–170.
3. Johansen KL, Finkelstein FO, Revicki DA, Gitlin M, Evans C, et al. (2011) Systematic review and meta-analysis of exercise tolerance and physical functioning in dialysis patients treated with erythropoiesis-stimulating agents. Am J Kidney Dis 55: 535–548.
4. Massimetti C, Pontillo D, Feriozzi S, Costantini S, Capezzuto A, et al. (1998) Impact of recombinant human erythropoietin treatment on left ventricular hypertrophy and cardiac function in dialysis patients. Blood Purif 16: 317–324.
5. Fishbane S, Berns JS (2005) Hemoglobin cycling in hemodialysis patients treated with recombinant human erythropoietin. Kidney Int 68: 1337–1343.
6. Berns JS, Elzein H, Lynn RI, Fishbane S, Meisels IS, et al. (2003) Hemoglobin variability in epoetin-treated hemodialysis patients. Kidney Int 64: 1514–1521.
7. Ebben JP, Gilbertson DT, Foley RN, Collins AJ (2006) Hemoglobin level variability: associations with comorbidity, intercurrent events, and hospitalizations. Clin J Am Soc Nephrol 1: 1205–1210.
8. Gilbertson DT, Ebben JP, Foley RN, Weinhandl ED, Bradbury BD, et al. (2008) Hemoglobin level variability: associations with mortality. Clin J Am Soc Nephrol 3: 133–138.
9. Gilbertson DT, Peng Y, Bradbury B, Ebben JP, Collins AJ (2009) Hemoglobin level variability: anemia management among variability groups. Am J Nephrol 30: 491–498.
10. Kainz A, Mayer B, Kramar R, Oberbauer R (2010) Association of ESA hypo-responsiveness and haemoglobin variability with mortality in haemodialysis patients. Nephrol Dial Transplant 25: 3701–3706.
11. Lau JH, Gangji AS, Rabbat CG, Brimble KS (2010) Impact of haemoglobin and erythropoietin dose changes on mortality: a secondary analysis of results from a randomized anaemia management trial. Nephrol Dial Transplant 25: 4002–4009.
12. Singh AK, Milford E, Fishbane S, Keithi-Reddy SR (2008) Managing anemia in dialysis patients: hemoglobin cycling and overshoot. Kidney Int 74: 679–683.
13. Brunelli SM, Lynch KE, Ankers ED, Joffe MM, Yang W, et al. (2008) Association of hemoglobin variability and mortality among contemporary incident hemodialysis patients. Clin J Am Soc Nephrol 3: 1733–1740.
14. Ishani A, Solid CA, Weinhandl ED, Gilbertson DT, Foley RN, et al. (2008) Association between number of months below K/DOQI haemoglobin target and risk of hospitalization and death. Nephrol Dial Transplant 23: 1682–1689.
15. Kainz A, Wilflingseder J, Fugger R, Kramar R, Oberbauer R (2012) Hemoglobin variability after renal transplantation is associated with mortality. Transpl Int 25: 323–327.
16. Weinhandl ED, Peng Y, Gilbertson DT, Bradbury BD, Collins AJ (2011) Hemoglobin variability and mortality: confounding by disease severity. Am J Kidney Dis 57: 255–265.
17. van der Putten K, van der Baan FH, Schellekens H, Gaillard CA (2009) Hemoglobin variability in patients with chronic kidney disease in the Netherlands. Int J Artif Organs 32: 787–793.
18. Selby NM, Fonseca SA, Fluck RJ, Taal MW (2012) Hemoglobin variability with epoetin beta and continuous erythropoietin receptor activator in patients on peritoneal dialysis. Perit Dial Int 32: 177–182.
19. Chen HC, Chen KH, Lin YJ, Chang CJ, Tian YC, et al. (2012) Hemoglobin variability does not predict mortality in peritoneal dialysis patients. Chang Gung Med J 35: 79–87.
20. Walker R, Pussell BA (2009) Fluctuations in haemoglobin levels in haemodialysis, pre-dialysis and peritoneal dialysis patients receiving epoetin alpha or darbepoetin alpha. Nephrology (Carlton) 14: 689–695.
21. Eckardt KU, Kim J, Kronenberg F, Aljama P, Anker SD, et al. (2010) Hemoglobin variability does not predict mortality in European hemodialysis patients. J Am Soc Nephrol 21: 1765–1775.
22. Beutler E, Waalen J (2006) The definition of anemia: what is the lower limit of normal of the blood hemoglobin concentration? Blood 107: 1747–1750.
23. Canavesi E, Alfieri C, Pelusi S, Valenti L (2012) Hepcidin and HFE protein: Iron metabolism as a target for the anemia of chronic kidney disease. World J Nephrol 1: 166–176.
24. Arneson TJ, Zaun D, Peng Y, Solid CA, Dunning S, et al. (2009) Comparison of methodologies to characterize haemoglobin variability in the US Medicare haemodialysis population. Nephrol Dial Transplant 24: 1378–1383.
25. Yang W, Israni RK, Brunelli SM, Joffe MM, Fishbane S, et al. (2007) Hemoglobin variability and mortality in ESRD. J Am Soc Nephrol 18: 3164–3170.
26. Ferrucci L, Balducci L (2008) Anemia of aging: the role of chronic inflammation and cancer. Semin Hematol 45: 242–249.
27. McCranor BJ, Langdon JM, Prince OD, Femnou LK, Berger AE, et al. (2013) Investigation of the role of interleukin-6 and hepcidin antimicrobial peptide in the development of anemia with age. Haematologica.
28. Kausz AT, Solid C, Pereira BJ, Collins AJ, St Peter W (2005) Intractable anemia among hemodialysis patients: a sign of suboptimal management or a marker of disease? Am J Kidney Dis 45: 136–147.
29. Lacson E, Jr., Rogus J, Teng M, Lazarus JM, Hakim RM (2008) The association of race with erythropoietin dose in patients on long-term hemodialysis. Am J Kidney Dis 52: 1104–1114.
30. Kaufman JS (2008) Racial differences in erythropoietin responsiveness. Am J Kidney Dis 52: 1035–1038.
31. Yeun JY, Kaysen GA (1997) Acute phase proteins and peritoneal dialysate albumin loss are the main determinants of serum albumin in peritoneal dialysis patients. Am J Kidney Dis 30: 923–927.
32. Yeun JY, Kaysen GA (1998) Factors influencing serum albumin in dialysis patients. Am J Kidney Dis 32: S118–125.
33. Kaysen GA, Dubin JA, Muller HG, Rosales LM, Levin NW (2000) The acute-phase response varies with time and predicts serum albumin levels in hemodialysis patients. The HEMO Study Group. Kidney Int 58: 346–352.
34. Kaysen GA, Chertow GM, Adhikarla R, Young B, Ronco C, et al. (2001) Inflammation and dietary protein intake exert competing effects on serum albumin and creatinine in hemodialysis patients. Kidney Int 60: 333–340.
35. Kaysen GA, Dubin JA, Muller HG, Mitch WE, Rosales LM, et al. (2002) Relationships among inflammation nutrition and physiologic mechanisms establishing albumin levels in hemodialysis patients. Kidney Int 61: 2240–2249.
36. Kaysen GA, Dubin JA, Muller HG, Rosales L, Levin NW, et al. (2004) Inflammation and reduced albumin synthesis associated with stable decline in serum albumin in hemodialysis patients. Kidney Int 65: 1408–1415.
37. Cooper AC, Mikhail A, Lethbridge MW, Kemeny DM, Macdougall IC (2003) Increased expression of erythropoiesis inhibiting cytokines (IFN-gamma, TNF-alpha, IL-10, and IL-13) by T cells in patients exhibiting a poor response to erythropoietin therapy. J Am Soc Nephrol 14: 1776–1784.
38. Faquin WC, Schneider TJ, Goldberg MA (1992) Effect of inflammatory cytokines on hypoxia-induced erythropoietin production. Blood 79: 1987–1994.
39. Yilmaz MI, Solak Y, Covic A, Goldsmith D, Kanbay M (2011) Renal anemia of inflammation: the name is self-explanatory. Blood Purif 32: 220–225.

40. Ashby DR, Gale DP, Busbridge M, Murphy KG, Duncan ND, et al. (2010) Erythropoietin administration in humans causes a marked and prolonged reduction in circulating hepcidin. Haematologica 95: 505–508.
41. Ashby DR, Gale DP, Busbridge M, Murphy KG, Duncan ND, et al. (2009) Plasma hepcidin levels are elevated but responsive to erythropoietin therapy in renal disease. Kidney Int 75: 976–981.
42. Bian XX, Yuan XS, Qi CP (2010) Effect of recombinant human erythropoietin on serum S100B protein and interleukin-6 levels after traumatic brain injury in the rat. Neurol Med Chir (Tokyo) 50: 361–366.
43. Shen Y, Wang Y, Li D, Wang C, Xu B, et al. (2010) Recombinant human erythropoietin pretreatment attenuates heart ischemia-reperfusion injury in rats by suppressing the systemic inflammatory response. Transplant Proc 42: 1595–1597.
44. Canavese C, Bergamo D, Barbieri S, Timbaldi M, Thea A, et al. (2002) Clinical relevance of hemochromatosis-related HFE C282Y/H63D gene mutations in patients on chronic dialysis. Clin Nephrol 58: 438–444.

The Burden of Nephrotoxic Drug Prescriptions in Patients with Chronic Kidney Disease

Ylenia Ingrasciotta[1], Janet Sultana[1], Francesco Giorgianni[1], Achille Patrizio Caputi[1], Vincenzo Arcoraci[1], Daniele Ugo Tari[2], Claudio Linguiti[2], Margherita Perrotta[2], Andrea Nucita[3], Fabio Pellegrini[4], Andrea Fontana[4], Lorenzo Cavagna[5], Domenico Santoro[1], Gianluca Trifirò[1]*

1 Department of Clinical and Experimental Medicine, University of Messina, Messina, Italy, **2** Caserta Local Health Service, Caserta, Italy, **3** Department of Cognitive Science, Educational and Cultural Studies (CSECS), University of Messina, Messina, Italy, **4** Unit of Biostatistics, IRCCS "Casa Sollievo della Sofferenza", San Giovanni Rotondo (FG), Italy, **5** Division of Rheumatology, University and IRCCS Foundation Policlinico S. Matteo, Pavia, Italy

Abstract

Background: The use of nephrotoxic drugs can further worsening renal function in chronic kidney disease (CKD) patients. It is therefore imperative to explore prescribing practices that can negatively affect CKD patients.

Aim: To analyze the use of nephrotoxic drugs in CKD patients in a general population of Southern Italy during the years 2006–2011.

Methods: The general practice "Arianna" database contains data from 158,510 persons, registered with 123 general practitioners (GPs) of Caserta. CKD patients were identified searching: CKD-related ICD-9 CM codes among causes of hospitalization; CKD-relevant procedures undergone in hospital (e.g. dialysis); drug prescriptions issued for a CKD-related indication. A list of nephrotoxic drugs was compiled and validated by pharmacologists and nephrologists. The summary of product characteristics was used to classify drugs as 'contraindicated' or 'to be used with caution' in renal diseases. Frequency of nephrotoxic drug use, overall, by drug class and single compounds, by GPs within one year prior or after first CKD diagnosis and within one year after dialysis entry was calculated.

Results: Overall, 1,989 CKD patients and 112 dialysed patients were identified. Among CKD patients, 49.8% and 45.2% received at least one prescription for a contraindicated nephrotoxic drug within one year prior or after first CKD diagnosis, respectively. In detail, 1,119 CKD patients (56.3%) had at least one nonsteroidal anti-inflammatory drugs (NSAIDs) prescription between CKD diagnosis and end of follow-up. A large proportion of CKD patients (35.6%) were treated with NSAIDs for periods exceeding 90 days. Contraindicated nephrotoxic drugs were used commonly in CKD, with nimesulide (16.6%) and diclofenac (11.0%) being most frequently used.

Conclusions: Contraindicated nephrotoxic drugs were highly prescribed in CKD patients from a general population of Southern Italy. CKD diagnosis did not seem to reduce significantly the prescription of nephrotoxic drugs, which may increase the risk of preventable renal function deterioration.

Editor: Shree Ram Singh, National Cancer Institute, United States of America

Funding: These authors have no support or funding to report.

Competing Interests: The authors have declared that no competing interests exist.

* E-mail: trifirog@unime.it

Introduction

Chronic kidney disease (CKD) is a progressive and widely prevalent disorder worldwide. In the past decade, prevalence of CKD has doubled in the general population [1]. Prevalence rates of moderate CKD (eGFR <60 ml/min per 1.73 m^2) were reported to range from 0.2% in 20–39 year-olds to 24.9% in > 70 year-olds in population-based studies from America [2], and similarly from Italy [3].

End stage renal disease (ESRD) requiring dialysis or kidney transplantation is a frequent outcome in patients with CKD stage 3 and 4 [4]. Over the last decade, the number of CKD patients requiring dialysis has increased annually by 6.1% in Canada [5], 11% in Japan [6] and 9% in Australia [7]. CKD may progress toward ESRD which results in a significant reduction of patient and relatives quality of life due to increasing morbidity and disability, in addition to increasing healthcare costs [8]. These observations underline the urgent need for strategies to prevent renal diseases [9]. Worsening of renal function is often due to the use (especially long term use at high dosage) of nephrotoxic drugs such as nonsteroidal anti-inflammatory drugs (NSAIDs) [10–12].

Nephrotoxic drugs should therefore be avoided or used with caution in patients with underlying CKD. Most of the drugs known to be nephrotoxic exert their toxic effects through different pathogenic mechanisms, such as altered intraglomerular hemodynamics, tubular cell toxicity, inflammation, crystal nephropathy, rhabdomyolysis, and thrombotic microangiopathy [13,14]. No population-based studies in Italy investigated the use of nephrotoxic drugs in CKD patients so far.

This study is aimed at addressing this research gap by exploring the use of nephrotoxic drugs in patients with CKD in a general population of Southern Italy in the years 2006–2011.

Methods

Data Source

Data were extracted from the Arianna database from the years 2005–2011. This database was set up by the Caserta Local Health Agency in Southern Italy in the year 2000 and currently contains information on a population of almost 400,000 inhabitants who are registered in the list of almost 300 general practitioners (GPs). Participating GPs record data during their daily clinical practice using dedicated software and send complete and anonymous clinical data of their patients to the Arianna Database on a monthly basis. The Arianna database can be linked to a hospital discharge registry through a unique and anonymous patient identifier. Quality and completeness of data out of the defined ranges were investigated and back-submitted to each participating GP in order to receive an immediate feedback. GPs failing to meet these standard quality criteria were excluded from the epidemiologic surveys according to the basic standards in the conduction of pharmacoepidemiological investigations. Of all the GPs in Caserta, 123 GPs covering a population of 158,510 inhabitants met these standard quality criteria for the considering period.

Information collected included patient demographics, prescriptions for drugs (coded according to the Anatomical Therapeutic Chemical classification system (ATC)) reimbursed by National Health System and their indications for use, and hospital admissions and procedures (coded by the ninth edition of International Classification of Diseases, Clinical Modification (ICD-9 CM)). So far, the Arianna database has been shown to provide accurate and reliable information for pharmacoepidemiological research, as documented elsewhere [15–21].

Nephrotoxic drugs assessment

Nephrotoxic drugs were identified through a stepwise procedure. A literature review was conducted by using specific MeSH terms 'nephrotoxic drug' and 'drug-induced renal failure', identifying the most relevant publications. The resulting literature review yielded a list of 127 potentially nephrotoxic drugs which was validated by two nephrologists (DS, VC) and two clinical pharmacologists (GT, VA). Finally, based on the Summary of Product Characteristic (SPC), we classified all these drugs as "contraindicated drugs" (see Table S1) or "drugs to be used with caution (i.e., precaution of use)" in renal diseases (see Table S2). For each contraindicated nephrotoxic drug we identified the specific contraindication as reported in the SPC (see Table S3).

Study population

For the evaluation of the nephrotoxic drugs prescription in CKD patients, we included all patients with a first-ever diagnosis of CKD during the study period 2006–2011 and with at least one year of database history prior to study entry. The year 2005 was considered as a run-in period to identify newly diagnosed CKD patients from 2006 onwards. The index date (ID) was defined as the date of first CKD diagnosis. We identified CKD patients as those with at least one of the specific codes among either primary/secondary causes of hospital admission, procedures or indication of use associated to the prescribed drugs (see Table S4). Of these, we also identified those requiring dialysis (see Table S4).

Statistical analysis

The assessment of the exposure to contraindicated drugs and drugs to be used with caution was carried out on all patients with incident CKD (N = 1,989, 1.25% of the total study population). We analyzed the frequency of CKD patients who received at least one prescription of nephrotoxic drug during three different time intervals, i.e. within one year prior and within one year after the first CKD diagnosis as well as within one year after entry in dialysis.

The frequency of CKD patients receiving at least one prescription of nephrotoxic drug by drug classes, was explored in the same three time intervals. Since NSAIDs were the most frequently prescribed drugs, a post-hoc frequency analysis by single compound for this class only was carried out. As low-dose acetylsalicylic acid (aspirin) is contraindicated only in severe renal disease even though it is frequently prescribed for cardiovascular prevention in CKD patients, we analyzed this drug separately.

A sensitivity analysis on the frequency of a limited number of CKD patients (identified by stage-specific codes) receiving at least one prescription of nephrotoxic drug was carried out.

Baseline CKD patients' characteristics were reported as mean and standard deviation (SD) and frequencies (percentages) for continuous and categorical variables, respectively. Age and sex adjusted multilevel logistic regressions [22] were performed to evaluate the proportion of CKD patients receiving at least one contraindicated nephrotoxic drug within one year prior and after CKD diagnosis. Multilevel methods allowed to appropriately model within- and between-patient variability [23], accounting for the multilevel nature of the data (patients clustered within GP), and to control simultaneously for the possible confounding effects of the different variables (e.g. patient's case-mix). Posterior means for the proportion of contraindicated nephrotoxic drug prescriptions, provided by each GP, were estimated from random intercepts, controlling for level-one patient's age and sex centered variables, and were graphically represented along with the observed frequencies of drug prescriptions.

To identify predictors of short- ($<$ 6 months) and long-term ($\geq$ 6 months) NSAIDs use, an ordinary and cumulative age-sex adjusted logistic regression models were performed using non users for NSAIDs as comparator. Cumulative logistic regressions models the patient's probability of being treated with NSAIDs during the entire follow-up ($<$180 days or more). Possible predictors of NSAID use, evaluated any time prior to the date of first registration of CKD diagnosis, were also considered. The risk of receiving short and long term therapy was reported as odds ratio (OR), along with their 95% confidence interval (95%CI). Two-sided p-values $<$0.05 were considered for statistical significance. All the analyses were performed using SAS Release 9.3 (SAS Institute, Cary, NC).

Results

A cohort of 2,128 patients with both prevalent and incident CKD was identified during the years 2006–2011. Of these, we included in the analysis 1,989 newly diagnosed CKD patients (1.25% of the total general population). Among incident CKD patients, 112 (5.6%) underwent dialysis during the observation period (Figure 1). The mean follow-up time of CKD patients between the index date and end of follow-up was 2.6 years. Figure 2 shows that 49.8% of incident CKD patients (N = 1,989) received at least one prescription for a contraindicated nephrotoxic drug within one year prior to the first CKD diagnosis with only a slight decrease of this proportion (45.2%) within one year after CKD diagnosis. A slightly lower proportion (33.9%) of CKD patients treated with contraindicated drugs was observed within one year after dialysis entry.

Overall, 41.2% of incident CKD patients received more than 5 different contraindicated nephrotoxic drugs and 64.6% of them received more than 5 prescriptions of these drugs during the entire follow-up. Drugs that should be used with caution in CKD were generally more commonly prescribed, with an increase in the proportion of patients receiving at least one prescription after the CKD diagnosis, as compared to the year prior to the diagnosis (85.4% vs. 80.7%). During the entire follow-up after CKD diagnosis, allopurinol (39.7%) and ramipril (26.7%) were the most commonly prescribed drugs to be used with caution.

The range of CKD patients who received at least one prescription of contraindicated nephrotoxic drugs from each individual GP, varied from 0 to 100%. Of note, 3 GPs continued to prescribe at least one contraindicated nephrotoxic drug to 100% of their CKD patients also within one year after CKD diagnosis. The cluster-adjusted results showed that all GPs prescribed nephrotoxic drugs to 27.7–74.5% of their patients before the CKD diagnosis and 21.8–76.6% after the CKD diagnosis, suggesting that the CKD diagnosis did not significantly alter the prescribing pattern (Figure 3).

Looking at individual drug classes, NSAIDs were the most commonly prescribed contraindicated nephrotoxic drugs to CKD patients during the study period, with a small decrease in the use from one year prior to one year after first CKD diagnosis, and much larger decrease after dialysis entry (47.3% vs. 42.0% vs. 29.5%) (Figure 4). The opposite trend was observed for the use of aminoglycosides (1.8% vs. 2.5% vs. 5.4%), which were in general much less prescribed as compared to NSAIDs (Figure 4). Among NSAIDs used in CKD patients, nimesulide, diclofenac and ibuprofen were the most frequently prescribed compounds, which all showed a small reduction in the use within the first year after CKD diagnosis, as compared to the previous year (Figure 5). A very large proportion of CKD patients received low dosage acetylsalicylic acid and this proportion was even higher after CKD diagnosis (43.5% vs. 41.4%). Overall, 1,119 CKD patients (56.3%) had at least one prescription of any NSAID between the index date and the end of follow-up. Of these, more than one third (35.6%) were treated with NSAIDs for periods exceeding 90 days and almost 16.5% for more than 6 months.

CKD stage-specific codes were reported for 518 (26.0%) CKD patients and in a sensitivity analysis, the 52% of CKD patients at stage IV and V received at least one prescription of contraindicated drug.

The most common reason for starting NSAID therapy was osteoarticular disease (mainly osteoarthrosis, arthralgia, rheumatoid arthritis) with 91.4% of NSAID users in long-term therapy (≥ 6 months) and 77.4% in short-term therapy (< 6 months) having this indication. Table 1 shows the characteristics of incident CKD patients who received short-term (< 6 months) or long-term therapy (≥ 6 months) with NSAIDs as compared to non-users, along with results from logistic regressions. NSAIDs were more likely to be used by female (65.4%) than male (34.6%) CKD patients who received the long-term therapy. Moreover, age-sex adjusted logistic regression showed an OR = 0.48 with 95% CI:

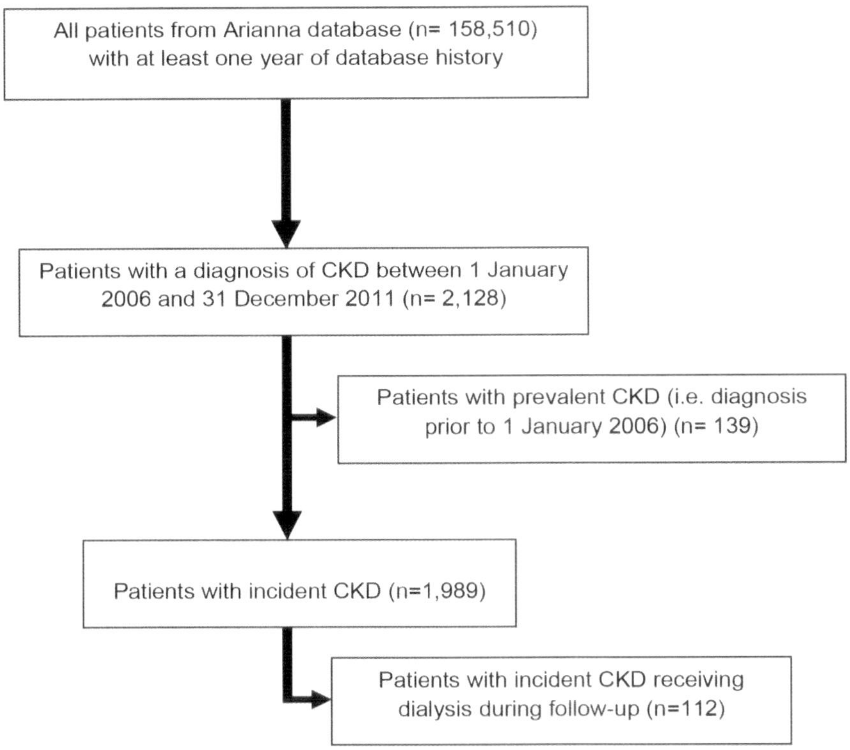

Figure 1. Flow chart of CKD patients included in the study.

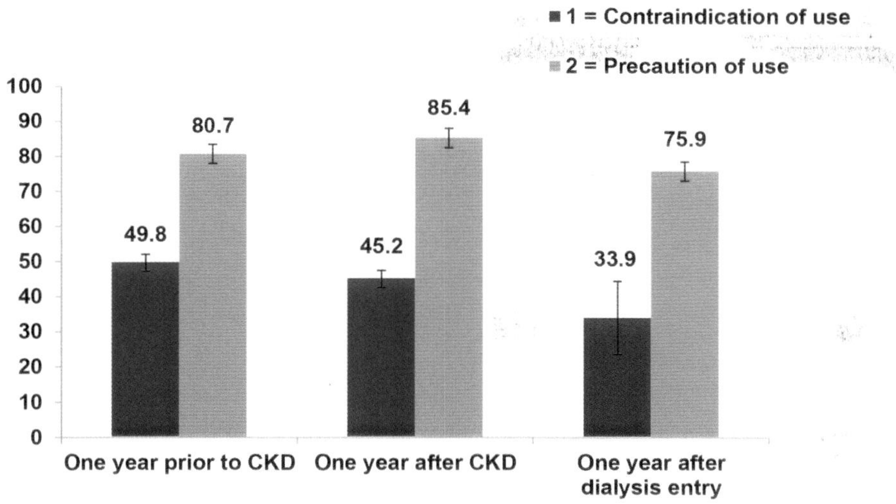

Figure 2. Proportion of incident CKD patients (N = 1,989) who received at least one prescription of nephrotoxic drug. Proportion of incident CKD patients (N = 1,989) who received at least one prescription of nephrotoxic drug within one year prior or after first CKD diagnosis, and within one year after dialysis entry (N = 112).

0.34–0.67. CKD patients receiving long-term therapy with NSAIDs were more likely to be between 65–80 years old as compared to <45 years old (Adjusted OR: 15.7; 95% CI: 2.2–114.9) and to be affected by osteoarticular diseases in general and by osteoarthritis in particular, as compared to non-users of NSAIDs. On the contrary CKD patients receiving both short and long -term therapy with NSAIDs were less likely to be affected by liver diseases (Adjusted OR: 0.53; 95% CI: 0.36–0.78 and OR: 0.49; 95% CI: 0.23–1.04 respectively).

Discussion

To our knowledge, this is the first population-based study exploring the use of nephrotoxic drugs in CKD patients in Italy. Our study shows that, although contraindicated, such nephrotoxic drugs (mostly NSAIDs) were highly prescribed to CKD patients from a general population of Southern Italy. The new diagnosis of CKD did not seem to reduce the prescription of potentially harmful nephrotoxic drugs, since an elevated number of patients continued to receive prescriptions of nephrotoxic drugs after CKD diagnosis. Substantial variability in the use of nephrotoxic drugs among 123 GPs was observed. Nimesulide was found to be the most commonly prescribed NSAIDs.

In general, use of contraindicated drugs exposes CKD patients to a high risk of worsening of renal function. The prescribing pattern of contraindicated nephrotoxic drugs was not substantially modified after CKD diagnosis or after dialysis entry. This may be justified because renal function is mostly lost by the time dialysis is required and is completely supplanted by the dialysis process. However, avoiding the use of nephrotoxic drugs such as NSAIDs, aminoglycosides etc. is not only a predialytic measure aimed at preventing kidney disease progression, but should also be a post-dialysis measured to preserve residual renal function [24].

An Australian longitudinal cohort study with 3,175 persons >18 years from the general population showed high use of NSAIDs in patients with renal disease as 31% of users of these drugs had stage 3 or higher CKD stage [25], similar to our study findings. Several nephrotoxic drugs, including NSAIDs, are known to exert nephrotoxic effects through renal vasoconstriction and clinically significant reduction in glomerular filtration rate (GFR) via renal prostaglandin inhibition, or through other mechanisms as occurs in interstitial nephritis, membranous glomerulonephropathy, type 4 renal tubular acidosis and acute and chronic renal papillary necrosis [26–28]. Long-acting NSAIDs or those having a half-life >12 hours should be avoided to prevent persistent and clinically significant GFR reduction induced by NSAIDs via inhibition of renal vasodilatory prostaglandins [29].

The most common reason for starting therapy with NSAIDs, in our study cohort, was the occurrence of osteoarticular disease (mainly osteoarthrosis, arthralgia, rheumatoid arthritis) with 91.4% of NSAID users in long-term therapy (≥ 6 months) having this indication. Pain, a common complaint in osteoarticular diseases [30], has been reported to be a common problem in end-stage renal disease (ESRD) patients [31]. Moreover, the overuse of over-the-counter NSAIDs is particularly common in rheumatic conditions such as osteoarthritis [32], thus further highlighting the importance of our results in CKD patients with such diseases who are already use prescription-only NSAIDs. Pain treatment in CKD still remains a primary issue for clinicians: while, in general, acetaminophen has been considered to be the safest non-narcotic analgesic in CKD patients it may be nephrotoxic with chronic use at high doses [33]. For treatment of moderate pain, the use of low-potency opioids is suggested unless CKD is very advanced [34]. Tramadol may be also used because it is not known to be nephrotoxic. Nonetheless, it must be noted that its systemic elimination is reduced with advanced CKD, thus requiring dose adjustment in patients with renal disease. Opioids without potential for accumulation such as fentanyl, buprenorphine and hydromorphone can be considered as valid option in case of severe pain [35,36].

Our results also show that low-dose acetylsalicylic acid for cardiovascular prevention is widely prescribed in elderly patients with CKD [37]. According to the Summary of Product Characteristics, low-dose acetylsalicylic acid is contraindicated in patients with severe CKD (GFR <30 ml/min). However, evidence suggests that early CKD increases risk of cardiovascular events and death [38–40]. As a result, the absolute benefits of aspirin might be greater for CKD patients than the risk of

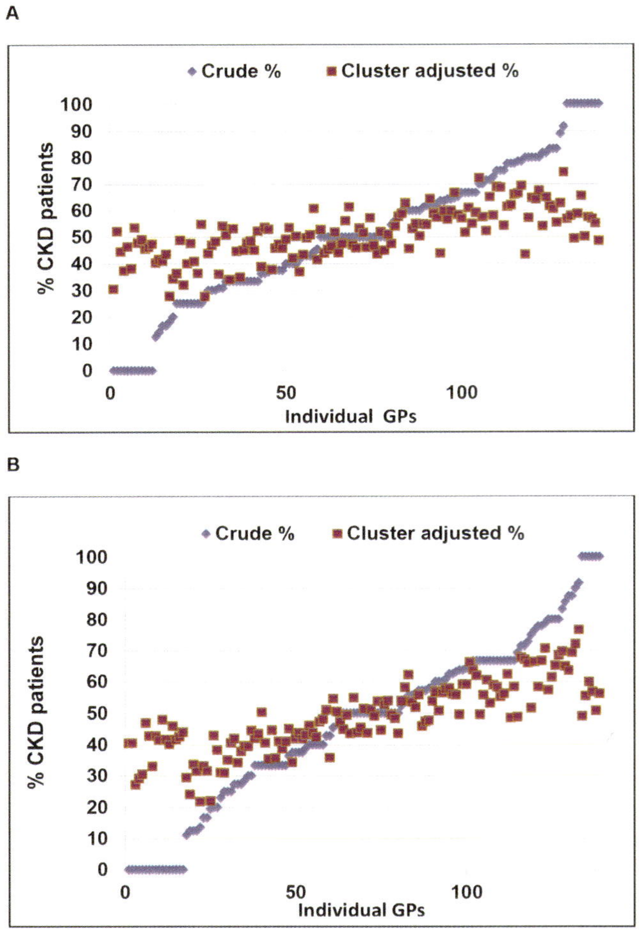

Figure 3. Crude and Cluster-adjusted analysis of CKD patients' CND prescription by GP. Distribution (%) of CKD patients who received at least one prescription of contraindicated nephrotoxic drugs (CND) within the year prior (A) and after (B) first CKD diagnosis, clustered by GP. The distribution was clustered by GP and the was adjusted also by sex and age. CND: contraindicated nephrotoxic drug.

worsening kidney function. On the other hand, CKD patients have abnormal platelet function, potentially leaving them at increased risk of hemorrhage when treated with anticoagulants or antiplatelet agents [41]. A meta-analysis of cardiovascular risk reduction with aspirin therapy suggests that aspirin reduces cardiovascular risk, both in primary and secondary prevention, but the protective effect on patients with renal dysfunction was unknown [42]. A randomised-controlled trial on 18,597 hypertensive patients investigating associations between the benefits of aspirin and glomerular filtration found that aspirin therapy prevented significantly more cardiovascular events and deaths, and all-cause deaths in CKD patients compared to those with normal kidney function [43]. Major cardiovascular events were reduced by 9%, 15% and 66% for patients with mild, moderate, and severe CKD respectively, even though the risk of major or minor bleeding in CKD subgroups was nearly 10 times higher than the general population. The overall benefits of aspirin seem to outweigh the risk of bleeding [44]. Finally, our findings show also a substantial increase in CKD patients treated with aminoglycosides after dialysis entry (5.4%), probably due to an increase in infections following use of central venous catheters or arteriovenous fistula for renal hemodialysis.

This study has several strengths as well as limitations. We included CKD patients on dialysis in our study, unlike other similar studies [45], which allowed us to investigate the prescription of nephrotoxic drugs even in these patients. In addition, the methodology used here has the advantages of an administrative database study: it is free from biases such as recall and selection bias. However, diagnoses recorded by GPs may not be accurate despite we used very specific codes for renal disease and related procedures. We cannot exclude a possible misclassification of acute kidney injury (AKI) as chronic kidney disease (CKD). However, for case ascertainment we considered only specific CKD codes and in presence of less specific codes, we considered these codes only if registered multiple times to ensure the disease was chronic. We cannot identify the exact date of onset of CKD as it was defined as the date of first registration of CKD-related primary/secondary hospital discharge diagnosis, procedure or indication of use for drug prescription. Nonetheless, the frequency of use of nephrotoxic drugs after CKD diagnosis is very high and only slightly lower as compared to the year prior to the diagnosis, thus confirming poor awareness of prescribers about possible detrimental effects of these drugs in CKD patients. Some drugs are specifically contraindicated in patients with severe renal disease (creatinine clearance < 30 ml/min) only. We could not identify the stage for most CKD patients due to lack of laboratory data (e.g. serum creatinine test, GFR value) and registration of CKD codes of unspecified stage. For this reason the rate of contraindicated nephrotoxic drug use may have been overestimated. However, CKD stage-specific codes were reported for 518 (26.0%) CKD patients and in a sensitivity analysis restricted to CKD stage IV and V patients, similar figures concerning contraindicated drug use were observed. We used outpatient prescription data and we had no information about actual filling of prescriptions and medication use. However, this study was primarily aimed at exploring the prescribing pattern of nephrotoxic drugs and it is unlikely that NSAIDs, generally prescribed as painkiller, were not ultimately taken by the patient. Furthermore, the traceability of some nephrotoxic drug prescriptions was incomplete as being administered in the hospital (e.g. oncology drugs, and partly, aminoglycosides) or used as OTC drugs (e.g. NSAIDs), as a consequence, the nephrotoxic drugs use could be underestimate. In addition, this study was carried out using outpatient data collected from a large general practice of Southern Italy. We therefore cannot exclude that these findings are not fully generalizable to the whole Italian general population. However, the applied methodology and the Arianna database have been shown to provide accurate and reliable information for pharmacoepidemiological research, as documented elsewhere [15–21].

Conclusions

This study shows that contraindicated nephrotoxic drugs (mostly NSAIDS) are frequently prescribed to CKD patients and the new diagnosis of CKD did not modify the prescription pattern. NSAIDs were most commonly used as analgesics in diseases such as osteoarthritis and rheumatic arthritis. Therapeutic alternatives such as acetaminophen and weak opioids can be used at the lowest dosages and shortest durations in patients whose CKD is not advanced. More awareness is needed about the safety issues of using nephrotoxic drugs in CKD. Intervention strategies to improve prescribing pattern in CKD patients should be mostly targeted to GPs who prescribe more frequently contraindicated nephrotoxic drugs.

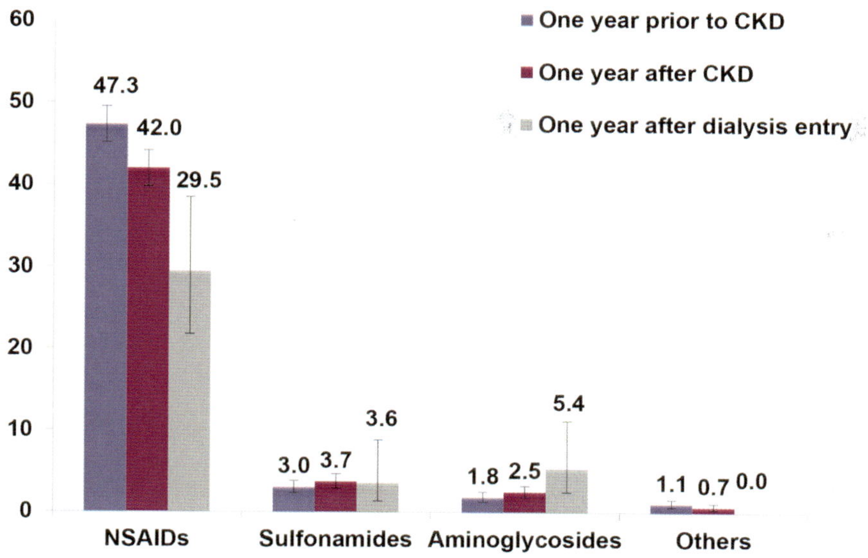

Figure 4. Proportion of CKD patients (N = 1,989) who received ≥ 1 prescription of CND, stratified by classes. Proportion of CKD patients (N = 1,989) who received at least one prescription of contraindicated nephrotoxic drugs, stratified by drug classes, within one year prior or after first CKD diagnosis, and within one year after the entry in dialysis (N = 112) within one year prior or after first CKD diagnosis, and within one year after the entry in dialysis (N = 112). Others: zoledronate, lithium, antineoplastic agents (methotrexate, interferon alfa-2B), gold preparations (auranofin), hydrochlorothiazide. Low dosage acetylsalicylic acid was not included among NSAIDs, but it was analysed in Figure 5, separately. CND: contraindicated nephrotoxic drug.

Supporting Information

Table S1 List of contraindicated nephrotoxic drugs in patients with renal disease on the basis of the summary of product characteristics (SPC).

Table S2 List of drugs to be used with caution in patients with renal disease on the basis of the summary of product characteristics (SPC).

Table S3 List of nephrotoxic drugs classified by CKD stage-specific contraindication as reported in Summary

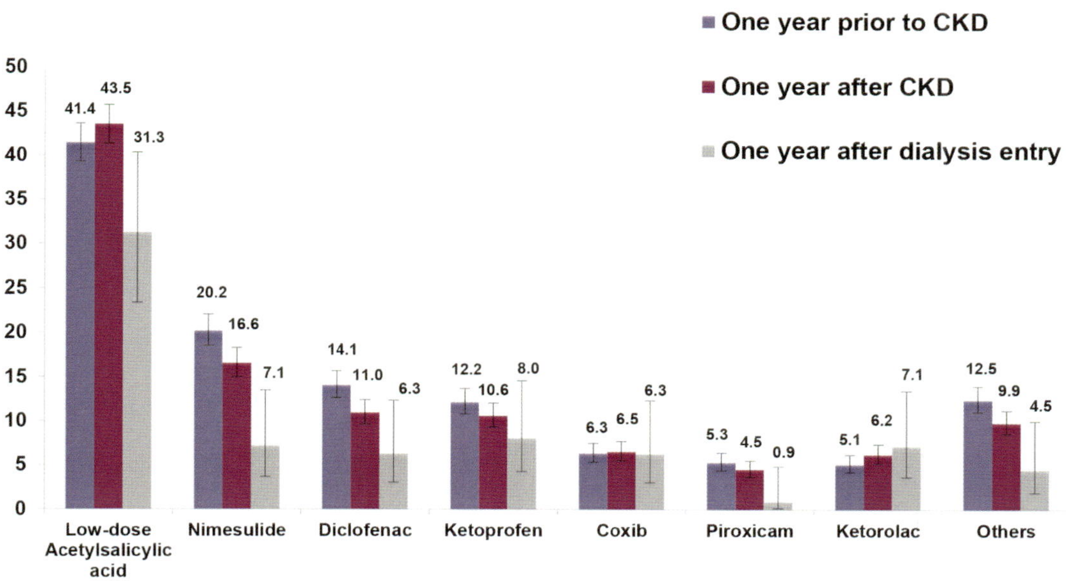

Figure 5. Proportion of CKD patients (N = 1,989) who received ≥ 1 prescription of NSAIDs. Proportion of CKD patients (N = 1,989) who received at least one prescription of individual NSAIDs within one year prior or after the first CKD diagnosis and within one year after the entry in dialysis (N = 112). Others (<5%): tenoxicam, meloxicam, aceclofenac, ibuprofen, dexibuprofen, tiaprofenic acid, naproxen, lornoxicam, acetylsalicylic acid, acetylsalicylic acid and ascorbic acid, niflumic acid, diclofenac sodium plus misoprostol. Coxib: celecoxib, etoricoxib.

Table 1. Characteristics of incident CKD patients, stratified by cumulative use of NSAIDs during the follow-up, and results from ordinary and cumulative logistic regressions.

	Non-use of NSAIDs N = 870 (%)	< 180 days of NSAID use N = 934 (%)	Adj. OR* (95% CI) <180 days of NSAID use vs. non-use	≥ 180 days of NSAID use N = 185 (%)	Adj. OR*(95% CI) ≥180 days of NSAID use vs. non-use	Cumulative logistic regression*
Sex						
Male	456 (52.4)	460 (49.3)	0.88(0.73–1.06)	64 (34.6)	0.48(0.34 –0.67)	0.74 (0.63–0.88)
Female	414 (47.6)	474 (50.7)	1	121 (65.4)	1	1
Mean age ± SD	72.6 ± 15.0	72.1 ± 12.3		72.2 ± 10.0		
Mean duration of follow-up (years)	1.8 (0 – 5.9)	3.0 (0 – 6.0)		4.0 (0.6 – 6.0)		
Age categories						
<45	55 (6.3)	26 (2.8)	1	1 (0.5)	1	1
45–64	148 (17.1)	197 (21.1)	2.81 (1.67 –4.7)	40 (21.6)	14.86 (1.99–110.75)	3.3 (2.03–5.49)
65–80	357 (41.0)	474 (50.7)	2.81(1.73 –4.57)	102 (55.1)	15.71 (2.19 –114.94)	3.39 (2.11–5.45)
>80	310 (35.6)	237 (25.4)	1.62 (0.98–2.66)	42 (22.8)	7.45 (1.00–55.27)	1.92 (1.18–3.13)
Comorbidities[1]						
Diabetes mellitus	296 (34)	358 (38.3)	1.20 (0.99–1.46)	71 (38.4)	1.15 (0.82–1.60)	1.17 (0.98–1.39)
Hypertension	736 (84.6)	819 (87.7)	1.39 (1.04–1.85)	159 (85.9)	1.09 (0.66–1.78)	1.26 (0.97–1.64)
Ischemicheartdisease	329 (37.8)	357 (38.2)	1.05 (0.86–1.27)	48 (25.9)	0.59 (0.41–0.85)	0.89 (0.74–1.06)
Cerebrovascular disease	153 (17.6)	133 (14.2)	0.78 (0.61–1.01)	26 (14.1)	0.75 (0.47–1.19)	0.79 (0.62–1.00)
Liver disease	76 (8.7)	45 (4.8)	0.53 (0.36–0.78)	8 (4.3)	0.49 (0.23–1.04)	0.53 (0.37–0.76)
Malignant neoplasm	101 (11.6)	101 (10.8)	0.95 (0.71–1.27)	10 (5.4)	0.46 (0.24–0.91)	0.82 (0.62–1.08)
Rheumatoid arthritis	13 (1.5)	21 (2.2)	1.50 (0.75–3.02)	8 (4.3)	2.78 (1.12–6.90)	1.89 (1.05–3.41)
Osteoarthritis	443 (50.9)	675 (72.3)	2.74 (2.23–3.36)	156 (84.3)	5.75 (3.68–8.97)	3.04 (2.51–3.69)
Enthesopathies	6 (0.7)	5 (0.5)	0.77 (0.23–2.53)	3 (1.6)	2.52 (0.61–10.41)	1.36 (0.49–3.75)
Gout	255 (29.3)	250 (26.8)	0.92 (0.72–1.18)	36 (19.4)	0.58 (0.35–0.96)	0.82 (0.65–1.04)
Dyslipidemia	251 (28.8)	319 (34.1)	1.29 (1.05–1.57)	54 (29.2)	1.01 (0.71–1.44)	1.18 (0.98–1.41)
Concomitant drugs[1]						
Corticosteroids	264 (30.3)	305 (32.7)	1.13 (0.92–1.38)	65 (35.1)	1.27 (0.91–1.79)	1.16 (0.96–1.39)
Vitamin A and/or D[†]	92 (10.6)	111 (11.9)	1.10 (0.82–1.49)	25 (13.5)	1.07 (0.66–1.75)	1.08 (0.82–1.41)
Opioids	134 (15.4)	135 (14.5)	0.92 (0.71–1.20)	27 (14.6)	0.85 (0.54–1.35)	0.91 (0.72–1.16)

SD = standard deviation; 95% CI = confidence interval; adj. OR = adjusted OR; mean duration of follow-up (years): mean follow-up between date of incident CKD diagnosis (i.e. index date) and end of the follow-up.
*The analysis was adjusted by sex and age.
[1] Co-morbidities and concomitant drugs have been evaluated any time prior to the index date and they are not mutually exclusive.
[†]Combination therapy consisting of vitamin A and D (ATC: A11CB) or vitamin D/vitamin D analogues (ATC: A11CC).

of Product Characteristics (SPC). CKD: chronic kidney disease; BUN: Blood Urea Nitrogen; GFR: glomerular filtration rate.

Table S4 Diagnosis or procedure codes to identify CKD and dialyzed patients. Patients identified through ICD9-CM code "583*" or "586*" were considered as CKD patients only if these codes were repeated more than twice during the study period to prevent the misclassification of patients with acute renal disease as CKD.

Author Contributions

Conceived and designed the experiments: GT DS. Performed the experiments: FG YI JS. Analyzed the data: FG GT AF FP. Contributed reagents/materials/analysis tools: GT VA. Wrote the paper: YI JS GT VA AN MP AF CL DUT APC LC.

References

1. Snively CS, Gutierrez C (2004) Chronic kidney disease: prevention and treatment of common complications. Am Fam Physician. 70(10): p. 1921–8.
2. Coresh J, Byrd-Holt D, Astor BC, Briggs JP, Eggers PW, et al. (2005) Chronic kidney disease awareness, prevalence, and trends among U.S. adults, 1999 to 2000. J Am Soc Nephrol. 16(1): p. 180–8.
3. Cirillo M, Laurenzi M, Mancini M, Zanchetti A, Lombardi C, et al. (2006) Low glomerular filtration in the population: prevalence, associated disorders, and awareness. Kidney Int. 70(4): p. 800–6.
4. De Nicola L, Chiodini P, Zoccali C, Borrelli S, Cianciaruso B, et al. (2011) Prognosis of CKD patients receiving outpatient nephrology care in Italy. Clin J Am Soc Nephrol. 6(10): p. 2421–8.
5. Ottawa V, Ontario (2001) Dialysis and renal transplantation, Canadian Organ Replacement Register. Canadian Institute for Health Information.
6. Usami T, Sato R, Yoshida A, Kimura G (2002) Regional variation in end-stage renal disease. Curr Opin Nephrol Hypertens. 11(3): p. 343–6.
7. Disney AP (1998) Some trends in chronic renal replacement therapy in Australia and New Zealand, 1997. Nephrol Dial Transplant. 13(4): p. 854–9.

8. Khan S, Amedia CA Jr (2008) Economic burden of chronic kidney disease. J Eval Clin Pract. 14(3): p. 422–34.
9. Obrador GT, García-García G, Villa AR, Rubilar X, Olvera N, et al. (2010) Prevalence of chronic kidney disease in the Kidney Early Evaluation Program (KEEP) Mexico and comparison with KEEP US. Kidney Int Suppl, (116): p. S2–8.
10. Delzell E, Shapiro S (1998) A review of epidemiologic studies of nonnarcotic analgesics and chronic renal disease. Medicine (Baltimore). 77(2): p. 102–21.
11. Kuo HW, Tsai SS, Tiao MM, Liu YC, Lee IM, et al. (2010) Analgesic use and the risk for progression of chronic kidney disease. Pharmacoepidemiol Drug Saf. 19(7): p. 745–51.
12. Pannu N, Nadim MK (2008) An overview of drug-induced acute kidney injury. Crit Care Med. 36(4 Suppl): p. S216–23.
13. Schetz M, Dasta J, Goldstein S, Golper T (2005) Drug-induced acute kidney injury. Curr Opin Crit Care. 11(6): p. 555–65.
14. Zager RA (1997), Pathogenetic mechanisms in nephrotoxic acute renal failure. Semin Nephrol. 17(1): p. 3–14.
15. Piacentini N, Trifiró G, Tari M, Moretti S, Arcoraci V, et al. (2005) Statin-macrolide interaction risk: a population-based study throughout a general practice database. Eur J Clin Pharmacol. 61(8): p. 615–20.
16. Trifirò G, Corrao S, Alacqua M, Moretti S, Tari M, et al. (2006) Interaction risk with proton pump inhibitors in general practice: significant disagreement between different drug-related information sources. Br J Clin Pharmacol. 62(5): p. 582–90.
17. Oteri A, Trifirò G, Gagliostro MS, Tari DU, Moretti S, et al. (2010) Prescribing pattern of anti-epileptic drugs in an Italian setting of elderly outpatients: a population-based study during 2004-07. Br J Clin Pharmacol. 70(4): p. 514–22.
18. Alacqua M, Trifirò G, Spina E, Moretti S, Tari DU, et al. (2009) Newer and older antiepileptic drug use in Southern Italy: a population-based study during the years 2003–2005. Epilepsy Res. 85(1): p. 107–13.
19. Alacqua M, Trifirò G, Cavagna L, Caporali R, Montecucco CM, et al. (2008) Prescribing pattern of drugs in the treatment of osteoarthritis in Italian general practice: the effect of rofecoxib withdrawal. Arthritis Rheum. 59(4): p. 568–74.
20. Trifirò G, Alacqua M, Corrao S, Moretti S, Tari DU, et al. (2008) Lipid-lowering drug use in Italian primary care: effects of reimbursement criteria revision. Eur J Clin Pharmacol. 64(6): p. 619–25.
21. Trifirò G, Savica R, Morgante L, Vanacore N, Tari M, et al. (2008) Prescribing pattern of anti-Parkinson drugs in Southern Italy: cross-sectional analysis in the years 2003–2005. Parkinsonism Relat Disord. 14(5): p. 420–5.
22. Snijders TAB, Bosker RJ (2012) Multilevel analysis. An introduction to basic and advanced multilevel modeling (2nd edition). London, Sage Publications.
23. De Berardis G, Pellegrini F, Franciosi M, Belfiglio M, Di Nardo B, et al. (2004) Quality of care and outcomes in type 2 diabetic patients: a comparison between general practice and diabetes clinics. Diabetes Care. 27(2): p. 398–406.
24. Radulescu D, Ferechide D (2009) The importance of residual renal function in chronic dialysed patients. J Med Life. 2(2): p. 199–206.
25. Adams RJ, Appleton SL, Gill TK, Taylor AW, Wilson DH, et al. (2011) Cause for concern in the use of non-steroidal anti-inflammatory medications in the community—a population-based study. BMC Fam Pract. 12: p. 70.
26. Whelton A, Hamilton CW (1991) Nonsteroidal anti-inflammatory drugs: effects on kidney function. J Clin Pharmacol. 31(7): p. 588–98.
27. Clive DM, Stoff JS (1984) Renal syndromes associated with nonsteroidal antiinflammatory drugs. N Engl J Med. 310(9): p. 563–72.
28. Singh AK, Colvin RB (2003) Case records of the Massachusetts General Hospital. Weekly clinicopathological exercises. Case 36-2003. A 68-year-old woman with impaired renal function. N Engl J Med. 349(21): p. 2055–63.
29. Henry D, Page J, Whyte I, Nanra R, Hall C (1997) Consumption of non-steroidal anti-inflammatory drugs and the development of functional renal impairment in elderly subjects. Results of a case-control study. Br J Clin Pharmacol. 44(1): p. 85–90.
30. Montecucco C (2009) Pain and rheumatology: An overview of the problem. Eur J Pain Supplements. 3: p. p.105–9.
31. Santoro D, Satta E, Messina S, Costantino G, Savica V, et al. (2013) Pain in end-stage renal disease: a frequent and neglected clinical problem. Clin Nephrol. 79 Suppl 1: p. S2–11.
32. Cavagna L, Caporali R, Trifiro G, Arcoraci V, Rossi S, et al. (2013) Overuse of prescription and OTC non-steroidal anti-inflammatory drugs in patients with rheumatoid arthritis and osteoarthritis. Int J Immunopathol Pharmacol. 26(1): p. 279–81.
33. Broadbent A, Khor K, Heaney A (2003) Palliation and chronic renal failure: opioid and other palliative medications-Dosage guidelines. ProgPalliat Care. 11: p. p. 183–190.
34. Niscola P (2011) Analgesici oppioidi in pazienti con Insufficienza Renale Cronica: principi d'impiego e Raccomandazioni correnti. G Ital Nefrol. 28(3): p.p. 269–277.
35. Trescot AM, Datta S, Lee M, Hansen H (2008) Opioid pharmacology. Pain Physician. 11(2 Suppl): p. S133–53.
36. Murtagh F (2007)Opioids in special circumstances. In Forbes K: Opioids in Cancer Pain. Oxford University Press. p. p. 131–43.
37. Nderitu P, Doos L, Jones PW, Davies SJ, Kadam UT (2013) Non-steroidal anti-inflammatory drugs and chronic kidney disease progression: a systematic review. Fam Pract. 30(3): p. 247–55.
38. Sarnak MJ, Levey AS, Schoolwerth AC, Coresh J, Culleton B, et al. (2003) Kidney disease as a risk factor for development of cardiovascular disease: a statement from the American Heart Association Councils on Kidney in Cardiovascular Disease, High Blood Pressure Research, Clinical Cardiology, and Epidemiology and Prevention. Hypertension. 42(5): p. 1050–65.
39. Go AS, Chertow GM, Fan D, McCulloch CE, Hsu CY (2004) Chronic kidney disease and the risks of death, cardiovascular events, and hospitalization. N Engl J Med. 351(13): p. 1296–305.
40. Ninomiya T, Perkovic V, de Galan BE, Zoungas S, Pillai A, et al. (2009) Albuminuria and kidney function independently predict cardiovascular and renal outcomes in diabetes. J Am Soc Nephrol. 20(8): p. 1813–21.
41. Weigert AL, Schafer AI (1998) Uremic bleeding: pathogenesis and therapy. Am J Med Sci. 316(2): p. 94–104.
42. Antithrombotic Trialists' (ATT) Collaboration, Baigent C, Blackwell L, Collins R, Emberson J, et al. (2009) Aspirin in the primary and secondary prevention of vascular disease: collaborative meta-analysis of individual participant data from randomised trials. Lancet. 373(9678): p. 1849–60.
43. Jardine MJ, Ninomiya T, Perkovic V, Cass A, Turnbull F, et al. (2010) Aspirin is beneficial in hypertensive patients with chronic kidney disease: a post-hoc subgroup analysis of a randomized controlled trial. J Am Coll Cardiol. 56(12): p. 956–65.
44. Antithrombotic Trialists' Collaboration (2002) Collaborative meta-analysis of randomised trials of antiplatelet therapy for prevention of death, myocardial infarction, and stroke in high risk patients. Bmj. 324(7329): p. 71–86.
45. Gooch K, Culleton BF, Manns BJ, Zhang J, Alfonso H, et al. (2007) NSAID use and progression of chronic kidney disease. Am J Med. 120(3): p. 280 e1–7.

14

P Wave Dispersion and Maximum P Wave Duration Are Associated with Renal Outcomes in Chronic Kidney Disease

Jiun-Chi Huang[1,3], Shu-Yi Wei[6,7], Szu-Chia Chen[1,3,4], Jer-Ming Chang[1,3,4], Chi-Chih Hung[1,4], Ho-Ming Su[2,3,4]*, Shang-Jyh Hwang[1,5], Hung-Chun Chen[1,5]

1 Division of Nephrology, Department of Internal Medicine, Kaohsiung Medical University Hospital, Kaohsiung Medical University, Kaohsiung, Taiwan, 2 Division of Cardiology, Department of Internal Medicine, Kaohsiung Medical University Hospital, Kaohsiung Medical University, Kaohsiung, Taiwan, 3 Department of Internal Medicine, Kaohsiung Municipal Hsiao-Kang Hospital, Kaohsiung Medical University, Kaohsiung, Taiwan, 4 Faculty of Medicine, College of Medicine, Kaohsiung Medical University, Kaohsiung, Taiwan, 5 Faculty of Renal Care, College of Medicine, Kaohsiung Medical University, Kaohsiung, Taiwan, 6 Department of Internal Medicine, Kaohsiung Municipal United Hospital, Kaohsiung, Taiwan, 7 Yuh-Ing Junior College of Health Care & Management, Kaohsiung, Taiwan

Abstract

P wave parameters measured by 12-lead electrocardiogram (ECG) are commonly used as a noninvasive tool to evaluate left atrial enlargement. This study was designed to assess whether P wave parameters were associated with renal outcomes in chronic kidney disease (CKD) patients. This longitudinal study enrolled 439 patients with CKD stages 3–5. Renal end points were defined as the commencement of dialysis or death. Change in renal function was measured using the estimated glomerular filtration rate (eGFR) slope. We measured two ECG P wave parameters corrected for heart rate, i.e., corrected P wave dispersion and corrected maximum P wave duration. The values of P wave dispersion and maximum P wave duration were 88.8±21.7 ms and 153.3±21.7 ms, respectively. During the follow-up period (mean, 25.2 months), 95 patients (21.6%) started hemodialysis and 30 deaths (6.8%) were recorded. Multivariate Cox regression analysis identified that increased P wave dispersion [hazard ratio (HR), 1.020; 95% confidence interval (CI), 1.009–1.032; $P<0.001$] and maximum P wave duration (HR, 1.013; 95% CI, 1.003–1.024; $P=0.012$) were associated with progression to renal end points. Furthermore, increased P wave dispersion (unstandardized coefficient $\beta=-0.016$; $P=0.037$) and maximum P wave duration (unstandardized coefficient $\beta=-0.014$; $P=0.040$) were negatively associated with the eGFR slope. We demonstrated that increased P wave dispersion and maximum P wave duration were associated with progression to the renal end points of dialysis or death and faster renal function decline in CKD patients. Screening CKD patients on the basis of P wave dispersion and maximum P wave duration may help identify patients at high risk for worse renal outcomes.

Editor: Martin H. de Borst, University Medical Center Groningen and University of Groningen, Netherlands

Funding: The authors have no support or funding to report.

Competing Interests: The authors have declared that no competing interests exist.

* Email: cobeshm@seed.net.tw

Introduction

Both traditional risk factors, such as hypertension, diabetes, and dyslipidemia, and non-traditional risk factors, such as cardiovascular disease contribute to the risk of progressive renal function loss [1,2]. Faster renal function decline has been significantly associated with high cardiovascular morbidity and mortality in patients with chronic kidney disease (CKD) [3,4]. It is therefore essential to identify those CKD patients with faster renal function decline in order to initiate aggressive treatment interventions and improve survival.

Echocardiographic measures of left ventricular function and structure as well as left atrial size have been reported to predict adverse renal outcomes [5–7]. This implies that patients with cardiac dysfunction and left atrial enlargement might have faster renal function decline and adverse renal outcome. However, structural and functional abnormalities of the heart are frequently evaluated using echocardiography, which may preclude its application if echocardiography or experienced operators are not available. 12-lead electrocardiogram (ECG) is a simple, inexpensive, and noninvasive clinical tool to assess structural and functional abnormalities of the heart [8]. P wave parameters measured by 12-lead ECG have been reported to be useful tools for assessing the risk of left atrial enlargement, left ventricular hypertrophy (LVH), and left ventricular diastolic dysfunction [9–17]. Furthermore, P wave parameters have been independently associated with increased risk of both atrial fibrillation and recurrent transient ischemic attacks [18,19]. However, there are limited studies evaluating whether P wave parameters are associated with progression to end-stage renal disease, decline in renal function, or death in CKD patients. The aim of this study in a cohort of patients with CKD stages 3–5 were to assess whether P wave parameters were associated with progression to the commencement of dialysis or death and whether these parameters were associated with the rate of renal function decline.

Subjects and Methods

Ethics statement

The study protocol was approved by the Institutional Review Board of the Kaohsiung Medical University Hospital (KMUH-IRB-20130305). Informed consent was obtained in written form from patients and all clinical investigations were conducted according to the principles of the Declaration of Helsinki. The patients gave consent for the publication of the clinical details.

Study patients

The study was conducted in a regional hospital in southern Taiwan. From January 2007 to May 2010, we consecutively enrolled 505 pre-dialysis patients with CKD stages 3–5, according to the National Kidney Foundation-Kidney Disease Outcomes Quality Initiative (K/DOQI) guidelines [20] from our Outpatient Department of Internal Medicine. Patients with evidence of kidney damage lasting for more than 3 months were classified as CKD stages 3, 4, and 5, on the basis of an estimated glomerular filtration rate (eGFR) level (mL/min/1.73 m^2) of 30–59, 15–29, and <15 respectively. Patients with atrial fibrillation, significant mitral valve disease, and inadequate ECG image visualization were excluded. Twenty-seven patients with less than three eGFR measurements during the follow-up period were excluded. Those patients who died (n = 9) or entered dialysis therapy (n = 30) within 3 months after enrollment were also excluded to avoid incomplete observation of changes in renal function. Finally, 439 patients (mean age, 66.0±12.0 years, 274 males) were included in this study.

Assessment of P wave parameters

A standard 12-lead surface ECG (25-mm/s, 1-mV/cm, and 100-Hz) was performed in all study patients. An image analysis software system (Image Tool 3.0) was used to perform quantitative assessments. We assessed the correlation of two P wave parameters, corrected P wave dispersion and corrected maximum P wave duration, with progression to dialysis or death and decline in renal function. P wave dispersion was calculated as the difference between maximum and minimum P wave duration [21]. Both the P wave measurements were corrected for heart rate using Bazett's formula, i.e., the corrected P wave parameters were equal to P wave parameters/$(RR)^{1/2}$ [22].

Definition of LVH

LVH was defined as Sokolow-Lyon voltage criteria via 12-lead ECG (sum of the amplitude of the S wave in lead V_1 and the R wave in lead V_5 or V_6 greater than 3.5 mV) [23].

Collection of demographic, medical, and laboratory data

Demographic and medical data including age, gender, smoking history (ever *versus* never), and comorbid conditions were obtained from medical records or patient interviews. The body mass index (BMI) was calculated as the ratio of weight in kilograms divided by square of height in meters. Laboratory data were measured from fasting blood samples using an autoanalyzer (Roche Diagnostics GmbH, D-68298 Mannheim COBAS Integra 400). Serum creatinine was measured by the compensated Jaffé (kinetic alkaline picrate) method in a Roche/Integra 400 Analyzer (Roche Diagnostics, Mannheim, Germany) using a calibrator traceable to isotope-dilution mass spectrometry [24]. The value of eGFR was calculated using the 4-variable equation in the Modification of Diet in Renal Disease (MDRD) study [25]. Dipsticks (Hema-Combistix, Bayer Diagnostics) were used to evaluate proteinuria. A dipstick test result of 1+ or more was defined as positive. Blood and urine samples were obtained within 1 month of study enrollment.

Definition of renal end points

Renal end points were defined as the commencement of dialysis or death. In patients reaching study end points, renal function data were censored at the start of renal replacement therapy or death. The remaining patients were followed until March 2011. The commencement of dialysis was determined according to the regulations of the National Health Insurance for dialysis therapy based on laboratory data, nutritional status, and uremic symptoms and signs. Renal end points-free survival was defined as the time from study enrollment to the commencement of dialysis or death.

Assessment of the rate of renal function decline

The rate of renal function decline was assessed by the eGFR slope, defined as the regression coefficient between eGFR and time in units of mL/min/1.73 m^2/year. At least three eGFR measurements following 12-lead ECG examination were required to estimate the eGFR slope. Faster renal function decline was defined as a greater value of decline in the eGFR slope.

Reproducibility

Thirty-five patients were randomly selected for evaluation of the interobserver variability of P wave dispersion and maximum P wave duration measurements by two independent observers. The same measurement was repeated twice, 1 week apart, to calculate the intraobserver variability. Mean percent error was calculated as the absolute difference divided by the average of the two observations.

Statistical analysis

Statistical analysis was performed using SPSS version 17.0 (SPSS Inc., Chicago, IL, USA) for Windows. Data were expressed as percentages, mean ± standard deviation, mean ± standard error of the mean for the eGFR slope, or median (25th–75th percentile) for triglycerides and number of serum creatinine measurements. The differences between groups were analyzed using the Chi-square test for categorical variables and using the independent *t*-test for continuous variables. Time to renal end points and covariates of risk factors were modeled using the Cox proportional hazards model. The survival curve for renal end points was derived using Kaplan–Meier analysis. Linear regression analysis was used to identify the factors associated with the eGFR slope. The association of P wave parameters with renal end points and the eGFR slope was assessed using a modified stepwise procedure in two modeling steps. The first model consisted of age and sex. In the second model, clinical and biochemical risk factors were added. A significant improvement in model prediction was found by calculating the improvement in −2 log likelihood or adjusted R square values. A difference was considered significant if the *P* value was less than 0.05.

Results

Four hundred and thirty-nine non-dialyzed CKD patients were included. The mean age was 66.0±12.0 years and there were 274 males and 165 females. The average number of serum creatinine measurements during the follow-up period was eight (25th–75th percentile: 6–12). The values of P wave dispersion and maximum P wave duration were 88.8±21.7 ms and 153.3±21.7 ms, respectively. The eGFR slope for all patients was −1.60±0.15 mL/min/1.73 m^2/year. The underlying etiology of CKD in our patients was diabetic kidney disease in 232 (52.8%), non-diabetic glomerular diseases in 128 (29.2%), tubulointerstitial diseases in 46 (10.5%), hypertension in 23 (5.2%), and other diseases in 10 (2.3%). The clinical characteristics of patients with and without renal end points are shown in Table 1. Compared with patients without renal end points, patients with renal end points were found to have higher P wave dispersion, higher maximum P wave duration, higher prevalence of LVH, females outnumbered males, higher prevalence of diabetes mellitus (DM) and hypertension, higher systolic blood pressure, lower BMI, more advanced CKD stage, lower albumin, higher fasting glucose, lower hemoglobin, lower baseline eGFR, higher calcium-phosphorus product, higher uric acid, and higher prevalence of proteinuria.

Risk of progression to renal end points

The mean follow-up period was 25.2±12.7 months (range, 3.3–50.0 months). During the follow-up period, ninety-five patients (21.6%) started hemodialysis and 30 deaths were recorded in the 439 patients. Causes of death included fatal cardiovascular events (n = 13), infectious disease (n = 13), and other (n = 4). Among the 13 fatal cardiovascular events, 4 were myocardial infarction, 3 were pulseless electrical activity, 3 were ventricular fibrillation and 3 were heart failure. The multivariate Cox proportional hazards regression analyses of P wave dispersion and maximum P wave duration for renal end points are shown in Table 2. In the first analysis, P wave dispersion was associated with progression to renal end points in the multivariable model after adjustment for age and sex [hazard ratio (HR), 1.024; 95% confidence interval (CI), 1.014–1.034; $P<0.001$). The relationship remained significant after further adjustment for smoking, DM, hypertension, coronary artery disease, cerebrovascular disease, LVH, systolic and diastolic blood pressure, BMI, albumin, fasting glucose, log triglycerides, total cholesterol, hemoglobin, baseline eGFR, calcium-phosphorus product, uric acid, and proteinuria (HR, 1.020; 95% CI, 1.009–1.032; $P<0.001$). In the second analysis, there was also a significant prognostic value of maximum P wave duration in relation to renal end points (HR, 1.013; 95% CI, 1.003–1.024; $P=0.012$) in multivariate analysis after adjustment for demographic, clinical, and biochemical factors. In addition, the commencement of dialysis and death were competitive risks for composite end points in this study. We also performed competing risk analysis and found that P wave dispersion ($P=0.046$) remained significantly associated with progression to dialysis after multivariate analysis, but maximum P wave duration did not ($P=0.14$).

Table 1. Comparison of baseline characteristics between patients with and without renal end points.

Characteristics	All patients (n = 439)	Patients without renal end points (n = 314)	Patients with renal end points (n = 125)	*P*
Electrocardiogram data				-
P wave dispersion (ms)	90 (76.5–100.8)	88.5 (73.7–97)	93.9 (84.1–105.9)	<0.001
Maximum P wave duration (ms)	154 (140.4–166.8)	151.5 (138–164)	157.3 (144.7–171.7)	0.002
LVH (%)	4.3	2.9	8.0	0.017
Age (year)	67.6 (57.1–76.3)	65.9 (56.9–76.2)	67.5 (57.6–76.4)	0.768
Male gender (%)	62.4	65.9	53.6	0.016
Smoking history (%)	31.0	30.6	32.0	0.770
Diabetes mellitus (%)	56.7	52.9	66.4	0.010
Hypertension (%)	82.2	79.0	90.4	0.005
Coronary artery disease (%)	11.6	10.8	13.6	0.413
Cerebrovascular disease (%)	15.3	14.0	18.7	0.249
Systolic BP (mmHg)	140 (129.5–153)	140 (126.5–150)	149 (130–163.8)	<0.001
Diastolic BP (mmHg)	80 (70–89)	80 (70–88)	79 (69–90)	0.397
Body mass index (kg/m^2)	25.2 (22.8–27.5)	25.4 (23.3–27.7)	24.4 (22.1–26.9)	0.020
CKD stage				<0.001
Stage 3 (%)	38.7	51.0	8.0	
Stage 4 (%)	31.4	36.0	20.0	
Stage 5 (%)	29.8	13.1	72.0	
Laboratory parameters				
Albumin (g/dL)	4.1 (3.9–4.2)	4.1 (4.0–4.3)	3.8 (3.5–4.1)	<0.001
Fasting glucose (mg/dL)	107 (93–139)	104 (91–138)	114 (97–142.8)	0.024
Triglyceride (mg/dL)	138.5 (97–201)	139 (99–199.5)	135 (96–221.75)	0.449
Total cholesterol (mg/dL)	189 (162–220)	188 (162–219)	190.5 (160.8–230.3)	0.693
Hemoglobin (g/dL)	11.6 (9.8–13.3)	12.2 (10.7–13.7)	9.6 (8.5–10.9)	<0.001
Baseline eGFR (mL/min/1.73 m^2)	25.2 (13.1–37.4)	30.4 (21.3–40.7)	11.1 (7.6–16.6)	<0.001
Calcium-phosphorus product (mg^2/dL^2)	37.4 (32.7–42.4)	36.2 (31.8–40.7)	41.9 (34.7–48.3)	<0.001
Uric acid (mg/dL)	7.9 (6.8–9.3)	7.8 (6.8–9.1)	8.4 (6.9–10.1)	0.001
Proteinuria (%)	65.2	55.1	90.4	<0.001

Abbreviations: LVH, left ventricular hypertrophy; BP, blood pressure; CKD, chronic kidney disease; eGFR, estimated glomerular filtration rate.

Table 2. Predictors of progression to renal end points of dialysis or death using Cox proportional hazards model.

	P wave dispersion		Maximum P wave duration	
	HR (95% CI)	*P*	HR (95% CI)	*P*
Unadjusted	1.024 (1.014–1.034)	<0.001	1.016 (1.008–1.025)	<0.001
Age and sex adjusted	1.024 (1.014–1.034)	<0.001	1.017 (1.008–1.025)	<0.001
Multivariate adjusted	1.020 (1.009–1.032)	<0.001	1.013 (1.003–1.024)	0.012

Values express as hazard ratios (HR) and 95% confidence interval (CI).
Multivariate model: adjusted for age, sex, smoking history, diabetes mellitus, hypertension, and coronary artery disease, cerebrovascular disease, left ventricular hypertrophy, systolic and diastolic blood pressure, body mass index, albumin, fasting glucose, log triglycerides, total cholesterol, hemoglobin, baseline eGFR, calcium-phosphorus product, uric acid, and proteinuria.

Figure 1 illustrates the Kaplan-Meier curves for renal end points-free survival in patients subdivided according to the tertiles of P wave dispersion (<83.2, 83.3–96.0, >96.0 ms; log-rank $P<0.001$). The unadjusted HR for tertile 2 *versus* tertile 1 was 1.834 (95% CI, 1.113–3.023, $P=0.017$) and for tertile 3 *versus* tertile 1 was 2.842 (95% CI, 1.173–4.555, $P<0.001$). Figure 2 illustrates the Kaplan–Meier curves for renal end points-free survival in patients subdivided according to the tertiles of maximum P wave duration (<145.0, 145.0–162.0, >162.0 ms; log-rank $P=0.003$). The unadjusted HR for tertile 2 *versus* tertile 1 was 1.385 (95% CI, 0.861–2.226, $P=0.179$) and for tertile 3 *versus* tertile 1 was 2.115 (95% CI, 1.350–3.314, $P=0.001$).

The addition of P wave dispersion and maximum P wave duration to a basic model (including age, sex, DM, hypertension, coronary artery disease, cerebrovascular disease, LVH, systolic and diastolic blood pressure, BMI, albumin, fasting glucose, log triglycerides, total cholesterol, hemoglobin, baseline eGFR, calcium-phosphorus product, uric acid, and proteinuria) significantly improved the prediction value for renal end points (difference in the −2 log likelihood value: 13.531, $P<0.001$ and 6.335, $P=0.012$, respectively).

Patients with CKD stage 5 (n = 131) were at an extremely high risk of reaching end-stage renal disease in a very short term. Therefore, we performed subgroup analysis after excluding those patients. The results were similar, i.e., patients with increased P wave dispersion (HR, 1.060; 95% CI, 1.031–1.089; $P<0.001$) and maximum P wave duration (HR, 1.048; 95% CI, 1.022–1.074; $P<0.001$) were significantly associated with progression to renal end points after multiple adjustments for demographic, clinical, and biochemical factors.

Risk of faster renal function decline

Table 3 shows the determinants of the eGFR slope. In the first multivariate analysis, P wave dispersion was negatively associated with the eGFR slope after adjustment for age and sex (unstandardized coefficient $\beta=-0.020$, $P=0.015$) and, further adjustment for smoking, DM, hypertension, coronary artery disease, cerebrovascular disease, LVH, systolic and diastolic blood pressure, BMI,

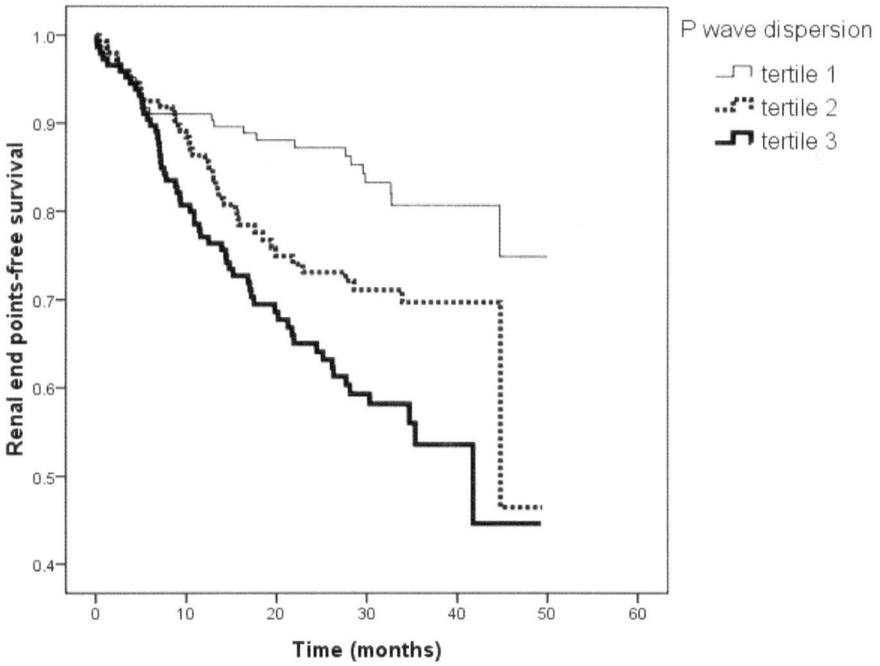

Figure 1. Kaplan-Meier analysis of renal end points-free survival according to the tertiles of P wave dispersion (log-rank *P*<0.001). The group with the highest two tertiles had a worse renal end points-free survival than that with the lowest tertile of P wave dispersion.

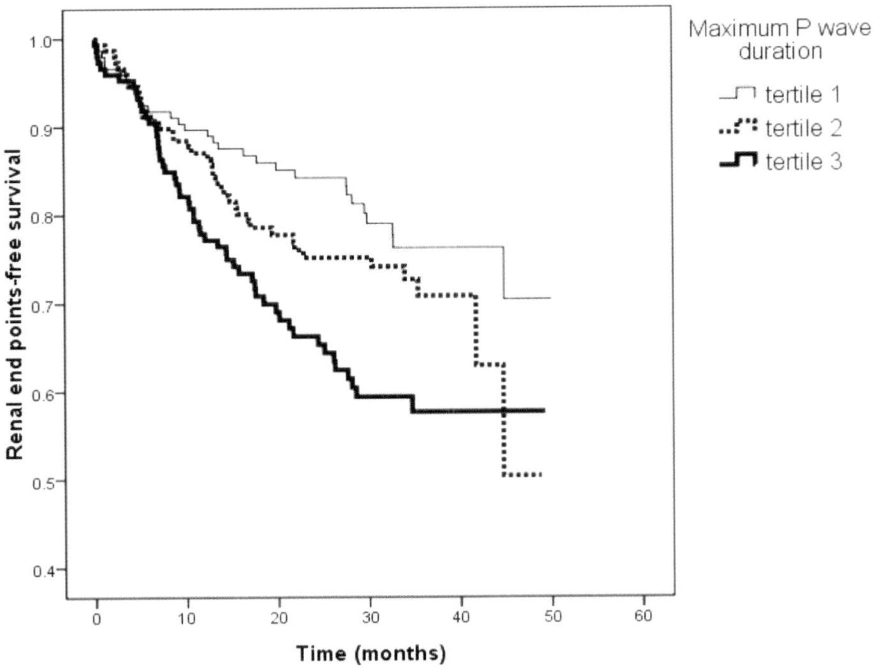

Figure 2. Kaplan-Meier analysis of renal end points-free survival according to the tertiles of maximum P wave duration (log-rank P=0.003). The group with the highest tertile had a worse renal end points-free survival than that with the lowest tertile of maximum P wave duration.

albumin, fasting glucose, log triglycerides, total cholesterol, hemoglobin, baseline eGFR, calcium-phosphorus product, uric acid, and proteinuria (unstandardized coefficient $\beta = -0.016$, $P = 0.037$). In the second multivariate analysis, maximum P wave duration was also negatively associated with the eGFR slope (unstandardized coefficient $\beta = -0.014$, $P = 0.040$) after adjustment for demographic, clinical, and biochemical factors.

The addition of P wave dispersion and maximum P wave duration to a basic model (including age, sex, DM, hypertension, coronary artery disease, cerebrovascular disease, LVH, systolic and diastolic blood pressure, BMI, albumin, fasting glucose, log triglycerides, total cholesterol, hemoglobin, baseline eGFR, calcium-phosphorus product, uric acid, and proteinuria) significantly improved the prediction value for renal function decline (difference in the adjusted R square value: 0.01, $P = 0.037$ and 0.009, $P = 0.040$, respectively).

Determinants of P wave dispersion and maximum P wave duration

In univariate analysis, P wave dispersion had a significant positive correlation with DM (unstandardized coefficient $\beta = 4.366$, $P = 0.020$). In addition, maximum P wave duration had a significant positive correlation with DM, fasting glucose, log triglycerides, and proteinuria. In multivariate analysis, maximum P wave duration was independently correlated with DM (unstandardized coefficient $\beta = 5.635$, $P = 0.015$).

Reproducibility of P wave measurements

The intraobserver mean percent errors for P wave dispersion and maximum P wave duration measurements were 8.6±7.8% and 4.0±3.0%, respectively. The interobserver mean percent errors for P wave dispersion and maximum P wave duration measurements were 10.4±7.3% and 5.0±3.5%, respectively.

Table 3. Determinants of the eGFR slope.

	P wave dispersion		Maximum P wave duration	
	unstandardized coefficient β (95% CI)	***P***	**unstandardized coefficient β (95% CI)**	***P***
Unadjusted	−0.020 (−0.036, −0.004)	0.017	−0.021 (−0.036, −0.007)	0.003
Age and sex adjusted	−0.020 (−0.036, −0.004)	0.015	−0.021 (−0.035, −0.006)	0.005
Multivariate adjusted	−0.016 (−0.031, 0)	0.037	−0.014 (−0.028, 0)	0.040

Abbreviations: eGFR, estimated glomerular filtration rate.
Values expressed as unstandardized coefficient β and 95% confidence interval (CI).
Multivariate model: adjusted for age, sex, smoking history, diabetes mellitus, hypertension, and coronary artery disease, cerebrovascular disease, left ventricular hypertrophy, systolic and diastolic blood pressure, body mass index, albumin, fasting glucose, log triglycerides, total cholesterol, hemoglobin, baseline eGFR, calcium-phosphorus product, uric acid, and proteinuria.

Discussion

In the present study, we evaluated the association of P wave parameters with kidney disease progression to dialysis or death and the rate of renal function decline in patients with CKD stages 3–5. Increased P wave dispersion and maximum P wave duration were associated with progression to dialysis or death and faster renal function decline. Furthermore, the addition of P wave dispersion and maximum P wave duration to a model of clinical features significantly improved the prediction value for progression to dialysis or death and faster renal function decline.

Paoletti et al. [26] studied the role of LVH in the prediction of progression to dialysis in 144 patients with CKD stages 3–4. They found that increased left ventricular mass index was independently associated with CKD progression to dialysis and with combined end points of dialysis or death. Shlipak et al. [27] demonstrated that decreased left ventricular systolic function was an independent predictor of rapid renal function decline (defined as an annual eGFR loss >3 mL/min/1.73 m^2) in the elderly. We recently reported that concentric LVH, increased left atrial diameter, and decreased left ventricular ejection fraction were associated with adverse renal outcomes [5,6]. This suggested that patients with structural or functional abnormalities of the heart might have a faster renal function decline and worse renal outcomes. The mechanisms of faster renal function decline in patients with cardiac abnormalities are multi-factorial, including chronic renal hypoperfusion, subclinical inflammation, endothelial dysfunction, accelerated atherosclerosis, increased renal vascular resistance, systemic neurohormonal factors, pharmacotherapies, and anemia [28,29]. Previous studies have reported that increased P wave dispersion and maximum P wave duration were correlated with left atrial enlargement, LVH, and left ventricular systolic and diastolic dysfunction [12,16,17]. Furthermore, we have previously reported that increased P wave dispersion and maximum P wave duration were associated with progression to the renal end point of ≥ 25% decline in eGFR in 166 patients with a mean eGFR of 57.0±17.2 mL/min/1.73 m^2 [17]. The present study also revealed that increased P wave dispersion and maximum P wave duration were associated with progression to dialysis or death and faster renal function decline in CKD stages 3–5 patients with a mean eGFR of 26.1±14.2 mL/min/1.73 m^2.

Diabetic nephropathy is one of the major complications of DM and one of the major causes of renal replacement therapy [30]. Cardiovascular disease is the leading cause of morbidity and mortality in patients with diabetic nephropathy [31]. This amplified cardiovascular risk is partly attributable to increased traditional risk factors among diabetic patients, along with the non-traditional risk factors among CKD patients, such as proteinuria, fluid retention, anemia, oxidative stress, and the presence of a chronic inflammatory state [31–33]. There are a number of hemodynamic and metabolic disturbances that affect the structure and function of the heart in patients with diabetic nephropathy. The major factors that contribute to further heart failure in diabetic patients include cardiac microangiopathy, neuropathy of the cardiac autonomic nervous system, disturbed metabolism, and fatty degeneration of the myocardium [34]. These patients were reported to have a high prevalence of decreased left ventricular systolic function and increased left ventricular mass index due to pressure and volume overload [35–37]. Our results demonstrated a significant association between P wave parameters and DM, which might be partially explained by ischemic or non-ischemic diabetic cardiomyopathy.

Our study had some limitations. The number and interval of serum creatinine measurements varied in each patient. We therefore excluded patients with less than three eGFR measurements during the follow-up period and those patients with a follow-up period of <3 months, in order to decrease the chance of not completely observing a change in renal function. In addition, P wave parameters cannot completely replace echocardiography because they do not provide a comprehensive examination of the heart. However, they can provide a simple and inexpensive method for detecting patients at risk of left atrial enlargement and left ventricular diastolic and systolic dysfunction.

In conclusion, our results demonstrated that increases in P wave dispersion and maximum P wave duration were independently associated with progression to the renal end points of dialysis or death and faster renal function decline in patients with CKD stages 3–5. Beyond conventional clinical features, measurement of P wave dispersion and maximum P wave duration offers an extra benefit in predicting the renal end points of dialysis or death and faster renal function decline. Screening CKD patients on the basis of P wave dispersion and maximum P wave duration, measured by 12-lead ECG, may help identify patients at high risk for worse renal outcomes.

Author Contributions

Conceived and designed the experiments: J-CH H-MS. Performed the experiments: J-CH S-YW S-CC H-MS. Analyzed the data: J-CH S-YW S-CC J-MC. Contributed reagents/materials/analysis tools: J-CH S-YW S-CC J-MC C-CH H-MS S-JH H-CC. Wrote the paper: J-CH H-MS.

References

1. Go AS, Chertow GM, Fan D, McCulloch CE, Hsu CY (2004) Chronic kidney disease and the risks of death, cardiovascular events, and hospitalization. N Engl J Med 351: 1296–1305.
2. Tonelli M, Wiebe N, Culleton B, House A, Rabbat C, et al. (2006) Chronic kidney disease and mortality risk: a systematic review. J Am Soc Nephrol 17: 2034–2047.
3. Kovesdy CP (2010) Rate of kidney function decline associates with increased risk of death. J J Am Soc Nephrol 21: 1814–1816.
4. Perkins RM, Bucaloiu ID, Kirchner HL, Ashouian N, Hartle JE, et al. (2011) GFR decline and mortality risk among patients with chronic kidney disease. Clin J Am Soc Nephrol 6: 1879–1886.
5. Chen SC, Lin TH, Hsu PC, Chang JM, Lee CS, et al. (2011) Impaired left ventricular systolic function and increased brachial-ankle pulse-wave velocity are independently associated with rapid renal function progression. Hypertens Res 34: 1052–1058.
6. Chen SC, Su HM, Hung CC, Chang JM, Liu WC, et al. (2011) Echocardiographic Parameters are Independently Associated with Rate of Renal Function Decline and Progression to Dialysis in Patients with Chronic Kidney Disease. Clin J Am Soc Nephrol 6: 2750–2758.
7. Furukawa M, Io H, Tanimoto M, Hagiwara S, Horikoshi S, et al. (2011) Predictive factors associated with the period of time before initiation of hemodialysis in CKD stages 4 and 5. Nephron Clin Pract 117: c341–347.
8. Alpert MA, Munuswamy K (1989) Electrocardiographic diagnosis of left atrial enlargement. Arch Intern Med 149: 1161–1165.
9. Birkbeck JP, Wilson DB, Hall MA, Meyers DG (2006) P-wave morphology correlation with left atrial volumes assessed by 2-dimensional echocardiography. J Electrocardiol 39: 225–229.
10. Kim DH, Kim GC, Kim SH, Yu HK, Choi WG, et al. (2007) The relationship between the left atrial volume and the maximum P-wave and P-wave dispersion in patients with congestive heart failure. Yonsei Med J 48: 810–817.
11. Truong QA, Charipar EM, Ptaszek LM, Taylor C, Fontes JD, et al. (2011) Usefulness of electrocardiographic parameters as compared with computed tomography measures of left atrial volume enlargement: from the ROMICAT trial. J Electrocardiol 44: 257–264.
12. Gunduz H, Binak E, Arinc H, Akdemir R, Ozhan H, et al. (2005) The relationship between P wave dispersion and diastolic dysfunction. Tex Heart Inst J 32: 163–167.
13. Yilmaz R, Demirbag R, Durmus I, Kasap H, Baykan M, et al. (2004) Association of Stage of Left Ventricular Diastolic Dysfunction with P Wave

Dispersion and Occurrence of Atrial Fibrillation after First Acute Anterior Myocardial Infarction. Ann Noninvasive Electrocardiol 9: 330–338.

14. Buxton AE, Josephson ME (1981) The role of P wave duration as a predictor of postoperative atrial arrhythmias. Chest 80: 68–73.
15. Soliman EZ, Prineas RJ, Case LD, Zhang Z-m, Goff DC, Jr (2009) Ethnic Distribution of ECG Predictors of Atrial Fibrillation and Its Impact on Understanding the Ethnic Distribution of Ischemic Stroke in the Atherosclerosis Risk in Communities (ARIC) Study. Stroke 40: 1204–1211.
16. Dagli N, Karaca I, Yavuzkir M, Balin M, Arslan N (2008) Are maximum P wave duration and P wave dispersion a marker of target organ damage in the hypertensive population? Clin Res Cardiol 97: 98–104.
17. Su HM, Tsai WC, Lin TH, Hsu PC, Lee WH, et al. (2012) P wave dispersion and maximum P wave duration are independently associated with rapid renal function decline. PloS one 7: e42815.
18. Koz C, Uzun M, Yokusoglu M, Ulas UH, Baysan O, et al. (2008) Echocardiographic, electrocardiographic, and clinical correlates of recurrent transient ischemic attacks: a follow-up study. South Med J 101: 246–251.
19. Magnani JW, Johnson VM, Sullivan LM, Gorodeski EZ, Schnabel RB, et al. (2011) P wave duration and risk of longitudinal atrial fibrillation in persons >/= 60 years old (from the Framingham Heart Study). Am J Cardiol 107: 917–921 e911.
20. (2002) K/DOQI clinical practice guidelines for chronic kidney disease: evaluation, classification, and stratification. Am J Kidney Dis 39: S1–266.
21. Dilaveris PE, Gialafos EJ, Sideris SK, Theopistou AM, Andrikopoulos GK, et al. (1998) Simple electrocardiographic markers for the prediction of paroxysmal idiopathic atrial fibrillation. Am Heart J 135: 733–738.
22. Bazett HC (1920) The time relations of the blood-pressure changes after excision of the adrenal glands, with some observations on blood volume changes. J Physiol 53: 320–339.
23. Sokolow M, Lyon TP (1949) The ventricular complex in left ventricular hypertrophy as obtained by unipolar precordial and limb leads. Am Heart J 37: 161–186.
24. Vickery S, Stevens PE, Dalton RN, van Lente F, Lamb EJ (2006) Does the ID-MS traceable MDRD equation work and is it suitable for use with compensated Jaffe and enzymatic creatinine assays? Nephrol Dial Transplant 21: 2439–2445.
25. Levey AS, Bosch JP, Lewis JB, Greene T, Rogers N, et al. (1999) A more accurate method to estimate glomerular filtration rate from serum creatinine: a new prediction equation. Modification of Diet in Renal Disease Study Group. Ann Intern Med 130: 461–470.
26. Paoletti E, Bellino D, Gallina AM, Amidone M, Cassottana P, et al. (2011) Is left ventricular hypertrophy a powerful predictor of progression to dialysis in chronic kidney disease? Nephrol Dial Transplant 26: 670–677.
27. Shlipak MG, Katz R, Kestenbaum B, Siscovick D, Fried L, et al. (2009) Rapid decline of kidney function increases cardiovascular risk in the elderly. J Am Soc Nephrol 20: 2625–2630.
28. Bock JS, Gottlieb SS (2010) Cardiorenal syndrome: new perspectives. Circulation 121: 2592–2600.
29. Ronco C (2010) Cardiorenal syndromes: definition and classification. Contrib Nephrol 164: 33–38.
30. Ritz E (2006) Diabetic nephropathy. Saudi J Kidney Dis Transpl 17: 481–490.
31. Ritz E (2006) Heart and kidney: fatal twins? Am J Med 119: S31–39.
32. Levin A, Singer J, Thompson CR, Ross H, Lewis M (1996) Prevalent left ventricular hypertrophy in the predialysis population: identifying opportunities for intervention. Am J Kidney Dis 27: 347–354.
33. Levin A, Thompson CR, Ethier J, Carlisle EJ, Tobe S, et al. (1999) Left ventricular mass index increase in early renal disease: impact of decline in hemoglobin. Am J Kidney Dis 34: 125–134.
34. Veves A, Akbari CM, Primavera J, Donaghue VM, Zacharoulis D, et al. (1998) Endothelial dysfunction and the expression of endothelial nitric oxide synthetase in diabetic neuropathy, vascular disease, and foot ulceration. Diabetes 47: 457–463.
35. Glowinska I, Grochowski J, Malyszko J (2008) Cardiovascular complications in patients with diabetic nephropathy receiving pharmacological versus renal replacement therapy. Pol Arch Med Wewn 118: 404–412.
36. Mataradzija A, Resic H, Rasic S, Kukavica N, Masnic F (2010) Risk factors for development of cardiovascular complications in patients with chronic renal disease and diabetic nephropathy. Bosn J Basic Med Sci 10 Suppl 1: S44–50.
37. Chen SC, Chang JM, Liu WC, Tsai YC, Tsai JC, et al. (2012) Stepwise increases in left ventricular mass index and decreases in left ventricular ejection fraction correspond with the stages of chronic kidney disease in diabetes patients. Exp Diabetes Res 2012: 789325.

15

The Association between Contrast Dose and Renal Complications Post PCI across the Continuum of Procedural Estimated Risk

Judith Kooiman[1], Milan Seth[2], David Share[3], Simon Dixon[4], Hitinder S. Gurm[2]*

1 Department of Thrombosis and Hemostasis and Department of Nephrology, Leiden University Medical Center, Leiden, Zuid-Holland, The Netherlands, **2** Department of Internal Medicine, Division of Cardiovascular Medicine, University of Michigan, Ann Arbor, Michigan, United States of America, **3** Blue Cross Blue Shield of Michigan, Detroit, Michigan, United States of America, **4** Beaumont Hospital, Royal Oak, Michigan, United States of America

Abstract

Background: Prior studies have proposed to restrict the contrast volume (CV) to <3x calculated creatinine clearance (CCC), to prevent contrast induced nephropathy (CIN) post percutaneous coronary interventions (PCI). The predictive value of this algorithm for CIN and therefore the benefit of this approach in high risk patients has been questioned. The aim of our study was to assess the association between contrast dose and the occurrence of CIN in patients at varying predicted risks of CIN and baseline CCC following contemporary PCI.

Methods: Consecutive patients undergoing PCI between 2010–2012 were included. Baseline risk of CIN was calculated using a previously validated risk tool. High contrast dose was defined as CV/CCC >3. Likelihood ratio tests were used to evaluate whether the effect of a high contrast dose on the risk of CIN and nephropathy requiring dialysis (NRD) varied across the spectrum of baseline predicted risk.

Results: Of the 82,120 PCI included in our analysis, 25% were performed using a high contrast dose. Patients treated with a high compared with a low contrast dose were at increased risks of CIN and NRD, throughout the entire range of baseline predicted risk and CCC in our population. The effect size of a high contrast dose on risks of both outcomes varied significantly with baseline predicted CIN risk and CCC (CIN $p = 0.004$, NRD $p < 0.001$ for adding interactions), and was largest for patients with predicted CIN risk <10% and pre-existing chronic kidney disease.

Conclusions: The use of a high contrast dose is associated with increased risks of CIN and NRD across the continuum of baseline predicted risk and CCC. Efforts to reduce contrast dose may therefore be effective in preventing renal complications in all patients undergoing PCI.

Editor: Davide Capodanno, Ferrarotto Hospital, University of Catania, Italy

Funding: The BMC2 registry is funded by Blue Cross Blue Shield of Michigan. Hitinder S. Gurm receives research funding from the National Institutes of Health and Agency for Healthcare Research and Quality. The funders had no role in study design, data collection and analysis, decision to publish, or preparation of the manuscript.

Competing Interests: One of the co-authors, Dr. Share is currently employed by Blue Cross Blue Shield of Michigan. Hitinder S. Gurm has, in the interim, consulted for Osprey medical, a company that is developing devices for prevention of contrast induced kidney injury. No compensation was received for this work but the company made a donation to a local non-profit of his choice. This does not alter the authors' adherence to all the PLOS ONE policies on sharing data and materials.

* E-mail: hgurm@med.umich.edu

Introduction

Contrast media induced renal complications are common among patients undergoing percutaneous coronary interventions (PCI) [1]. Contrast induced nephropathy (CIN) and the need for dialysis (NRD) post PCI have been associated with increased early and long-term mortality rates, and add significantly to healthcare expenses [1,2]. Current guidelines support multiple strategies for prophylaxis of CIN including adequate hydration, minimization of contrast dose and the use of iso-osmolar or certain low-osmolar contrast media[3–7].

Use of renal function based contrast dosing with the total contrast volume (CV) restricted to less than thrice the calculated creatinine clearance (CCC) has been suggested as a practical strategy to reduce the risk of CIN [3]. However, the predictive value of this dosing algorithm for CIN and hence the benefit of this approach in patients at high risk of renal complications post PCI has been debated [8].

We recently reported an accurate prediction model for the risk of renal complications in patients undergoing PCI [9]. This model estimates the risk of CIN and NRD based on pre-procedural variables, has a higher discriminative power than other commonly used prediction models, and can therefore be used to study the effect of a high contrast dose on the occurrence of CIN in patients with varying baseline risks of renal complications.

The aim of our current study was to assess the impact of high contrast dose (CV/CCC >3) on the risk of renal complications across the continuum of pre-procedural predicted risk of CIN in a large cohort of patients undergoing contemporary PCI.

Methods

Our study population comprised consecutive patients undergoing PCI between January 2010 and September 2012 across 47 hospitals in Michigan participating in the Blue Cross Blue Shield of Michigan Cardiovascular Consortium (BMC2). Hence, this cohort consists of patients other than the population in which the effect of renal function-based contrast dosing on the risk of renal complications was originally assessed (who underwent PCI between 2007 and 2008) [3]. BMC2 is a quality improvement collaborative that tracks the inpatient outcome of consecutive patients undergoing PCI at all non-federal hospitals in the State of Michigan. The details of the BMC2 and its data collection and auditing process have been described previously [10,11]. Procedural data on all consecutive patients undergoing PCI at participating hospitals are collected using standardized data collection forms. Collected data include clinical and demographic patient characteristics, procedural, and angiographic characteristics, as well as medications used before, during, and after PCI, and in-hospital outcomes. All data elements have been prospectively defined, and the protocol is approved by local institutional review boards at each of the participating hospitals. In addition to a random audit in 2% of all PCI procedures, medical records of all patients undergoing multiple procedures or coronary artery bypass grafting and of patients who died in the hospital are reviewed routinely to ensure data accuracy.

Patients who were already on dialysis at the time of PCI, those with missing serum creatinine values pre or post procedurally, and those who died in the catheterization laboratory were excluded from outcome analysis. Patients with missing values for weight, gender, or CV were also excluded as these variables were needed to determine whether a patient received a high contrast dose. The type and volume of contrast media and hydration protocols used were as per the operator preference guided by institutional policy and practice.

Study Endpoints

CIN was defined as an acute decline in renal function post PCI resulting in an absolute increase in serum creatinine ≥0.5 mg/dL from baseline [12]. Baseline creatinine values were collected within a month prior to PCI. Among patients who had multiple assessments of serum creatinine in the month prior to PCI, the value closest to the time of the procedure was considered as the baseline value. Peak creatinine was defined as the highest value of creatinine in the week following the procedure or during the hospitalization following PCI and was ascertained as per local clinical practice. Time between PCI and peak creatinine was at least 1 day, and varied depending on length of hospital stay. The secondary endpoint for the study was NRD defined as a new, unplanned need for dialysis during hospitalization due to progression of chronic kidney disease post PCI.

High contrast dose was defined as administration of a CV thrice the CCC. CCC was calculated using the Cockgroft-Gault equation [13].

Statistical Analyses

Continuous variables are presented as mean with standard deviation and categorical variables as percentages, with standardized differences between groups presented for both types of variables as percentages. Unless otherwise stated, student t-tests for continuous and Chi-squared tests for categorical variables were utilized for univariate comparisons.

Baseline estimated risk of CIN was calculated using the BMC2 CIN prediction tool [9]. Multivariate logistic regression models with CIN and NRD as outcomes were developed including high contrast dose, baseline estimated CIN risk, CCC, and other baseline clinical covariates as main effect terms. To investigate potential effect modification of baseline predicted CIN risk on CIN and NRD rates associated with a high contrast dose, regression models adding two and three way interaction terms involving baseline estimated CIN risk (logit transformed linear and quadratic terms) and CCC with high contrast dose were fitted to the data. A stepwise selection algorithm optimizing the Akaike Information Criteria was used to select an optimal model. The selected models including interactions were then compared to the base model using likelihood ratio tests to assess whether inclusion of interactions significantly improved the fit of the model.

Model predicted relative risks for CIN and NRD comparing high with low contrast dosages were plotted over a range of CCC and baseline predicted risk of CIN, to demonstrate the extent and implications of effect modification.

All analyses were performed in R version 2.14.1 using freely distributed contributed packages [14,15].

Results

Our study cohort comprised 82,120 (85%) of the 96,753 PCI procedures performed across Michigan between January 2010 through December 2012. Of the 14,633(15%) procedures that were excluded from the analysis, 2,251 (15%) patients were already on dialysis at the time of the procedure, 11,997 (82%) had missing serum creatinine values prior to (n = 2,229 (15%)) or following PCI (n = 9,907 (68%)), with 139 patients missing both pre and post procedural creatinine values. Additionally, 466 patients lacked information on CV, 99 on bodyweight, and 1 patient on gender. As all of these variables were needed to determine whether a patient received a high contrast dose, patients missing one or more of these data elements were excluded.

Table 1 reports characteristics at baseline of study patients categorized to the use of either a low or a high contrast dose at time of PCI (CV/CCC < = 3 and CV/CCC >3). In this cohort, 20,915(25.3%) patients received a high contrast dose who had a greater burden of comorbidities, a higher baseline estimated CIN risk, and were more likely to have preexisting chronic kidney disease.

The median predicted risk of CIN of the cohort was 0.54% (range = 0–80.4%, IQR = 0.08%–2.43%), and 90% of patients had a predicted risk of less than 7.92%. Patients at higher predicted risk of CIN were more likely to be treated with a high contrast dose ($p<0.001$, Figure 1).

CIN occurred in 2,146/82,120 (2.61%, 95% CI 2.51–2.72%) patients, and NRD in 308/82,120 (0.37%, 95% CI 0.33–0.42%). The median baseline CIN risk estimate, calculated using the risk tool, was 11.6% (IQR 3.1–25.5%) among patients developing CIN, and 24.9% (10.9–36.6%) among those with NRD. Of patients with CIN, 1,144/2,146 (53.3%, 95% CI 51.2–55.4%) received a high contrast doses, as did 211/308 (68.5%, 95% CI 63.0–73.7%) patients with NRD.

In regression models adjusting for baseline predicted CIN risk and CCC, high contrast dose was significantly associated with increased rates of both CIN (OR = 1.61, 95% CI 1.46–1.79, P< .001) and NRD (OR = 1.65, 95% CI 1.24–2.21, P<.001), indicating that high contrast dose is an independent predictor of these outcomes. Within a multivariate model adjusting for baseline

Table 1. Baseline characteristics of patients treated with high versus low contrast dose.

Characteristic	CV/CCC ≤3	CV/CCC >3	P-value	Standardized difference (%)
N (procedures)	61.205 (74.5%)	20.915 (25.5%)	NA	NA
BMI	31.48±7.83	27.89±5.63	<0.001	52.54
Age	62.16±11.36	73.26±10.53	<0.001	101.28
Creatinine clearance (CCC)	106.24±42.83	59.10±22.87	<0.001	137.31
Contrast volume (ml)	17[illegible].84±63.15	248.90±88.46	<0.001	100.28
Predicted CIN risk (%)	2.10±4.99	5.23±8.91	<0.001	43.32
Female gender	18.338/61.205 (30.8%)	9.039/20.915 (43.2%)	<0.001	25.98
Race - White	53.502/61.205 (87.4%)	17.725/20.915 (84.7%)	<0.001	7.71
Race - Black or African American	6.139/61.205 (10.1%)	2.655/20.915 (12.7%)	<0.001	8.13
Current/recent smoker (w/in 1 year)	20.138/61.178 (32.9%)	4.099/20.906 (19.6%)	<0.001	30.60
Hypertension	51.108/61.185 (83.5%)	18.726/20.905 (89.6%)	<0.001	17.79
Prior MI	20.910/61.196 (34.2%)	7.645/20.910 (36.6%)	<0.001	5.01
Prior heart failure	7.924/61.185 (13.0%)	4.696/20.907 (22.5%)	<0.001	25.11
Prior PCI	27.440/61.200 (44.8%)	9.087/20.913 (43.5%)	<0.001	2.79
Prior CABG	9.642/61.187 (15.8%)	5.668/20.912 (27.1%)	<0.001	27.92
Cerebrovascular disease	7.821/61.187 (12.8%)	4.652/20.907 (22.3%)	<0.001	25.11
Peripheral arterial disease	8.447/61.190 (13.8%)	4.937/20.909 (23.6%)	<0.001	25.35
Diabetes mellitus	22.697/61.198 (37.1%)	7.715/20.912 (36.9%)	0.614	0.40
CAD presentation/Evaluation				
No symptom. no angina	4.172/61.185 (6.8%)	1.329/20.906 (6.4%)	0.021	1.86
Symptom unlikely ischemic	1.352/61.185 (2.2%)	494/20.906 (2.4%)	0.197	1.03
Stable angina	9.701/61.185 (15.9%)	3.215/20.906 (15.4%)	0.102	1.31
Unstable angina	24.129/61.185 (39.4%)	7.957/20.906 (38.1%)	<0.001	2.82
Non-STEMI	12.223/61.185 (20.0%)	4.619/20.906 (22.1%)	<0.001	5.20
STEMI or equivalent	9.608/61.185 (15.7%)	3.292/20.906 (15.7%)	0.881	0.12
Cardiogenic shock w/in 24 hours	759/61.187 (1.2%)	592/20.909 (2.8%)	<0.001	11.28
Cardiac arrest w/in 24 hours	1.037/61.166 (1.7%)	460/20.901 (2.2%)	<0.001	3.66
PCI Indication				
Immediate PCI for STEMI	8.451/61.195 (13.8%)	2.912/20.909 (13.9%)	0.672	0.34
PCI for STEMI (unstable. >12 hrs from Sx onset)	421/61.195 (0.7%)	223/20.909 (1.1%)	<0.001	4.06
PCI for STEMI (Stable. >12 hrs from Sx onset)	218/61.195 (0.4%)	85/20.909 (0.4%)	0.301	0.82
Staged PCI	4.222/61.195 (6.9%)	870/20.909 (4.2%)	<0.001	12.00

Data are presented as mean (SD), or N (%) unless stated otherwise.
Abbreviations: BMI = body mass index, CIN = contrast induced nephropathy, CV/CCC = contrast volume/calculated creatinine clearance, MI = myocardial infarction, PCI = percutaneous coronary intervention, CABG = coronary artery bypass graft, CAD = coronary artery disease, STEMI = ST-elevation myocardial infarction.

clinical covariates (age, gender, recent heart failure, cardiogenic shock, cardiac arrest, CAD presentation, PCI status and indications), the effect of high contrast dose on the risk of CIN and NRD was consistent for both outcomes (CIN OR = 1.77, 95% CI 1.58–1.98, $P<.001$, NRD OR = 1.92, 95% CI 1.13–2.16, $P<0.01$).

Regression models were developed to investigate potential effect modification of baseline predicted CIN risk and baseline CCC on the association between high contrast dose and the risks of CIN and NRD. The fit of the models were significantly improved compared with the base models after adding of interaction terms involving baseline estimated CIN risk and CCC (Likelihood ratio test: LR 28 on 11 df, $p = 0.004$ for CIN, LR = 29 on 6 df, $p<0.001$ for NRD). This indicates that the effect of high contrast dose on the risks of both CIN and NRD varied significantly across the spectrum of predicted CIN risk and baseline CCC.

Figure 2 depicts the model predicted relative risk of CIN (Figure 2A) and NRD (Figure 2B) for high versus a low contrast dose across the spectrum of baseline predicted risk and CCC. Both figures demonstrate an increased risk of renal complications post PCI associated with a high contrast dose regardless of a patient's baseline predicted risk or CCC, although the effect of a high contrast dose was most pronounced in those at lower predicted risk. The points on the graphed surfaces highlighted in red represent the estimated relative risks of high versus a low contrast dose at the median baseline risk and creatinine clearance values for patients with CIN (risk: 11.6%, CCC: 57 ml/min) and NRD (risk: 24.9%, CCC: 42.6 ml/min). The relative risk associated with

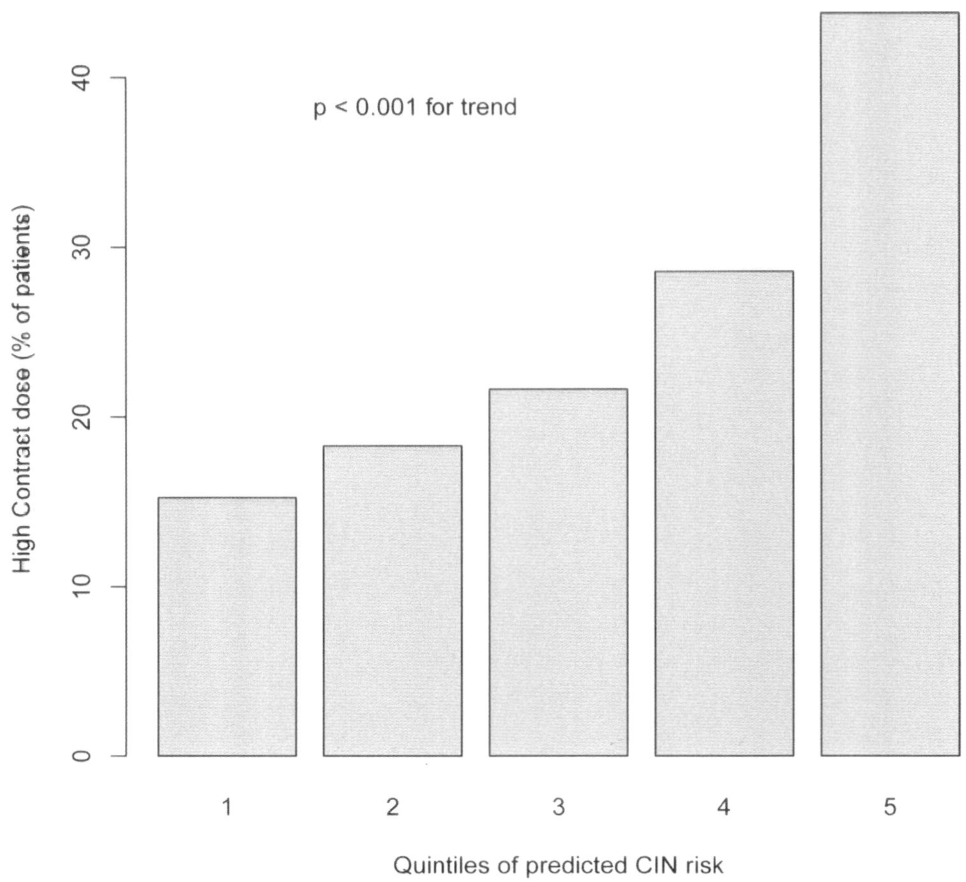

Figure 1. Proportions of patients treated with high dose contrast (Contrast volume/calculated creatinine clearance >3) across the quintiles of predicted risk of contrast induced nephropathy.

high a contrast dose at this point is 1.56 (95% CI 1.37–1.76) for CIN, and 2.05 (95% CI 1.35–2.75) for NRD.

Discussion

The key finding of our study is that the use of a high contrast dose is associated with increased risks of CIN and NRD across the

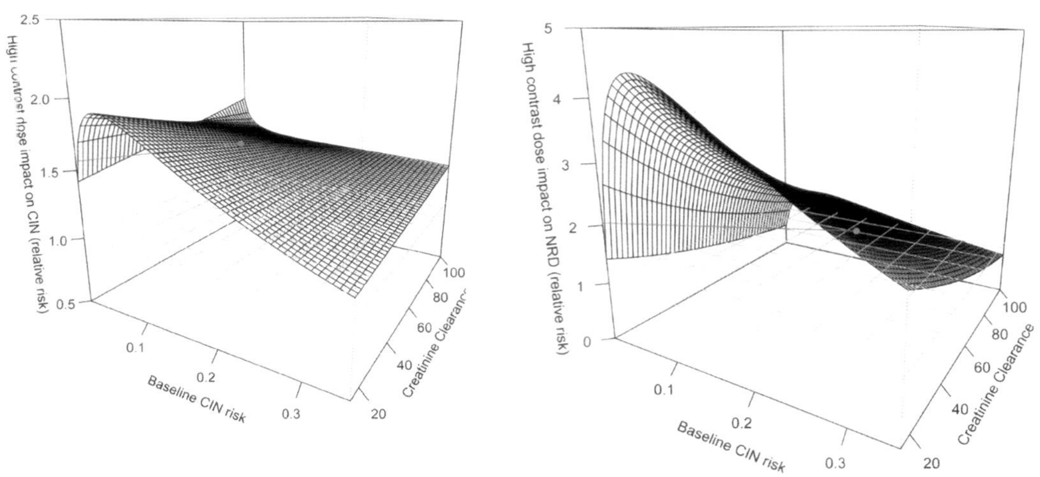

Figure 2. A. The relative risk of contrast induced nephropathy in association with high contrast dose across the continuum of predicted risk of contrast induced nephropathy among patients undergoing PCI. **B.** The relative risk of nephropathy requiring dialysis in association with high contrast dose across the continuum of predicted risk of contrast induced nephropathy among patients undergoing PCI.

continuum of predicted risk and CCC. Efforts to reduce the contrast dose may therefore be effective in preventing renal complications in all patients undergoing PCI. Especially in patients with pre-existing renal failure, restricting the contrast dose might result in lower rates of NRD.

Our findings significantly add to extend prior observations in this field. Work from many groups including ours has highlighted the role of high contrast dose as a risk factor for CIN and NRD in patients undergoing invasive cardiac procedures [3,16,17]. We have now demonstrated that regardless of baseline CCC and predicted risk of renal complications, the use of a high contrast dose is associated with increased risks of CIN and NRD post PCI. These results are in line with the results of two previous smaller studies concluding a high contrast dose to be associated with an increased risk of CIN throughout the continuum of baseline renal function [18,19]. These studies however, did not analyze the effect of baseline predicted risk on the association between a high contrast dose and renal complications post PCI. Our results demonstrated the effect of a high contrast dose on the risk of CIN and NRD to be most pronounced in those at lower predicted risk.

Efforts to improve outcomes of patients undergoing PCI for acute myocardial infarction or cardiogenic shock have traditionally focused on enhancing myocardial perfusion and hemodynamic support [20,21]. Restriction of contrast dose might be another important strategy to improve patient outcome after PCI, as our study findings suggest that the use of high contrast dosages is associated with an increased risk of CIN in all patients undergoing PCI. Limiting the CV to less than thrice the CCC may be even more important in patients at high risk of CIN, in terms of an absolute risk reduction, but also in those with pre-existing chronic kidney disease (i.e. eGFR <60 ml/min) in whom the effect of a high contrast dose on the risks of CIN was more profound compared to those without renal impairment. Our study findings also suggest that efforts to limit contrast dose in patients undergoing PCI may be helpful in reducing the risk of NRD, a complication which although rare, has not declined in the last few years among patients undergoing PCI, regardless of the introduction of less nephrotoxic contrast agents.

Patients at high predicted risk of CIN were more likely to receive a high contrast dose in our study. These patients might more frequently have comorbidity than patients receiving a low contrast dose, like peripheral artery disease, or an altered coronary vasculature due to prior PCI or prior coronary artery bypass graft resulting in more complex PCI procedures, requiring higher contrast volumes. Additionally, as a high contrast dose (CV/CCC >3) is also driven by impaired renal function, the frequent use of a high contrast dose in patients at high risk might also be explained by comorbidity associated with chronic kidney disease, increasing the baseline predicted risk of CIN. Measures to reduce contrast dose are well recognized in literature but most of the work on contrast preservation has been performed in elective or stable patients, not those with acute myocardial infarction. Therefore, further research of the preventive effect of contrast preservation on the risk of renal complications in patients undergoing emergent PCI is warranted [22].

Our study findings must, however, be interpreted with certain qualifications. Our study associations, while strong do not support causality. However, it is unlikely that a randomized trial would ever be performed to evaluate the impact of high versus low contrast dose on the risk of renal complications. Since the findings appear biologically plausible and statistically robust, measures to limit contrast dose especially in high risk patients should be considered to reduce the risk of CIN and NRD. We have used the term CIN, although the role of contrast media in all patients who develop acute kidney injury after PCI remains debatable. It is likely that acute kidney injury after PCI is multifactorial and it may be preferable to use terms that do not assume that all renal dysfunction after PCI is secondary to contrast media. However, regardless of the term used, our study suggests that there is strong association between a high contrast dose and acute renal failure post PCI, even in high risk patients, implying that contrast media have an important contributory role towards the development of acute renal failure post PCI observed in this population. Only one post -procedure creatinine value was available and no follow up beyond the initial hospitalization was performed. Moreover, we lacked information on the timing of post-procedure serum creatinine measurements. No data on the type and amount of hydration used were available and this likely varied across institutions. However, we believe this makes our findings more generalizable to routine clinical care since it reflects observations from contemporary practice across multiple institutions.

To conclude, the use of a high contrast dose at time of PCI is associated with increased risks of CIN and NRD in all patients, regardless of their baseline predicted risk of these complications and renal function. Future research is needed to study whether the use of CV restricting measures decrease the risk of renal complications post PCI in patients with acute myocardial infarction. Until then, efforts to reduce CVs to less than thrice a patient's CCC should be encouraged for all patients undergoing PCI.

Author Contributions

Conceived and designed the experiments: HG JK MS. Analyzed the data: MS. Wrote the paper: JK. Provided critical review on study design and revision of the manuscript: SD DS.

References

1. Rihal CS, Textor SC, Grill DE, Berger PB, Ting HH, et. al. Incidence and prognostic importance of acute renal failure after percutaneous coronary intervention. Circulation 105: 2259–2264.
2. Gupta R, Gurm HS, Bhatt DL, Chew DP, Ellis SG (2005) Renal failure after percutaneous coronary intervention is associated with high mortality. Catheter Cardiovasc Interv 64: 442–448. 10.1002/ccd.20316 [doi].
3. Gurm HS, Dixon SR, Smith DE, Share D, Lalonde T, et al. (2011) Renal function-based contrast dosing to define safe limits of radiographic contrast media in patients undergoing percutaneous coronary interventions. J Am Coll Cardiol 58: 907–914. S0735–1097(11)02052–3 [pii];10.1016/j.jacc.2011.05.023 [doi].
4. Meier P, Ko DT, Tamura A, Tamhane U, Gurm HS (2009) Sodium bicarbonate-based hydration prevents contrast-induced nephropathy: a meta-analysis. BMC Med 7: 23. 1741-7015-7-23 [pii];10.1186/1741-7015-7-23 [doi].
5. Reed M, Meier P, Tamhane UU, Welch KB, Moscucci M, et al. (2009) The relative renal safety of iodixanol compared with low-osmolar contrast media: a meta-analysis of randomized controlled trials. JACC Cardiovasc Interv 2: 645–654. S1936-8798(09)00322-7 [pii];10.1016/j.jcin.2009.05.002 [doi].
6. Reed MC, Moscucci M, Smith DE, Share D, Lalonde T, et al. (2010) The relative renal safety of iodixanol and low-osmolar contrast media in patients undergoing percutaneous coronary intervention. Insights from Blue Cross Blue Shield of Michigan Cardiovascular Consortium (BMC2). J Invasive Cardiol 22: 467–472.
7. Stacul F, van der Molen AJ, Reimer P, Webb JA, Thomsen HS, et al. (2011) Contrast induced nephropathy: updated ESUR Contrast Media Safety Committee guidelines. Eur Radiol 21: 2527–2541. 10.1007/s00330-011-2225-0 [doi].
8. Kalra N, Fenster P (2012) Is renal function-based contrast dosing of radiographic contrast media in patients undergoing percutaneous coronary intervention sufficient to delineate safe limits of contrast dose? J Am Coll Cardiol 59: 432–433. S0735-1097(11)04825-X [pii];10.1016/j.jacc.2011.09.060 [doi].
9. Gurm HS, Seth M, Kooiman J, Share D (2013) A novel tool for reliable and accurate prediction of renal complications in patients undergoing percutaneous coronary intervention. J Am Coll Cardiol 61: 2242–2248. S0735-1097(13)01348-X [pii];10.1016/j.jacc.2013.03.026 [doi].

10. Kline-Rogers E, Share D, Bondie D, Rogers B, Karavite D, et al. (2002) Development of a multicenter interventional cardiology database: the Blue Cross Blue Shield of Michigan Cardiovascular Consortium (BMC2) experience. J Interv Cardiol 15: 387–392.
11. Moscucci M, Rogers EK, Montoye C, Smith DE, Share D, et.al. (2006) Association of a continuous quality improvement initiative with practice and outcome variations of contemporary percutaneous coronary interventions. Circulation 113: 814–822. CIRCULATIONAHA.105.541995 [pii];10.1161/CIRCULATIONAHA.105.541995 [doi].
12. Slocum NK, Grossman PM, Moscucci M, Smith DE, Aronow HD, et al. (2012) The changing definition of contrast-induced nephropathy and its clinical implications: insights from the Blue Cross Blue Shield of Michigan Cardiovascular Consortium (BMC2). Am Heart J 163: 829–834. S0002-8703(12)00095-6 [pii];10.1016/j.ahj.2012.02.011 [doi].
13. Cockcroft DW, Gault MH (1976) Prediction of creatinine clearance from serum creatinine. Nephron 16: 31–41.
14. Liaw A, Wiener M (2002) Classification and Regression by random Forest. R News 2: 18–22.
15. Robin X, Turck N, Hainard A, Tiberti N, Lisacek F, et.al. (2011) pROC: an open-source package for R and S+ to analyze and compare ROC curves. BMC Bioinformatics 12: 77. 1471-2105-12-77 [pii];10.1186/1471-2105-12-77 [doi].
16. Marenzi G, Assanelli E, Campodonico J, Lauri G, Marana I, et al. (2009) Contrast volume during primary percutaneous coronary intervention and subsequent contrast-induced nephropathy and mortality. Ann Intern Med 150: 170–177. 150/3/170 [pii].
17. Freeman RV, O'Donnell M, Share D, Meengs WL, Kline-Rogers E, et al. (2002) Nephropathy requiring dialysis after percutaneous coronary intervention and the critical role of an adjusted contrast dose. Am J Cardiol 90: 1068–1073. S0002914902027716 [pii].
18. Nyman U, Bjork J, Aspelin P, Marenzi G (2008) Contrast medium dose-to-GFR ratio: a measure of systemic exposure to predict contrast-induced nephropathy after percutaneous coronary intervention. Acta Radiol 49: 658–667. 792395239 [pii];10.1080/02841850802050762 [doi].
19. Brown JR, Robb JF, Block CA, Schoolwerth AC, Kaplan AV, et. al. (2010) Does safe dosing of iodinated contrast prevent contrast-induced acute kidney injury? Circ Cardiovasc Interv 3: 346–350. CIRCINTERVENTIONS.109.910638 [pii];10.1161/CIRCINTERVENTIONS.109.910638 [doi].
20. Mehran R, Aymong ED, Nikolsky E, Lasic Z, Iakovou I, et.al. (2004) A simple risk score for prediction of contrast-induced nephropathy after percutaneous coronary intervention: development and initial validation. J Am Coll Cardiol 44: 1393–1399. S0735-1097(04)01445-7 [pii];10.1016/j.jacc.2004.06.068 [doi].
21. McCullough PA (2008) Contrast-induced acute kidney injury. J Am Coll Cardiol 51: 1419–1428. S0735-1097(08)00353-7 [pii];10.1016/j.jacc.2007.12.035 [doi].
22. Nayak KR, Mehta HS, Price MJ, Russo RJ, Stinis CT, et al. (2010) A novel technique for ultra-low contrast administration during angiography or intervention. Catheter Cardiovasc Interv 75: 1076–1083. 10.1002/ccd.22414 [doi].

16

Clinical Analysis of Cause, Treatment and Prognosis in Acute Kidney Injury Patients

Fan Yang, Li Zhang, Hao Wu, Hongbin Zou, Yujun Du*

Department of Nephrology, The First Bethune Hospital of Jilin University, Jilin, China

Abstract

Acute kidney injury (AKI) is characterized by an abrupt decline in renal function, resulting in an inability to secrete waste products and maintain electrolyte and water balance, and is associated with high risks of morbidity and mortality. This study retrospectively analyzed clinical data, treatment, and prognosis of 271 hospitalized patients (172 males and 99 females) diagnosed with AKI from December, 2008 to December, 2011. In addition, this study explored the association between the cause of AKI and prognosis, severity and treatment of AKI. The severity of AKI was classified according to the Acute Kidney Injury Network (AKIN) criteria. Renal recovery was defined as a decrease in a serum creatinine level to the normal value. Prerenal, renal, and postrenal causes accounted for 36.5% (99 patients), 46.5% (126 patients) and 17.0% (46 patients), respectively, of the incidence of AKI. Conservative, surgical, and renal replacement treatments were given to 180 (66.4%), 30 (11.1%) and 61 patients (22.5%), respectively. The overall recovery rate was 21.0%, and the mortality rate was 19.6%. Levels of Cl^-, Na^+ and carbon dioxide combining power decreased with increasing severity of AKI. Cause and treatment were significantly associated with AKI prognosis. Likewise, the severity of AKI was significantly associated with cause, treatment and prognosis. Multivariate logistic regression analysis found that respiratory injury and multiple organ dysfunction syndrome (MODS) were associated with AKI patient death. Cause, treatment and AKIN stage are associated with the prognosis of AKI. Respiratory injury and MODS are prognostic factors for death of AKI patients.

Editor: Cephas Tagumirwa Musabayane, University of KwaZulu-Natal, South Africa

Funding: The authors have no support or funding to report.

Competing Interests: The authors have declared that no competing interests exist.

* E-mail: kjkduyujun@126.com

Introduction

The kidney is critical in maintaining a stable internal environment by regulating the body fluid volume, maintaining electrolyte balance, and excreting potentially metabolic toxic end products. Glomerular filtration, tubular reabsorption, and tubular secretion are involved in forming urine. Glomerular infiltration involves the ultrafiltration of plasma in the glomerulus, and the filtrates, including water, salts, glucose and urea, are accumulated in the urinary space of Bowman's capsule. Tubular reabsorption involves reabsorption of approximately 99% of the infiltrates into the blood, while tubular secretion involves the transport of substances such as K^+, H^+, ammonium, creatinine, and urea into the urine. The volume of urine formed is approximately 1.5 liter per day for an adult".

Acute kidney injury (AKI), previously called acute renal failure, is characterized by an abrupt decline in renal function, resulting in an inability to secrete wastes and maintain electrolyte and water balance. [1] AKI has clinical manifestations ranging from a small elevation in serum creatinine (SCr) levels to anuric renal failure. [2] The severity of AKI is defined by Risk Injury Failure Loss End-Stage (RIFLE) and Acute Kidney Injury Network (AKIN) criteria, which are based on the presence of increased SCr levels and/or a decreased urine output. [1,3] The AKIN definition also emphasizes the change in SCr levels over a short period of time (within 48 h). This serious disorder may aggravate pre-existing kidney disease, thus leading to a rapid loss of renal function. Several studies have shown that AKI is associated with an increased risk of morbidity and mortality.[4–6] The most important factor contributing to mortality after AKI is the underlying cause of AKI. [7,8].

To reduce the severity of and improve recovery from AKI, it is important to identify the underlying cause of AKI. The etiologies of AKI are commonly categorized into prerenal, renal or postrenal. Prerenal AKI is due to impaired blood flow to the kidneys as a result of decreased blood volume, low circulating volume to the kidneys, and agents that reduce renal blood flow. Renal AKI is due to damage to the renal parenchyma, such as glomeruli, renal tubules and interstitium. Postrenal AKI is due to the obstruction of the urinary tract. The most common causes of AKI are frequently associated with infection, renal ischemia, and nephrotoxic drugs. [7,9].

Successful management of AKI requires correction of underlying causes, management of complications, including hyperkalemia and acidosis, and timely renal replacement therapies (RRT). [9] Restoration of normal renal perfusion with intravenous fluids is the primary therapy for prerenal AKI. Relief of the obstruction is necessary to prevent irreversible kidney damage. Surgical intervention may be used to permanently remove any obstruction. In addition, fluid replacement therapy, nutritional support, avoidance of nephrotoxic agents and pharmacological intervention are used to treat AKI patients. [9,10] RRT, such as intermittent hemodialysis (IHD), continuous renal replacement therapies (CRRT) and peritoneal dialysis (PD), have been used for AKI

Table 1. The baseline characteristics of the 271 AKI patients.

Characteristics	**Patients (n = 271)**
sex	
Male n (%)	172 (63.5%)
female n (%)	99 (36.5%)
length of hospital stay (interquartile range)	8 days (3–16 days)
Patients in department of hospitalization	
Department of Internal Medicine (%)	142 (52.4%)
Department of Surgery (%)	90 (33.2%),
ICU (%)	39 (14.4%)
Division of Nephrology (%)	40 (14.8%)
History	
Allergy (%)	15 (5.5%)
Smoking n (%)	88 (32.5%),
Drinking alcohol (%)	49 (18.1%)
SCr levels (μmol/l)	
First abnormal median SCr (interquartile range)	303.2 (167.4-553.5)
Median SCr levels at peak (interquartile range)	491.0 (323.8–716.0)
Median SCr levels at charge (interquartile range)	235.0 114.0–488.0)
BUN levels (mmol/l)	
First abnormal median BUN (interquartile range)	17.7 (10.9–27.22)
Median BUN levels at peak (interquartile range)	28.1 (19.06–36.83)
Median BUN levels at charge (interquartile range)	15.92 (8.0–27.0)

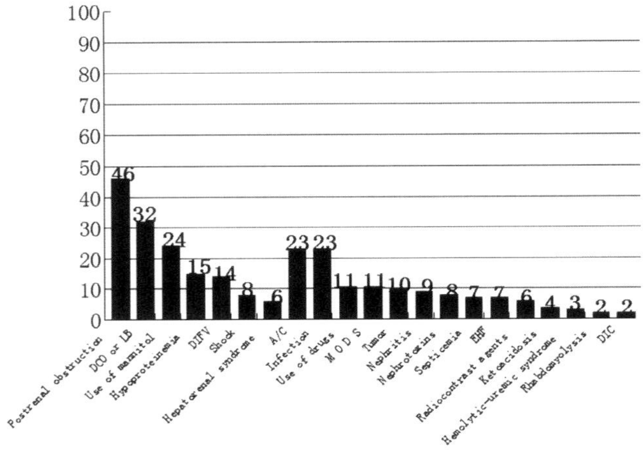

Figure 2. Causes of AKI in patients. From left to right:postrenal obstruction; prerenal causes, including decreased cardiac output or loss of blood (DCO or LB), use of mannitol, hypoproteinemia, decreased intravascular fluid volume (DIFV), shock, and hepatorenal syndrome; renal causes, including AKI in chronic kidney disease (A/C), infection, use of drugs, multiple organ dysfunction syndrome (MODS), tumors, nephritis, nephrotoxins, septicemia, epidemic hemorrhagic fever (EHF), radiocontrast agents, ketoacidosis, hemolytic-uremic syndrome, rhabdomyolysis, and disseminated intravascular coagulation (DIC).

patients with complications such as hyperkalemia, metabolic acidosis, acute pulmonary edema and uremic symptoms. [9,11].

Despite significant advances in supportive care, the mortality rate of AKI has not significantly improved over the past several decades. The in-hospital mortality rate is approximately 20% to 50% and may exceed 75% in critically ill patients or patients with sepsis.[12–14] The rate of renal recovery varies in the literature, possibly because of the lack of a consistent definition for renal recovery. Some studies reported that recovery rates ranged from 36% to 99%, based on the definition of recovery as dialysis independence at discharge. [4,15,16] Ali *et al.* [*17*] reported a rate of 68% for complete recovery and 5% for partial recovery, based on the definition of recovery as a decrease in SCr levels to baseline levels.

In this study, we retrospectively investigated 271 patients with AKI from December, 2008 to December, 2011. We categorized our patients according to the severity of AKI based on the AKIN criteria. The purpose of this study was to analyze clinical data, cause, treatment and prognosis of AKI patients with different AKI stages.

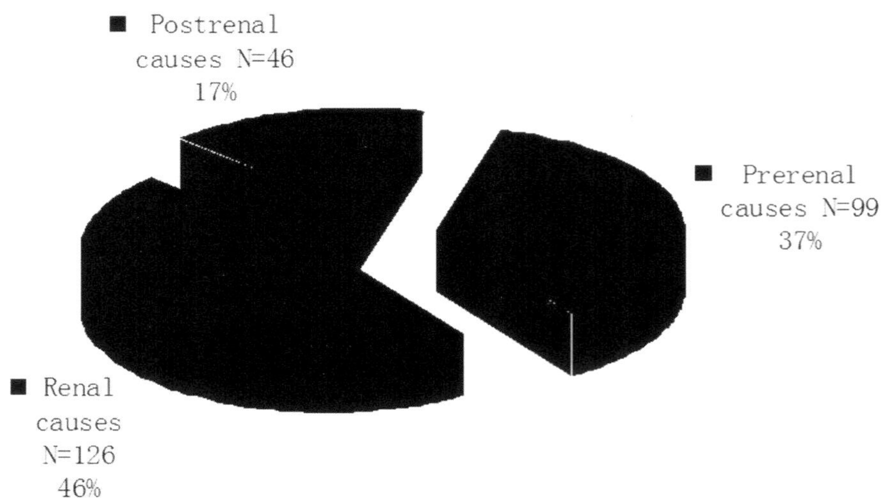

Figure 1. Etiologies of AKI patients. Causes of AKI were categorized into prerenal, renal, and postrental.

Table 2. Correlation between the cause of AKI and prognosis and treatment.

	Prognosis n (%)				
	Complete recovery	**Partial Recovery**	**No recovery**	**Discharge without treatment**	**Death**
Causes					
Prerenal (n = 99)	24 (24.2)	29 (29.3)	10 (10.1)	9 (9.1)	27 (27.3)
Renal (n = 126)	18 (14.3)	47 (37.3)	12 (9.5)	25 (19.8)	24 (19.2)
Postrenal (n = 46)	15 (32.6)	26 (56.5)	0 (0.0)	3 (6.5)	2 (4.4)
Treatment					
Conservative	41 (22.8)	39 (21.7)	19 (10.6)	33 (18.3)	48 (26.7)
Surgical	11(36.7)	19 (63.3)	0 (0.0)	0 (0.0)	0 (0.0)
RRT	5 (8.2)	44 (72.1)	3 (4.9)	4 (6.6)	5 (8.2)

RRT: renal replacement therapy. For cause: $x^2 = 32.08$: $P<0.0001$ (chi square). For treatment: $x^2 = 73.57$, $P<0.0001$ (chi square).

Materials and Methods

Patients

The study was approved by the ethics committee of The First Bethune Hospital of JiLin University, JiLin, China. All data used in this retrospective study were collected during the course of routine medical care in the hospital, and patients were not asked to give informed consent at the time of these clinical encounters. Since the study was retrospective and patient data were all de-identified, the Ethics Committee waived the need for written informed consent (No. 2011–12). All the data used in this study were previously collected, and use of these data did not pose any additional risks to the patients. This retrospective study included 271 patients (172 males and 99 females) admitted to our hospital and diagnosed with AKI from December, 2008 to December, 2011. We included all patients with AKI except those who had only one SCr measurement. Clinical data such as age, gender, admission and discharge times, days of hospitalization, and history of allergies, smoking, and drinking were recorded for all patients. We also evaluated other clinical information, including the department in charge of hospitalization, primary diagnosis, etiology, treatment, complications, and prognosis. Laboratory tests including SCr, blood urine nitrogen (BUN), Ca^{2+}, K^+, Na^+, Cl^-, carbon dioxide combining power (CO_2CP), hemoglobin (HGB), hematocrit (HCT), serum albumin (ALB), urine blood (BLO) and urine protein (Pro) were reviewed. These biological parameters were measured using an automatic biochemistry analyzer (Hitachi 76000, Japan). The laboratory data at the first or latest abnormal SCr were used for analysis. BUN and SCr levels at peak and at discharge were also recorded. Kidney size was calculated from radiological imaging after AKI diagnosis was analyzed. The normal kidney size in Chinese patients was 10.5–11.5 cm (length)×5.0–7.2 cm (width)×2.0–3.0 cm (thickness). Enlarged kidney was defined as a length >11.5, a width > 7.2 cm, or a thickness >3.0 cm. A reduced-sized kidney was defined as a length <10.5, a width <5.0 cm, or a thickness < 2.0 cm.

Definition and Criteria of AKI

AKI was defined as an absolute increase in SCr of at least 26.5 μmol/l (0.3 mg/dl) or a 50% or above increase in SCr from baseline according to the AKIN criteria. [3] The severity of AKI was defined by the AKIN staging criteria as follows: Stage I, SCr increase to 1.5–2 fold of baseline; Stage II, SCr increase to 2–3 fold of baseline; and Stage III, SCr increase to >3 fold of baseline or an absolute increase of >356.6 μmol/l (4.0 mg/dl) with an acute increase of at least 44.2 μmol/l (0.5 mg/dl). All patients who needed dialysis were categorized into Stage III. [3] AKI was classified as prerenal, renal or postrenal AKI according to the identified causes. The prerenal causes were categorized as follows: (a) decreased cardiac output or loss of blood due to myocardial infarction, arrhythmia, ischemic heart diseases, cardiomyopathy, hypertensive diseases or corpumonale; (b) decreased intravascular fluid volume due to diarrhea, vomiting, severe burn, or pancreatitis; (c) hypoproteinemia; (d) shock; (e) hepatorenal syndrome; and (f) use of mannitol. The renal causes were categorized as follows: (a) AKI in chronic kidney disease (A/C); (b) infection; (c) drugs; (d) multiple organ dysfunction syndrome

Table 3. AKI stage in 271 patients with AKI.

AKI Stage: n (%)	Median age (years)	Length of hospital stay (days)
Stage I 86 (33.7)	59 (46–72)	10 (3–21)
Stage II 44 (16.2)	57 (38.5–68)	8.5 (2.5–15)
Stage II1 141 (52.0)	50 (37–64)	7 (4–14)
P value	0.13	0.21
H value	8.66	3.14

Table 4. Association* of AKI stage with department of hospitalization.

	Department of Hospitalization n(%)			
AKI stages	**Internal departments#**	**Surgery**	**ICU**	**Nephrology**
Stage I	47 (54.7)	17 (19.8)	13 (15.1)	9 (10.5)
Stage II	20 (45.5)	16 (36.4)	3 (6.8)	5 (11.4)
Stage III	35 (24.8)	57 (40.4)	23 (16.3)	26(18.4)

Department of Internal Medicine excluding the Division of Nephrology.
*Chi square test, P = 0.003, $x^2 = 25.36$.

(MODS); (e) tumor; (f) interstial nephritis; (g) nephrotoxin exposure; (h) septicemia; (i) epidemic hemorrhagic fever (EHF); (j radiocontrast agents; (k) ketoacidosis; (l) hemolytic-uremic syndrome; (m) rhabdomyolysis; and (n) disseminated intravascular coagulation (DIC). The postrenal causes included obstructions distal to the collecting systems due to tumors, stones, urethral structure, prostate hypertrophy, or neurogenic bladder.

Treatment of AKI

Patients were categorized according to the treatment for AKI as follows: conservative treatment; surgical treatment; and renal replacement therapy (RRT). RRT included intermittent hemodialysis (IHD), continuous renal replacement therapy (CRRT) and peritoneal dialysis (PD). Surgical treatment included surgical removal of obstructive tumors, stones, or prostate hypertrophy. Patients without RRT and surgical treatment were included in the conservative treatment group. Treatment included correction of the primary cause of AKI, fluid replacement therapy, and nutritional support. IfAKI was due to serious trauma, heart failure and acute hemorrhage, patients were administered normal saline to correct intravascular volume depletion. In AKI patients with severe hyperkalemia, 5–10 units of insulin and 50% dextrose were used to promote uptake of potassium into cells. Supportive therapies such as antibiotics and adequate nutrition were given according to standard management practice. All medications that could potentially affect renal function were discontinued.

Outcome of AKI

Renal recovery was defined according to the SCr levels at discharge as follows: 1) complete recovery, defined as a decrease in SCr levels to the baseline value; 2) partial recovery, defined as a decrease in SCr levels compared with peak SCr, but the final Scr level was above baseline; and 3) no recovery, defined by no decrease in SCr levels compared with peak SCr. The outcomes of patients were classified as follows: (a) complete recovery; (b) partial recovery; (c) no recovery; (d) discharge without treatment, defined as discharge without comprehensive treatment in the hospital; and (e) death during hospitalization.

Statistical Analysis

Analyses were performed using SPSS 17.0 software (SPSS, Chicago, IL, USA). Quantitative data with normal distribution were expressed as means ± SD and analyzed using analysis of variance (ANOVA). Quantitative data without normal distribution were expressed as median and interquartile range and analyzed using the rank sum test. Categorical data were expressed as frequency and percentage and analyzed using a chi square analysis. Ranked data were expressed as frequency and composition and analyzed using a Wilcoxon rank sum test. Spearman's partial correlation tests were used to analyze the association between AKI causes and the prognosis and treatment after adjusting for age and sex. Multivariate logistic regression was used when more than one independent variable was involved. Any variable having a significant univariate test was selected as a candidate for the multivariate analysis. $P<0.05$ was considered statistically significant.

Results

Clinical Characteristics of AKI Patients

The baseline characteristics of the 271 AKI patients are shown in Table 1. 172 (63.5%) were male and 99 (36.5%) were female. The median age was 54 years (interquartile range, 39–68 years). The median length of hospital stay was 8 days (interquartile range, 3–16 days). Hospitalization occurred in the Department of Internal Medicine, Department of Surgery, ICU and Division of Nephrology for 142 (52.4%), 90 (33.2%), 39 (14.4%), and 40 (14.8%) patients, respectively. The number of patients with a history of allergy, smoking, or drinking alcohol was 15 (5.5%), 88 (32.5%), or 49 (18.1%), respectively.

When the first abnormal SCr values occurred, the median BUN and SCr levels were 17.7 mmol/l (interquartile range, 10.9–27.22 mmol/l) and 303.2 μmol/l (interquartile range, 167.4–553.5 μmol/l), respectively. There were 210 (71.8%) and 222 (77.4%) patients who had hematuria and proteinuria, respectively. Median SCr levels at peak and at discharge were 491.0 μmol/l (interquartile range, 323.8–716.0 μmol/l) and 235.0 μmol/l (interquartile range, 114.0–488.0 μmol/l), respectively. Median BUN levels at peak and at discharge were28.1 mmol/l(interquartile range, 19.06–36.83 mmol/l)and15.92 mmol/l (interquartile range, 8.0–27.0 mmol/l), respectively.

Kidney size was examined in 107 (39.5%) of 271 patients after AKI diagnosis. The number of patients with normal-sized, enlarged or reduced-size kidneys or with only one kidney were 85 (79.4%), 16 (15.0%), 6 (5.6%) or 6 (5.6%), respectively.

Table 5. Association of AKI stage with laboratory tests.

	Stages			
	Stage I	**Stage II**	**Stage III**	**P Value**
HCT	0.36 (0.30–0.41)	0.37 (0.31–0.42)	0.34 (0.27–0.40)	0.11
HGB (g/l)	122±32	124±29	118±32	0.42
Ca^{2+}(×10^{-3} mmol)	5.275 (4.7–5.7)	5.225 (4.725–5.55)	5.075 (4.725–5.575)	0.33
K^+ (×10^{-3} mmol)	10.55 (9.325–11.575)	10.6 (8.775–11.7)	10.675 (9.55–12.425)	0.21
Na^+ (×10^{-3} mmol)	343.0 (331.0–352.5)	337.5 (325.75–352.75)	335 (320.25–344.5)	0.01
Cl^- (×10^{-3} mmol)	255 (240.25–269.0)	249.75 (235.5–265.25)	247.25 (232.25–257.5)	0.01
CO_2CP (×10^{-3} mmol)	54±16.75	54.25±13.75	49.5±14.25	0.04
ALB (g/l)	28.7±8.4	27.8±9.2	28.6±6.9	0.81

These biological parameters were measured using an automatic biochemistry analyzer (Hitachi 76000, Japan).
HCT: H = 4.38 (rank sum test); Ca^{2+}: H = 2.21 (rank sum test); K^+: H = 3.13 (rank sum test); Na^+: H = 10.49 (rank sum test); Cl^-: H = 10.34(rank sum test); HGB: F = 0.88 (ANOVA); CO_2CP: F = 03.25 (ANOVA); ALB: F = 0.22 (ANOVA).

Table 6. Association of AKI stages with BUN and SCr levels.

	Stage			
	Stage I	**Stage II**	**Stage III**	**P value***
First abnormality				
BUN (mmol/l)	11.1 (8.1–15.5)	15.2 (10.9–22.5)	24.8 (16.9–33.8)	<0.0001
SCr (µmol/l)	148.1 (132.0–178.0)	260.2 (237.1–305.1)	536.3 (381.1–804.0)	<0.0001
Peak				
BUN (mmol/l)	23.9 (14.6–34.1)	24.2 (15.4–33.4)	31.0 (22.8–40.6)	<0.0001
SCr (µmol/l)	290.0 (203.6–399.9)	392.6 (267.5–543.2)	670.7 (488.7–917.8)	<0.0001
Discharge				
BUN (mmol/l)	12.5 (7.3–29.0)	18.5 (7.6–26.8)	15.8 (8.4–25.9)	0.65
SCr (µmol/l)	185.0 (101.0–323.0)	244.6 (106.0–440.1)	299.0 (135.1–540.0)	0.001

These biological parameters were measured using an automatic biochemistry analyzer (Hitachi 76000, Japan).
*P for trend among AKI stage I to III.
BUN at first abnormality: H = 71.42 (rank sum test); BUN at peak: H = 19.19 (rank sum test); BUN at discharge: H = 0.85 (rank sum test); SCr at first abnormality: H = 169.62 (rank sum test); SCr at peak: H = 114.82 (rank sum test); SCr at discharge: H = 14.41, (rank sum test).

Analysis of Causes, Treatment and Prognosis of AKI

The causes of AKI are summarized in Figures 1 and 2. Renal causes occurred in 126 (46.5%) patients and were the leading cause of AKI. The most frequent renal cause for AKI was chronic kidney disease (A/C) and infection (Fig. 2). Prerenal causes occurred in 99 (36.5%) patients, most commonly due to decreased cardiac output or loss of blood, which occurred in 32 patients. Mannitol also caused AKI in 24 patients. Postrenal causes were found in 46 (17.0%) patients. Of the 271 AKI patients, 30 (11.1%) underwent surgical treatment and 61 (22.5%) received RRT. The majority (66.4%) of patients received conservative treatment. After treatment, the majority of patients achieved complete recovery (57 cases; 21.0%) or partial recovery (102 cases; 37.6%). No recovery, discharge without treatment and death occurred in 22 patients (8.1%), 37 patients (13.7%) and 53 patients (19.6%), respectively.

The cause of AKI significantly correlated with the prognosis ($r = -0.17$, $p = 0.005$) and the treatment ($r = 0.21$, $p < 0.001$) after adjustment for age and sex. In addition, the prognosis of AKI patients was significantly associated with the treatment ($r = -0.19$, $P = 0.002$). Postrenal causes were associated with a significantly higher recovery rate compared with prerenal and renal causes ($P < 0.0002$; Table 2). The prerenal causes of AKI were associated with the highest death rate. In addition, the complete and partial recovery rates were significantly higher in patients with surgical treatment compared to those with conservative treatment and RRT treatment ($P < 0.0001$; Table 2).

Analysis of AKI According to AKI Stage

Table 3 summarizes the AKI stages in the cohort of 271 patients. The majority of AKI patients were Stage III (52.0%) and the minority of patients were Stage II (16.2%). No significant differences in patient age or the length of hospital stay were found among Stage I, Stage II and Stage III patients ($P > 0.05$). However, the number of patients in different hospitalized departments was significantly different among patients with different AKI stages ($P < 0.01$; Table 4). There were significantly more Stage III patients from the Department of Surgery, ICU and Division of Nephrology. However, more Stage I patients were hospitalized in other divisions of the Department of Internal Medicine besides Nephrology.

Table 5 summarizes the association of severity of AKI with laboratory tests. No significant association of AKI stage was found with HCT, HGB, Ca^{2+}, K^+ or ALB levels ($P > 0.05$). However, we found that Cl^-, Na^+ and CO_2CP levels were significantly different among patients who were in different stages of AKI. There was a tendency toward a decrease in Cl^-, Na^+ and CO_2CP with increased severity of AKI. The Na^+ concentration was elevated from $337.55 \pm 28.15 \times 10^{-3}$ mmol before conservative treatment to $340.48 \pm 36.20 \times 10^{-3}$ mmolafter conservative treatment, from $336.30 \pm 11.73 \times 10^{-3}$ mmol before surgical treatment to $347.78 \pm 13.55 \times 10^{-3}$ mmol after surgical treatment, and from $335.95 \pm 22.58 \times 10^{-3}$ mmol before PPT to $342.05 \pm 16.23 \times 10^{-3}$ mmol after PPT. There was no significant differences in the Na^+ concentration before and after conservative treatment (paired t test, $t = 0.96$, $p = 0.34$) and PPT (paired t test, $t = 1.88$, $p = 0.07$). Moreover, the Na^+ concentration was significantly increased after surgical treatment (paired t test, $t = 3.28$, $p = 0.004$). In addition, SCr levels at first abnormality, at peak, and at discharge were significantly higher with increased severity of AKI. BUN levels at first abnormality and at peak, but not at discharge, were significantly higher with an increased severity of AKI (Table 6).

The causes of AKI were significantly associated with the severity of AKI ($P < 0.01$; Table. 7). Prerenal and renal causes were significantly associated with Stage I and II compared with postrenal causes. In addition, postrenal causes were more highly associated with Stage III compared with Stage I and Stage II patients.

Treatment of AKI was significantly associated with the severity of AKI ($P < 0.0001$; Table 7). Since patients who received dialysis were categorized as Stage III, no Stage I or II patients were categorized in the RRT group. Stage I and II patients received primarily conservative treatment. The incidence of surgical treatment was significantly higher in Stage III patients compared with Stage I and II patients.

The outcome of AKI was also significantly associated with the severity of AKI ($P < 0.0001$; Table 7). Rates of complete recovery and rates of death were significantly higher, and rates of partial recovery were significantly lower in Stage I patients compared with Stage III patients. In addition, univariate analysis found that respiratory injury, DIC, shock and MODS were associated with

Table 7. Association of AKI stage with the causeof AKI, treatment, and prognosis.

	Causes n (%)				Treatment n (%)				Outcomes n (%)					
AKI stages	**Prerenal**	**Renal**	**Postrenal**	**P value***	**Conservative**	**Surgery**	**RRT**	**P value**	**Complete Recovery**	**Partial recovery**	**No Recovery**	**Discharge without treatment**	**Death**	**P value***
Stage I	40 (46.5)	41 (47.7)	5 (5.8)	0.0002	82 (95.4)	4 (4.65)	0 (0.00)	<0.0001	23 (26.7)	13 (15.1)	6 (7.0)	10 (11.6)	34 (39.6)	<0.0001
Stage II	21 (47.7)	19 (43.2)	4 (9.1)		41 (93.2)	3 (6.82)	0 (0.00)		13 (29.5)	10 (22.8)	7 (15.9)	7 (15.9)	7 (15.9)	
Stage III	38 (26.9)	66 (46.8)	37 (26.3)		57 (40.4)	23 (16.3)	61 (43.3)		21 (14.9)	79 (56.0)	9 (6.4)	12 (8.5)	12 (8.5)	

*p for variation among sub-groups.
RRT: renal replacement therapy. For causes: $\chi^2 = 22.59$ (chi square). For treatment: $\chi^2 = 93.58$ (chi square). For prognosis: $\chi^2 = 63.28$ (chi square).

the prognosis of AKI (Table 8). Multivariate logistic regression analysis found that respiratory injury (odds ratio, 21.4) and MODS (odds ratio, 19.1) were associated with the incidence of death of AKI patients (both $p<0.05$).

Discussion

AKI is associated with a high risk of mortality and morbidity, especially in critically ill patients. AKI is common in the clinic, occurring in 8% of all in-hospital patients and in approximately 50% of ICU patients. [18] The definition of AKI according to the AKIN criteria is an absolute increase of more than 0.3 mg/dl or at least a 50% increase in SCr levels from baseline. Our study used this definition to diagnose AKI.

Of the 271 AKI patients, the majority of patients were over 50 years of age (mean age of 54 years). However, there was no association of patient age with the severity of AKI. Since AKI was defined by an abrupt increase in SCr levels within 48 h, the potential age-related and chronic effects on AKI were excluded. Of 107 patients whose kidney size was examined after AKI diagnosis, 85 (79.4%) patients had normal-sized kidneys, 16 (15.0%) patients had enlarged kidneys and 6 (5.6%) patients had reduced-size kidneys. Our finding that only 15.0% of AKI patients had an enlarged kidney suggests that AKI does not necessarily lead to an enlarged kidney. The fractional excretion of Na^+ (FENa) is a good measure to evaluate the underlying causes of kidney enlargement in AKI patients. However, since the urinary concentrations of Na^+ and Cr in these AKI patients were not measured in our AKI patients, we could not retrospectively calculate FENa evaluate whether the enlargement was associated with glomerular thickening. In addition, more Stage I and II patients were hospitalized in other divisions of the Departments of Internal Medicine other than the Division of Nephrology, and more Stage III patients were hospitalized at the Division of Nephrology, ICU and Department of Surgery. The cases of AKI in the Division of Nephrology were mainly associated with chronic kidney diseases, those in the Department of Surgery with obstruction, and those in the ICU with MODS or toxic agents. The cases of AKI in these departments were serious and associated with a rapid decline in kidney function, and often required dialysis. Thus, AKI patients in these departments were categorized as Stage III. In contrast, AKI in other departments was usually caused by low blood volume or the use of mannitol or radiocontrast agents. In these patients, SCr levels were transient without a rapid decline within 48 h. Thus, these patients were categorized as Stage I or II.

Prerenal, renal and postrenal causes occurred in 99 (36.5%), 126 (46.5%) and 46 (17.0%) patients, respectively. The most frequent causes for AKI in our study were postrenal obstruction (46 cases), decreased cardiac output or loss of blood (32 cases), use of mannitol (24 cases), A/C (23 cases), and infection (23 cases). The high incidence of postrenal causes of AKI in this study waspossibly due to a high incidence of kidney stones in our local area and a large number of patients with kidney stones in the Department of Surgery. Decreased cardiac output or loss of blood volume was mostly due to trauma, surgery or postpartum hemorrhage. "Osmotic nephrosis" induced by an overdose of mannitol, which is commonly used for lowering intracranial pressure, was likely the major reason for the high incidence of AKI in our study.[19–21] Sepsis has been reported to occur in approximately 19% of patients with moderate AKI and 23% of patients with severe AKI. [22] Consistent with a previous report, [22] we also found a relatively high incidence of infection-

Table 8. Prognostic factors for AKI.

	Prognosis n (%)				
	Complete recovery	**Partial recovery**	**No recovery**	**Discharge without treatment**	**Death**
Cardiac injury	3 (10.3)	8 (27.6)	3 (10.3)	6 (20.7)	9 (31.0)
Hepatic injury	3 (9.38)	11 (34.4)	4 (12.5)	5 (15.6)	9(28.1)
Respiratory injury*	2 (6.25)	6 (18.8)	5 (15.6)	6 (18.8)	13 (40.6)
shock△	4 (14.81)	1 (3.70)	1 (3.70)	6 (22.2)	15 (55.6)
MODS△	2 (11.8)	2 (11.8)	0 (0.00)	2 (11.8)	11 (64.7)
DIC*	0 (0.00)	0 (0.00)	1 (25.0)	0 (0.00)	3 (75.0)
Severe infection	7 (18.4)	11 (29.0)	5 (13.2)	8 (21.1)	7 (18.4)
Septicemia	1 (12.5)	1 (12.5)	0 (0.00)	2 (25.0)	4 (50.0)
Gastrointestinal bleeding	1 (14.3)	3 (42.9)	0 (0.00)	1 (14.3)	2 (28.6)
Malignant tumors	8 (26.7)	8 (26.7)	6 (20.0)	4 (13.3)	4 (13.3)
History of allergy	4 (26.7)	6 (40.0)	0 (0.00)	1 (6.67)	4 (26.7)
History of smoking	16 (18.2)	40(45.5)	4 (4.55)	11 (12.5)	17 (19.3)
History of drinking	7 (14.3)	23 (46.9)	2 (4.08)	7 (14.3)	10 (20.4)
Anemia	21 (18.0)	45 (38.5)	8 (6.84)	19 (16.2)	24 (20.5)
Renal diseases	5 (21.7)	9 (39.1)	2 (8.70)	2 (8.70)	5 (21.7)

*$P<0.05$;
△$P<0.0001$ (chi square).

associated AKI. Infection has been reported to be associated with a high risk of mortality. [12].

AKI patients were categorized according to the AKIN criteria. [1,3] Stage III patients accounted for more than half (52.0%) of our patients. The large number of Stage III patients was likely due to the inclusion of all patients with dialysis according to the AKIN criteria. [1,3] SCr and BUN levels were also significantly elevated with increasing severity of AKI. Although SCr and BUN levels are affected by many factors, such as high protein diet, high metabolism rate, and inflammation, our results suggest that SCr and BUN levels are still good indicators for the diagnosis of AKI. In addition, Cl^-, Na^+, and CO_2CP levels were also lower with increasing severity of AKI, suggesting that AKI with greater severity is likely associated with complications such as hypochloremia, hyponatremia and metabolic acidosis.

The cause of AKI was significantly associated with the severity of AKI. Prerenal and renal causes were significantly associated with Stage I and II, while postrenal causes were associated with Stage III. Since prerenal causes such as low blood volume and decreased cardiac output can induce compensatory regulation in the body, prerenal AKI can be mild, especially within a short period of time (within 48 h), and thus is categorized as Stage I according to the AKIN criteria. In contrast, postrenal obstruction produces a rapid and serious kidney injury within a short period of time without compensatory regulation, and is thus categorized as Stage III. Dialysis is often used in renal AKI caused by nephritis, nephrotoxins and rhabdomyolysis, and are categorized as Stage III. [3] Therefore, renal and postrenal causes are the major causes for Stage III AKI patients. In this study, treatment and severity of AKI were significantly associated. Stage I and II patients primarily received conservative treatment, and rarely had surgery. Surgical treatment was significantly increased in Stage III patients.

In-hospital death occurred in 53 patients (19.6%). This mortality rate is similar or lower than the mortality rate of approximately 20%–50% of the reports in the literature.[12–14] Prerenal causes were associated with the highest death rate. The high mortality was possibly due to serious pre-existing diseases such as shock, low blood volume after a major operation, and hepatorenal syndrome. Pre-existing comorbidities have been reported to be associated with mortality after AKI. [23] Postrenal AKI was associated with a higher recovery rate, most likely because kidney damage caused by obstruction is transient and mild and is reversible after removal of obstruction.

Using multivariate logistic regression analysis, we further found that respiratory injury and MODS were prognostic factors for death in AKI patients. Oxygen is critical for the maintenance of normal function of vital organs including the kidneys. The kidneys have a very rich blood supply and are very sensitive to ischemia and hypoxia. Therefore, the kidneys are susceptible to damage in patients with respiratory injury, and thus AKI patients with respiratory injury show a poor prognosis. In addition, long-term respiratory failure can lead to multiple organ failures due to insufficient oxygen supply. MODS can also be caused by severe trauma, septic shock, and accidents. With the increase in the number of failed organs, the mortality rate increases. [24] It has been reported that mortality rate is significantly increased in the presence of MODS. [25,26] In agreement with these reports, we also found that MODS was a prognostic factor for death in AKI patients.

In summary, we retrospectively studied 217 hospitalized patients with a diagnosis of AKI. Prerenal causes were the leading cause for AKI in this study. The majority of patients received conservative treatment, and only 22.5% of patients received RRT. The recovery rate was 21.0% and the mortality rate was 19.6%. Both cause and treatment were significantly associated with the prognosis of AKI. Similarly, the severity of AKI was significantly associated with cause, treatment and prognosis. Respiratory injury and MODS are prognostic factors for death in AKI patients.

Author Contributions

Conceived and designed the experiments: YJD. Performed the experiments: FY LZ. Analyzed the data: FY LZ HW HBZ. Wrote the paper: FY.

References

1. Ricci Z, Cruz DN, Ronco C (2011) Classification and staging of acute kidney injury: beyond the RIFLE and AKIN criteria. Nat Rev Nephrol 7: 201–208.
2. Hoste EA, Kellum JA (2006) Acute kidney injury: epidemiology and diagnostic criteria. Curr Opin Crit Care 12: 531–537.
3. Mehta RL, Kellum JA, Shah SV, Molitoris BA, Ronco C, et al. (2007) Acute Kidney Injury Network: report of an initiative to improve outcomes in acute kidney injury. Crit Care 11: R31.
4. Coca SG, Yusuf B, Shlipak MG, Garg AX, Parikh CR (2009) Long-term risk of mortality and other adverse outcomes after acute kidney injury: a systematic review and meta-analysis. Am J Kidney Dis 53: 961–973.
5. Lafrance JP, Miller DR (2010) Acute kidney injury associates with increased long-term mortality. J Am Soc Nephrol 21: 345–352.
6. Waikar SS, Liu KD, Chertow GM (2008) Diagnosis, epidemiology and outcomes of acute kidney injury. Clin J Am Soc Nephrol 3: 844–861.
7. Barretti P, Soares VA (1997) Acute renal failure: clinical outcome and causes of death. Ren Fail 19: 253–257.
8. Woodrow G, Turney JH (1992) Cause of death in acute renal failure. Nephrol Dial Transplant 7: 230–234.
9. Akcay A, Turkmen K, Lee D, Edelstein CL (2010) Update on the diagnosis and management of acute kidney injury. Int J Nephrol Renovasc Dis 3: 129–140.
10. Lameire NH, De Vriese AS, Vanholder R (2003) Prevention and nondialytic treatment of acute renal failure. Curr Opin Crit Care 9: 481–490.
11. Pannu N, Klarenbach S, Wiebe N, Manns B, Tonelli M (2008) Renal replacement therapy in patients with acute renal failure: a systematic review. JAMA 299: 793–805.
12. Brady HR, Singer GG (1995) Acute renal failure. Lancet 346: 1533–1540.
13. Hilton R (2006) Acute renal failure. BMJ 333: 786–790.
14. Waikar SS, Curhan GC, Wald R, McCarthy EP, Chertow GM (2006) Declining mortality in patients with acute renal failure, 1988 to 2002. J Am Soc Nephrol 17: 1143–1150.
15. Ishani A, Xue JL, Himmelfarb J, Eggers PW, Kimmel PL, et al. (2009) Acute kidney injury increases risk of ESRD among elderly. J Am Soc Nephrol 20: 223–228.
16. Wald R, Quinn RR, Luo J, Li P, Scales DC, et al. (2009) Chronic dialysis and death among survivors of acute kidney injury requiring dialysis. JAMA 302: 1179–1185.
17. Ali T, Khan I, Simpson W, Prescott G, Townend J, et al. (2007) Incidence and outcomes in acute kidney injury: a comprehensive population-based study. J Am Soc Nephrol 18: 1292–1298.
18. Hoste EA, Schurgers M (2008) Epidemiology of acute kidney injury: how big is the problem? Crit Care Med 36: S146–151.
19. Fang L, You H, Chen B, Xu Z, Gao L, et al. (2010) Mannitol is an independent risk factor of acute kidney injury after cerebral trauma: a case-control study. Ren Fail 32: 673–679.
20. Moran M, Kapsner C (1987) Acute renal failure associated with elevated plasma oncotic pressure. N Engl J Med 317: 150–153.
21. Visweswaran P, Massin EK, Dubose TD Jr (1997) Mannitol-induced acute renal failure. J Am Soc Nephrol 8: 1028–1033.
22. Schrier RW, Wang W (2004) Acute renal failure and sepsis. N Engl J Med 351: 159–169.
23. Pereira MB, Zanetta DM, Abdulkader RC (2012) The real importance of pre-existing comorbidities on long-term mortality after acute kidney injury. PLoS One 7: e47746.
24. Chen YC, Chen CY, Tien YC, Fang JT, Huang CC (2001) Organ system failures prediction model in intensive care patients with acute renal failure treated with dialysis. Ren Fail 23: 207–215.
25. Bernieh B, Al Hakim M, Boobes Y, Siemkovics E, El Jack H (2004) Outcome and predictive factors of acute renal failure in the intensive care unit. Transplant Proc 36: 1784–1787.
26. Mataloun SE, Machado FR, Senna AP, Guimaraes HP, Amaral JL (2006) Incidence, risk factors and prognostic factors of acute renal failure in patients admitted to an intensive care unit. Braz J Med Biol Res 39: 1339–1347.

17

High-Sensitivity C-Reactive Protein Predicts Mortality and Technique Failure in Peritoneal Dialysis Patients

Shou-Hsuan Liu[1], Yi-Jung Li[1,2], Hsin-Hsu Wu[1,2], Cheng-Chia Lee[1], Chan-Yu Lin[1], Cheng-Hao Weng[1,2], Yung-Chang Chen[1], Ming-Yang Chang[1], Hsiang-Hao Hsu[1], Ji-Tseng Fang[1], Cheng-Chieh Hung[1], Chih-Wei Yang[1], Ya-Chung Tian[1]*

1 Kidney Research Center, Department of Nephrology, Lin-Kou Chang Gung Memorial Hospital and Department of Medicine, Chang Gung University, Tao Yuan, Taiwan,
2 Graduate Institute of Clinical Medical Sciences, Chang Gung University, Tao Yuan, Taiwan

Abstract

Introduction: An elevated level of serum C-reactive protein (CRP) is widely considered an indicator of an underlying inflammatory disease and a long-term prognostic predictor for dialysis patients. This cross-sectional cohort study was designed to assess the correlation between the level of high-sensitivity CRP (HS-CRP) and the outcome of peritoneal dialysis (PD) patients.

Methods: A total of 402 patients were stratified into 3 tertiles (lower, middle, upper) according to serum HS-CRP level and and followed up from October 2009 to September 2011. During follow-up, cardiovascular events, infection episodes, technique failure, and mortality rate were recorded.

Results: During the 24-month follow-up, 119 of 402 patients (29.6%) dropped out from PD, including 28 patients (7.0%) who died, 81 patients (20.1%) who switched to hemodialysis, and 10 patients (2.5%) who underwent kidney transplantation. The results of Kaplan–Meier analysis and log-rank test demonstrated a significant difference in the cumulative patient survival rate across the 3 tertiles (the lowest rate in upper tertile). On multivariate Cox regression analysis, only higher HS-CRP level, older age, the presence of diabetes mellitus (DM), lower serum albumin level, and the occurrence of cardiovascular events during follow-up were identified as independent predictors of mortality. Every 1 mg/L increase in HS-CRP level was independently predictive of a 1.4% increase in mortality. Multivariate Cox regression analysis also showed that higher HS-CRP level, the presence of DM, lower hemoglobin level, lower serum albumin level, higher dialysate/plasma creatinine ratio, and the occurrence of infective episodes and cardiovascular events during follow-up were independent predictors of technique failure.

Conclusions: The present study shows the importance of HS-CRP in the prediction of 2-year mortality and technique survival in PD patients independent of age, diabetes, hypoalbuminemia, and the occurrence of cardiovascular events.

Editor: Leighton R. James, University of Florida, United States of America

Funding: The authors have no support or funding to report.

Competing Interests: The authors have declared that no competing interests exist.

* E-mail: dryctian@adm.cgmh.org.tw

Introduction

An elevated level of serum C-reactive protein (CRP), an acute-phase reactant, has been found to predict the clinical outcome of various cardiovascular diseases such as myocardial infarction and stroke in the general population and in patients with chronic kidney disease and those undergoing dialysis [1,2]. Some studies reported that CRP itself is pro-inflammatory as it has the ability to bind damaged cells and activate complements [3,4]. A high CRP level is widely considered an indicator of an underlying inflammatory disease or a high oxidative stress condition, and a long-term prognostic predictor for patients undergoing dialysis [5–7]. A high-sensitivity CRP (HS-CRP) test is more sensitive than conventional CRP detection tests and can detect levels of CRP within the reference range [8].

Many studies have recognized uremic milieu as a state of chronic inflammation [9–12]. Even after dialysis, patients remain in an inflammatory status because the serum level of pro-inflammatory cytokines such as interleukin-1 (IL-1), IL-6, and tumor necrosis factor-α are elevated in dialysis patients [13–17]. It has been reported that up to 30–50% of peritoneal dialysis (PD) patients have increased CRP levels [7,18,19]. Although several studies have reported that the elevation of CRP is a useful predictor of the occurrence of cardiovascular events and mortality [7,13,20,21], some demonstrate that CRP is not significantly associated with all-cause mortality [19,22,23]. It has been reported that the characteristics of membrane transporter status and residual renal function affect the serum CRP level [24,25]. Therefore, this discrepancy may be attributed to the sample size, analyzed parameters, and study period.

Table 1. Demographic and laboratory characteristics of the PD patients stratified according to serum HS-CRP levels.

HS-CRP (mg/L)	Total (n=402) 9.57±16.35	Lower tertile (n=134) 0.90±0.43 (<1.77)	Middle tertile (n=134) 3.90±1.69 (1.77–7.51)	Upper tertile (n=134) 23.90±22.09 (>7.51)	P
Male	148 (36.8%)	43 (32.1%)	53 (39.6%)	52 (38.8%)	0.38
Age (years)	48.6±14.6	44.3±15.3	49.1±13.0	52.4±14.3	<0.001
Body mass index (kg/m^2)	22.4±3.6	21.1±2.9	22.8±3.6	23.4±3.9	<0.001
Diabetes mellitus	71 (17.7%)	11 (8.2%)	23 (17.2%)	37 (27.6%)	<0.001
PD duration (months)	73.6±41.0	66.9±35.7	76.1±40.4	77.8±45.8	0.07
Residual urine	254 (63.2%)	103 (76.9%)	80 (59.7%)	71 (53.0%)	<0.001
WBC count (1000/μL)	7.655±2.523	6.400±1.959	7.679±2.058	8.866±2.840	<0.001
Hemoglobin (g/dL)	10.06±1.56	10.24±1.56	10.18±1.45	9.66±1.61	<0.001
Platelet count (1000/μL)	257.81±82.63	247.65±79.33	258.69±77.09	266.92±90.35	0.17
AST (U/L)	20.1±11.9	20.3±12.6	19.4±9.3	20.6±13.4	0.73
ALT (U/L)	20.2±18.4	20.3±20.5	19.9±12.2	20.5±21.2	0.9
Total bilirubin (mg/dL)	0.30±0.12	0.28±0.13	0.36±0.12	0.25±0.08	0.20
Albumin (g/dL)	3.96±0.46	4.07±0.38	3.98±0.43	3.85±0.55	<0.001
Total cholesterol (mg/dL)	202.3±49.0	205.6±44.6	203.2±49.5	198.3±52.5	0.48
HDL (mg/dL)	47.4±15.1	55.2±16.0	45.0±13.4	40.9±11.5	<0.001
LDL (mg/dL)	119.7±40.8	121.6±40.6	119.2±41.4	117.9±40.8	0.82
Triglyceride (mg/dL)	190.3±129.3	149.3±79.4	195.4±132.8	224.6±152.5	<0.001
Total patients					
Fasting sugar (mg/dL)	114.7±53.4	103.5±43.7	110.6±40.3	129.9±68.6	<0.001
HbA1c %	5.66±1.03	5.43±0.85	5.61±0.89	5.96±1.23	<0.001
Diabetic patients					
Fasting sugar (mg/dL)	187.4±90.1	194.9±114.9	172.9±61.6	193.8±97.4	0.67
HbA1c %	7.31±1.50	7.81±1.34	7.02±1.36	7.33±1.61	0.40
Non-diabetic patients					
Fasting sugar (mg/dL)	98.8±17.8	94.9±10.2	98.1±16.7	104.5±24.3	<0.001
HbA1c %	5.33±0.38	5.22±0.36	5.35±0.42	5.42±0.33	<0.001
Creatinine (mg/dL)	11.32±3.01	11.73±3.23	11.40±2.83	10.82±2.89	0.046
Uric acid (mg/dL)	6.81±1.32	6.76±1.25	6.73±1.24	6.95±1.45	0.35
Calcium (mg/dL)	10.01±1.00	9.96±1.00	10.12±0.98	9.95±0.99	0.30
Phosphorus (mg/dL)	4.94±1.32	5.09±1.28	4.90±1.27	4.83±1.42	0.26
PTH (pg/mL)	329.0±388.8	332.8±391.3	285.8±318.3	367.2±443.4	0.25
Transferrin saturation	0.272±0.127	0.295±0.118	0.276±0.134	0.244±0.122	0.01
Ferritin (μg/L)	329.1±510.9	261.9±435.2	371.9±667.9	352.6±382.4	0.20

Note:
Continuous variables given as mean ± standard deviation, and categorical variables, as number (percentage).
Abbreviations: HS-CRP, high-sensitivity C-reactive protein; PD, peritoneal dialysis; WBC, white blood cell; AST, aspartate transaminase; ALT, alanine transaminase; HDL, high-density lipoprotein; LDL, low-density lipoprotein; HbA1c, glycated hemoglobin; iPTH, intact parathyroid hormone.

In addition to predicting mortality, an elevated CRP level has been shown to be linked to technique failure. Nevertheless, only a few studies have assessed the impact of baseline serum CRP level on technique failure, and the association between baseline serum CRP level and subsequent technique failure is still inconclusive. Some studies demonstrated that serum CRP level was independently associated with technique failure [26], whereas others found that serum CRP level was not a predictor for technique failure [27,28]. Therefore, it would be interesting to know whether serum CRP level is correlated with technique failure in PD patients.

Both residual renal function and peritoneal clearance have been reported to be inversely associated with serum CRP level [24,25], whereas some studies demonstrate that serum CRP is not influenced by peritoneal solute transport rate and residual renal function [22,29]. As these 2 factors have also been shown to be predictive markers for mortality and technique failure in PD patients and are associated with CRP, it would be crucial to elucidate whether HS-CRP can predict the clinical outcome in PD patients independently of residual renal function and peritoneal clearance.

Table 2. Peritoneal membrane characteristics of the PD patients stratified according to HS-CRP levels.

	Total	Lower tertile	Middle tertile	Upper tertile	
	(n = 402)	**(n = 134)**	**(n = 134)**	**(n = 134)**	
HS-CRP (mg/L)	**9.57±16.35**	**0.90±0.43**	**3.90±1.69**	**23.90±22.09**	**P**
		(<1.77)	**(1.77–7.51)**	**(>7.51)**	
Dialysate/plasma creatinine	0.64±0.12	0.62±0.12	0.65±0.10	0.66±0.13	0.01
Peritoneal equilibration test					<0.001
High	28 (7.0%)	5 (3.7%)	6 (4.5%)	17 (12.7%)	
High average	152 (37.8%)	41 (30.6%)	63 (47.0%)	48 (35.8%)	
Low average	179 (44.5%)	66 (49.3%)	55 (41.0%)	58 (43.3%)	
Low	43 (10.7%)	22 (16.4%)	10 (7.5%)	11 (8.2%)	
Weekly CCr (normalized)	59.6±13.9	58.8±13.8	60.3±14.9	59.7±13.1	0.70
Weekly CCr (total)	54.1±14.5	52.0±14.6	55.5±14.9	54.7±13.9	0.12
Weekly CCr (PD)	45.1±12.1	41.0±12.0	47.1±10.6	47.3±12.6	<0.001
Weekly CCr (renal)	8.9±15.2	11.0±13.9	8.2±16.8	7.4±14.6	0.12

Note:
Continuous variables given as mean ± standard deviation, and categorical variables, as number (percentage).
Abbreviations: PD, peritoneal dialysis; HS-CRP, high-sensitivity C-reactive protein; CCr, creatinine clearance.

The aim of this cross-sectional cohort study was to investigate whether serum HS-CRP level was independently associated with mortality and technique failure in PD patients.

Materials and Methods

This cross-sectional cohort study complied with the guidelines of the Declaration of Helsinki and approved by the Medical Ethics Committee of Chang Gung Memorial Hospital, a tertiary referral center located in the northern part of Taiwan. Since this study involved retrospective review of existing data, the Institutional Review Board approval was obtained, but without specific informed consent from patients. In addition, all individual information was securely protected (by delinking identifying information from main data set) and available to investigators only. Furthermore, all the data were analyzed anonymously. The Institutional Review Board of Chang Gung Memorial Hospital has approved this study and no informed consent was requested by the Committee. Finally, all primary data were collected according to strengthening the reporting of observational studies in epidemiology guidelines.

Study Population and Follow-up

This cohort observational study was conducted in the PD unit of Linkou Chang-Gung Memorial Hospital from October 2009 to September 2011 to determine the impact of HS-CRP on the patients' outcome. All the data were obtained from the record of the routine examination. Among 445 patients, 43 patients were excluded owing to recent episodes of peritonitis, active infection, chronic liver disease, autoimmune disease, malignant diseases, or acute myocardial infarction within 3 months. The remaining 402

Table 3. Clinical outcomes in the PD patients stratified according to HS-CRP levels.

	Total	Lower tertile	Middle tertile	Upper tertile	
	(n = 402)	**(n = 134)**	**(n = 134)**	**(n = 134)**	
HS-CRP (mg/L)	**9.57±16.35**	**0.90±0.43**	**3.90±1.69**	**23.90±22.09**	**P**
		(<1.77)	**(1.77–7.51)**	**(>7.51)**	
Outcomes					
Death	28 (7.0%)	0 (0.0%)	4 (3.0%)	24 (17.9%)	<0.001
Transfer to HD	81 (20.1%)	25 (18.7%)	25 (18.7%)	31 (23.1%)	0.575
Transplantation	10 (2.5%)	3 (2.2%)	4 (3.0%)	3 (2.2%)	0.903
Technique survival	283 (70.4%)	106 (79.1%)	101 (75.4%)	76 (56.7%)	<0.001
Infection episodes	192 (47.8%)	55 (41.0%)	66 (49.3%)	71 (53.0%)	0.14
Cardiovascular events	72 (17.9%)	17 (12.7%)	21 (15.7%)	34 (25.4%)	0.02

Note:
Continuous variables given as mean ± standard deviation, and categorical variables, as number (percentage).
Abbreviations: PD, peritoneal dialysis; HS-CRP, high-sensitivity C-reactive protein; HD, hemodialysis.

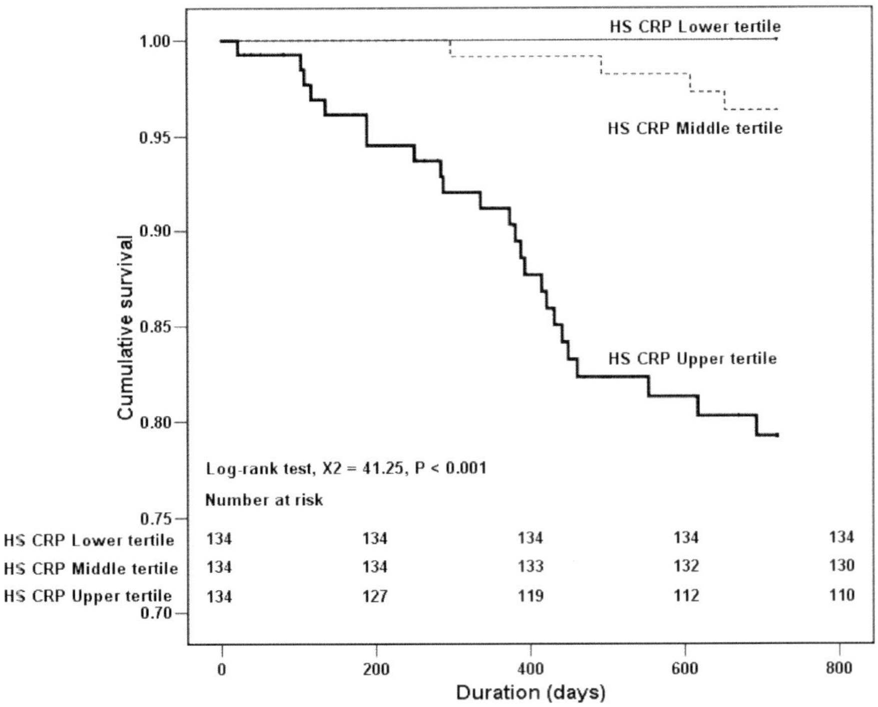

Figure 1. Kaplan–Meier survival curves based on serum HS-CRP levels among PD patients in the 2-year follow-up.

patients were enrolled in this study. All patients had been undergoing PD for >3 months and were observed during a period of 24 months. Patients were categorized into 3 tertiles according to the baseline HS-CRP level in October 2009.

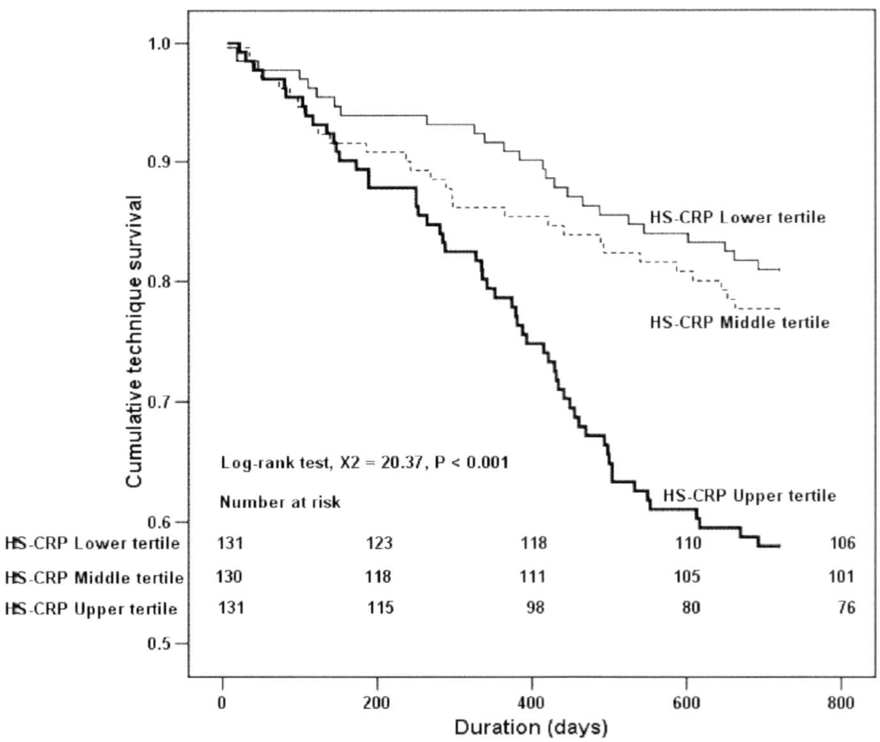

Figure 2. Kaplan–Meier technique survival (transplantation censored) curves based on serum HS-CRP levels among PD patients in the 2-year follow-up.

Table 4. Relative risk of mortality in univariate Cox regression analysis.

		Univariate analysis	
	RR	HR (95% CI)	P
HS-CRP (mg/L)	1.025	1.014–1.035	<0.001
Male	1.692	0.719–3.981	0.23
Age	1.067	1.036–1.098	<0.001
Body mass index (kg/m^2)	1.051	0.954–1.158	0.32
Diabetes mellitus	5.979	2.846–12.560	<0.001
PD duration (months)	0.993	0.982–1.004	0.20
Residual urine	0.700	0.331–1.480	0.35
White blood cell count (1000/μL)	1.158	1.046–1.281	0.01
Hemoglobin (g/dL)	0.859	0.684–1.079	0.19
Platelet count (1000/μL)	1.000	0.996–1.005	0.9
AST (U/L)	1.018	0.996–1.041	0.12
ALT (U/L)	1.003	0.983–1.023	0.80
Total bilirubin (mg/dL)	0.168	0.000–231.652	0.67
Albumin (g/dL)	0.194	0.110–0.341	<0.001
Total cholesterol (mg/dL)	0.996	0.988–1.004	0.31
HDL (mg/dL)	1.002	0.964–1.042	0.9
LDL (mg/dL)	0.991	0.974–1.008	0.28
Triglyceride (mg/dL)	1.001	0.999–1.004	0.34
Sugar (mg/dL)	1.008	1.004–1.012	<0.001
HbA1c %	1.532	1.232–1.905	<0.001
Creatinine (mg/dL)	0.730	0.620–0.858	<0.001
Uric acid (mg/dL)	0.746	0.541–1.028	0.07
Calcium (mg/dL)	0.653	0.476–0.896	0.01
Phosphorus (mg/dL)	0.674	0.488–0.931	0.02
iPTH (pg/mL)	0.999	0.998–1.000	0.11
Transferrin saturation	3.398	0.259–44.651	0.35
Ferritin (μg/L)	1.000	1.000–1.001	0.19
Dialysate/plasma creatinine	19.269	0.942–394.309	0.06
Peritoneal equilibration test (%)	1.612	0.995–2.613	0.05
Weekly CCr (normalized)	0.996	0.969–1.024	0.77
Weekly CCr (total)	0.992	0.966–1.018	0.54
Weekly CCr (PD)	1.003	0.973–1.034	0.85
Weekly CCr (renal)	0.990	0.961–1.019	0.49
Infection episodes	2.434	1.122–5.279	0.02
Cardiovascular events	5.979	2.847–12.557	<0.001

Note:
Abbreviations: RR, relative risk; HR, hazard ratio; CI, confidence interval; HS-CRP, high-sensitivity C-reactive protein; PD, peritoneal dialysis; AST, aspartate transaminase; ALT, alanine transaminase; HDL, high-density lipoprotein; LDL, low-density lipoprotein; HbA1c, glycated hemoglobin; iPTH, intact parathyroid hormone; CCr, creatinine clearance.

Baseline demographic and clinical data, including age, sex, body mass index (BMI), presence of diabetes, duration of PD at the entry of this study, residual renal function, hemogram, and biochemical parameters, were recorded. PD membrane characteristics, including the dialysate/plasma creatinine ratio (D/P_{Cr}) and peritoneal equilibrium test (PET) results, were assessed. All of these data were obtained during routine clinical practice. During the 24-month follow-up, cardiovascular events, infection episodes, technique failure, and mortality rate were recorded. A cardiovascular event was defined as acute myocardial infarction, intervention of coronary artery disease with angioplasty or stenting, cerebral vascular accident, and peripheral vascular occlusion requiring intervention. An infection episode was defined as PD-related infection or non-PD-related infection.

No patient was lost to follow-up. Patient deaths were recorded, and those patients who underwent kidney transplantation or were transferred to hemodialysis were censored when they received alterative renal replacement therapy.

Table 5. Relative risk of mortality in multivariate Cox regression analysis.

	Multivariate analysis		
	RR	HR (95% CI)	P
HS-CRP (mg/L)	1.014	1.003–1.026	0.02
Age	1.042	1.011–1.074	0.01
Diabetes mellitus	3.381	1.578–7.243	0.002
Albumin (g/dL)	0.289	0.156–0.535	<0.001
Cardiovascular events	2.839	1.309–6.160	0.008

Note:
Abbreviations: RR, relative risk; HR, hazard ratio; CI, confidence interval; HS-CRP, high-sensitivity C-reactive protein.

Laboratory Parameters

Blood specimens were collected within a few days of clinical examination during stable PD routine examination to minimize the effect of any acute event. Blood was drawn immediately, centrifuged, and then stored at −70°C until used in assays. Serum HS-CRP was analyzed by using immunonephelometry (Nanopia CRP; Daiichi, Tokyo, Japan). Serum intact parathyroid hormone (iPTH) was determined by using a chemiluminometric immunoassay (ADVIA Centaur iPTH; Siemens Medical Solutions Diagnostics, New York, NY, USA) with a reference range of 7–53 pg/mL. All other biochemical parameters were obtained with standard laboratory procedures by using an automatic analyzer.

Peritoneal Dialysis Membrane Characteristics

The adequacy of dialysis was determined by measuring the total weekly creatinine clearance (CCr), which was normalized to 1.73 m^2 of the body surface area. Residual renal CCr was calculated as an average of the 24-h urine urea and CCr. Dialysate creatinine concentration was corrected for interference by glucose. The dialysate/plasma creatinine ratio (D/P_{Cr}) was calculated from the concentrations of creatinine in the 24-h dialysate and the plasma.

Statistical Analysis

Continuous variables are expressed as means and standard deviations, and categorical variables as numbers and percentages in brackets. All data were tested for normality of distribution and equality of standard deviations before analysis. For comparisons between patient groups, one-way ANOVA was used for quantitative variables, whereas chi-square or Fisher's exact test was used for categorical variables. P values were calculated, and the null hypothesis was rejected if the P value was <0.05. The independent links between HS-CRP and variables were analyzed further with simple and stepwise backward multiple linear regression analyses, adjusting for other factors linked with HS-CRP. Mortality was examined by using Kaplan–Meier analysis. Differences in the survival curves among the 3 groups were evaluated by using the log-rank test. An initial univariate Cox regression analysis was performed to compare the frequency of possible risk factors associated with mortality. To control for possible confounding factors, a multivariate Cox regression analysis (stepwise backward approach) was performed to analyze the significant factors ($P<0.05$) on the univariate analysis that met the assumptions of a proportional hazard model. The criterion for significance was a 95% confidence interval to reject the null hypothesis ($P<0.05$). All analyses were performed by using SPSS 12.0 for Windows (SPSS Inc., Chicago, IL, USA).

Results

Baseline Patient Characteristics of Demography and Biochemistry

Of the 402 patients in this cohort observational study, 148 (36.8%) were men and 254 (63.2%) were women. Their mean age was 48.6±14.6 years. The mean duration of PD was 73.6±41.0 months. Table 1 shows the baseline characteristics and laboratory parameters of these 402 patients stratified into 3 tertiles according to the serum HS-CRP level. The mean HS-CRP value in the study patients was 9.57 mg/L. The mean HS-CRP values were 0.90 mg/L (0–1.77 mg/L) in the lower tertile (T1), 3.90 mg/L (1.77–7.51 mg/L) in the middle tertile (T2), and 23.90 mg/L (7.51–45.85 mg/L) in the upper tertile (T3). Among the 3 tertiles, there was no significant difference in sex and PD duration. There was a significant increase ($P<0.001$) in the mean age across HS-CRP tertiles: 44.3 years in T1, 49.1 years in T2, and 52.4 years in T3. The percentages of patients with diabetes were significantly increased: 8.2% in T1, 17.2% in T2, and 27.6% in T3. A significant increase in the BMI values was also found across the 3 tertiles. Up to 76.9% of patients in T1 had residual renal function, whereas 59.7% of patients in T2 and 53.0% of patients in T3 had residual renal function ($P<0.001$). The white blood cell count was significantly increased and the hemoglobin level was reduced, whereas the platelet count was not different across these groups. Liver biochemistry test showed no difference in serum aspartate transaminase, alanine transaminase, and total bilirubin levels across the HS-CRP tertiles. The serum albumin level was in inverse proportion to the HS-CRP level, with the lowest level in T3. The examination of lipid profiles revealed a significant decrease in high-density lipoprotein (HDL) levels and an increase in triglyceride levels across the 3 tertiles of increasing HS-CRP, whereas total cholesterol and low-density lipoprotein (LDL) levels were not different across these tertiles. Fasting blood sugar and glycated hemoglobin (HbA1c) levels were examined in every patient, and the results showed a significant increase in these 2 parameters across the 3 tertiles of increasing HS-CRP. Surprisingly, further analysis revealed that in patients without diabetes, fasting blood sugar and HbA1c levels were increased across the 3 tertiles of increasing HS-CRP, whereas in patients with diabetes, blood sugar and HbA1c levels varied and were not different across the HS-CRP tertiles. Compared with patients in the other tertiles, the serum creatinine level was lowest in the patients in T3. Serum uric acid, calcium, phosphorus, and iPTH levels were not significantly different across the HS-CRP tertiles. Transferrin saturation was significantly decreased across the 3 tertiles of increasing HS-CRP. There was a trend toward the higher ferritin

Table 6. Relative risk of technique failure in univariate Cox regression analysis.

	Univariate analysis		
	RR	HR (95% CI)	P
HS-CRP (mg/L)	1.016	1.009–1.023	<0.001
Male	0.364	0.814–1.750	0.36
Age	1.020	1.006–1.034	0.01
Body mass index (kg/m^2)	1.028	0.976–1.082	0.30
Diabetes mellitus	2.902	1.946–4.330	<0.001
PD duration (months)	0.995	0.990–1.001	0.08
Residual urine	0.656	0.449–0.958	0.03
White blood cell count (1000/μL)	1.077	1.011–1.147	0.02
Hemoglobin (g/dL)	0.831	0.742–0.931	0.001
Platelet count (1000/μL)	1.001	0.999–1.003	0.23
AST (U/L)	1.008	0.993–1.022	0.30
ALT (U/L)	1.004	0.995–1.013	0.42
Total bilirubin (mg/dL)	0.139	0.000–178.189	0.59
Albumin (g/dL)	0.326	0.233–0.455	<0.001
Total cholesterol (mg/dL)	0.996	0.992–1.000	0.06
HDL (mg/dL)	1.002	0.981–1.024	0.86
LDL (mg/dL)	0.994	0.986–1.003	0.20
Triglyceride (mg/dL)	1.002	0.999–1.003	0.23
Sugar (mg/dL)	1.006	1.004–1.008	<0.001
HbA1c %	1.360	1.193–1.550	<0.001
Creatinine (mg/dL)	0.901	0.839–0.967	0.004
Uric acid (mg/dL)	0.953	0.816–1.113	0.54
Calcium (mg/dL)	0.830	0.691–0.997	0.05
Phosphorus (mg/dL)	0.797	0.681–0.933	0.01
iPTH (pg/mL)	1.000	0.999–1.000	0.21
Transferrin saturation	0.416	0.078–2.207	0.30
Ferritin (μg/L)	1.000	1.000–1.000	0.56
Dialysate/plasma creatinine	19.105	4.168–87.571	<0.001
Peritoneal equilibration test (%)	1.579	1.237–2.014	<0.001
Weekly CCr (normalized)	1.000	0.987–1.014	0.9
Weekly CCr (total)	1.000	0.988–1.013	0.9
Weekly CCr (PD)	1.017	1.001–1.033	0.04
Weekly CCr (renal)	0.988	0.973–1.004	0.13
Infection episodes	5.153	3.225–8.232	<0.001
Cardiovascular events	2.886	1.921–4.275	<0.001

Note:
Abbreviations: RR, relative risk; HR, hazard ratio; CI, confidence interval; HS-CRP, high-sensitivity C-reactive protein; PD, peritoneal dialysis; AST, aspartate transaminase; ALT, alanine transaminase; HDL, high-density lipoprotein; LDL, low-density lipoprotein; HbA1c, glycated hemoglobin; iPTH, intact parathyroid hormone; CCr, creatinine clearance.

level in the upper tertiles, although it did not reach statistical significance.

Baseline Peritoneal Membrane Characteristics

Table 2 outlines the peritoneal membrane characteristics of the PD patients. Among the 3 tertiles of increasing HS-CRP, the value of D/P_{Cr} was significantly increased. According to the results of PET, the peritoneal transport status in the 3 tertiles was significantly different, as 12.7% of patients in T3 were high transporters and 8.2% of patients were low transporters, whereas 3.7% of patients in T1 were high transporters and 16.4% of patients were low transporters. There was no significant difference for the weekly CCr (total) in the 3 tertiles, whereas the weekly CCr (PD) in T1 was significantly lower than that in the other 2 tertiles ($P<0.001$). There was also a trend toward a lower value of weekly CCr (renal) in T3.

Table 7. Relative risk of technique failure in multivariate Cox regression analysis.

		Multivariate analysis	
	RR	HR (95% CI)	P
HS-CRP (mg/L)	1.009	1.001–1.017	0.03
Diabetes mellitus	2.170	1.424–3.306	<0.001
Hemoglobin (g/dL)	0.877	0.774–0.994	0.04
Albumin (g/dL)	0.631	0.418–0.953	0.03
Dialysate/plasma creatinine	6.133	1.152–32.656	0.03
Infection episodes	4.775	2.931–7.778	<0.001
Cardiovascular events	1.896	1.228–2.927	0.004

Note:
Abbreviations: RR, relative risk; HR, hazard ratio; CI, confidence interval; HS-CRP, high-sensitivity C-reactive protein.

Patient Survival, Technique Survival, Cardiovascular Events, and Infection Episodes during the 24-month Follow-up

During the 24-month follow-up, 119 of 402 patients (29.6%) dropped out from PD, including 28 patients who died (7.0%), 81 patients (20.1%) who switched to hemodialysis, and 10 patients (2.5%) who underwent kidney transplantation (Table 3). There were significant differences in the mortality and technique failure in the three tertiles, whereas there was no significant difference in the number of patients transferring to HD and receiving transplantation among three groups (Table 3).

The results of the Kaplan–Meier analysis and log-rank test also demonstrated that there was significant difference in the cumulative patient survival rate between T3 vs T1 (P<0.001) and T3 vs T2 (P<0.001) (Fig. 1). Nevertheless, despite a trend towards a higher patient survival rate in T1 than that in T2, the difference did not reach statistically significant. In addition, the Kaplan–Meier analysis and log-rank test also revealed that the cumulative technique survival rate in T3 was significantly lower than T1 and T2 (T3 *vs.* T1, P<0.001; T3 *vs.* T2, P<0.001) (Fig. 2), whereas the comparison of the cumulative technique survival rate between T1 and T2 was not statistically different.

During the 24-month follow-up, there was no difference in the episodes of PD-related and non-PD-related infection across the 3 tertiles. Because serum CRP level has been identified as a cardiovascular factor, we examined the predictive value of serum HS-CRP level for subsequent cardiovascular events during the 24-month follow-up. More patients (25.4%) in T3 had cardiovascular events during the follow-up period than patients in T2 (15.7%) and T1 (12.7%) (P = 0.018). These results suggest that patients in the high HS-CRP tertiles are at risk of developing cardiovascular events in the following 24 months.

HS-CRP Level is an Independent Predictor of Mortality and Technique Failure

To further assess the independent predictors of mortality, Cox regression analysis was used. The results of univariate Cox regression analysis revealed that higher HS-CRP level, older age, the presence of DM, higher white blood cell count, lower serum albumin level, higher plasma sugar level and HbA1c value, lower serum creatinine level, lower calcium and phosphorus levels, and the occurrence of infection episodes and cardiovascular events during the 24-month follow-up were risk factors for mortality (Table 4). On multivariate Cox regression analysis, only higher HS-CRP level, older age, the presence of DM, lower serum albumin level, and the occurrence of cardiovascular events during follow-up were identified as independent predictors of mortality (Table 5). Every 1 mg/L increase in HS-CRP level was independently predictive of a 1.4% increase in mortality.

To identify the risk factors for technique failure (death or transfer to hemodialysis), univariate and multivariate Cox regression analyses were applied. The results of univariate Cox regression analysis demonstrated that higher HS-CRP level, older age, the presence of DM, the existence of residual urine, higher white blood cell count, lower hemoglobin level, lower serum albumin level, higher plasma sugar level and HbA1c value, lower serum creatinine level, lower serum phosphorus levels, higher dialysate/plasma creatinine ratio, peritoneal equilibration test, higher weekly CCr (PD), and the occurrence of infection episodes and cardiovascular events during follow-up were significant risk factors for technique failure (Table 6). Multivariate Cox regression analysis showed that higher HS-CRP level, the presence of DM, lower hemoglobin level, lower serum albumin level, higher dialysate/plasma creatinine ratio, and the occurrence of infection episodes and cardiovascular events during follow-up were independent predictors of technique failure (Table 7).

Discussion

This study is a cross-sectional cohort study that enrolled 402 patients to assess the impact of serum HS-CRP levels on mortality and technique survival in PD patients. The major causes of death and technique failure in PD patient is attributed to cardiovascular disease, infection, and loss of dialysis adequacy, all of which are associated with inflammation. Our results demonstrate that HS-CRP as an inflammatory marker predicts mortality and technique survival, supporting the hypothesis that inflammation has an adverse effect on the clinical outcome. Our study demonstrates that 42% of PD patients had serum HS-CRP levels more than 5 mg/L, slightly higher than those reported in Chinese PD patients (36%) [7]. In this study, the patients in the high HS-CRP tertile have a higher mortality rate and a lower technique survival rate during the 24-month follow-up. Relatively small number of patient deaths may contribute to insignificant difference in mortality and technique survival rate between T1 (none of patients) vs T2 (4 patients). In accordance, the results of multivariate logistical regression analysis also showed that HS-CRP is an independent predictor of both mortality and technique failure.

During the past decade, CRP has emerged as a powerful predictor of mortality in dialysis patients [10,30–34]. Our study also verifies the importance of HS-CRP in predicting the subsequent survival of PD patients. CRP is the most used inflammatory marker. It has been associated with the nutrition status and its markers, including serum albumin level [35,36]. In accordance, our study also showed that serum albumin level was significantly reduced across the 3 tertiles of increasing HS-CRP. Serum albumin level is an important predictor of all-cause mortality in both PD and hemodialysis patients [37,38]. As frequently there is a reciprocal interaction between serum albumin and CRP levels, some studies have shown that on multivariate Cox regression analysis, serum CRP level instead of serum albumin level remains significant in predicting mortality [39]. In contrast, our study showed that both serum HS-CRP and albumin levels were independent risk factors for mortality and technique failure. This discrepancy may be attributed to the low percentage (17.7%) of patients with diabetes in our study, as serum albumin level has been reported to be lower in diabetic PD patients and may become a confounding factor in studies recruiting a high population of diabetic patients. CRP has been shown to be strongly associated with diabetes in recent years [40,41]. Oh et al. reported that diabetic PD patients had a higher serum HS-CRP level, suggesting an interrelation between diabetes and HS-CRP. Our study demonstrates that on multivariate Cox regression analysis, serum HS-CRP, albumin level, and diabetes all remain independent factors for predicting mortality and technique failure in PD patients.

Both peritoneal clearance and residual renal function are major determinants of survival in PD patients [42–44]. In addition, these 2 factors have been shown to be linked with serum CRP level. Some studies reported that a reduction of residual renal function and peritoneal clearance led to an elevated serum CRP level [24,25,45–47], whereas other studies did not find this correlation [19,22,29,48]. There is therefore a controversy about whether CRP predicts the clinical outcome of PD patients independent of peritoneal clearance and residual renal function. Our study demonstrated that peritoneal clearance was decreased across the 3 tertiles of increasing HS-CRP, whereas there was no significant difference in the CCr of residual renal function across the 3 tertiles. On multivariate logistic regression analysis, serum HS-CRP level instead of peritoneal clearance and residual renal function was a negative predictive marker for both mortality and technique failure. The CANUSA study showed that there was a 12% decrease in the relative risk (RR) of death (RR, 0.88; 95% confidence interval [CI], 0.83 to 0.94) for each 5 L/wk per 1.73 m2 increment in glomerular filtration rate [49]. Compared with the patients in the CANUSA study, our patients had less residual renal function (37.7 L/wk in CANUSA study *vs.* 8.9 L/wk in our study). Thus, our study might underestimate the contribution of residual renal function to mortality and technique failure.

Technique failure in PD patients is frequently caused by peritonitis or high peritoneal membrane solute transport [42,43,48,50,51]. Our data showed that the patients in the high HS-CRP tertile had a higher value of D/P_{Cr} and a larger proportion of high transporters than those in the other tertiles. In addition, despite having no role in predicting mortality, a high D/P_{Cr} value is indeed a high risk factor for technique failure. Furthermore, high HS-CRP level predicted subsequent technique failure independent of D/P_{Cr}. Being a high transporter has been shown to be a significant risk factor for PD failure in a large-scale study [48], and associated with a trend to higher technique failure in a meta-analysis report [43]. In addition, Fine et al. have demonstrated that being a high transporter predicts an increase in serum CRP level [45]. Whether the association between a high transporter status and serum HS-CRP level is a causal relation or an epiphenomenon remains elusive.

Cardiovascular events are the most common cause of death in dialysis patients [52,53]. It may be related to uremic toxins, volume status, vascular calcification, anemia, hypoalbuminemia, and chronic inflammation [52,54,55]. An elevated CRP level has been reported to be an independent predictor of myocardial infarction and cardiovascular mortality in PD patients [7,15,19,20]. Our study further demonstrated that although the incidence of cardiovascular events was significantly increased across the increasing HS-CRP tertiles, both HS-CRP and cardiovascular events were independent predictive markers for all-cause mortality on multivariate Cox regression analysis.

Our study also verified some well-established factors associated with HS-CRP (Table 1), including age, DM, BMI, existence of residual urine, white blood cell count, hemoglobin, albumin, HDL, triglycerides, fasting sugar, HbA1c level, and transferrin saturation. Among these factors, it is of interest that fasting sugar and HbA1c levels were significantly increased across the 3 tertiles in non-diabetic patients, whereas it lost statistical significance in diabetic patients. In addition to blood sugar control, chronic inflammation and oxidant stress have been found to be elevated in diabetic dialysis patients. Our finding may suggest that other factors, such as oxidative stress and chronic inflammation, in diabetic PD patients may surpass the influence of blood sugar control on serum HS-CRP level, whereas blood sugar level is still associated with the elevated serum HS-CRP level in nondiabetic PD patients. Nevertheless, except HS-CRP, age, DM, and hypoalbuminemia, all of these factors, including fasting sugar and HbA1c level, failed to predict mortality and technique failure on multivariate logistical regression analysis.

This study has several limitations. First, this study was restricted to a single-center observation. Second, this study is cross-sectional and includes prevalent patients. As HS-CRP is associated with high mortality in PD patients, this study enrolled only prevalent patients and may have underestimated the impact of HS-CRP on mortality owing to censoring bias. Nevertheless, the large number of PD patients and the extensive analysis of possible parameters that can affect clinical outcome in this study reduce these limitations.

In conclusion, the present study shows the importance of HS-CRP in predicting the 2-year mortality and technique survival in PD patients independent of age, diabetes, hypoalbuminemia, and the occurrence of cardiovascular events.

Acknowledgments

The authors thank all the members of the PD unit, Chang Gung Memorial Hospital, Linkou, for their invaluable help.

Author Contributions

Conceived and designed the experiments: SHL YCT. Performed the experiments: SHL YCT. Analyzed the data: SHL YCT. Contributed reagents/materials/analysis tools: YJL HHW CCL CYL CHW YCC MYC HHH JTF CCH CWY. Wrote the paper: SHL YCT.

References

1. Yeun JY, Levine RA, Mantadilok V, Kaysen GA (2000) C-Reactive protein predicts all-cause and cardiovascular mortality in hemodialysis patients. Am J Kidney Dis 35: 469–476.

2. Ridker PM, Cushman M, Stampfer MJ, Tracy RP, Hennekens CH (1997) Inflammation, aspirin, and the risk of cardiovascular disease in apparently healthy men. N Engl J Med 336: 973–979.

3. Volanakis JE, Narkates AJ (1981) Interaction of C-reactive protein with artificial phosphatidylcholine bilayers and complement. J Immunol 126: 1820–1825.
4. Torzewski J, Torzewski M, Bowyer DE, Frohlich M, Koenig W, et al. (1998) C-reactive protein frequently colocalizes with the terminal complement complex in the intima of early atherosclerotic lesions of human coronary arteries. Arterioscler Thromb Vasc Biol 18: 1386–1392.
5. Windgassen EB, Funtowicz L, Lunsford TN, Harris LA, Mulvagh SL (2011) C-reactive protein and high-sensitivity C-reactive protein: an update for clinicians. Postgrad Med 123: 114–119.
6. Chen HY, Chiu YL, Hsu SP, Pai MF, Lai CF, et al. (2010) Elevated C-reactive protein level in hemodialysis patients with moderate/severe uremic pruritus: a potential mediator of high overall mortality. QJM 103: 837–846.
7. Wang AY, Woo J, Lam CW, Wang M, Sea MM, et al. (2003) Is a single time point C-reactive protein predictive of outcome in peritoneal dialysis patients? J Am Soc Nephrol 14: 1871–1879.
8. Corrado E, Novo S (2007) [High sensitivity of C-reactive protein in primary prevention]. G Ital Cardiol (Rome) 8: 327–334.
9. Panichi V, Migliori M, De Pietro S, Taccola D, Bianchi AM, et al. (2000) C-reactive protein as a marker of chronic inflammation in uremic patients. Blood Purif 18: 183–190.
10. Meuwese CL, Stenvinkel P, Dekker FW, Carrero JJ (2011) Monitoring of inflammation in patients on dialysis: forewarned is forearmed. Nat Rev Nephrol 7: 166–176.
11. Filiopoulos V, Vlassopoulos D (2009) Inflammatory syndrome in chronic kidney disease: pathogenesis and influence on outcomes. Inflamm Allergy Drug Targets 8: 369–382.
12. Wanner C, Drechsler C, Krane V (2009) C-reactive protein and uremia. Semin Dial 22: 438–441.
13. Choi HY, Lee JE, Han SH, Yoo TH, Kim BS, et al. (2010) Association of inflammation and protein-energy wasting with endothelial dysfunction in peritoneal dialysis patients. Nephrol Dial Transplant 25: 1266–1271.
14. Honda H, Qureshi AR, Heimburger O, Barany P, Wang K, et al. (2006) Serum albumin, C-reactive protein, interleukin 6, and fetuin a as predictors of malnutrition, cardiovascular disease, and mortality in patients with ESRD. Am J Kidney Dis 47: 139–148.
15. Wang AY, Lam CW, Chan IH, Wang M, Lui SF, et al. (2009) Long-term mortality and cardiovascular risk stratification of peritoneal dialysis patients using a combination of inflammation and calcification markers. Nephrol Dial Transplant 24: 3826–3833.
16. Filiopoulos V, Hadjiyannakos D, Takouli L, Metaxaki P, Sideris V, et al. (2009) Inflammation and oxidative stress in end-stage renal disease patients treated with hemodialysis or peritoneal dialysis. Int J Artif Organs 32: 872–882.
17. Stenvinkel P, Ketteler M, Johnson RJ, Lindholm B, Pecoits-Filho R, et al. (2005) IL-10, IL-6, and TNF-alpha: central factors in the altered cytokine network of uremia the good, the bad, and the ugly. Kidney Int 67: 1216–1233.
18. Yeun JY, Kaysen GA (1997) Acute phase proteins and peritoneal dialysate albumin loss are the main determinants of serum albumin in peritoneal dialysis patients. Am J Kidney Dis 30: 923–927.
19. Herzig KA, Purdie DM, Chang W, Brown AM, Hawley CM, et al. (2001) Is C-reactive protein a useful predictor of outcome in peritoneal dialysis patients? J Am Soc Nephrol 12: 814–821.
20. Ducloux D, Bresson-Vautrin C, Kribs M, Abdelfatah A, Chalopin JM (2002) C-reactive protein and cardiovascular disease in peritoneal dialysis patients. Kidney Int 62: 1417–1422.
21. Avram MM, Fein PA, Paluch MM, Schloth T, Chattopadhyay J (2005) Association between C-reactive protein and clinical outcomes in peritoneal dialysis patients. Adv Perit Dial 21: 154–158.
22. Oh KH, Moon JY, Oh J, Kim SG, Hwang YH, et al. (2008) Baseline peritoneal solute transport rate is not associated with markers of systemic inflammation or comorbidity in incident Korean peritoneal dialysis patients. Nephrol Dial Transplant 23: 2356–2364.
23. Cho JH, Hur IK, Kim CD, Park SH, Ryu HM, et al. (2010) Impact of systemic and local peritoneal inflammation on peritoneal solute transport rate in new peritoneal dialysis patients: a 1-year prospective study. Nephrol Dial Transplant 25: 1964–1973.
24. Perez-Flores I, Coronel F, Cigarran S, Herrero JA, Calvo N (2007) Relationship between residual renal function, inflammation, and anemia in peritoneal dialysis. Adv Perit Dial 23: 140–143.
25. Chung SH, Heimburger O, Stenvinkel P, Bergstrom J, Lindholm B (2001) Association between inflammation and changes in residual renal function and peritoneal transport rate during the first year of dialysis. Nephrol Dial Transplant 16: 2240–2245.
26. Zalunardo NY, Rose CL, Ma IW, Altmann P (2007) Higher serum C-reactive protein predicts short and long-term outcomes in peritoneal dialysis-associated peritonitis. Kidney Int 71: 687–692.
27. Westhuyzen J, Mills K, Healy H (2005) Predicting clinical outcomes in peritoneal dialysis patients using small solute modeling. Ann Clin Lab Sci 35: 46–53.
28. Noh H, Lee SW, Kang SW, Shin SK, Choi KH, et al. (1998) Serum C-reactive protein: a predictor of mortality in continuous ambulatory peritoneal dialysis patients. Perit Dial Int 18: 387–394.
29. Wang T, Heimburger O, Cheng HH, Bergstrom J, Lindholm B (1999) Does a high peritoneal transport rate reflect a state of chronic inflammation? Perit Dial Int 19: 17–22.
30. Kaysen GA (2009) Biochemistry and biomarkers of inflamed patients: why look, what to assess. Clin J Am Soc Nephrol 4 Suppl 1: S56–63.
31. Pecoits-Filho R, Stenvinkel P, Wang AY, Heimburger O, Lindholm B (2004) Chronic inflammation in peritoneal dialysis: the search for the holy grail? Perit Dial Int 24: 327–339.
32. Wanner C, Metzger T (2002) C-reactive protein a marker for all-cause and cardiovascular mortality in haemodialysis patients. Nephrol Dial Transplant 17 Suppl 8: 29–32; discussion 39–40.
33. Stenvinkel P, Lindholm B (2005) C-reactive protein in end-stage renal disease: are there reasons to measure it? Blood Purif 23: 72–78.
34. Lacson E, Jr., Levin NW (2004) C-reactive protein and end-stage renal disease. Semin Dial 17: 438–448.
35. Don BR, Kaysen GA (2000) Assessment of inflammation and nutrition in patients with end-stage renal disease. J Nephrol 13: 249–259.
36. Kaysen GA, Dubin JA, Muller HG, Rosales LM, Levin NW (2000) The acute-phase response varies with time and predicts serum albumin levels in hemodialysis patients. The HEMO Study Group. Kidney Int 58: 346–352.
37. Jones CH, Newstead CG, Wills EJ, Davison AM (1997) Serum albumin and survival in CAPD patients: the implications of concentration trends over time. Nephrol Dial Transplant 12: 554–558.
38. Owen WF, Jr., Lew NL, Liu Y, Lowrie EG, Lazarus JM (1993) The urea reduction ratio and serum albumin concentration as predictors of mortality in patients undergoing hemodialysis. N Engl J Med 329: 1001–1006.
39. Kang SH, Cho KH, Park JW, Yoon KW, Do JY (2012) Risk factors for mortality in stable peritoneal dialysis patients. Ren Fail 34: 149–154.
40. Kaul K, Hodgkinson A, Tarr JM, Kohner EM, Chibber R (2010) Is inflammation a common retinal-renal-nerve pathogenic link in diabetes? Curr Diabetes Rev 6: 294–303.
41. Calle MC, Fernandez ML (2012) Inflammation and type 2 diabetes. Diabetes Metab.
42. Churchill DN, Thorpe KE, Nolph KD, Keshaviah PR, Oreopoulos DG, et al. (1998) Increased peritoneal membrane transport is associated with decreased patient and technique survival for continuous peritoneal dialysis patients. The Canada-USA (CANUSA) Peritoneal Dialysis Study Group. J Am Soc Nephrol 9: 1285–1292.
43. Brimble KS, Walker M, Margetts PJ, Kundhal KK, Rabbat CG (2006) Meta-analysis: peritoneal membrane transport, mortality, and technique failure in peritoneal dialysis. J Am Soc Nephrol 17: 2591–2598.
44. Liao CT, Chen YM, Shiao CC, Hu FC, Huang JW, et al. (2009) Rate of decline of residual renal function is associated with all-cause mortality and technique failure in patients on long-term peritoneal dialysis. Nephrol Dial Transplant 24: 2909–2914.
45. Fine A (2002) Relevance of C-reactive protein levels in peritoneal dialysis patients. Kidney Int 61: 615–620.
46. Chung SH, Heimburger O, Stenvinkel P, Qureshi AR, Lindholm B (2003) Association between residual renal function, inflammation and patient survival in new peritoneal dialysis patients. Nephrol Dial Transplant 18: 590–597.
47. Ates K, Ates A, Ekmekci Y, Nergizoglu G (2005) The time course of serum C-reactive protein is more predictive of mortality than its baseline level in peritoneal dialysis patients. Perit Dial Int 25: 256–268.
48. Rumpsfeld M, McDonald SP, Johnson DW (2006) Higher peritoneal transport status is associated with higher mortality and technique failure in the Australian and New Zealand peritoneal dialysis patient populations. J Am Soc Nephrol 17: 271–278.
49. Bargman JM, Thorpe KE, Churchill DN (2001) Relative contribution of residual renal function and peritoneal clearance to adequacy of dialysis: a reanalysis of the CANUSA study. J Am Soc Nephrol 12: 2158–2162.
50. Mujais S, Story K (2006) Peritoneal dialysis in the US: evaluation of outcomes in contemporary cohorts. Kidney Int Suppl: S21–26.
51. Kavanagh D, Prescott GJ, Mactier RA (2004) Peritoneal dialysis-associated peritonitis in Scotland (1999–2002). Nephrol Dial Transplant 19: 2584–2591.
52. Krediet RT, Balafa O (2010) Cardiovascular risk in the peritoneal dialysis patient. Nat Rev Nephrol 6: 451–460.
53. Li PK, Chow KM (2005) The clinical and epidemiological aspects of vascular mortality in chronic peritoneal dialysis patients. Perit Dial Int 25 Suppl 3: S80–83.
54. Johnson DW, Craven AM, Isbel NM (2007) Modification of cardiovascular risk in hemodialysis patients: an evidence-based review. Hemodial Int 11: 1–14.
55. Nolan CR (2005) Strategies for improving long-term survival in patients with ESRD. J Am Soc Nephrol 16 Suppl 2: S120–127.

18

Correlations of *MTHFR* 677C>T Polymorphism with Cardiovascular Disease in Patients with End-Stage Renal Disease

Xian-Hui Gao[1]*, Guo-Yi Zhang[1], Ying Wang[2], Hui-Ying Zhang[3]

1 Laboratory of Preventive Medicine, School of Public Health, Liaoning Medical University, Jinzhou, China, **2** Department of Toxicology, School of Public Health, Liaoning Medical University, Jinzhou, China, **3** Sleep Monitoring Center, First Affiliated Hospital of Liaoning Medical University, Jinzhou, China

Abstract

Objective: This meta-analysis was conducted to evaluate the correlations of a common polymorphism (677C>T) in the methylenetetrahydrofolate reductase (*MTHFR*) gene with risk of cardiovascular disease (CVD) in patients with end-stage renal disease (ESRD).

Method: The following electronic databases were searched without language restrictions: Web of Science (1945~2013), the Cochrane Library Database (Issue 12, 2013), MEDLINE (1966~2013), EMBASE (1980~2013), CINAHL (1982~2013) and the Chinese Biomedical Database (CBM) (1982~2013). Meta-analysis was performed using STATA statistical software. Odds ratios (ORs) with their 95% confidence intervals (95%CIs) were calculated.

Results: Eight cohort studies met all inclusion criteria and were included in this meta-analysis. A total of 2,292 ESRD patients with CVD were involved in this meta-analysis. Our meta-analysis results revealed that the *MTHFR* 677C>T polymorphism might increase the risk of CVD in ESRD patients (TT vs. CC: OR = 2.75, 95%CI = 1.35~5.59, $P = 0.005$; CT+TT vs. CC: OR = 1.39, 95%CI = 1.09~1.78, $P = 0.008$; TT vs. CC+CT: OR = 2.52, 95%CI = 1.25~5.09, $P = 0.010$; respectively). Further subgroup analysis by ethnicity suggested that the *MTHFR* 677C>T polymorphism was associated with an elevated risk for CVD in ESRD patients among Asians (TT vs. CC: OR = 3.38, 95%CI = 1.11~10.28, $P = 0.032$; CT+TT vs. CC: OR = 1.44, 95%CI = 1.05~1.97, $P = 0.022$; TT vs. CC+CT: OR = 3.15, 95%CI = 1.02~9.72, $P = 0.046$; respectively), but not among Africans or Caucasians (all $P > 0.05$).

Conclusion: Our findings indicate that the *MTHFR* 677C>T polymorphism may be associated with an elevated risk for CVD in ESRD patients, especially among Asians.

Editor: Yan Gong, University of Florida, United States of America

Funding: The authors have no support or funding to report.

Competing Interests: The authors have declared that no competing interests exist.

* Email: gaoxianhui16@126.com

Introduction

Hemodialysis (HD) is a common form of dialysis therapy for kidney disease by achieving the extracorporeal removal of waste products such as creatinine, urea and free water from the blood [1]. HD is the most common procedure performed for patients with end-stage renal disease (ESRD), with an estimation of 1.5 million ESRD patients receiving HD worldwide [2]. Despite its important role in treating ESRD, HD also serves as a multiplier for other vascular risk factors, contributing to an increased incidence of cardiovascular disease, such as atrial fibrillation and myocardial ischemia [3,4]. Moreover, it has been reported that mortality caused by cardiovascular disease (CVD) in ESRD patients is 25% higher than that in the general population [5,6]. Therefore, the assessment and prevention of CVD are major considerations for dealing patients with HD [7]. Generally, CVD refers to any disease that affects the cardiovascular system, principally cardiac disease, vascular diseases of the brain and kidney, and peripheral arterial disease [8]. Clinically, traditional CVD risk factors include old age, male sex, diabetes mellitus, and systolic hypertension and so on [9]. Over past few decades, studies have demonstrated that the severity and extent of cardiovascular complications in ESRD patients is disproportionate to the number and severity of traditional risk factors [10,11]. In recent years, nontraditional risk factors such as hemoglobin levels, inflammation, oxidative stress, and particularly epigenetic mechanisms of gene regulation have been emphasized as factors that may play an important role in the development of cardiovascular disease in patients with HD [12]. In addition, genetic polymorphisms have received considerable attention as a competitive candidate for the risk of CVD in ESRD patients [13].

Methylene tetrahydrofolate reductase (MTHFR), encoded by the *MTHFR* gene, is a key enzyme in folate metabolism which plays a critical role in the synthesis and methylation of DNA encoding for an enzyme responsible for re-methylation of homocysteine (Hcy) to methionine [14–16]. Actually, Hazra et al. confirmed that the functional polymorphism in MTHFR

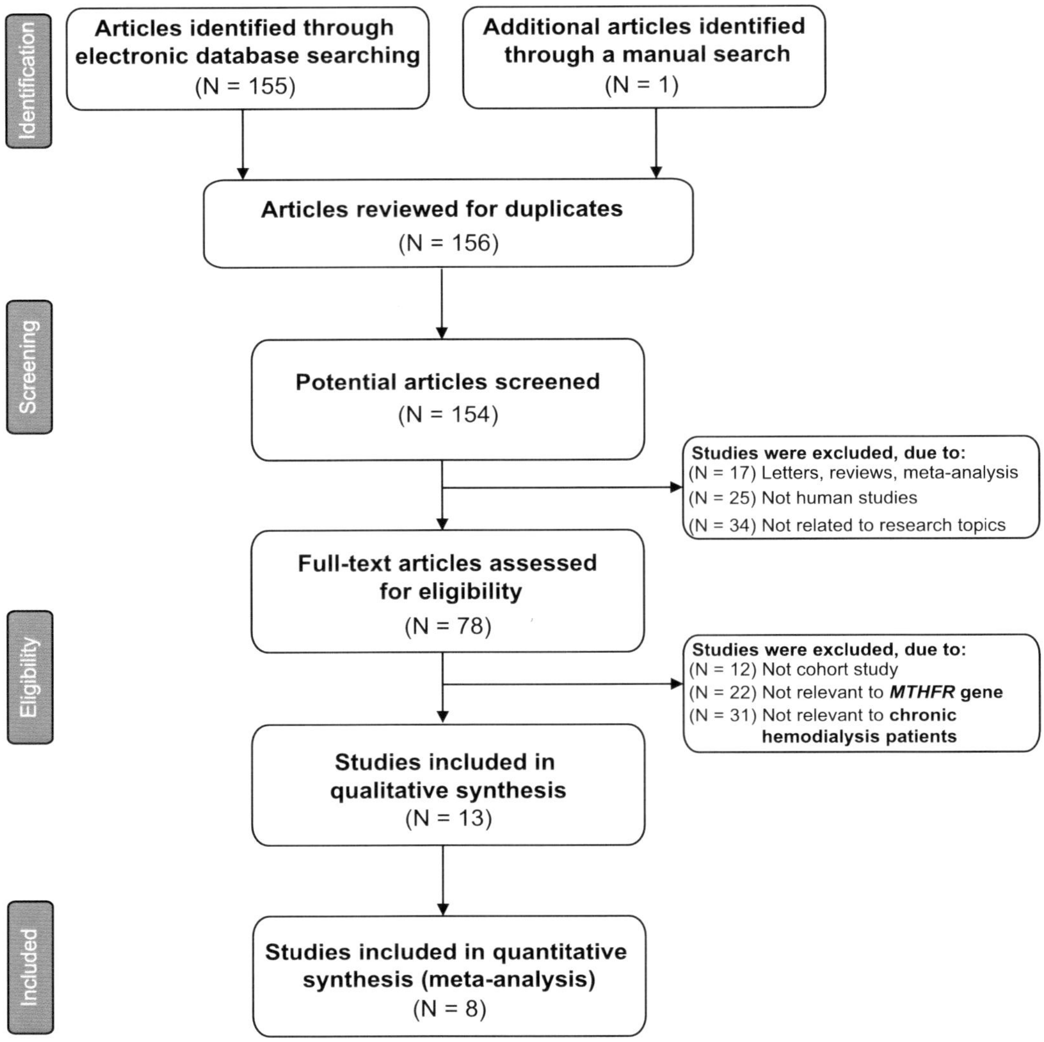

Figure 1. Flow chart shows study selection procedure. Eight cohort studies were included in this meta-analysis.

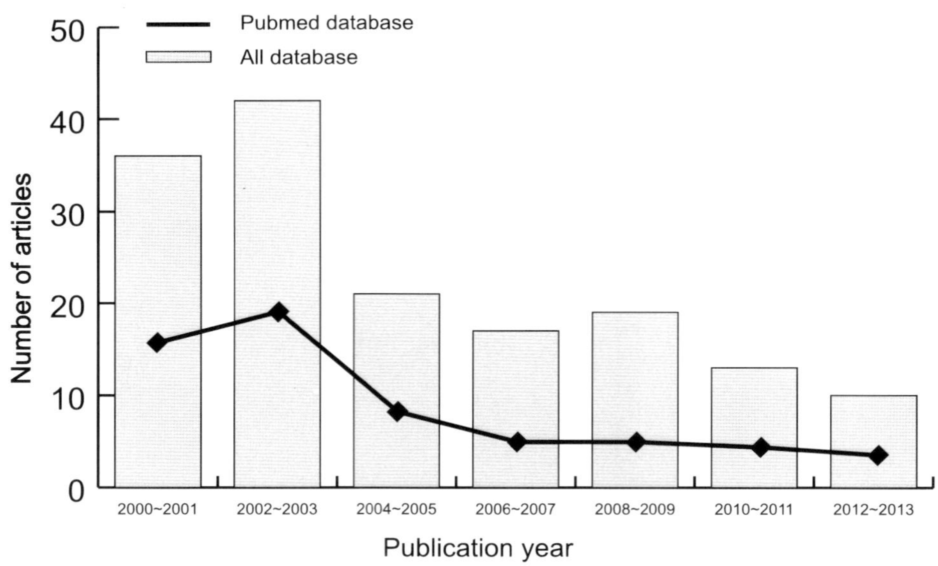

Figure 2. The distribution of the number of topic-related literatures in the electronic database over the last decade.

Table 1. Baseline characteristics and methodological qualities of all included studies.

First author	Year	Country	Ethnicity	Case number	Gender (M/F)	Age (years)	Genotyping method	Genotype frequency			HWE test	NOS score
								CC	CT	TT	(*P* value)	
Lee et al [21]	2011	Korea	Asians	152	83/69	56.8±13.6	PCR-RFLP	44	72	36	0.538	7
Ibrahim et al [30]	2009	Egypt	Africans	50	29/21	41.6±11.8	Direct sequencing	30	16	4	0.385	6
Aucella et al [28]	2005	Italy	Caucasians	461	217/244	58.8±15.6	PCR-RFLP	134	220	86	0.801	8
Fukasawa et al [23]	2003	Japan	Asians	337	196/141	61.5±13.7	Direct sequencing	111	158	68	0.390	8
Morimoto et al [32]	2002	Japan	Asians	168	87/81	60.7±13.1	PCR-RFLP	78	67	23	0.167	7
Haviv et al [29]	2002	USA	Caucasians	120	72/48	48.0±13.0	PCR-RFLP	40	60	19	0.656	7
Wrone et al [24]	2001	USA	Caucasians	459	230/226	-	Direct sequencing	216	184	59	0.049	7
Kimura et al [31]	2000	Japan	Asians	545	319/226	58.7±12.5	PCR-RFLP	199	251	95	0.303	8

Legend: M – male; F – female; SNP - single nucleotide polymorphism; HWE - Hardy-Weinberg equilibrium; NOS - Newcastle-Ottawa Scale; PCR-RFLP - polymerase chain reaction-restriction fragment length polymorphism.

Ala222Val (also reported as MTHFR C677T), rs1801133, on chromosome 1 was associated with plasma homocysteine in a healthy population [17]. The human *MTHFR* gene is located on the short arm of chromosome 1 (1p36.3), is comprised of 11 exons and 10 introns, and is 19.3 kb in length [17]. Currently, multiple researchers have demonstrated that genetic variations in the *MTHFR* gene might alter its production and function, thereby affecting individual prevalence rates of some diseases and even cancers [18,19]. More specifically, multiple polymorphic sites such as 677C>T (rs1801133) and 1298A>C (rs1801131) within the *MTHFR* promoter region have been reported in previous studies, of which 677C>T has been suggested to be implicated in the susceptibility to CVD in ESRD patients [20,21]. It should be noted that plasma Hcy levels have been found to be an important risk factor for the development of CVD in ESRD patients [22]. However, polymorphism at nucleotide 677C>T may reduce the activation and thermo-stability of MTHFR, and subsequently inhibit the generation of 5-Methylenetetrahydrofolate and interfere with the normal metabolism and re-methylation of Hcy, thereby resulting in the accumulation of Hcy and an elevated plasma Hcy concentration in individuals; however, contradictory results have also been reported [23,24]. Given the conflicting evidence on this issue, we conducted a meta-analysis of all available cohort studies to determine whether *MTHFR* genetic polymorphisms contribute to the pathogenesis of CVD in ESRD patients.

Methods

Publication search

The following electronic databases were searched without language restrictions: Web of Science (1945~2013), the Cochrane Library Database (Issue 12, 2013), MEDLINE (1966~2013), EMBASE (1980~2013), CINAHL (1982~2013) and the Chinese Biomedical Database (CBM) (1982~2013). We used the following keywords and MeSH terms in conjunction with a highly sensitive search strategy: ["SNP" or "mutation" or "genetic polymorphism" or "variation" or "polymorphism" or "single nucleotide polymorphism" or "variant"] and ["cardiovascular disease" or "CVD" or "cardiovascular risk" or "Hemodialysis" or "HD"] and ["methylenetetrahydrofolate reductase" or "MTHFR" or "methylene tetrahydrofolate reductase" or "5,10-methylenetetrahydrofolate reductase"]. We also conducted a manual search to find other potential articles based on references identified in retrieved articles.

Inclusion and exclusion criteria

The following criteria were used to determine the eligibility of included studies: (1) the study design must be a clinical cohort study; (2) the study must relate to the relationships of *MTHFR* 677C>T polymorphisms with the risk of CVD in ESRD patients; (3) all patients met the diagnostic criteria for HD; (4) the study must provide sufficient information about the frequencies of the *MTHFR* 677C>T polymorphism. If a study could not meet the inclusion criteria, it was excluded. The most recent or the largest sample size publication was included when the authors published several studies using the same subjects. The supporting PRISMA checklist is available as Checklist S1.

Data extraction

Data were systematically extracted by two authors from each included study using a standardized form. The form used for data extraction documented the most relevant items including publication year, language of publication, the first author's surname,

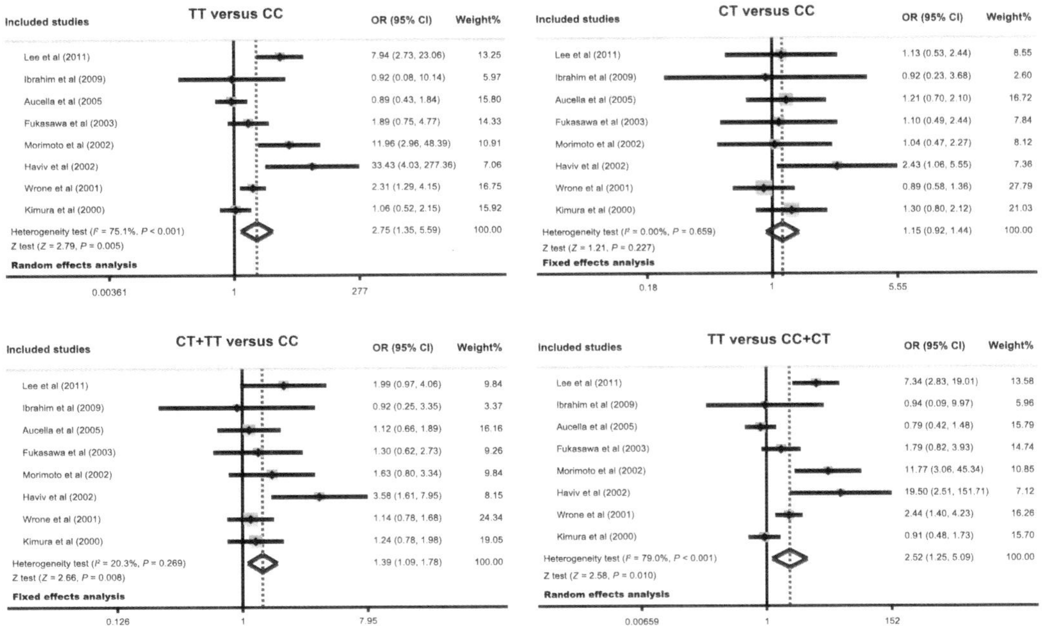

Figure 3. Forest plots for the relationships between the *MTHFR* 677C>T polymorphism and the risk of cardiovascular disease in chronic hemodialysis patients.

geographical location, sample size, design of study, the source of the subjects, source of samples, allele frequencies, genotyping method of SNP, evidence of HWE in healthy controls, etc.

Methodological assessment

Methodological quality was independently assessed by two observers according to the Newcastle-Ottawa Scale (NOS) criteria [25]. The NOS criteria includes three aspects: (1) subject selection: 0~4 points; (2) comparability of subject: 0~2 points; (3) clinical outcome: 0~3 points. NOS scores range from 0 to 9 with a score ≥7 indicating good quality. The supporting NOS score criteria are available in Supplement S1.

Statistical analysis

Meta-analysis was performed with the use of the STATA statistical software (Version 12.0, Stata Corporation, College Station, TX, USA). Odds ratios (ORs) with their 95% confidence intervals (95%CIs) were calculated as estimates of relative risk for CVD in ESRD patients. The *Z* test was used to estimate the statistical significance of pooled ORs. Heterogeneity among studies was estimated by the Cochran's *Q*-statistic and I^2 tests [26]. If a *Q*-test shows a $P<0.05$ or $I^2>50\%$, indicating significant heterogeneity, the random-effects model was conducted; otherwise the fixed-effects model was used. We also explored reasons for heterogeneity using meta-regression and subgroup analyses. In order to evaluate the influence of single studies on the overall estimate, a sensitivity analysis was performed. Funnel plots and Egger's linear regression test were applied to investigate publication bias [27].

Results

Eligible studies

Initially, the highly sensitive search strategy identified 156 articles. After screening the titles and abstracts of all retrieved articles, 78 articles were excluded. Then full texts were reviewed and 65 articles were further excluded. Another 5 studies were also excluded due to lack of data integrity (Figure 1). Finally, 8 cohort studies were included in this meta-analysis [21,23,24,28–32]. Publication years of the eligible studies ranged from 2000 to 2011. Figure 2 shows the distribution of the number of topic-related literatures in electronic databases over the last decade. A total of 2,292 ESRD patients with CVD were involved in this meta-analysis. Four studies were conducted among Asians, three studies among Caucasians, and one study among Africans. The polymerase chain reaction-amplified genes with restriction endonucleases (PCR-RFLP) was performed in 5 studies, while 3 studies used the direct DNA sequencing method. The genotype frequencies of controls were all in HWE (all $P>0.05$). The NOS scores of all included studies were ≥6. The main characteristics of all eligible studies are listed in Table 1.

Quantitative data synthesis

Meta-analysis findings on the relationship between the *MTHFR* 677C>T polymorphism and susceptibility to CVD in ESRD patients is shown in Table 2. The random-effects model was conducted due to significant heterogeneity between studies. Our meta-analysis results revealed that the *MTHFR* 677C>T polymorphism might increase the risk of CVD in ESRD patients (TT vs. CC: OR = 2.75, 95%CI = 1.35~5.59, $P=0.005$; CT+TT vs. CC: OR = 1.39, 95%CI = 1.09~1.78, $P=0.008$; TT vs. CC+CT: OR = 2.52, 95%CI = 1.25~5.09, $P=0.010$; respectively) (Figure 3).

Subgroup and meta-regression analysis were conducted based on ethnicity to investigate potential sources of heterogeneity. Our results suggested that the *MTHFR* 677C>T polymorphism was associated with the incidence of CVD in ESRD patients among Asians (TT vs. CC: OR = 3.38, 95%CI = 1.11~10.28, $P=0.032$; CT+TT vs. CC: OR = 1.44, 95%CI = 1.05~1.97, $P=0.022$; TT vs. CC+CT: OR = 3.15, 95%CI = 1.02~9.72, $P=0.046$; respectively), but not among Africans or Caucasians (all $P>0.05$). Further subgroup analyses based on genotyping method suggested

Table 2. Meta-analysis of the relationships between the *MTHFR* 677 C>T polymorphism and the risk of cardiovascular disease in patients with end-stage renal disease.

	Sample size	TT vs. CC			CT vs. CC			CT+TT vs. CC			TT vs. CC+CT		
		OR	95%CI	*P*	OR	95%CI	*P*	OR	95%CI	*P*	OR	95%CI	*P*
Overall		2.75	1.35–5.59	0.005	1.15	0.92–1.44	0.227	1.39	1.09–1.78	0.008	2.52	1.25–5.09	0.010
Ethnicity													
Asians (n = 4)	1202	3.38	1.11–10.28	0.032	1.18	0.85–1.65	0.327	1.44	1.05–1.97	0.022	3.15	1.02–9.72	0.046
Africans (n = 1)	50	0.92	0.08–10.14	0.943	0.92	0.23–3.68	0.902	0.92	0.25–3.35	0.895	0.94	0.09–9.97	0.962
Caucasians (n = 3)	1040	2.72	0.76–9.78	0.125	1.25	0.75–2.07	0.389	1.52	0.84–2.73	0.165	2.35	0.69–7.96	0.171
Genotyping method													
PCR-RFLP (n = 5)	1446	4.00	1.19–13.53	0.025	1.31	0.98–1.74	0.065	1.61	1.11–2.32	0.012	3.42	1.04–11.23	0.043
Direct sequencing (n = 3)	846	2.11	1.30–3.42	0.003	0.93	0.65–1.34	0.695	1.16	0.83–1.61	0.394	2.14	1.37–3.33	0.001

Legend: OR - odds ratio; 95%CI - 95% confidence interval; PCR-RFLP - polymerase chain reaction-restriction fragment length polymorphism.

that the *MTHFR* 677C>T polymorphism was closely linked to an increased risk of CVD in the majority of subgroups (as shown in Table 2).

Meta-regression analysis confirmed that none of the considered factors was the main source of heterogeneity (as shown in Table 3). Sensitivity analysis suggested that no single study could influence the overall pooled estimates (Figure 4). We found no evidence of obvious asymmetry in the funnel plots (Figure 5). Egger's test also did not display strong statistical evidence for publication bias (all $P>0.05$).

Discussion

MTHFR can catalyze a rate-limiting reaction in the transformation of methionine into Hcy and back exclusively through the transfer of the methyl group to and from methyl-tetrahydrofolate, separately [33–35]. It is well documented that an elevated level of the sulphur amino-acid Hcy in plasma is an independent risk factor for atherosclerosis, coronary heart disease, stroke and other CVDs [36,37]. Meanwhile, the increased fasting level of total Hcy was found to establish an independent contribution to the excess incidence of fatal and non-fatal cardiovascular outcomes [38]. Indeed, the formation of hyperhomocysteinemia (HHcy) was closely associated with folic acid, Vitamin B_6 and B_{12} supplementation [39], but also correlated with sulfur amino acid metabolism [40]. As for *MTHFR*, since the methyl groups for Hcy mediated DNA-methylation to methionine are related to the provision of 5-methylenetetrahydrofolate, which can be irreversibly transferred from 5 to 10-methylenetetrahydrofolate through MTHFR catalysis, the *MTHFR* gene probably plays a crucial role in the re-methylation of Hcy [41]. On the other hand, it has been estimated by statistical data in clinical studies that HD patients suffering from mild to moderate HHcy account for a great proportion of the high-risk population for CVD [42]. Therefore, it was hypothesized that common polymorphisms in the *MTHFR* gene could be functional and associated with the development and progression of CVD in ESRD patients. Recently, the usage of human *MTHFR* gene mutations in predicting the increased Hcy levels and susceptibility to CVD has been widely adopted [13,34]. In particular, a relatively common functional polymorphism in *MTHFR* rs1801133 (677C>T) in exon 4 may influence the plasma Hcy in ESRD patients. Abundant evidence has supported the view that a half reduction in enzymatic capability might lead to a mild Hcy, as well as total elevation of plasma Hcy concentrations in individuals, both of which might contribute to the genetic predisposition to CVD [30,43].

We undertook the present meta-analysis to elucidate the association of genetic mutations in the *MTHFR* gene with the incidence of CVD in ESRD patients. Our meta-analysis results showed that the *MTHFR* 677C>T polymorphism was associated with an increased risk of CVD in ESRD patients, indicating that variants in the *MTHFR* gene may play a pivotal role in the pathology of CVD in ESRD patients. Although the mechanism by which *MTHFR* genetic polymorphisms lead to the development of CVD in ESRD patients still remains partially understood, a possible explanation is that the *MTHFR* 677C>T polymorphism may lead to a mild decrease in MTHFR activity which plays a crucial role in the remethylation of Hcy to methionine, resulting in elevated total plasma Hcy levels which may contribute independently to the excess incidence of fatal and nonfatal CVD. Haviv YS et al. have suggested a major role for plasma Hcy level as a determinant of CVD in ESRD patients, whereby the *MTHFR* variants and low serum folate are important determinants of plasma Hcy level and therefore may also have an indirect impact

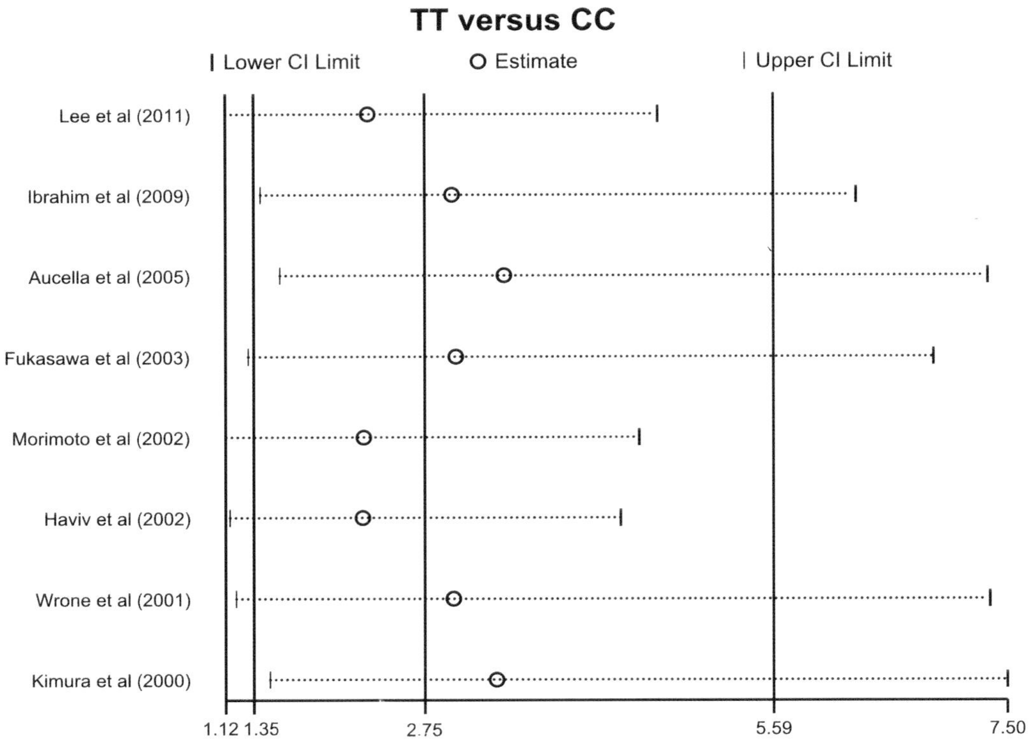

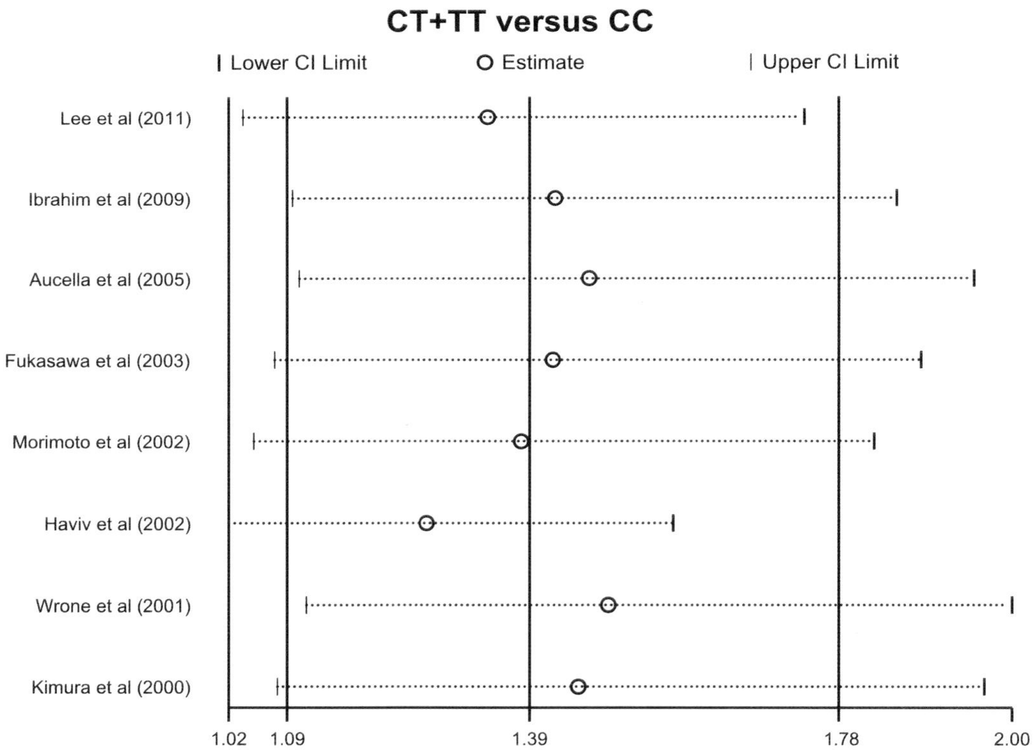

Figure 4. Sensitivity analysis of the summary odds ratio coefficients on the relationships between the *MTHFR* 677C>T polymorphism and the risk of cardiovascular disease in chronic hemodialysis patients.

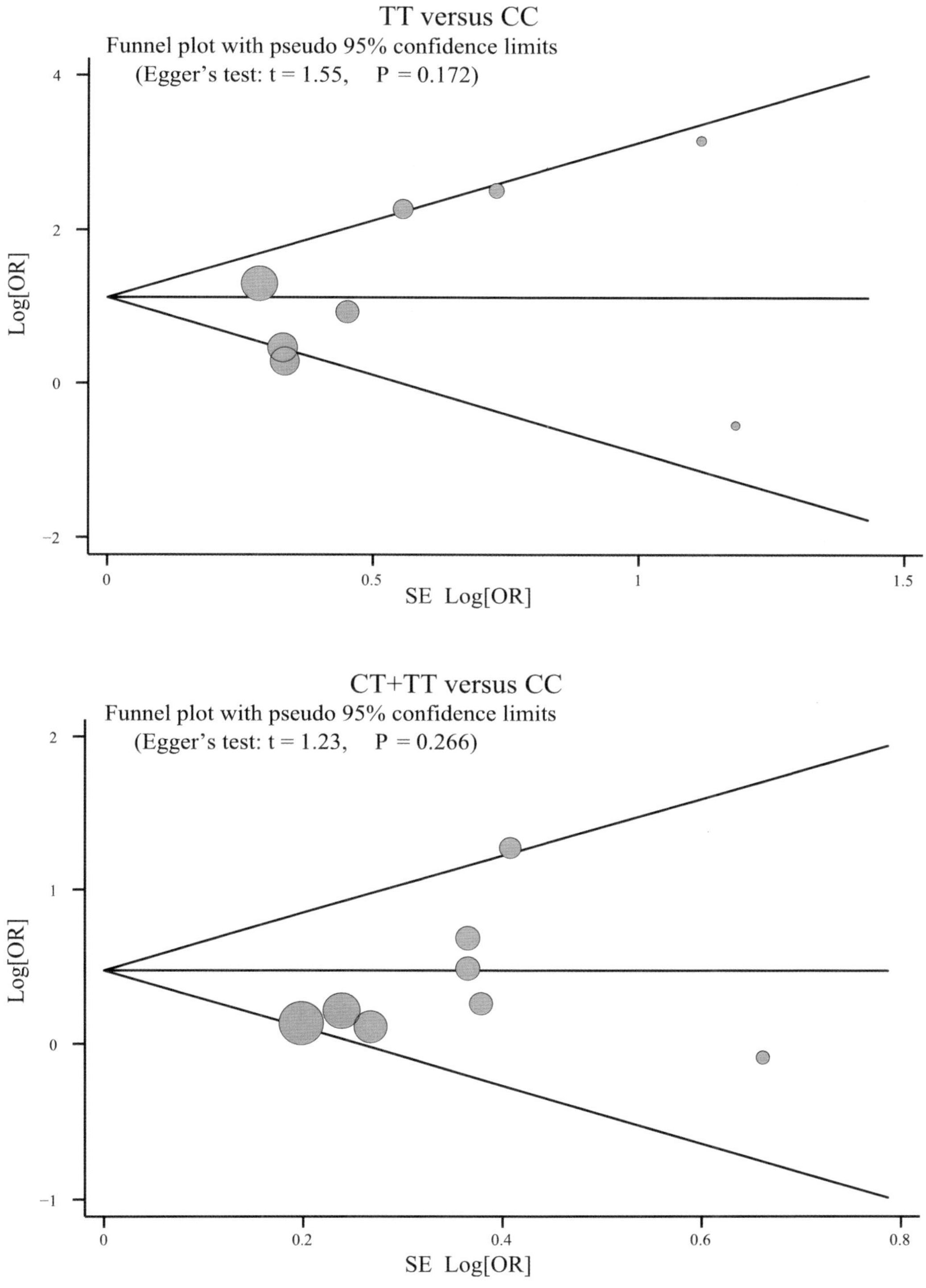

Figure 5. Funnel plot of publication biases on the relationships between the *MTHFR* 677C>T polymorphism and the risk of cardiovascular disease in chronic hemodialysis patients.

on the cardiovascular status [29]. Since heterogeneity obviously existed in our meta-analysis, we performed stratified analyses based on ethnicity and genotyping method. Subgroup analysis by ethnicity indicated that there were marked associations between the *MTHFR* 677C>T polymorphism and an increased risk of CVD in ESRD patients among Asians. In short, our findings were in accordance with previous studies that found that the *MTHFR* 677C>T polymorphism may alter the risk of developing CVD in ESRD patients, suggesting that these polymorphisms may be useful as biomarkers for the early diagnosis of CVD in ESRD patients.

Table 3. Univariate and multivariate meta-regression analyses of potential source of heterogeneity.

Heterogeneity factors	Coefficient	SE	Z	P	95%CI	
					LL	UL
Publication year						
Univariate	0.028	0.122	0.23	0.820	−0.212	0.267
Multivariate	−0.078	0.067	−1.17	0.241	−0.209	0.053
Ethnicity						
Univariate	−0.439	0.697	−0.63	0.528	−1.806	0.927
Multivariate	−0.132	0.339	−0.39	0.697	−0.796	0.532
Genotyping method						
Univariate	−0.769	0.922	−0.83	0.405	−2.577	1.039
Multivariate	0.562	0.372	1.51	0.131	−0.167	1.291

Legend: SE - standard error; 95%CI - 95% confidence interval; UL - upper limit; LL - lower limit.

As the first meta-analysis focused on the relationships between the *MTHFR* 677C>T polymorphism and the risk of CVD in ESRD patients, our study has some limitations. First, our results lacked sufficient statistical power to assess correlations between the *MTHFR* 677C>T polymorphism and susceptibility to CVD in ESRD patients due to a relatively small sample size. Second, as a retrospective study, our meta-analysis may have been influenced by subject selection bias, thereby affecting the reliability of our results. Third, our meta-analysis failed to obtain original data from the included studies, which may have limited further evaluation of the potential roles of the *MTHFR* 677C>T polymorphism in the development and progression of CVD in ESRD patients. Importantly, the inclusion criteria of cases and controls were not well defined in all included studies, which might also have influenced our results.

In conclusion, our findings indicate that the *MTHFR* 677C>T polymorphism may contribute to increased CVD risk in ESRD patients. Thus, the *MTHFR* 677C>T polymorphism may be a useful and promising biomarker for the early detection and prognosis of CVD in ESRD patients. However, due to the limitations mentioned above, more research studies with larger sample sizes are still needed to provide a more representative statistical analysis.

Acknowledgments

We would like to acknowledge the helpful comments on this paper received from our reviewers.

Author Contributions

Conceived and designed the experiments: XHG. Performed the experiments: XHG HYZ. Analyzed the data: XHG YW. Contributed reagents/materials/analysis tools: GYZ YW. Wrote the paper: XHG.

References

1. Mehrotra R, Chiu YW, Kalantar-Zadeh K, Bargman J, Vonesh E (2011) Similar outcomes with hemodialysis and peritoneal dialysis in patients with end-stage renal disease. Arch Intern Med, 171(2): 110–118.
2. Palacio S, Gonzales NR, Sangha NS, Birnbaum LA, Hart RG (2011) Thrombolysis for acute stroke in hemodialysis: international survey of expert opinion. Clin J Am Soc Nephrol, 6(5): 1089–1093.
3. Winkelmayer WC, Patrick AR, Liu J, Brookhart MA, Setoguchi S (2011) The increasing prevalence of atrial fibrillation among hemodialysis patients. J Am Soc Nephrol, 22(2): 349–357.
4. McIntyre CW (2010) Haemodialysis-induced myocardial stunning in chronic kidney disease - a new aspect of cardiovascular disease. Blood Purif, 29(2): 105 110.
5. Weiner DE, Scott TM, Giang LM, Agganis BT, Sorensen EP, et al (2011) Cardiovascular disease and cognitive function in maintenance hemodialysis patients. Am J Kidney Dis, 58(5): 773–781.
6. Matias PJ, Jorge C, Ferreira C, Borges M, Aires I, et al (2010) Cholecalciferol supplementation in hemodialysis patients: effects on mineral metabolism, inflammation, and cardiac dimension parameters. Clin J Am Soc Nephrol, 5(5): 905–911.
7. Shiotsu Y, Mori Y, Nishimura M, Sakoda C, Tokoro T, et al (2011) Plasma S100A12 level is associated with cardiovascular disease in hemodialysis patients. Clin J Am Soc Nephrol, 6(4): 718–723.
8. Anderson JL, May HT, Horne BD, Bair TL, Hall NL, et al (2010) Relation of vitamin D deficiency to cardiovascular risk factors, disease status, and incident events in a general healthcare population. Am J Cardiol, 106(7): 963–968.
9. Stenvinkel P, Carrero JJ, Axelsson J, Lindholm B, Heimburger O, et al (2008) Emerging biomarkers for evaluating cardiovascular risk in the chronic kidney disease patient: how do new pieces fit into the uremic puzzle? Clin J Am Soc Nephrol, 3(2): 505–521.
10. Kendrick J, Chonchol MB (2008) Nontraditional risk factors for cardiovascular disease in patients with chronic kidney disease. Nat Clin Pract Nephrol, 4(12): 672–681.
11. Chonchol M, Kendrick J, Targher G (2011) Extra-skeletal effects of vitamin D deficiency in chronic kidney disease. Ann Med, 43(4): 273–282.
12. Cozzolino M, Biondi ML, Galassi A, Cusi D, Brancaccio D, et al (2010) Vascular calcification and cardiovascular outcome in dialysis patients: the role of gene polymorphisms. Blood Purif, 29(4): 347–351.
13. Fung MM, Salem RM, Lipkowitz MS, Bhatnagar V, Pandey B, et al (2012) Methylenetetrahydrofolate reductase (MTHFR) polymorphism A1298C (Glu429Ala) predicts decline in renal function over time in the African-American Study of Kidney Disease and Hypertension (AASK) Trial and Veterans Affairs Hypertension Cohort (VAHC). Nephrol Dial Transplant, 27(1): 197–205.
14. Spellicy CJ, Northrup H, Fletcher JM, Cirino PT, Dennis M, et al (2012) Folate metabolism gene 5,10-methylenetetrahydrofolate reductase (MTHFR) is associated with ADHD in myelomeningocele patients. PLoS One, 7(12): e51330.
15. Garner JL, Niles KM, McGraw S, Yeh JR, Cushnie DW, et al (2013) Stability of DNA methylation patterns in mouse spermatogonia under conditions of MTHFR deficiency and methionine supplementation. Biol Reprod, 89(5): 125.
16. Field MS, Shields KS, Abarinov EV, Malysheva OV, Allen RH, et al (2013) Reduced MTHFD1 activity in male mice perturbs folate- and choline-

dependent one-carbon metabolism as well as transsulfuration. J Nutr, 143(1): 41–45.
17. Hazra A, Kraft P, Lazarus R, Chen C, Chanock SJ, et al (2009) Genome-wide significant predictors of metabolites in the one-carbon metabolism pathway. Hum Mol Genet, 18(23): 4677–4687.
18. Abbas S, Raza ST, Ahmed F, Ahmad A, Rizvi S, et al (2013) Association of Genetic polymorphism of PPARgamma-2, ACE, MTHFR, FABP-2 and FTO genes in risk prediction of type 2 diabetes mellitus. J Biomed Sci, 20(1): 80.
19. Zhang J, Qiu LX, Wang ZH, Wu XH, Liu XJ, et al (2010) MTHFR C677T polymorphism associated with breast cancer susceptibility: a meta-analysis involving 15,260 cases and 20,411 controls. Breast Cancer Res Treat, 123(2): 549–555.
20. Perna AF, Lanza D, Sepe I, Conzo G, Altucci L, et al (2013) Altered folate receptor 2 expression in uraemic patients on haemodialysis: implications for folate resistance. Nephrol Dial Transplant, 28(5): 1214–1224.
21. Lee SY, Kim HY, Park KM, Hong SG, Kim HJ, et al (2011) MTHFR C677T polymorphism as a risk factor for vascular calcification in chronic hemodialysis patients. J Korean Med Sci, 26(3): 461–465.
22. Heinz J, Kropf S, Luley C, Dierkes J (2009) Homocysteine as a risk factor for cardiovascular disease in patients treated by dialysis: a meta-analysis. Am J Kidney Dis, 54(3): 478–489.
23. Fukasawa M, Matsushita K, Kamiyama M, Mikami Y, Araki I, et al (2003) The methylentetrahydrofolate reductase C677T point mutation is a risk factor for vascular access thrombosis in hemodialysis patients. Am J Kidney Dis, 41(3): 637–642.
24. Wrone EM, Zehnder JL, Hornberger JM, McCann LM, Coplon NS, et al (2001) An MTHFR variant, homocysteine, and cardiovascular comorbidity in renal disease. Kidney Int, 60(3): 1106–1113.
25. Stang A (2010) Critical evaluation of the Newcastle-Ottawa scale for the assessment of the quality of nonrandomized studies in meta-analyses. Eur J Epidemiol, 25(9): 603–605.
26. Zintzaras E, Ioannidis JP (2005) HEGESMA: genome search meta-analysis and heterogeneity testing. Bioinformatics, 21(18): 3672–3673.
27. Peters JL, Sutton AJ, Jones DR, Abrams KR, Rushton L (2006) Comparison of two methods to detect publication bias in meta-analysis. JAMA, 295(6): 676–680.
28. Aucella F, Margaglione M, Grandone E, Vigilante M, Gatta G, et al (2005) The C677T methylenetetrahydrofolate reductase gene mutation does not influence cardiovascular risk in the dialysis population: results of a multicentre prospective study. Nephrol Dial Transplant, 20(2): 382–386.
29. Haviv YS, Shpichinetsky V, Goldschmidt N, Atta IA, Ben-Yehuda A, et al (2002) The common mutations C677T and A1298C in the human methylenetetrahydrofolate reductase gene are associated with hyperhomocysteinemia and cardiovascular disease in hemodialysis patients. Nephron, 92(1): 120–126.
30. Ibrahim S, El Dessokiy O (2009) Prevalence of methylenetetrahydrofolate gene (MTHFR) C677T polymorphism among chronic hemodialysis patients and its association with cardiovascular disease: a cross-sectional analysis. Clin Exp Nephrol, 13(5): 501–507.
31. Kimura H, Gejyo F, Suzuki S, Miyazaki R (2000) The C677T methylenetetrahydrofolate reductase gene mutation in hemodialysis patients. J Am Soc Nephrol, 11(5): 885–893.
32. Morimoto K, Haneda T, Okamoto K, Ishida H, Kikuchi K (2002) Methylenetetrahydrofolate reductase gene polymorphism, hyperhomocysteinemia, and cardiovascular diseases in chronic hemodialysis patients [PMID: 11744804]. Nephron, 90(1): 43–50.
33. Yang Q, Bailey L, Clarke R, Flanders WD, Liu T, et al (2012) Prospective study of methylenetetrahydrofolate reductase (MTHFR) variant C677T and risk of all-cause and cardiovascular disease mortality among 6000 US adults. Am J Clin Nutr, 95(5): 1245–1253.
34. Clarke R, Bennett DA, Parish S, Verhoef P, Dotsch-Klerk M, et al (2012) Homocysteine and coronary heart disease: meta-analysis of MTHFR case-control studies, avoiding publication bias. PLoS Med, 9(2): e1001177.
35. Pereira TV, Rudnicki M, Pereira AC, Pombo-de-Oliveira MS, Franco RF (2006) 5,10-Methylenetetrahydrofolate reductase polymorphisms and acute lymphoblastic leukemia risk: a meta-analysis. Cancer Epidemiol Biomarkers Prev, 15(10): 1956–1963.
36. Yun KU, Ryu CS, Oh JM, Kim CH, Lee KS, et al (2013) Plasma homocysteine level and hepatic sulfur amino acid metabolism in mice fed a high-fat diet. Eur J Nutr, 52(1): 127–134.
37. Benight NM, Stoll B, Chacko S, da Silva VR, Marini JC, et al (2011) B-vitamin deficiency is protective against DSS-induced colitis in mice. Am J Physiol Gastrointest Liver Physiol, 301(2): G249–259.
38. Di Minno MN, Tremoli E, Coppola A, Lupoli R, Di Minno G (2010) Homocysteine and arterial thrombosis: Challenge and opportunity. Thromb Haemost, 103(5): 942–961.
39. Stanger O, Fowler B, Piertzik K, Huemer M, Haschke-Becher E, et al (2009) Homocysteine, folate and vitamin B12 in neuropsychiatric diseases: review and treatment recommendations. Expert Rev Neurother, 9(9): 1393–1412.
40. Stipanuk MH, Ueki I (2011) Dealing with methionine/homocysteine sulfur: cysteine metabolism to taurine and inorganic sulfur. J Inherit Metab Dis, 34(1): 17–32.
41. Safarinejad MR, Shafiei N, Safarinejad S (2011) Genetic susceptibility of methylenetetrahydrofolate reductase (MTHFR) gene C677T, A1298C, and G1793A polymorphisms with risk for bladder transitional cell carcinoma in men. Med Oncol, 28 Suppl 1: S398–412.
42. Shemin D, Bostom AG, Selhub J (2001) Treatment of hyperhomocysteinemia in end-stage renal disease. Am J Kidney Dis, 38(4 Suppl 1): S91–94.
43. Rubino E, Ferrero M, Rainero I, Binello E, Vaula G, et al (2009) Association of the C677T polymorphism in the MTHFR gene with migraine: a meta-analysis. Cephalalgia, 29(8): 818–825.

Resistance to Erythropoiesis Stimulating Agents in Patients Treated with Online Hemodiafiltration and Ultrapure Low-Flux Hemodialysis

Neelke C. van der Weerd[1,2]*, Claire H. Den Hoedt[3,4], Peter J. Blankestijn[3], Michiel L. Bots[5], Marinus A. van den Dorpel[4], Renée Lévesque[6], Albert H. A. Mazairac[3], Menso J. Nubé[2,7], E. Lars Penne[2,8], Pieter M. ter Wee[2,7], Muriel P. C. Grooteman[2,7], CONTRAST Investigators¶

1 Department of Nephrology, Academic Medical Center, Amsterdam, The Netherlands, 2 Department of Nephrology, VU Medical Center, Amsterdam, The Netherlands, 3 Department of Nephrology, University Medical Center Utrecht, Utrecht, The Netherlands, 4 Department of Internal Medicine, Maasstad Hospital, Rotterdam, The Netherlands, 5 Julius Center for Health Sciences and Primary Care, University Medical Center Utrecht, Utrecht, The Netherlands, 6 Department of Nephrology, Centre Hospitalier de l'Université de Montréal, St-Luc Hospital, Québec, Canada, 7 Institute for Cardiovascular Research VU Medical Center (ICaR-VU), VU Medical Center, Amsterdam, The Netherlands, 8 Department of Internal Medicine, Medical Center Alkmaar, Alkmaar, The Netherlands

Abstract

Resistance to erythropoiesis stimulating agents (ESA) is common in patients undergoing chronic hemodialysis (HD) treatment. ESA responsiveness might be improved by enhanced clearance of uremic toxins of middle molecular weight, as can be obtained by hemodiafiltration (HDF). In this analysis of the randomized controlled CONvective TRAnsport STudy (CONTRAST; NCT00205556), the effect of online HDF on ESA resistance and iron parameters was studied. This was a pre-specified secondary endpoint of the main trial. A 12 months' analysis of 714 patients randomized to either treatment with online post-dilution HDF or continuation of low-flux HD was performed. Both groups were treated with ultrapure dialysis fluids. ESA resistance, measured every three months, was expressed as the ESA index (weight adjusted weekly ESA dose in daily defined doses [DDD]/hematocrit). The mean ESA index during 12 months was not different between patients treated with HDF or HD (mean difference HDF versus HD over time 0.029 DDD/kg/Hct/week [−0.024 to 0.081]; P = 0.29). Mean transferrin saturation ratio and ferritin levels during the study tended to be lower in patients treated with HDF (−2.52% [−4.72 to −0.31]; P = 0.02 and −49 ng/mL [−103 to 4]; P = 0.06 respectively), although there was a trend for those patients to receive slightly more iron supplementation (7.1 mg/week [−0.4 to 14.5]; P = 0.06). In conclusion, compared to low-flux HD with ultrapure dialysis fluid, treatment with online HDF did not result in a decrease in ESA resistance.

Trial Registration: ClinicalTrials.gov NCT00205556

Editor: Robert K. Hills, Cardiff University, United Kingdom

Funding: CONTRAST is financially supported by a grant from the Dutch Kidney Foundation (Nierstichting Nederland, grant C02.2019) and unrestricted grants from Fresenius Medical Care (The Netherlands) and Gambro Lundia AB (Sweden). Additional support was received from the Dr. E.E. Twiss Fund, Roche Netherlands, the International Society of Nephrology/Baxter Extramural Grant Program, and the Dutch Organization for Health Research and Development (ZonMW, grant 17088.2802). The funders had no role in study design, data collection and analysis, decision to publish, or preparation of the manuscript.

Competing Interests: As can be seen at the Financial Disclosure section, funding for the CONTRAST study was obtained from commercial sources (Fresenius Medical Care, Gambro Lundia AB and Roche Netherlands). However, this does not alter the authors' adherence to all the PLOS ONE policies on sharing data and materials.

* E-mail: n.c.vanderweerd@amc.uva.nl

¶ Membership of the CONTRAST Investigators is provided in the Acknowledgments.

Introduction

In chronic hemodialysis (HD) patients, renal anemia is generally treated with erythropoiesis stimulating agents (ESA) and iron supplements. Although treatment with ESA has been shown to improve left ventricular mass index [1] and quality of life [2], ESA treatment has not been associated with a survival benefit, neither in HD patients [3] nor in patients with chronic kidney disease not yet on dialysis [4,5,6]. In many HD patients, target hemoglobin levels are not reached due to a varying degree of ESA resistance. A diminished response to ESA has been associated with various factors, including (functional) iron deficiency, an impaired nutritional state and the presence of (micro)inflammation [7,8]. Furthermore, the microbiological purity of the dialysis fluid [9], the presence of hyperparathyroidism [10] and low dialysis adequacy [11] have been associated with ESA resistance.

Hemodiafiltration (HDF) is an extracorporeal renal replacement therapy that combines diffusive and convective solute removal. In comparison with conventional HD, removal of substances in the middle molecular weight (MMW) range (0.5–

40 kilodalton) is enhanced. Several observational studies showed a survival benefit in patients treated with HDF [12,13,14,15], whereas in the randomized controlled CONvective TRAnsport STudy (CONTRAST) study and the Turkish Online Hemodiafiltration Study, survival was similar in patients treated with online HDF and conventional HD [16,17]. The recently published randomized On-Line Hemodiafiltration Survival Study (ESHOL) did show a survival advantage for patients treated with HDF, however [18].

It has been suggested that adding convective solute removal improves ESA resistance, and hence the degree of anemia, possibly by removing MMW toxins with erythropoiesis inhibiting properties [19,20], increasing red blood cell life span [21,22] and/or improving iron utilization [23]. Clinical data on the effect of HDF on ESA resistance, however, are conflicting (table 1).

Anemia management and ESA resistance were predefined secondary endpoints of the CONTRAST study [16,24]. In the present analysis of this randomized controlled trial (RCT), the effect of online post-dilution HDF and ultrapure low-flux HD on hemoglobin levels, ESA resistance and iron parameters was evaluated over a 12 month period.

Materials and Methods

Patients and study design

In the CONTRAST study (clinicaltrials.gov identifier NCT00205556; first registration on September 2005), 714 chronic HD patients were randomized either to switch to online HDF or to continue low-flux HD. The protocol for this trial and supporting CONSORT checklist are available as supporting information; see Checklist S1 and Protocol S1. The study was conducted in accordance with the Declaration of Helsinki and was approved by a central medical ethics committee and by all local medical ethics review boards. Written informed consent was obtained from all patients prior to enrolment. Central approval was obtained by the Medical Ethical Committee of the VU University Medical Center. Local approval was obtained from the Medical Ethical Committees of all participating centers, which are listed in the acknowledgements. The enrolment period started in June 2004 and ended on January 1st 2010. The study stopped on January 1st 2011. For the present analysis, all available data on anemia management and ESA resistance until 12 months of follow-up were evaluated. Anemia management and ESA resistance was a pre-specified secondary endpoint of the study and as such registered on clinicaltrials.gov. The trial registration date of the study was slightly after enrolment started due to logistic reasons. The authors confirm that all related trials for this treatment intervention are registered.

The rationale and the design of the CONTRAST study have been described before [24]. Primary endpoint of the study is all cause mortality [16]. Patients were recruited from 26 dialysis centers in The Netherlands, 2 centers in Canada and 1 center in Norway and randomized centrally into a 1:1 ratio for treatment with online HDF or continuation of low-flux HD, stratified per participating center. Patients were eligible for inclusion if they were treated two or three times per week with HD for at least two months. Exclusion criteria were age below 18 years, treatment with hemo(dia)filtration or high-flux HD in six months prior to randomization, a life expectancy less than three months due to non-renal disease, participation in another clinical intervention trial evaluating cardiovascular outcomes and severe incompliance regarding frequency and/or duration of dialysis treatment.

Treatment protocol

Upon randomization, all patients were stable with a minimum dialysis $spKt/V_{urea}$ of 1.2 per treatment. Treatment times were fixed at baseline and could only be increased during follow-up when the spKt/V dropped below 1.2. Online HDF was performed in post-dilution mode with a target dose for convection flow of 100 mL/min and high-flux synthetic dialyzers were used (UF coefficient 55–85 ml/mmHg/h: FX80, FX100 and Optiflux F200NR [Fresenius Medical Care, Bad Homburg, Germany] and Polyflux170H and Polyflux210H [Gambro Corporation AB, Lund, Sweden]). Conventional HD was performed with low-flux synthetic dialyzers (UF coefficient 10–18 ml/mmHg/h: F6HPS, F8HPS and Optiflux18NR [Fresenius] and Polyflux14L and Polyflux17L [Gambro]). Routine patient care was performed according to the opinion of the attending nephrologist and based

Table 1. Studies on the effect of HDF versus HD on ESA resistance.

	Design	N	Conventional treatment; ultrapure dialysis fluid?[a]	Mean convection volume (L/session)	Outcome
Bonforte 2002 [37]	Observational	32	Low-flux HD; no	19.5; post-dilution	↓ ESA resistance
Lin 2002 [23]	Cross-over	92	High-flux HD; yes	21; post-dilution	↓ ESA resistance
Vaslaki 2006 [36]	Randomized cross-over	129	Low-flux HD; no	20.2; post-dilution	↓ ESA resistance
Schiffl 2007 [35]	Randomized cross-over	76	Low-flux HD; no	20.3; post-dilution	↓ ESA resistance
Turkish online HDF study 2013 [17]	RCT	782	High-flux HD; no	21.0; post-dilution	↓ ESA resistance
Vilar 2009 [15]	Observational	858 (232 HDF)	High-flux HD; yes	Not available	No difference
Oates 2011 [38]	Observational	34 HDF, 44 HD	High-flux HD; yes	>16; post-dilution	No difference
Ward 2000 [39]	RCT	44	High-flux HD; yes	18.0; post-dilution	No difference
Wizemann 2000 [40]	RCT	44	Low-flux HD; yes	60; mid-dilution	No difference
Locatelli 2012 [41]	RCT	146	Low-flux HD; yes	HF: 60.4, HDF: 39.9; pre-dilution	No difference
ESHOL 2013 [18]	RCT	906	High-flux HD; yes	23.4; post-dilution	No difference
CONTRAST 2013	RCT	714	Low-flux HD; yes	20.3; post-dilution	No difference

[a]Ultrapure dialysis fluid is defined as <0.1 colony forming units per ml and <0.03 endotoxin units per ml [28].

or the Quality of Care Guidelines of the Dutch Federation of Nephrology. The Dutch Guideline on Anemia Management is derived from the European Best Practice Guidelines [25] and the KDOQI guidelines [26,27].

ESA and iron supplements were administered via the venous blood line at the end of a dialysis session. Both HDF and HD patients were treated with ultrapure dialysis fluids, containing less than 0.1 colony forming units per mL and less than 0.03 endotoxin units per mL [28,29]. The quality of the dialysis solutions was regularly monitored as part of the Quality of Care Guideline on water quality of the Dutch Federation of Nephrology [29].

Data collection

At baseline, data on demography, cause of renal failure, history of cardiovascular disease, diabetes mellitus, type of vascular access, dialysis vintage and treatment parameters were collected. Subsequent study visits were performed at three month intervals. During these visits, information on ESA and iron doses at the time of the visit date was collected.

ESA was prescribed as epoetin α or β (IU) or darbepoetin α (μg). To compare the different types of ESA, weekly prescribed dosages were converted to daily defined doses (DDD), using conversion factors as provided by the World Health Organization (WHO) Drug Classification (http://www.whocc.no/atcddd). DDD represents the assumed average maintenance dose per day for a drug used for its main indication in adults. For darbepoetin α (ATC code B03XA02) DDD is 4.5 μg and for epoetin α and β (ATC code B03XA01) DDD is 1000 IU.

ESA resistance was expressed as an ESA index: the weekly weight adjusted ESA dose (DDD) divided by the haematocrit (Hct) [30]. Iron supplements were prescribed as iron sucrose or iron dextran (in mg/week), both with an equal amount of elemental iron per mg.

At each study visit, with a window of two weeks around the exact visit date, blood samples were drawn prior to dialysis for routine laboratory assessments. All laboratory samples were analysed in the local hospitals by standard laboratory techniques. Ferritin levels (μg/L) and the transferrin saturation ratio (TSAT) were used as indices of iron stores. TSAT values were either reported directly or calculated as serum iron divided by the serum total-iron-binding capacity (TIBC), which was considered to represent serum transferrin level [31].

Serum albumin was measured with either the bromcresol green or bromcresol purple method and bromcresol purple concentrations were converted to bromcresol green [32]. The second generation Daugirdas formula was used to calculate $spKt/V_{urea}$ [33]. In patients treated with HDF, the average achieved convection volume per session was calculated as the sum of the intradialytic weight loss and the infusion volume (substitution volume). The HDF treatment was quantified by the convection volume and pre-dialysis levels of β2-microglobulin (β2M; mg/L) over time [34].

Statistical analysis

All analyses were conducted according to an intention-to-treat principle. Patient data were censored at the date of death or date of the last study visit if the patient stopped with the study. All variables were reported as proportions or means ± standard deviation (SD) or 95% confidence interval (CI), or medians with 25th–75th percentiles when appropriate.

Laboratory parameters, ESA dose and -index and iron supplementation over time were evaluated with linear mixed-effects models, as repeated measurements over time were assumed to be related within participants. All available measurements until 12 months of follow-up were entered into the models. For each individual, a mean level of the laboratory parameters during the follow-up was estimated. Subsequently, the difference in the mean levels between the treatment groups was calculated, adjusted for the baseline levels.

To evaluate a possible dose-response relation in HDF patients, the effect of treatment on change in ESA index was explored in different tertiles of convection volume during 12 months of follow-up. Low-flux HD was regarded as the reference category. The choice for tertiles was based on the reasonable sample size in each of the tertiles.

To evaluate whether the treatment effect on mean ESA index was modified by the stratum of ESA resistance at baseline, the possibility of effect modification was explored by adding an interaction term (ESA index×treatment modality) to the linear mixed-effects model.

Since a total of nine parameters were evaluated, we applied a Bonferroni adjustment for multiple testing and considered a two sided p-value<0.006 as statistically significant. Statistical analyses were performed with SPSS software (version 20, 2011, IBM SPSS Statistics) and R (version 2.9.2; 2009 The R Foundation for Statistical Computing).

Results

Patient characteristics and clinical parameters at baseline

In total, 714 patients were included in the study, 358 were allocated to HDF and 356 to HD. The two groups were well balanced with respect to baseline characteristics (table 2). During 12 months of follow-up, 62 patients in the HDF group and 74 in the HD group were censored because they died, received a kidney transplant, switched to peritoneal dialysis, moved to another center or for other reasons (figure 1).

Clinical parameters during follow-up

For patients treated with HDF, the mean (± SD) achieved convection volume during one year of follow-up was 20.3±4.8 liters per session. During the study, the mean dialysis single pool Kt/V urea ($spKt/V_{urea}$) was higher in in the HDF group (mean [95% CI] difference HDF vs. HD 0.17 [0.07 to 0.27; P<0.001]). The mean β2M level during follow-up was significantly lower in the HDF group (mean difference HDF vs. HD −7.8 mg/L [−10.5 to −4.9; P<0.001]). Furthermore, albumin levels were equal in both groups during follow-up (mean difference HDF vs. HD −0.02 g/dL [−0.06 to 0.02; P=0.35]).

Hemoglobin and ESA resistance. Anemia parameters during follow-up are listed in table 3. Hemoglobin levels were not different between both groups. Furthermore, there was no difference in mean ESA index and ESA dose between the treatment groups during follow-up (table 3, figure 2).

To explore a possible effect of the HDF dose, expressed as the average achieved convection volume during follow-up, the change in ESA index was analyzed separately within tertiles of convection volume. Within each tertile of achieved convection volume, the ESA index did not change and was not different compared to HD (data not shown).

Iron parameters and iron therapy. Ferritin levels at baseline were not different between both groups (HDF: (median [interquartile range]: 314 ng/mL [191–567]; HD 367 ng/mL [196–606]; P=0.16). During one year of follow-up, mean ferritin and TSAT levels tended to be marginally lower in the HDF group as compared to HD (mean difference HDF vs. HD −49 ng/mL [−103 to 4; P=0.06] and −2.5% [−4.7 to −0.3; P=0.02] respectively; table 3).

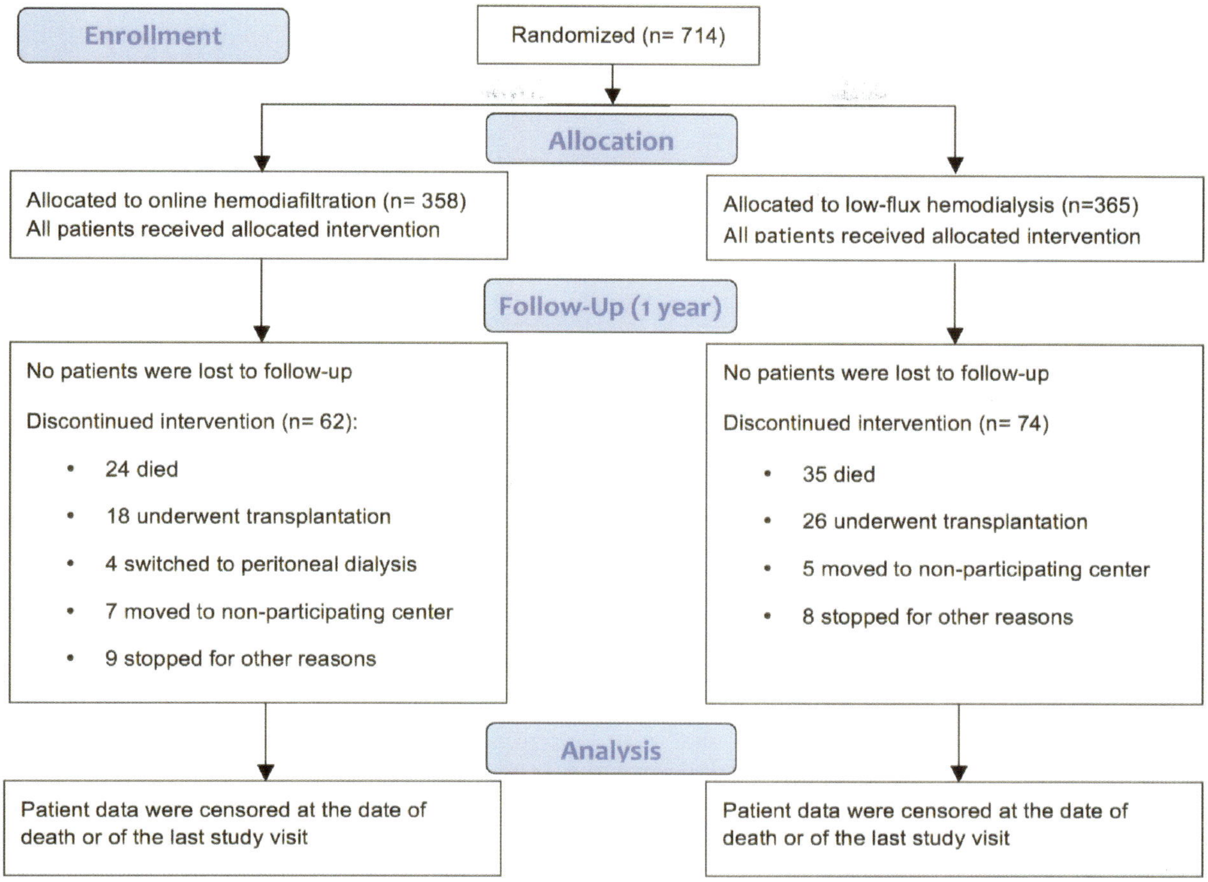

Figure 1. CONSORT flow chart of patient inclusion.

The mean dose of iron supplementation during follow-up tended to be slightly higher in the HDF group as compared to HD (mean difference HDF vs. HD 7.1 mg/week [−0.4 to 14.5; P = 0.06]).

Sub-analysis: ESA resistance over time in different groups of ESA index at baseline. The effect of HDF versus HD on mean ESA index over time was not modified by the ESA index at baseline (P-value for the interaction term = 0.15).

Discussion

The present secondary analysis of a RCT showed that ESA resistance over a 12 months' period, as measured by the mean ESA index over time, was not different between patients treated with online HDF or HD. In the HDF group, iron parameters (ferritin and TSAT) tended to be slightly lower during follow up whereas there was a trend towards more intravenous iron supplementation in this group.

As mentioned before, studies on the effect of HDF on ESA resistance have been conflicting (table 1). Our overall results are in contrast with results of two cross-over studies [35,36], two observational studies [23,37] and one RCT [17] in which ESA dose and/or ESA resistance decreased and/or hemoglobin levels increased in patients treated with online HDF. On the contrary, in two non-randomized studies [15,38] and two small [39,40] and two large RCTs [18,41], no difference between treatment with HDF or HD in either ESA dose or hemoglobin levels was shown either. Remarkably, in virtually all studies in which a beneficial effect of HDF on ESA resistance was shown, the dialysis fluid applied in the conventional HD group was not ultrapure according to the generally accepted definition (<0.1 colony forming units per ml and <0.03 endotoxin units per ml) [28]. In contrast, in the studies that did not show a difference, ultrapure dialysis fluid was used for both treatment with HD and HDF (table 1). A recent meta-analysis has shown that the use of ultrapure dialysis fluid resulted in increased hemoglobin levels and diminished ESA requirements [9]. Furthermore, in a recently published RCT in 704 patients, it was shown that ultrapure dialysis fluid as compared to standard dialysis fluid resulted in reduced ESA doses and ESA resistance despite equal hemoglobin and ferritin levels [42]. Therefore, we hypothesized that the use of ultrapure dialysis fluid may be of predominant importance with respect to erythropoiesis and ESA responsiveness as compared to increasing MMW clearance by adding convection [43,44,45].

Another possible explanation for the absent effect of HDF on ESA resistance may be that with HDF, besides removal of ESA or erythropoiesis inhibiting toxins, erythropoiesis stimulating substances are removed as well. However, we have no data to support this hypothesis.

We postulated that the amount of convection volume, being a key quantifier for HDF treatment according to a recent position statement by the HDF working group (EUDIAL) of the European Renal Association-European Dialysis and Transplant Association [34], might affect ESA responsiveness. In an on-treatment analysis

Table 2. Baseline characteristics[a].

	Online HDF (n = 358)	Low-flux HD (n = 356)
Gender (no. [%] male)	214 (60)	231 (65)
Age (years)	64.1 ± 14.0	64.0 ± 13.4
Caucasian race (no. [%])	304 (85)	296 (83)
Dialysis vintage (years)	1.8 (1.0–3.7)	2.1 (1.0–4.0)
Cause of ESRD (no. [])		
- vascular	104 (29)	96 (27)
- diabetes mellitus	76 (21)	60 (17)
- glomerulonephritis	36 (10)	53 (15)
- interstitial nephropathy	35 (10)	31 (9)
- multisystem disease	15 (4)	11 (3)
- cystic disease	27 (7)	26 (7)
- other/unknown	65 (18)	79 (22)
Diabetes mellitus (no. [%])	92 (26)	78 (22)
History of cardiovascular disease (no. [%])[b]	141 (42)	162 (46)
Body weight after dialysis (kg)[c]	71.6 ± 15.0	73.3 ± 13.6
BMI after dialysis (kg/m^2)	25.2 ± 5.0	25.6 ± 4.6
Residual kidney function (no. [%])[d]	186 (52)	190 (53)
eGFR (ml/min/1.73 m^2)[e]	0.32 (0–3.30)	0.30 (0–3.35)
Treatment frequency (no. [%])		
- 2×/week	26 (7)	18 (5)
- 3×/week	332 (93)	338 (95)
Duration of a dialysis session (min)	226 ± 26	227 ± 22
Bloodflow (mL/min)	302 ± 39	299 ± 41
Dialysis access (no. [%])		
- AV fistula	279 (78)	288 (81)
- graft	57 (16)	43 (12)
- central catheter	22 (5)	25 (7)
$spKt/V_{urea}$	1.42 ± 0.25	1.38 ± 0.20
Hemoglobin (g/dL)	11.9 ± 1.3	11.8 ± 1.1
Hematocrit	0.36 ± 0.04	0.36 ± 0.04
Ferritin (ng/mL)		
- Median (interquartile range)	314 (191–567)	367 (196–606)
- Mean ± SD	423 ± 347	442 ± 322
TSAT (%)	23.9 ± 11.1	24.4 ± 11.7
Albumin (g/dL)	3.66 ± 0.45	3.70 ± 0.46
Parathyroid hormone (pg/ml)	193.7 (94.0–322.9)	194.7 (104.5–355.2)
β2-microglobulin (mg/L)	30.7 ± 14.2	32.3 ± 13.6
ESA treatment (no. [%])	311 (87)	320 (90)
Type of ESA (no [%])		
- Darbepoetin α	226 (73)	231 (72)
- Epoetin β	64 (20)	71 (22)
- Epoetin α	21 (7)	18 (6)
ESA dose (DDD/week)		
- Median (interquartile range)	8.0 (4.0–13.3)	7.6 (4.4–13.3)
- Mean ± SD	9.7 ± 9.0	9.8 ± 8.1
ESA index (DDD/kg/Hct/week)		
- Median (interquartile range)	0.31 (0.14–0.59)	0.30 (0.15–0.55)
- Mean ± SD	0.40 ± 0.39	0.40 ± 0.37
Iron replacement (no. [%])	236 (66)	231 (65)

Table 2. Cont.

	Online HDF (n = 358)	Low-flux HD (n = 356)
Type of iron replacement (no. [%])		
- Ironsucrose	215 (91)	213 (92)
- Irondextran	21 (9)	18 (8)
Iron dose (mg/week)		
- Median (interquartile range)	23.3 (0–100)	23.3 (0–100)
- Mean ± SD	48±51	43±42

[a]Values represent mean ± SD, median (interquartile range) or proportion (%).
[b]History of cardiovascular disease was defined as history of angina pectoris or myocardial infarction and/or a previous coronary bypass graft and/or percutaneous coronary intervention and/or stroke or transient ischemic attack and/or peripheral vascular disease.
[c]Weight after dialysis (dry weight) defined as the mean of three consecutive values.
[d]Defined as >100 mL per day.
[e]eGFR (estimated glomerular filtration rate) calculated as mean of creatinine and urea clearance in 24 h urine collection adjusted for body surface area [48].
Conversion factors for units: hemoglobin in g/dL to mmol/L, ×0.62; albumin in g/dL to g/L, ×10; parathyroid hormone pg/ml to pmol/l ×0.11; no conversion necessary for ferritin in ng/mL and μg/L.

of both CONTRAST and the Turkish HDF study, a survival benefit for HDF patients treated with the highest convection volumes was observed [16,17]. In the ESHOL study, in which an overall survival benefit for HDF was shown, convection volumes were higher (23.4 L per session versus 19.8 L and 21.04 in CONTRAST and the Turkish study, respectively) [18]. Considering convection volume and ESA resistance, it was shown in a study in 37 chronic dialysis patients that a switch from treatment with low-volume HDF (mean substitution volume 4.0 L/session) to high-volume online HDF (mean substitution volume 22.5 L/session) resulted in increased hemoglobin levels and decreased ESA doses. In our study, however, we could not identify such a dose-response effect with respect to ESA resistance.

Concerning iron therapy, it was previously reported that ferritin and TSAT levels decreased in HDF patients despite a lower ESA dose and a higher haematocrit, suggesting improved iron utilization [23]. As mentioned, in our study, HDF patients tended to receive slightly more intravenous iron than HD patients which might be partially explained by relatively low ferritin levels in HDF patients at baseline, suggesting that overall, patients randomized to HDF were more iron deplete at the time of enrolment. This relative iron deplete state seemed to remain present during the study. Other potential explanations for the relative iron deplete state in the HDF group despite slightly more iron supplementation might be loss of ascorbic acid (vitamin C) [46], since this vitamin enhances iron availability [47,48], and blood loss due to clotting in the extracorporeal circuit as a result of increased pro-coagulatory activity during HDF [49].

We restricted the analysis to one year of follow-up since previous studies already showed an effect of HDF on ESA resistance after 3 to 6 months [36,37]. A limitation of our study is the conversion of ESA dose to DDD, which may be an oversimplification, as a non-linear conversion factor, dependent upon the actual ESA dose, has been described [50]. An additional drawback is the lack of a specific treatment protocol for ESA and iron administration. However, as the treatment allocation was

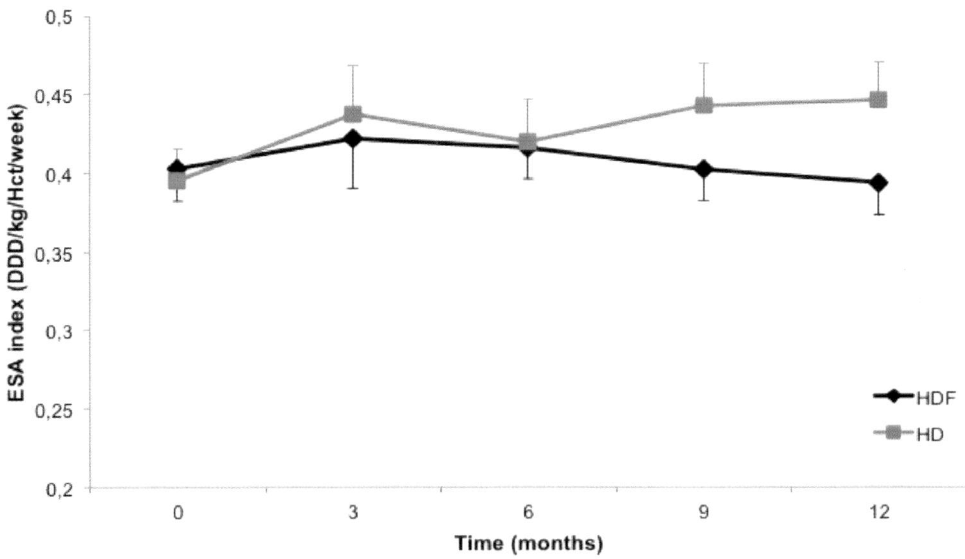

Figure 2. Change in ESA index for HDF and HD. Crude means (SE) at time of visit are depicted. P-value for mean difference in ESA index over time (HDF vs. HD) = 0.29 (based on a linear mixed-effects model including all 3122 measurements during 12 months of follow-up).

Table 3. Mean of the parameters of anemia management during follow-up period, by treatment assignment.

	Online HDF[a]	Low-flux HD[a]	Difference HDF vs HD[b]	
	Mean value (95% CI)	Mean value (95% CI)	Mean value (95% CI)	P-value
Hemoglobin (g/dL)	11.9 (11.8 to 12.0)	11.7 (11.6 to 11.8)	0.1 (−0.2 to 0.3)	0.63
Hematocrit	0.36 (0.35 to 0.36)	0.35 (0.35 to 0.36)	0.003 (−0.004 to 0.010)	0.48
Ferritin (ng/mL)	441 (409 to 473)	472 (440 to 504)	−49 (−103 to 4)	0.06
TSAT (%)	23.1 (22.1 to 24.1)	24.3 (23.4 to 25.3)	−2.5 (−4.7 to −0.3)	0.02
ESA index (DDD/kg/Hct/week)	0.41 (0.38 to 0.45)	0.43 (0.39 to 0.47)	0.03 (−0.02 to 0.08)	0.29
ESA dose (DDD/week)	10.1 (9.3 to 10.9)	10.4 (9.5 to 11.2)	0.9 (−0.2 to 2.0)	0.12
Iron dose (mg/week)	45 (41 to 49)	35 (32 to 38)	7.1 (−0.4 to 14.5)	0.06

[a]Crude mean (95% CI) of values at 3, 6, 9 and 12 months.
[b]Difference in mean values during the follow-up period between groups as a result from a linear mixed-effects model adjusted for the value at baseline, including all measurements at 3, 6, 9 and 12 months.

stratified per participating center, the effect on the study outcome will probably be limited. Moreover, our study reflects usual care in the Netherlands. In our study, HDF was compared with low-flux HD although at present, the majority of patients is treated with high-flux dialyzers as recommended in current guidelines [51]. Since we observed no difference between HDF and low-flux HD concerning ESA resistance, it is highly unlikely that there would be a difference when HDF and high-flux HD (which can be considered as a form of "low-volume HDF") were compared. Furthermore, in the ESHOL study, no effect of HDF versus high-flux HD on ESA resistance was observed either [18]. A final limitation is the handling of missing data due to drop out. These data might be missing in a non-randomly fashion.

The strength of our study is the large sample size and its randomized design with an accurate prospective data collection. Furthermore, all available measurements during follow-up (at 3, 6, 9 and 12 months) were included in the analysis.

In conclusion, this multicenter randomized controlled study showed that ESA resistance was not different between patients treated with online HDF or ultrapure low-flux HD during 12 months of follow-up. These data indicate that when considering ESA resistance, online HDF has no benefit over low-flux ultrapure HD. Whether other factors are involved, such as the quality of the dialysis fluid, remains to be determined.

Acknowledgments

The authors are grateful to all patients and nursing staff participating in this project.

The members of the CONTRAST executive committee are: P.J. Blankestijn (chair), University Medical Center Utrecht, Utrecht; M.L. Bots, Julius Centrum for Health Sciences and Primary Care, University Medical Center Utrecht, Utrecht; M.A. van den Dorpel, Maasstad Hospital, Rotterdam, M.P.C. Grooteman, VU Medical Center, Amsterdam; M.J. Nubé, VU Medical Center, Amsterdam; P.M. ter Wee (chair), VU Medical Center, Amsterdam; The Netherlands.

CONTRAST investigators in Canada: Georges-L. Dumont Regional Hospital, Moncton: M. Dorval; CHUM St. Luc Hospital, Montréal: R. Lévesque. In the Netherlands: Academic Medical Center, Amsterdam: M.G. Koopman; Catharina Hospital, Eindhoven: C.J.A.M. Konings; Dialysis Clinic Noord, Beilen: W.P. Haanstra; Dianet Dialysis Centers, Utrecht: M. Kooistra and B. van Jaarsveld; Fransiscus Hospital, Roosendaal: T. Noordzij; Gelderse Vallei Hospital, Ede: G.W. Feith; Groene Hart Hospital, Gouda: H.G. Peltenburg; Haga Hospital, The Hague: M. van Buren; Isala Clinics, Zwolle: J.J.G. Offerman; Jeroen Bosch Hospital, Hertogenbosch: E.K. Hoogeveen; Maasland Hospital, Sittard: F. de Heer; Maasstad Hospital, Rotterdam: P.J. van de Ven; Martini Hospital, Groningen: T.K. Kremer Hovinga; Medical Center Alkmaar: W.A. Bax; Onze Lieve Vrouwe Gasthuis, Amsterdam: J.O. Groeneveld; Oosterschelde Hospital, Goes: A.T.J. Lavrijssen; Rijnland Hospital, Leiderdorp: A.M. Schrander-Van der Meer; Rijnstate Hospital, Arnhem: L.J.M. Reichert; Slingeland Hospital, Doetinchem: J. Huussen; St. Elisabeth Hospital, Tilburg: P.L. Rensma; St. Fransiscus Gasthuis, Rotterdam: Y. Schrama; University Medical Center St. Radboud, Nijmegen: H.W. van Hamersvelt; University Medical Center Utrecht, Utrecht: W.H. Boer; VieCuri Medical Center, Venlo: W.H. van Kuijk; VU University Medical Center, Amsterdam: M.G. Vervloet; Zeeuws-Vlaanderen Hospital, Terneuzen: I.M.P.M.J. Wauters. In Norway: Haukeland University Hospital, Bergen: I. Sekse.

Author Contributions

Conceived and designed the experiments: NCW PJB MLB MAD MJN PMW MPG. Performed the experiments: NCW CHH RL AHM ELP MPG. Analyzed the data: NCW CHH MLB MPG. Wrote the paper: NCW MJN PMW MPG.

References

1. Frank H, Heusser K, Hoffken B, Huber P, Schmieder RE, et al. (2004) Effect of erythropoietin on cardiovascular prognosis parameters in hemodialysis patients. Kidney Int 66: 832–840.
2. Foley RN, Curtis BM, Parfrey PS (2009) Erythropoietin therapy, hemoglobin targets, and quality of life in healthy hemodialysis patients: a randomized trial. ClinJAmSocNephrol 4: 726–733.
3. Besarab A, Bolton WK, Browne JK, Egrie JC, Nissenson AR, et al. (1998) The effects of normal as compared with low hematocrit values in patients with cardiac disease who are receiving hemodialysis and epoetin. NEnglJMed 339: 584–590.
4. Drueke TB, Locatelli F, Clyne N, Eckardt KU, Macdougall IC, et al. (2006) Normalization of hemoglobin level in patients with chronic kidney disease and anemia. NEnglJMed 355: 2071–2084.
5. Pfeffer MA, Burdmann EA, Chen CY, Cooper ME, de ZD, et al. (2009) A trial of darbepoetin alfa in type 2 diabetes and chronic kidney disease. NEnglJMed 361: 2019–2032.

6. Singh AK, Szczech L, Tang KL, Barnhart H, Sapp S, et al. (2006) Correction of anemia with epoetin alfa in chronic kidney disease. NEnglJMed 355: 2085–2098.
7. Kalantar-Zadeh K, McAllister CJ, Lehn RS, Lee GH, Nissenson AR, et al. (2003) Effect of malnutrition-inflammation complex syndrome on EPO hyporesponsiveness in maintenance hemodialysis patients. AmJKidney Dis 42: 761–773.
8. Locatelli F, Andrulli S, Memoli B, Maffei C, Del VL, et al. (2006) Nutritional-inflammation status and resistance to erythropoietin therapy in haemodialysis patients. NephrolDialTransplant 21: 991–998.
9. Susantitaphong P, Riella C, Jaber BL (2013) Effect of ultrapure dialysate on markers of inflammation, oxidative stress, nutrition and anemia parameters: a meta-analysis. Nephrol Dial Transplant 28: 438–446.
10. Lee CT, Chou FF, Chang HW, Hsu YH, Lee WC, et al. (2003) Effects of parathyroidectomy on iron homeostasis and erythropoiesis in hemodialysis patients with severe hyperparathyroidism. Blood Purif 21: 369–375.
11. Movilli E, Cancarini GC, Zani R, Camerini C, Sandrini M, et al. (2001) Adequacy of dialysis reduces the doses of recombinant erythropoietin independently from the use of biocompatible membranes in haemodialysis patients. NephrolDialTransplant 16: 111–114.
12. Bosch JP, Lew SQ, Barlee V, Mishkin GJ, von AB (2006) Clinical use of high-efficiency hemodialysis treatments: long-term assessment. HemodialInt 10: 73–81.
13. Canaud B, Bragg-Gresham JL, Marshall MR, Desmeules S, Gillespie BW, et al. (2006) Mortality risk for patients receiving hemodiafiltration versus hemodialysis: European results from the DOPPS. Kidney Int 69: 2087–2093.
14. Jirka T, Cesare S, Di BA, Perera CM, Ponce P, et al. (2006) Mortality risk for patients receiving hemodiafiltration versus hemodialysis. Kidney Int 70: 1524–1525.
15. Vilar E, Fry AC, Wellsted D, Tattersall JE, Greenwood RN, et al. (2009) Long-term outcomes in online hemodiafiltration and high-flux hemodialysis: a comparative analysis. ClinJAmSocNephrol 4: 1944–1953.
16. Grooteman MP, van den Dorpel MA, Bots ML, Penne EL, van der Weerd NC, et al. (2012) Effect of Online Hemodiafiltration on All-Cause Mortality and Cardiovascular Outcomes. J Am Soc Nephrol 23: 1087–1096.
17. Ok E, Asci G, Toz H, Ok ES, Kircelli F, et al. (2013) Mortality and cardiovascular events in online haemodiafiltration (OL-HDF) compared with high-flux dialysis: results from the Turkish OL-HDF Study. Nephrol Dial Transplant 28: 192–202.
18. Maduell F, Moreso F, Pons M, Ramos R, Mora-Macia J, et al. (2013) High-efficiency postdilution online hemodiafiltration reduces all-cause mortality in hemodialysis patients. J Am Soc Nephrol 24: 487–497.
19. Macdougall IC (2001) Role of uremic toxins in exacerbating anemia in renal failure. Kidney IntSuppl 78: S67–S72.
20. Rioux JP, Chan CT (2010) Nocturnal home hemodialysis and its impact on erythropoietin responsiveness. Clin Nephrol 74: 167–172.
21. Kruse A, Uehlinger DE, Gotch F, Kotanko P, Levin NW (2008) Red blood cell lifespan, erythropoiesis and hemoglobin control. ContribNephrol 161: 247–254.
22. Ly J, Marticorena R, Donnelly S (2004) Red blood cell survival in chronic renal failure. Am J Kidney Dis 44: 715–719.
23. Lin CL, Huang CC, Yu CC, Wu CH, Chang CT, et al. (2002) Improved iron utilization and reduced erythropoietin resistance by on-line hemodiafiltration. Blood Purif 20: 349–356.
24. Penne EL, Blankestijn PJ, Bots ML, van den Dorpel MA, Grooteman MP, et al. (2005) Effect of increased convective clearance by on-line hemodiafiltration on all cause and cardiovascular mortality in chronic hemodialysis patients - the Dutch CONvective TRAnsport STudy (CONTRAST): rationale and design of a randomised controlled trial [ISRCTN38365125]. CurrControl Trials CardiovascMed 6: 8.
25. Locatelli F, Aljama P, Barany P, Canaud B, Carrera F, et al. (2004) Revised European best practice guidelines for the management of anaemia in patients with chronic renal failure. NephrolDialTransplant 19 Suppl 2: ii1–47.
26. (2006) KDOQI Clinical Practice Guidelines and Clinical Practice Recommendations for Anemia in Chronic Kidney Disease. AmJKidney Dis 47: S11–145.
27. (2007) KDOQI Clinical Practice Guideline and Clinical Practice Recommendations for anemia in chronic kidney disease: 2007 update of hemoglobin target. AmJKidney Dis 50: 471–530.
28. Ledebo I, Nystrand R (1999) Defining the microbiological quality of dialysis fluid. Artif Organs 23: 37–43.
29. Penne EL, Visser L, van den Dorpel MA, van der Weerd NC, Mazairac AH, et al. (2009) Microbiological quality and quality control of purified water and ultrapure dialysis fluids for online hemodiafiltration in routine clinical practice. Kidney Int 76: 665–672.
30. Kaysen GA, Muller HG, Ding J, Chertow GM (2006) Challenging the validity of the EPO index. AmJKidney Dis 47: 166.
31. Gambino R, Desvarieux E, Orth M, Matan H, Ackattupathil T, et al. (1997) The relation between chemically measured total iron-binding capacity concentrations and immunologically measured transferrin concentrations in human serum. ClinChem 43: 2408–2412.
32. Clase CM, St Pierre MW, Churchill DN (2001) Conversion between bromcresol green- and bromcresol purple-measured albumin in renal disease. Nephrol Dial Transplant 16: 1925–1929.
33. Daugirdas JT (1993) Second generation logarithmic estimates of single-pool variable volume Kt/V: an analysis of error. JAmSocNephrol 4: 1205–1213.
34. Tattersall JE, Ward RA (2013) Online haemodiafiltration: definition, dose quantification and safety revisited. Nephrol Dial Transplant 28: 542–550.
35. Schiffl H (2007) Prospective randomized cross-over long-term comparison of online haemodiafiltration and ultrapure high-flux haemodialysis. EurJMedRes 12: 26–33.
36. Vaslaki L, Major L, Berta K, Karatson A, Misz M, et al. (2006) On-line haemodiafiltration versus haemodialysis: stable haematocrit with less erythropoietin and improvement of other relevant blood parameters. Blood Purif 24: 163–173.
37. Bonforte G, Grillo P, Zerbi S, Surian M (2002) Improvement of anemia in hemodialysis patients treated by hemodiafiltration with high-volume on-line-prepared substitution fluid. Blood Purif 20: 357–363.
38. Oates T, Pinney JH, Davenport A (2011) Haemodiafiltration versus High-Flux Haemodialysis: Effects on Phosphate Control and Erythropoietin Response. AmJNephrol 33: 70–75.
39. Ward RA, Schmidt B, Hullin J, Hillebrand GF, Samtleben W (2000) A comparison of on-line hemodiafiltration and high-flux hemodialysis: a prospective clinical study. JAmSocNephrol 11: 2344–2350.
40. Wizemann V, Lotz C, Techert F, Uthoff S (2000) On-line haemodiafiltration versus low-flux haemodialysis. A prospective randomized study. NephrolDialTransplant 15 Suppl 1: 43–48.
41. Locatelli F, Altieri P, Andrulli S, Sau G, Bolasco P, et al. (2012) Predictors of haemoglobin levels and resistance to erythropoiesis-stimulating agents in patients treated with low-flux haemodialysis, haemofiltration and haemodiafiltration: results of a multicentre randomized and controlled trial. Nephrol Dial Transplant 27: 3594–3600.
42. Asci G, Tz H, Ozkahya M, Duman S, Demirci MS, et al. (2013) The Impact of Membrane Permeability and Dialysate Purity on Cardiovascular Outcomes. J Am Soc Nephrol.
43. Hsu PY, Lin CL, Yu CC, Chien CC, Hsiau TG, et al. (2004) Ultrapure dialysate improves iron utilization and erythropoietin response in chronic hemodialysis patients - a prospective cross-over study. JNephrol 17: 693–700.
44. Johnson DW, Pollock CA, Macdougall IC (2007) Erythropoiesis-stimulating agent hyporesponsiveness. Nephrology(Carlton) 12: 321–330.
45. Sitter T, Bergner A, Schiffl H (2000) Dialysate related cytokine induction and response to recombinant human erythropoietin in haemodialysis patients. NephrolDialTransplant 15: 1207–1211.
46. Morena M, Cristol JP, Bosc JY, Tetta C, Forret G, et al. (2002) Convective and diffusive losses of vitamin C during haemodiafiltration session: a contributive factor to oxidative stress in haemodialysis patients. NephrolDialTransplant 17: 422–427.
47. Deved V, Poyah P, James MT, Tonelli M, Manns BJ, et al. (2009) Ascorbic acid for anemia management in hemodialysis patients: a systematic review and meta-analysis. AmJKidney Dis 54: 1089–1097.
48. Fouque D, Vennegoor M, ter WP, Wanner C, Basci A, et al. (2007) EBPG guideline on nutrition. NephrolDialTransplant 22 Suppl 2: ii45–ii87.
49. Klingel R, Schaefer M, Schwarting A, Himmelsbach F, Altes U, et al. (2004) Comparative analysis of procoagulatory activity of haemodialysis, haemofiltration and haemodiafiltration with a polysulfone membrane (APS) and with different modes of enoxaparin anticoagulation. NephrolDialTransplant 19: 164–170.
50. Bock HA, Hirt-Minkowski P, Brunisholz M, Keusch G, Rey S, et al. (2008) Darbepoetin alpha in lower-than-equimolar doses maintains haemoglobin levels in stable haemodialysis patients converting from epoetin alpha/beta. NephrolDialTransplant 23: 301–308.
51. Tattersall J, Canaud B, Heimburger O, Pedrini L, Schneditz D, et al. (2010) High-flux or low-flux dialysis: a position statement following publication of the Membrane Permeability Outcome study. Nephrol Dial Transplant 25: 1230–1232.

The Associations between the Family Education and Mortality of Patients on Peritoneal Dialysis

Zhi-Kai Yang[1], Qing-Feng Han[2], Tong-Ying Zhu[3], Ye-Ping Ren[4], Jiang-Hua Chen[5], Hui-Ping Zhao[6], Meng-Hua Chen[7], Jie Dong[1]*, Yue Wang[2], Chuan- Ming Hao[3], Rui Zhang[4], Xiao-Hui Zhang[5], Mei Wang[6], Na Tian[7], Hai-Yan Wang[1]

1 Renal Division, Department of Medicine, Peking University First Hospital, Institute of Nephrology, Peking University, Key Laboratory of Renal Disease, Ministry of Health, Key Laboratory of Renal Disease, Ministry of Education, Beijing, China, **2** Department of Nephrology, Peking University Third Hospital, Beijing, China, **3** Department of Nephrology, Huashan Hospital of Fudan University, Shanghai, China, **4** Department of Nephrology, Second Affiliated Hospital of Harbin Medical University, Heilongjiang, China, **5** Kidney Disease Center, The First Affiliated Hospital, College of Medicine, Zhejiang University, Hangzhou, China, **6** Department of Nephrology, Peking University People's Hospital, Beijing, China, **7** Department of Nephrology, General Hospital of Ningxia Medical University, Ningxia, China

Abstract

Aims: To investigate whether education level of family members predicts all-cause and cardiovascular death and initial-episode peritonitis in patients on peritoneal dialysis (PD).

Methods: A total of 2264 patients on chronic PD were collected from seven centers affiliated with the Socioeconomic Status on the Outcome of Peritoneal Dialysis (SSOP) Study. All demographic, socioeconomic and laboratory data of patients and the education level of all family members were recorded at baseline. Multivariate Cox regression was used to calculate the hazard ratio (HR) of all-cause and cardiovascular mortality, and initial-episode peritonitis with adjustments for recognized traditional factors.

Results: There were no significant differences in baseline characteristics between patients with (n = 1752) and without (n = 512) complete education information. According to the highest education level of patients' family, included 1752 patients were divided into four groups, i.e. elementary or lower (15%), middle (27%), high (24%) and more than high school (34%). The family highest education (using elementary school or lower group as reference, hazard ratio and 95% confidence interval of middle school group, high school group and more than high school group was 0.68[0.48–0.96], 0.64[0.45–0.91], 0.66[0.48–0.91], respectively) rather than their average education level or patients' or spouse's education was significantly associated with the higher mortality. Neither patients' nor family education level did correlate to the risk for cardiovascular death or initial-episode peritonitis.

Conclusions: Family members' education level was found to be a novel predictor of PD outcome. Family, as the main source of health care providers, should be paid more attention in our practice.

Editor: Hamid Reza Baradaran, Iran University of Medical Sciences, Iran (Islamic Republic Of)

Funding: This study is in part supported by New Century Excellent Talents from Education Department, China, Baxer Clinical Research Award from Baxter Corp, China and ISN Research Award from ISN GO R&P Committee. The funders had no role in study design, data collection and analysis, decision to publish, or preparation of the manuscript.

Competing Interests: This study is in part supported by New Century Excellent Talents from Education Department, China, Baxer Clinical Research Award from Baxter Corp, China and ISN Research Award from ISN GO R&P Committee. The funders had no role in study design, data collection and analysis, decision to publish, or preparation of the manuscript. The authors confirm that this does not alter their adherence to PLOS ONE policies on sharing data and materials.

* E-mail: dongjie@medmail.com.cn

Introduction

Peritoneal dialysis (PD) has been utilized as one of the main renal replacement therapies since the 1980s. Although the number of PD patients has markedly increased in both developing and developed countries[1], PD outcomes, such as mortality, technique failure, and hospitalization, have not markedly improved. Potential risk factors for poor outcome have been continuously explored in recent years. Among these, socioeconomic status (SES) has been indicated as a key predictor through multi-center PD cohort studies from various countries. These studies indicate that SES evaluated by individual education[2] and income[3], housing status[4], remote location[5,6], or social support[7–11] play the critical role in the outcomes of dialysis patients. Based on the inverse relationship between individual SES and mortality from our large-scale multi-center retrospective PD cohort study[3], we would further explore the association of social support and PD outcome.

Social support is the intricate network in which patients with various chronic illnesses may give and receive information and aid and have emotional needs met[12], which is mainly sourced from family members including a spouse, children and relatives, friends, and colleagues. For patients who receive long-term home care therapy, family members are the most important healthcare providers. At the start of dialysis, family members the main drivers for choosing PD or hemodialysis (HD) as a treatment[13,14]. Family members are also involved in the accommodation of lifestyle and living environment changes, and helping patients to improve their compliance to a therapy regime. For elderly or disabled patients, family members are more likely to take more responsibility for PD-associated care, such as performing the PD exchange and exit-site care, monitoring symptoms and signs daily, and contributing to food preparation and nutrition provision. All of the above are dependent on a strong education base[15]. Hence, it is hypothesized that the education level of family members may play a key role in the quality of therapy and PD outcome. To date, social support as a general index of SES rather than family members' education status has been investigated with respect to its impact on dialysis outcome in previous studies[7–11].

Therefore, we aimed to investigate associations between education level of PD patients' family members and outcome events, including all-cause and cardiovascular death and first-episode peritonitis through a large-scale multi-center retrospective cohort study, which will be helpful for unpacking the black box of the family education-outcome puzzle for PD population.

Methods

This is an affiliated study with the Socioeconomic Status on the Outcome of Peritoneal Dialysis (SSOP) study, which is a retrospective multi-center cohort study as described in detail in our previous paper[3]. The ethics committee of Peking University First Hospitl, China approved this study. Written consent was given by the patients for their information to be stored in the hospital database and used for research.

Center Enrollment

Centers with professional PD doctors and nurses and well-developed databases maintained for least 3 years, recording baseline characteristics and follow-up data every 1 to 3 months, participated in this study voluntarily. Nine centers were qualified, and seven of these, accounting for about 70% of all incident patients attending the nine centers, agreed to participate. The included PD centers were located in five different provinces and four geographical regions (north, northeast, northwest, and east) of China. Data from each center were collected within a strict quality control framework and further inspected and optimized to ensure the integrity and accuracy of the database. All study investigators and staff members completed a training program that taught them the methods and processes of the study. A manual of detailed instructions for data collection was distributed.

Subject Selection

All incident patients receiving chronic PD between the date of intact database creation and August 2011 were enrolled into this study. After starting PD, each patient signed informed consent agreeing to the use of their demographic and laboratory data in future studies. Those without information of education levels of family members were excluded. All subjects began the PD program within 1 month after catheter implantation and were given lactate-buffered glucose dialysate with a twin-bag connection system (Baxter Healthcare, Guangzhou, China).

Data collection

Demographic and clinical data including age, gender, body mass index (BMI), primary renal disease, history of cardiovascular disease (CVD), and presence of diabetes mellitus (DM) were collected at baseline. CVD was recorded if one of the following conditions was present: angina, class III/IV congestive heart failure (New York Heart Association), transient ischemic attack, history of myocardial infarction or cerebro-vascular accident, or peripheral arterial disease[16]. Baseline biochemistry data including hemoglobin, serum albumin, calcium, phosphate and intact parathyroid hormone (iPTH) were examined using an automatic Hitachi chemistry analyzer and then calculated as the mean of measurements made during the first 3 months. Dialysis adequacy and residual renal function (RRF) were measured during the first 6 months. RRF was defined as the mean of residual creatinine clearance and residual urea clearance. Dialysis adequacy was determined from the total Kt/V and total creatinine clearance (Ccr). Center size was also recorded according to the number of enrolled patients from each center.

The education level of patients and each family member, including spouses of those who are married was recorded from 1 to 4 as ordinal categorical variables according to diploma obtained based on school level: elementary school or lower = 1; middle school = 2; high school = 3; and more than high school = 4. Average education of a whole family except for the patient was calculated as the arithmetic mean of the education levels of all family members. The highest education of any one family member was recorded as the maximum education level of family members.

Family income was defined as the yearly household income per person and was divided into low (<¥20,000, <$3160,), medium (¥20,000–40,000, $3160–6320) and high (>¥40,000, >$6320) according to average income for urban information in 2011 from the bureau of statistics (http://www.bjstats.gov.cn/nj/main/2011-tjnj/index.htm) since most subjects were from urban. Information of reimbursement type and family residence was also collected. The frequent visitor was defined as someone visiting doctors at least one time every 3 months. Whether medical expenses are covered by national health care system was also recorded

Definition of Outcome Events

The Primary outcome was defined as all-cause death and cardiovascular death. Cardiovascular death was defined as death due to myocardial infarction, congestive heart failure, cerebral bleeding, cerebral infarction, arrhythmia, peripheral arterial disease, and sudden death. The secondary outcome was initial peritonitis, which was diagnosed according to International Society for Peritoneal Dialysis 2010 guidelines[17]. In all analyses, data of transferring to hemodialysis (HD), loss to follow-up, renal transplantation or till the end of the study (November 1, 2011) were censored.

Statistical Analysis

Continuous data were presented as mean with standard deviation except that RRF was presented as the median (inter-quartile range) because of high skew. Categorical variables were presented as proportions. Relevant characteristics were compared between different education groups, respectively. Patient data were compared using the one-way ANOVA for normally distributed continuous variables, or the Kruskall–Wallis H test for skewed continuous variables, and the Chi-square test for categorical variables. Spearman correlations were explored to identify correlation among various indices of education level and family income. To determine predictive effect of education level of the patient and family (couple education, average education and the highest education) on the outcome events, stratified multivariable Cox regression models were explored, adjusted by age, gender, BMI, presence of DM, CVD history, baseline albumin, hemoglobin, RRF, and family income, and center size was as the stratified factor to adjust for center effects. The center effect was reflected not only in disparity of center size (ranging from 78 patients to 815 patients), which has been demonstrated to be an independent predictor of PD outcome[18–20], but also in differences in practice patterns and biochemical assays between centers. We reported the multivariable adjusted hazard ratios (HRs) with 95% confidence interval (CI). All probabilities were two- tailed, and the level of significance was set at 0.05. Statistical analyses were performed using SPSS for Windows software version 15.0 (SPSS Inc., Chicago, IL).

Results

Baseline characteristics

Data from 2,264 patients were collected. Five hundred and twelve patients were excluded due to missing family education data. In the final cohort, the included 1,752 patients had a mean age of 57.93±15.30 years, with male patients accounting for 49.9%. Overall, 38.8% were diabetic and cerebrovascular disease (CVD) was present in 43.4% of subjects at baseline. The total follow-up duration was 27.6 (14.3–45.4) months. Chronic glomerulonephritis (CGN) was the most common cause of end-stage renal disease (ESRD) (34.4%), followed by diabetic nephropathy (29.7%) and hypertensive nephropathy (16.4%). There were no significant differences in age, gender, body mass index (BMI), or distribution of education level of patients and their family members between the included and excluded subjects ($P>0.05$).

Education levels of PD patients and their family members

The constitutions of education levels of the patients and their partners were nearly equivalent; e.g. elementary school 26.7% and 25.9%, middle school 30.0% and 34.5%, high school 23.3% and 22.2%, and more than high school 20.0% and 17.4%, respectively. As for the highest education level of the family members, 33.7% had more than high school level (**Figure 1**).

Comparing patients according to their family's highest level of education showed significant differences in age (over 65 years or not), gender, education and income level, reimbursement type (healthcare or not), or the percentage of rural residence ($P<0.001$ or 0.05; **Table 1**). Patients whose family's highest education was elementary or lower were more likely to be the eldest male patients from a rural area. They were also less likely to be covered by national healthcare, and had lower family income and lower education level. These patients also had the lowest plasma albumin at baseline. There were no significant differences in the presence of diabetes mellitus (DM), CVD history, percentage of frequent visitor, total Kt/V and Ccr, RRF, BMI, or hemoglobin ($P>0.05$).

Education levels of patients, their spouses, and the average and highest level of education of their family members, had positive correlations ($r=0.241\sim0.695$; $P<0.001$ for all). Likewise, each education level was correlated with yearly personal income ($r=0.241\sim0.265$; $P<0.001$ for all; **Table 2**).

Follow-up and outcomes

Among the 497 patients who died, 190 deaths (38.2%) were due to CVD and 120 (24.1%) infection; other causes were malignancy, gastrointestinal bleeding, malnutrition, miscellaneous, and undefined. One hundred and forty-eight patients were transferred to HD, most due to PD-associated infection (67 cases, 45.3%).

The time to first-episode peritonitis was 20.88 (9.73–35.23) months. Among 392 episodes of initial peritonitis during the study period, there were 139 episodes (35.5%) due to Gram-positive organisms, while 84 (21.4%) were due to Gram-negative organisms and 7 (1.8%) fungi.

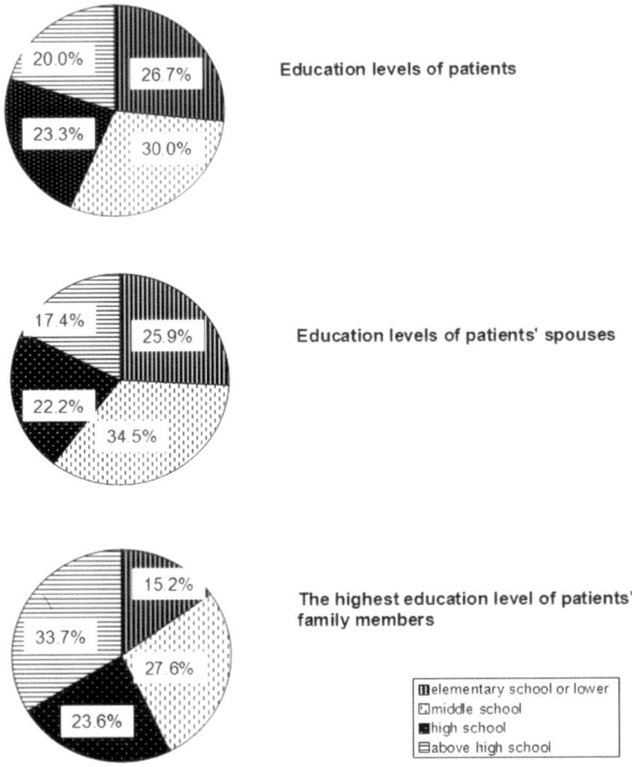

Figure 1. Education levels of PD patients and their family members.

Associations of education levels with outcome

By multivariable Cox regression analysis (**Table 3**), similar to our previous report[3], patient education level did not predict patient survival after adjusting for age, gender, BMI, presence of DM, CVD history, baseline albumin, hemoglobin, RRF, and family income, and using center size as a stratified factor to adjust for center effects. However, the highest education of family members was significantly associated with higher mortality. As compared to the family's highest education of elementary school or lower group, middle, high and more than high school education decreased the risk of death by 32%, 36%, and 34%, respectively. There also a trend that each increase of 1 in average education level decreased mortality by 11% ($P=0.05$). As for spouse's education, middle education rather than high school or more than high school also predicted a lower mortality. For cardiovascular death and initial-episode peritonitis, neither PD patients nor their family members' education level were associated with the higher risk after adjusting for the abovementioned covariates. No interactions between education level and age, gender, DM, or CVD history were found for predicting all-cause mortality, CV death, or initial-episode peritonitis.

Discussion

In this large-scale multi-center retrospective study, the highest educationof family members were identified as independent predictive factors of PD outcome; however, no such effects were detected for CV death or occurrence of the first episode of peritonitis after adjustment for well-recognized confounders. The education level of a PD patient was not found to contribute to any outcome events, similar to our previous reports[3]. To our

Table 1. The baseline characteristics and clinical data of PD patients according to their family's highest education level.

	The highest education level of patients' family members				
	elementary school or lower	middle school	high school	above high school	*P*
Age>65 yrs (%)	50.38	38.30	29.30	38.47	<0.001
Male(%)	55.26	52.80	47.22	46.95	0.048
BMI (Kg/m2)	22.63±3.88	22.93±3.51	23.05±3.59	22.81±3.39	0.47
DM (%)	39.02	40.22	36.39	39.18	0.70
CVD (%)	43.68	39.28	41.83	47.20	0.06
Family income					<0.001
Low (%)	61.89	53.11	48.54	34.92	
Medium (%)	30.57	38.59	39.08	34.92	
High (%)	7.55	8.30	12.38	30.15	
Education levels of patients					<0.001
Elementary school or lower (%)	53.01	27.44	21.31	18.00	
Middle school (%)	27.82	41.37	28.33	22.75	
High school (%)	12.03	22.25	32.93	22.54	
Above high school (%)	7.14	8.94	17.43	36.67	
Education levels of patients' spouse					NA
Elementary school or lower (%)	100.00	14.14	12.39	12.03	
Middle school (%)	0.00	85.86	18.13	17.15	
High school (%)	0.00	0.00	69.49	17.15	
Above high school (%)	0.00	0.00	0.00	53.67	
Average education level	1.00±0.00	1.88±0.22	2.65±0.44	3.38±0.63	<0.001
Rural residence (%)	34.2	23.8	21.1	8.6	<0.001
Health care (%)#	59.4	68.7	73.5	84.1	<0.001
Frequent visitors (%)□	85.71	88.54	86.68	90.15	0.19
Hemoglobin (g/L)	98.76±18.16	101.82±19.39	101.45±17.51	101.52±17.16	0.07
Serum albumin (g/L)	34.32±5.76	34.80±5.21	35.45±5.25	35.29±5.13	0.023
Calcium(mmol/L)	2.16±0.25	2.17±0.23	2.19±0.25	2.20±0.24	0.08
Phosphate(mmol/L)	1.53±0.47	1.58±0.50	1.54±0.46	1.56±0.42	0.36
iPTH (pg/ml)	179.2(78~343)	180.9(93.05~327.15)	192(87.7~338.5)	148(64.57~313.15)	0.07
Total Kt/V	2.03±0.66	2.05±0.63	2.12±0.67	2.02±.64	0.13
Total Ccr (L/w/1.73 m^2)	77.25±41.43	77.9±47.99	76.9±30.9	74.78±29.9	0.64
RRF (ml/min)	3.02(1.30–5.62)	3.30(1.76–5.40)	3.72(1.94–5.57)	3.51(1.93–5.50)	0.26

Abbreviations: BMI, body mass index; DM, diabetes mellitus; CVD, cardiovascular disease; iPTH, intact parathyroid hormone; Kt/V, urea clearance; Ccr, creatinine clearance; RRF, residual renal function.

#Healthcare % represents the percentage of patients whose medical expenses are covered more than 90% by the national healthcare system.

□Frequent visitor was defined as someone visiting doctors at least once every 3 months.

Table 2. Coefficient correlations between the education levels of PD patients and their family members and family income#.

	Patients' education	Spouse's education	The highest education	Average education	Family income
Patients' education	NA				
Spouse's education	0.566	NA			
The highest education	0.335	0.695	NA		
Average education	0.428	0.825	0.874	NA	
Family income	0.265	0.281	0.241	0.262	NA

Abbreviation: NA, non analysis.

#All *P* values for the correlation analyses were <0.001.

Table 3. The predictive role of education level of patients and their family members by multivariable Cox regression analysis.

	Death				Cardiovascular death				Initial- episode peritonitis			
	HR	95% CI		*P*	HR	95% CI		*P*	HR	95% CI		P
Patients' education												
Low	ref			0.47	ref			0.95	ref			0.85
Middle	0.81	0.61	1.09	0.17	0.93	0.57	1.50	0.77	0.93	0.69	1.25	0.63
High	0.87	0.63	1.21	0.40	0.88	0.52	1.49	0.64	0.91	0.66	1.27	0.59
>high	1.00	0.71	1.41	0.99	0.85	0.48	1.52	0.59	0.86	0.60	1.24	0.86
The highest education												
Low	ref			0.04	ref			0.49	ref			0.26
middle	0.68	0.48	0.96	0.03	0.74	0.42	1.33	0.31	0.85	0.58	1.26	0.43
High	0.64	0.45	0.91	0.01	0.62	0.34	1.13	0.12	1.08	0.74	1.59	0.67
>high	0.66	0.48	0.91	0.01	0.75	0.44	1.29	0.30	1.14	0.79	1.64	0.49
Spouse's education												
Low	ref			0.07	ref			0.18	ref			0.06
middle	0.69	0.49	0.97	0.03	0.69	0.41	1.17	0.17	0.90	0.62	1.29	0.56
High	0.72	0.49	1.07	0.10	0.62	0.33	1.17	0.14	1.39	0.95	2.05	0.09
>high	0.98	0.67	1.43	0.92	1.08	0.60	1.97	0.79	1.19	0.79	1.81	0.41
Average education	0.89	0.78	1.00	0.05	0.94	0.77	1.14	0.52	1.07	0.95	1.22	0.28

Notes:All models are adjusted for age, gender, BMI, presence of DM, CVD history, baseline albumin, hemoglobin, RRF and family income, and center size was used as a stratified factor to adjust for center effects.
The HRs and 95%CI for all-cause death, cardiovascular death, and initial-episode peritonitis are shown respectively using low level (elementary school or lower) as the reference. The HR and 95% of average education level as a continuous variable is also shown.

knowledge, this is the first study to offer insight into the impact of family members' education status on PD patient outcomes.

Most patients with chronic kidney disease will develop ESRD and sooner or later require renal replacement therapy. This is unpleasant and has a great impact on both the patients and their family members. Undoubtedly, the patients' illness affects the physical and mental health of families in this population[21–23]. On the other hand, family members as a primary source of social support can make great contributions to patients' disease management. To date, only a few studies have shown that spouse's behavior and attitude can affect patient management of diabetes[24,25], stroke[26], and osteoarthritis[27] rehabilitation therapy. For the dialysis population, although previous studies have indicated the significant impact of social support on satisfaction, psychological status, quality of life, hospitalization, and mortality for PD and HD patients[7–11], the association between a specific aspect of family members, such as education status and PD outcome has rarely been explored.

Our novel findings presented here revealed a close relationship between education level of family members and poor PD outcome. There are several reasons for these results. Firstly, for patients with ESRD, medical decisions are largely dependent on consultation with family members. Family members with high education backgrounds are more likely to get access to healthcare and offer better information sharing and advice. Such good social support from family probably leads to early referral to nephrologists, appropriate choice of dialysis modality, and timely preparation with dialysis access[28]. Secondly, once a dialysis program starts, the whole family has to strive to adapt to the changes in their daily lives, including dietary, complex medication regimens, some social isolation, frequent clinic visits, and hospitalization. Care giving activities, including appraising, advocating, and coaching, provided by family members is dependent on a strong knowledge base[15]. Family members with higher education levels can understand all the changes easily and are apt to adjust patients' lifestyles as suggested. As shown in a previous study, there is a very strong correlation between coherence and functionality of the non-chronically-ill spouse, social support, and compliance to chronic illness to his or her situation[29]. Besides the family-unit therapy nature of PD, according to our practice, deep-rooted family conception of Chinese patients may reveal the unnegligible affection from the whole family to the patient, hence patients' own education levels seemed less important. However, there was not such a linear trend that the family highest education level of middle school and above would be more benefit for patients' mortality. Though educated family would be expected to have better adherence to treatment and adaptation to daily life change, they also bear heavier mental pressure and endure more fierce decision conflict when accidents happen. Leadership, the role most likely played by person with the highest family education, might be important at such a difficult point to decision making, which would affect patients' outcomes.In addition, although close relationships among family's education level, income level, rural residence, and less healthcare were found, multivariate analysis could not validate that the predicting role of family's education level is confounded by these factors. Future studies should focus on the effect of improved social support from family members on the physical or psychosocial well-being of patients[30].

It is interesting that higher education level of the spouse did not decrease the death risk for PD patients despite the fact that the spouse has the closest relationship with patients acting as a caregiver, confidant, and primary source of emotional support. The cause for this phenomenon is not clear. However, recent studies have suggested that the quality of marriage rather than the presence of a marriage significantly influences the outcome for dialysis patients. Low patient marital satisfaction evaluated by the Dyadic Adjustment Scale is found to be associated with poorer psychological status of the partners and higher mortality[31]. Whether or how the education level of a spouse correlates to the quality of marriage and family support needs to be explored.

Based on our data, the education level of patients and their family members has no impact on initial-episode peritonitis. One possible explanation for this is that selected centers were equipped with professional PD clinicians and well-developed training programs[32]. In most centers, patients and their homecare helpers were often and repeatedly trained and examined for proper techniques with respect to bag exchange. Under these circumstances, it is likely that biological factors leading to the occurrence of peritonitis may outweigh the effects of education level of patients and their family members.

This study has several strengths. First, this is the only study to disclose the impact of education levels of both PD patients and their family members on PD outcomes with large sample sizes. The detailed information on the education status offers us a valuable chance to reveal a family education-outcome relationship. Our results alert clinicians to highlight the importance of family factors on the therapeutic effects of family-based treatment, such as in PD. In addition, the baseline education level is a fixed variable for the majority adult patients and their family. As compared to social support, a variable index during long-term follow up, baseline education status as a potential prognostic factor is more appropriate to be explored.

There are some limitations to this study. First, potential mechanisms for the association of family members' education and PD outcome are not clear since we did not evaluate a patient's satisfaction with care providers, perception of accessibility of care or to therapy for patients from less-educated families. Until such research is conducted, a determination of whether and how family members' education directly affects quality of therapy and PD outcome is difficult to make. Secondly, we should be aware of the possibility of residual confounding and recall bias because of the retrospective nature of this study. However, if confounding occurred, it would result in underestimation of the association but not change our main findings at all. In addition, we should be aware of the possibilities of ascertainment bias (totally 22.6% eligible patients were not included). Finally, as an observational study, a cause-effect relationship could not be established.

In conclusion, PD patients with well-educated family members have a lower death risk. This novel finding is helpful for us to understand the key role that family support plays in the quality of PD therapy, such a home-based therapy. Further research focusing on family-unit therapy and individualized care based on family education background should be designed to investigate their potential benefits for PD patients. The issues raised by the present study also highlight some challenges for caring practices in home-based therapy for conditions like PD.

Acknowledgments

The authors express their appreciation to the patients, doctors, and nursing staff of the peritoneal dialysis center of Peking University First Hospital, Division of Nephrology of Peking University Third Hospital, Division of Nephrology of Huashan Hospital, Fudan University, Division of Nephrology of the second affiliated hospital of Harbin Medical University, Division of Nephrology of Peking University People's Hospital, Division of Nephrology of the first affiliated hospital of Zhejiang University School of Medicine, Division of Nephrology of General Hospital of NingXia Medical University, for their participation in this study.

Author Contributions

Conceived and designed the experiments: JD HYW. Performed the experiments: QFH TYZ YPR JHC HPZ MHC JD YW CMH RZ XHZ MW NT. Analyzed the data: ZKY JD. Wrote the paper: ZKY JD.

References

1. Jain AK, Blake P, Cordy P, Garg AX (2012) Global trends in rates of peritoneal dialysis. J Am Soc Nephrol 23: 533–544.
2. Martin LC, Caramori JC, Fernandes N, Divino-Filho JC, Pecoits-Filho R, et al. (2011) Geographic and educational factors and risk of the first peritonitis episode in Brazilian Peritoneal Dialysis study (BRAZPD) patients. Clin J Am Soc Nephrol 6: 1944–1951.
3. Xu R, Han QF, Zhu TY, Ren YP, Chen JH, et al. (2012) Impact of individual and environmental socioeconomic status on peritoneal dialysis outcomes: a retrospective multicenter cohort study. PLoS One 7: e50766.
4. Farias MG, Soucie JM, McClellan W, Mitch WE (1994) Race and the risk of peritonitis: an analysis of factors associated with the initial episode. Kidney Int 46: 1392–1396.
5. Tonelli M, Hemmelgarn B, Culleton B, Klarenbach S, Gill JS, et al. (2007) Mortality of Canadians treated by peritoneal dialysis in remote locations. Kidney Int 72: 1023–1028.
6. Mehrotra R, Story K, Guest S, Fedunyszyn M (2012) Neighborhood location, rurality, geography, and outcomes of peritoneal dialysis patients in the United States. Perit Dial Int 32: 322–331.
7. Thong MS, Kaptein AA, Krediet RT, Boeschoten EW, Dekker FW (2007) Social support predicts survival in dialysis patients. Nephrol Dial Transplant 22: 845–850.
8. Szeto CC, Chow KM, Kwan BC, Law MC, Chung KY, et al. (2008) The impact of social support on the survival of Chinese peritoneal dialysis patients. Perit Dial Int 28: 252–258.
9. Plantinga LC, Fink NE, Harrington-Levey R, Finkelstein FO, Hebah N, et al. (2010) Association of social support with outcomes in incident dialysis patients. Clin J Am Soc Nephrol 5: 1480–1488.
10. Untas A, Thumma J, Rascle N, Rayner H, Mapes D, et al. (2011) The associations of social support and other psychosocial factors with mortality and quality of life in the dialysis outcomes and practice patterns study. Clin J Am Soc Nephrol 6: 142–152.
11. Ye XQ, Chen WQ, Lin JX, Wang RP, Zhang ZH, et al. (2008) Effect of social support on psychological-stress-induced anxiety and depressive symptoms in patients receiving peritoneal dialysis. J Psychosom Res 65: 157–164.
12. Patel SS, Peterson RA, Kimmel PL (2005) The impact of social support on end-stage renal disease. Semin Dial 18: 98–102.
13. Oliver MJ, Garg AX, Blake PG, Johnson JF, Verrelli M, et al. (2010) Impact of contraindications, barriers to self-care and support on incident peritoneal dialysis utilization. Nephrol Dial Transplant 25: 2737–2744.
14. Griva K, Li ZH, Lai AY, Choong MC, Foo MW (2013) Perspectives of patients, families, and health care professionals on decision-making about dialysis modality—the good, the bad, and the misunderstandings! Perit Dial Int 33: 280–289.
15. Beanlands H, Horsburgh ME, Fox S, Howe A, Locking-Cusolito H, et al. (2005) Caregiving by family and friends of adults receiving dialysis. Nephrol Nurs J 32: 621–631.
16. Smith SC, Jr., Jackson R, Pearson TA, Fuster V, Yusuf S, et al. (2004) Principles for national and regional guidelines on cardiovascular disease prevention: a scientific statement from the World Heart and Stroke Forum. Circulation 109: 3112–3121.
17. Li PK, Szeto CC, Piraino B, Bernardini J, Figueiredo AE, et al. (2010) Peritoneal dialysis-related infections recommendations: 2010 update. Perit Dial Int 30: 393–423.
18. Afolalu B, Troidle L, Osayimwen O, Bhargava J, Kitsen J, et al. (2009) Technique failure and center size in a large cohort of peritoneal dialysis patients in a defined geographic area. Perit Dial Int 29: 292–296.
19. Mujais S, Story K (2006) Peritoneal dialysis in the US: evaluation of outcomes in contemporary cohorts. Kidney Int Suppl: S21–26.
20. Schaubel DE, Blake PG, Fenton SS (2001) Effect of renal center characteristics on mortality and technique failure on peritoneal dialysis. Kidney Int 60: 1517–1524.
21. Sezer S, Uyar ME, Bal Z, Tutal E, Ozdemir Acar FN (2013) The influence of socioeconomic factors on depression in maintenance hemodialysis patients and their caregivers. Clin Nephrol 80: 342–348.
22. Schipper K, Abma TA (2011) Coping, family and mastery: top priorities for social science research by patients with chronic kidney disease. Nephrol Dial Transplant 26: 3189–3195.
23. Tsai TC, Liu SI, Tsai JD, Chou LH (2006) Psychosocial effects on caregivers for children on chronic peritoneal dialysis. Kidney Int 70: 1983–1987.
24. Stephens MA, Franks MM, Rook KS, Iida M, Hemphill RC, et al. (2013) Spouses' attempts to regulate day-to-day dietary adherence among patients with type 2 diabetes. Health Psychol 32: 1029–1037.
25. Khan CM, Stephens MA, Franks MM, Rook KS, Salem JK (2013) Influences of spousal support and control on diabetes management through physical activity. Health Psychol 32: 739–747.
26. Molloy GJ, Johnston M, Johnston DW, Pollard B, Morrison V, et al. (2008) Spousal caregiver confidence and recovery from ambulatory activity limitations in stroke survivors. Health Psychol 27: 286–290.
27. Stephens MA, Fekete EM, Franks MM, Rook KS, Druley JA, et al. (2009) Spouses' use of pressure and persuasion to promote osteoarthritis patients' medical adherence after orthopedic surgery. Health Psychol 28: 48–55.
28. Cohen SD, Sharma T, Acquaviva K, Peterson RA, Patel SS, et al. (2007) Social support and chronic kidney disease: an update. Adv Chronic Kidney Dis 14: 335–344.
29. Horsburgh ME, Rice VH, Matuk L (1998) Sense of coherence and life satisfaction: patient and spousal adaptation to home dialysis. ANNA J 25: 219–228; discussion 229–230.
30. Tong A, Sainsbury P, Craig JC (2008) Support interventions for caregivers of people with chronic kidney disease: a systematic review. Nephrol Dial Transplant 23: 3960–3965.
31. Kimmel PL, Peterson RA, Weihs KL, Shidler N, Simmens SJ, et al. (2000) Dyadic relationship conflict, gender, and mortality in urban hemodialysis patients. J Am Soc Nephrol 11: 1518–1525.
32. Xu R, Zhuo M, Yang Z, Dong J (2012) Experiences with assisted peritoneal dialysis in China. Perit Dial Int 32: 94–101.

Single Nucleotide Variants in the Protein C Pathway and Mortality in Dialysis Patients

Gürbey Ocak[1]*, Christiane Drechsler[2,3,4], Carla Y. Vossen[1], Hans L. Vos[5,6], Frits R. Rosendaal[1,5,6], Pieter H. Reitsma[5,6], Michael M. Hoffmann[7], Winfried März[8], Willem H. Ouwehand[9,10], Raymond T. Krediet[11], Elisabeth W. Boeschoten[12], Friedo W. Dekker[1], Christoph Wanner[2,3], Marion Verduijn[1]

1 Department of Clinical Epidemiology, Leiden University Medical Center, Leiden, The Netherlands, **2** Department of Medicine, Division of Nephrology, University Hospital, Würzburg, Germany, **3** Comprehensive Heart Failure Center, University of Wuerzburg, Wuerzburg, Germany, **4** Institute of Clinical Epidemiology and Biometry, University of Wuerzburg, Wuerzburg, Germany, **5** Department of Thrombosis and Haemostasis, Leiden University Medical Center, Leiden, The Netherlands, **6** Einthoven Laboratory for Experimental Vascular Medicine, Leiden University Medical Center, Leiden, The Netherlands, **7** Institute of Clinical Chemistry and Laboratory Medicine, University Medical Center, Freiburg, Germany, **8** Department of Public Health, Social and Preventive Medicine, University of Heidelberg, Mannheim, Germany, **9** Department of Hematology, University of Cambridge and National Health Service Blood and Transplant, Cambridge, United Kingdom, **10** Department of Human Genetics, Wellcome Trust Sanger Institute, Cambridge, United Kingdom, **11** Department of Nephrology, Academic Medical Center, Amsterdam, The Netherlands, **12** Hans Mak Institute, Naarden, The Netherlands

Abstract

Background: The protein C pathway plays an important role in the maintenance of endothelial barrier function and in the inflammatory and coagulant processes that are characteristic of patients on dialysis. We investigated whether common single nucleotide variants (SNV) in genes encoding protein C pathway components were associated with all-cause 5 years mortality risk in dialysis patients.

Methods: Single nucleotides variants in the factor V gene (*F5* rs6025; factor V Leiden), the thrombomodulin gene (*THBD* rs1042580), the protein C gene (*PROC* rs1799808 and 1799809) and the endothelial protein C receptor gene (*PROCR* rs867186, rs2069951, and rs2069952) were genotyped in 1070 dialysis patients from the NEtherlands COoperative Study on the Adequacy of Dialysis (NECOSAD) cohort) and in 1243 dialysis patients from the German 4D cohort.

Results: Factor V Leiden was associated with a 1.5-fold (95% CI 1.1–1.9) increased 5-year all-cause mortality risk and carriers of the AG/GG genotypes of the PROC rs1799809 had a 1.2-fold (95% CI 1.0–1.4) increased 5-year all-cause mortality risk. The other SNVs in *THBD*, *PROC*, and *PROCR* were not associated with 5-years mortality.

Conclusion: Our study suggests that factor V Leiden and PROC rs1799809 contributes to an increased mortality risk in dialysis patients.

Editor: Nandita Mitra, University of Pennsylvania, United States of America

Funding: The NECOSAD was supported in part by unrestricted grants from the Dutch Kidney Foundation. No additional funding was received for this study. The funders had no role in study design, data collection and analysis, decision to publish, or preparation of the manuscript.

Competing Interests: The authors have declared that no competing interests exist.

* E-mail: g.ocak@lumc.nl

Introduction

The protein C pathway plays an important role in endothelial barrier function and in inflammatory and anticoagulant processes [1]. Protein C activation occurs on the endothelial cell membrane by thrombin bound to thrombomodulin and this is enhanced when protein C is bound to the endothelial protein C receptor. Activated protein C together with its cofactor protein S inactivates the procoagulant factors Va and VIIIa. Activated protein C resistance is often caused by a variant of factor V (factor V Leiden), that abrogates one of the inactivation sites in factor Va [2]. Besides anticoagulant properties, activated protein C has direct cytoprotective effects on endothelial cells that include anti-inflammatory actions, anti-apoptotic activities, and stabilization of endothelial barriers. These effects are largely mediated by activation of protease activated receptors [3–7].

The crucial role of the protein C pathway in endothelial function, coagulation, and inflammation became evident in several studies [8–12]. The importance of the protein C system is most clearly demonstrated by the massive thrombotic complications occurring in infants with severe protein C deficiency due to genetic abnormalities [8] and the increased risk of venous thrombosis in adults with a genetic defect resulting in decreased protein C levels [9]. In severe sepsis patients with a high mortality risk treatment with activated protein C reduced mortality, probably through its anti-inflammatory and anticoagulant activities [10]. In addition, low plasma protein C levels have been shown to increase the risk of ischemic stroke [11]. Finally, particular combinations of variants in the thrombomodulin, protein C, and factor V genes seem to increase the risk of cardiovascular events in the general population [12].

Patients on dialysis have a high mortality risk due to endothelial damage and subsequent cardiovascular diseases [13]. Dialysis patients also have a high risk of dying from dialysis treatment failure [13], which is associated with thrombotic events (i.e. vascular access thrombosis and catheter thrombosis) and infections [13]. Genetic variation in the protein C pathway could influence the mortality risk by changing processes related to endothelial damage, by influencing inflammatory response, and by increasing or decreasing the chance of thrombotic events associated with treatment failure. We hypothesized that single nucleotide variants encoding protein C pathway components or targets might influence mortality rates in dialysis patients.

We selected seven single nucleotide variants (SNVs) that are known to influence levels or activity of proteins in the protein C pathway or have been associated with venous thrombosis, arterial thrombosis or mortality in the general population: factor V (*F5*) rs6025 (factor V Leiden) [2], thrombomodulin (*THBD*) rs1042580 [12,14], protein C (*PROC*) rs1799809 and rs1799808 [15], and protein C receptor (*PROCR*) rs867186, rs2069952, and rs2069952.[16] We investigated the association between these SNVs and all-cause and cause-specific (cardiovascular and non-cardiovascular) mortality in the NEtherlands COoperative Study on the Adequacy of Dialysis (NECOSAD) cohort and the German Diabetes Dialysis Study (4D-study).

Methods and Materials

Patients

The Netherlands Cooperative Study on the Adequacy of Dialysis (NECOSAD) is a prospective multicenter cohort study in which incident adult dialysis patients from 38 dialysis centers in the Netherlands were included. The Medical Review Ethics Committee of the Leiden University Medical Center approved the study. All patients gave written informed consent. Eligibility criteria included age older than 18 years, and no previous renal replacement therapy (transplantation or dialysis). For the current analyses, we used data from patients who were included between June 1997 and June 2007 in 23 dialysis centers that approved DNA analysis. Information was gathered from patients until date of death or date of censoring, i.e. transfer to a nonparticipating dialysis center, withdrawal from the study, transplantation, or end of the follow-up period in June 2009, whichever occurred first.

Demographic and clinical data

Data on age, sex, primary kidney disease, and cardiovascular disease were collected at the start of dialysis treatment. Pre-existing cardiovascular disease was defined as a history of angina pectoris, myocardial infarction, heart failure, ischemic stroke, or claudication at the time of inclusion.

Single nucleotide variants

Blood samples were collected for DNA analysis. We genotyped one SNV in the factor V gene (*F5* rs6025; factor V Leiden), one SNV in the thrombomodulin gene (*THBD* rs1042580), two SNVs in the protein C gene (*PROC* rs1799809 and rs1799808), and three SNVs in the protein C receptor gene (*PROCR* rs867186, rs2069951, and rs2069952) using TaqMan SNV Genotyping Assays (Applied Biosystems, Foster City, CA, USA) as described previously [14–17].

Mortality

We classified causes of death according to the codes of the European Renal Association-European Dialysis and Transplantation Association (ERA-EDTA) which is a standardized classification of death causes in dialysis patients [18]. We grouped death causes into cardiovascular and non-cardiovascular mortality. Cardiovascular mortality was defined as death due to myocardial ischemia and infarction (code 11); cardiac arrest/sudden death (code 15); cardiac failure/fluid overload/pulmonary edema (codes 14,16,18); hyperkalemia/hypokalemia (code 12,17); pulmonary embolism (code 21); cerebrum-vascular accident (code 22); hemorrhage from ruptured vascular aneurysm (code 26); mesenteric infarction (code 29); cause of death uncertain/unknown (code 0). All other deaths were designated as non-cardiovascular mortality.

Replication

For independent replication of the results of the NECOSAD study, we analyzed data from the German Diabetes Dialysis Study (4D-study). Methods of the 4D-study have been described in detail previously [19]. Briefly, the 4D-study was a double-blind, randomized trial on the effect of atorvastatin in hemodialysis patients with type 2 diabetes mellitus who had less than two years of previous hemodialysis treatment. The primary endpoint of was a composite of cardiac death, non-fatal myocardial infarction and stroke, whichever occurred first. Patients were randomly assigned to either 20 mg of atorvastatin or placebo once daily until the date of death, censoring, or the end of study in March 2004. Atorvastatin showed no effect on the composite primary end point [19]. The genotyping of the SNV in the factor V gene (*F5* rs6025; factor V Leiden), the SNV in the thrombomodulin gene (*THBD* rs1042580), the two SNVs in the protein C gene (*PROC* rs1799809 and rs1799808), and the three SNVs in the protein C receptor gene (*PROCR* rs867186, rs2069951, and rs2069952) were the same as described above for the NECOSAD cohort. The SNV in the factor V gene (*F5* rs6025; factor V Leiden), the SNV in the thrombomodulin gene (*THBD* rs1042580), and the SNV in the protein C receptor gene (*PROCR* rs867186) were genotyped earlier than the other SNVs, therefore the numbers vary for these SNVs as compared with the other SNVs. Mortality was also categorized into cardiovascular and non-cardiovascular deaths.

Statistical analysis

The baseline characteristics are presented as median and 5th–95th percentiles for continuous variables, and as percentages for categorical variables. Distributions of genotypes were compared by the chi-square test to test for Hardy-Weinberg equilibrium. We calculated pooled hazard ratios (HRs) with 95% confidence intervals (95% CIs) for all-cause, cardiovascular, and non-cardiovascular mortality by Cox's regression analysis to study the effect of the seven SNVs on 5-year mortality from start of dialysis in the NECOSAD and 4D-study together. Moreover, we investigated the effect on mortality of combinations of *THBD* rs1042580 and single nucleotide variants that increased the mortality risk of dialysis patients in our study, since a previous study found associations between the combination of single nucleotide variants in the protein C pathway and THBD rs1042580 in the risk of cardiovascular diseases [12]. Furthermore, we calculated HRs with 95% CIs separately for the NECOSAD cohort and 4D-study. In addition, we repeated the analyses in the NECOSAD cohort for only hemodialysis patients with diabetes mellitus, since the 4D-study consists of only hemodialysis patients with diabetes mellitus. HRs were calculated for homozygous or heterozygous carriers of the rare alleles (except for rs2069952 for which the risk allele was the common major allele) of the SNVs compared to non-carriers. We reported unadjusted HRs, since adjustment in genetic association studies could potentially introduce interference in the causal pathway and thereby bias through overadjustment [20]. We used SPSS statistical software (version 17.0; SPSS, Chicago) for all statistical analyses.

Results

A total of 1070 patients from the NECOSAD cohort and 1243 patients from the 4D cohort were genotyped for the seven SNVs. Baseline characteristics of the 1070 patients from the NECOSAD cohort and 1243 patients from the 4D cohort are shown in Table 1. In contrast to the NECOSAD cohort, the 4D cohort consisted only of hemodialysis patients with diabetes mellitus. In the NECOSAD cohort, 140 hemodialysis patients (20.7%) had diabetes mellitus.

Table 2 shows the genotype and allele frequencies for the seven SNVs. All SNVs in the NECOSAD cohort were in Hardy-Weinberg equilibrium, except *PROC* rs1799809 (p-value 0.002). In the 4D cohort, *F5* rs6025 (factor V Leiden) (p-value<0.001), *PROC* rs1799808 (p-value <0.036), and *PROCR* rs2069952 (p-value 0.001) were not in Hardy-Weinberg equilibrium (Table 2).

Of the 1070 patients from the NECOSAD cohort, 401 died within 5 years of follow-up; 185 patients due to cardiovascular causes and 216 due to non-cardiovascular causes. In the 4D cohort, 594 patients died within 5 years of follow-up (297 patients due to cardiovascular causes and 297 due to non-cardiovascular causes).

Factor V (Leiden) rs6025

Factor V Leiden was associated with a 1.5-fold (95% CI 1.1–1.9) increased year all-cause mortality risk in the pooled results. The hazard ratios were 1.4 (95% CI 0.9–2.1) in the total NECOSAD cohort and 1.6 (95% CI 1.1–2.2) in the 4D-study (Table 3). Restricting the analyses to diabetic patients with hemodialysis in the NECOSAD study (similar to the 4D study which only includes diabetic hemodialysis patients), factor V Leiden was associated with a 2.1-fold (95% CI 1.0–4.5) increased 5-year all-cause mortality risk (Table 3).

As compared with *THBD* rs1042580 AA genotype in the absence of factor V Leiden, the combination of factor V Leiden and *THBD* rs1042580 AA genotype resulted in a 1.5-fold (95% CI 0.9–2.4) increased mortality risk, the combination of *THBD* rs1042580 AA genotype in the absence of factor V Leiden resulted in a 1.0-fold (95% CI 0.9–1.1) increased mortality risk, and the combination of factor V Leiden and *THBD* rs1042580 AG/GG genotypes resulted in a 1.4-fold (95% CI 1.0–2.0) mortality risk.

Thrombomodulin, protein C and protein C receptor variants

As compared to the AA genotype in *PROC* rs1799809, carriers of the AG/GG genotypes had a 1.2-fold (95% CI 1.0–1.4) increased 5-year all-cause mortality risk (Table 3). As compared with *PROC* rs1799809 AA genotype and *THBD* rs1042580 AA genotype, the combination of *PROC* rs1799809 AG/GG genotypes and *THBD* rs1042580 AA genotype resulted in a 1.1-fold (95% CI 0.9–1.4) increased mortally risk, the combination of *PROC* rs1799809 AA genotype and *THBD* rs1042580 AG/GG genotypes resulted in a 0.9-fold (95% CI 0.7–1.2) increased mortally risk, and the combination of *PROC* rs1799809 AG/GG genotype and *THBD* rs1042580 AG/GG genotype resulted in a 1.2-fold (95% CI 0.9–1.5) increased mortally risk.

PROC rs1799809, *THBD* rs1042580, *PROC* rs1799808, *PROCR* rs867186, *PROCR* rs2069951, and *PROCR* rs2069952 were not associated with all-cause mortality in the NECOSAD and the 4D cohorts (Table 3).

Discussion

This candidate-gene study assessed the 5-years mortality risk while on dialysis treatment for seven genetic variants that influence levels or activity of proteins in the protein C pathway: one SNV in the factor V gene (factor V Leiden), two SNVs in the protein C gene (*PROC*), one SNV in the thrombomodulin gene (*THBD*) and three SNVs (tagging three haplotypes) in the protein C receptor gene (*PROCR*). We found that factor V Leiden was associated with a 1.5-fold (95% CI 1.1–1.9) increased 5-year all-cause mortality risk and that *PROC* rs1799809 was associated with a 1.2-fold (95% CI 1.0–1.4) increased 5-year all-cause mortality risk. Furthermore, we showed that *THBD* rs1042580, *PROC* rs1799808, *PROCR* rs867186, *PROCR* rs2069951, and *PROCR* rs2069952 were not associated with an increased mortality risk.

Studies in the general population have shown an association between factor V Leiden and an increased risk of different adverse outcomes, including venous thrombosis [17], ischemic stroke [21], and myocardial infarction [22]. We showed in the current study that factor V Leiden was associated with increased all-cause mortality in dialysis patients. Other studies did not find an increased all-cause mortality risk for factor V Leiden in the general population and in thrombophilic families [23,24]. However, it could be the interaction between dialysis and factor V Leiden that

Table 1. Baseline characteristics.

	NECOSAD N = 1070		4D-study N = 1243	
Age (years), median (5th-95th percentile)	62.2	(33.0–80.2)	66.0	(51.0–78.0)
Males, %	62.9		54.1	
Body mass index (kg/m^2), median (5th–95th percentile)	24.3	(19.2–33.2)	26.7	(20.7–36.3)
Dialysis duration (months), median (5th–95th percentile)	0		6.0	(1.1–22.5)
Dialysis modality,%				
Hemodialysis	63.4		100	
Peritoneal dialysis	36.6		0	
History of diabetes mellitus, %	20.7		100	
Cardiovascular disease,%	35.2		29.5	

Table 2. Distribution of single nucleotide variants.

Gene	SNV / Location	Genotype	NECOSAD N = 1070 N	%	HW equilibrium	4D-STUDY N = 1243 N	%	HW equilibrium
Factor V (Leiden)	rs6025	GG	984	(94.7)	$p = 0.157$	837	(94.2)	$p < 0.001$
	exon	AG	53	(5.1)		48	(5.4)	
		AA	2	(0.2)		4	(0.4)	
		Allele frequency A		2.7%			3.1%	
Thrombomodulin	rs1042580	AA	404	(38.8)	$p = 0.443$	321	(36.1)	$p = 0.397$
	3'UTR	AG	479	(46.1)		437	(49.1)	
		GG	157	(15.1)		132	(14.8)	
		Allele frequency G		38.1%			39.4%	
Protein C	rs1799808	CC	431	(41.1)	$p = 0.681$	491	(39.7)	$p = 0.036$
	promoter	CT	478	(45.6)		604	(48.8)	
		TT	140	(13.3)		143	(11.6)	
		Allele frequency T		36.1%			35.9%	
Protein C	rs1799809	AA	368	(35.2)	$p = 0.002$	402	(32.5)	$p = 0.363$
	promoter	AG	461	(44.3)		620	(50.1)	
		GG	215	(20.6)		215	(17.4)	
		Allele frequency G		42.7%			42.4%	
Protein C receptor	rs867186	AA	834	(79.8)	$p = 0.084$	667	(75.1)	$p = 0.136$
	exon	AG	193	(18.5)		211	(23.8)	
		GG	18	(1.7)		10	(1.1)	
		Allele frequency G		11.0%			13.0%	
Protein C receptor	rs2069951	GG	919	(87.1)	$p = 0.549$	1129	(91.1)	$p = 0.372$
	intron	GA	130	(12.3)		106	(8.6)	
		AA	6	(0.6)		4	(0.3)	
		Allele frequency A		6.7%			4.6%	
Protein C receptor	rs2069952	CC	164	(15.8)	$p = 0.798$	263	(21.2)	$p = 0.001$
	intron	CT	493	(47.4)		552	(44.6)	
		TT	383	(36.8)		424	(34.2)	
		Allele frequency C		39.5%			43.5%	

Table 3. Effect of single nucleotide variants on 5-year mortality.

			POOLED RESULTS		NECOSAD		NECOSAD HD and DM*		4D-STUDY	
			N = 2313		N = 1070		N = 140		N = 1243	
Gene/SNV	**Genotype**	**Mortality**	**HR**	**(95% CI)**	**HR**	**(95% CI)**	**HR**	**(95% CI)**	**HR**	**(95% CI)**
Factor V	GG		1	(reference)	1	(reference)	1	(reference)	1	(reference)
(Leiden)/rs6025	AG/AA	All-cause	1.5	(1.1–1.9)	1.4	(0.9–2.1)	2.1	(1.0–4.5)	1.6	(1.1–2.2)
		CV	1.5	(1.0–2.2)	1.3	(0.7–2.4)	0.5	(0.1–3.9)	1.6	(1.0–2.6)
		Non-CV	1.5	(1.0–2.2)	1.4	(0.8–2.5)	4.0	(1.7–9.5)	1.6	(0.9–2.6)
Thrombomodulin/	AA		1	(reference)	1	(reference)	1	(reference)	1	(reference)
rs1042580	AG/GG	All-cause	1.0	(0.9–1.1)	1.0	(0.8–1.2)	1.2	(0.8–1.9)	1.0	(0.8–1.2)
		CV	1.0	(0.8–1.2)	0.9	(0.7–1.2)	1.0	(0.5–1.9)	1.0	(0.8–1.3)
		Non-CV	1.0	(0.8–1.2)	1.0	(0.8–1.4)	1.4	(0.7–2.8)	1.0	(0.8–1.3)
Protein C/	CC		1	(reference)	1	(reference)	1	(reference)	1	(reference)
rs1799808	CT/TT	All-cause	1.0	(0.9–1.2)	1.1	(0.9–1.3)	1.1	(0.7–1.7)	1.0	(0.8–1.2)
		CV	1.0	(0.8–1.2)	0.9	(0.7–1.3)	0.8	(0.4–1.5)	1.0	(0.8–1.3)
		Non-CV	1.0	(0.9–1.2)	1.2	(0.9–1.5)	1.5	(0.8–3.0)	1.0	(0.8–1.2)
Protein C/	AA		1	(reference)	1	(reference)	1	(reference)	1	(reference)
rs1799809	AG/GG	All-cause	1.2	(1.0–1.4)	1.2	(0.9–1.5)	0.9	(0.5–1.4)	1.2	(1.0–1.4)
		CV	1.2	(1.0–1.5)	1.2	(0.9–1.6)	1.0	(0.5–2.0)	1.3	(1.0–1.6)
		Non-CV	1.2	(1.0–1.4)	1.2	(0.9–1.6)	0.8	(0.4–1.5)	1.1	(0.9–1.5)
Protein C	AA		1	(reference)	1	(reference)	1	(reference)	1	(reference)
receptor/	AG/GG	All-cause	1.0	(0.8–1.1)	0.9	(0.7–1.2)	1.3	(0.8–2.2)	1.0	(0.8–1.2)
rs867186		CV	0.8	(0.6–1.0)	0.7	(0.5–1.0)	1.0	(0.4–2.1)	0.8	(0.6–1.1)
		Non-CV	1.2	(1.0–1.5)	1.2	(0.9–1.6)	1.7	(0.9–3.4)	1.2	(0.9–1.5)
Protein C	GG		1	(reference)	1	(reference)	1	(reference)	1	(reference)
receptor/	AG/AA	All-cause	1.1	(0.9–1.4)	1.1	(0.8–1.5)	1.0	(0.5–1.9)	1.2	(0.9–1.6)
rs2069951		CV	1.2	(0.9–1.5)	1.0	(0.7–1.6)	1.3	(0.5–3.1)	1.4	(0.9–1.9)
		Non-CV	1.1	(0.8–1.4)	1.2	(0.8–1.7)	0.6	(0.2–2.0)	1.0	(0.7–1.5)
Protein C	CC		1	(reference)	1	(reference)	1	(reference)	1	(reference)
receptor/	CT/TT	All-cause	1.0	(0.8–1.1)	0.9	(0.7–1.2)	2.3	(1.2–4.5)	1.1	(0.9–1.3)
rs2069952		CV	1.0	(0.8–1.2)	0.9	(0.6–1.3)	1.5	(0.7–3.4)	1.1	(0.8–1.4)
		Non-CV	1.0	(0.8–1.2)	1.0	(0.7–1.4)	4.1	(1.3–13.4)	1.0	(0.8–1.4)

*hemodialysis patients with diabetes mellitus

could lead to an increased mortality, which is not present in the general population. Previous studies on factor V in the dialysis population have been focused on arteriovenous access failure. A recent study showed that a factor V gene SNV (rs6019) was associated with arteriovenous graft failure in dialysis patients suggesting an association between factor V SNVs and adverse outcomes in dialysis patients [25], which is in line with our study.

Factor V Leiden represents a single nucleotide variant in the Factor V gene, encoding a change in the protein from an arginine at position 506 to a glutamine. Since this amino acid is normally the cleavage site for activated protein C, the mutation prevents efficient inactivation of factor V. When factor V remains active, it facilitates overproduction of thrombin leading to a procoagulant state. Several mechanisms might provide plausible explanations for the higher mortality risk in dialysis patients associated with factor V Leiden. First, factor V Leiden in combination with pre-existing and highly prevalent endothelial damage could lead to excess mortality from cardiovascular events. Second, factor V Leiden has been associated with venous thrombosis [14,16,17,26]. The excess mortality could have been caused by fatal pulmonary embolisms due to the procoagulant changes due to factor V Leiden in combination with the start of dialysis which is also associated with an increased risk of venous thrombosis [27,28]. Arguing against this explanation is that in our study confirmed pulmonary embolism was the cause of death in only three patients, but pulmonary embolisms as cause of death might have gone undetected or misclassified as for example sudden cardiac death. Third, one of the main complications in dialysis therapy is clot formation and thrombosis in vascular accesses [29]. Factor V Leiden is associated with procoagulant changes and could therefore lead to treatment failure in dialysis patients. Previous studies have reported an increased risk of arteriovenous access failure in patients with factor V SNVs [30,31].

THBD rs1042580 AG/GG genotypes have been associated with venous thrombosis in the general population [14]. In addition, the combination of *THBD* rs1042580 with different Factor V SNVs was associated with an increased risk of cardiovascular events [12]. Other *THBD* SNVs have also been associated with cardiovascular outcomes when combined with *PROC* SNVs or factor V Leiden in the general population [12]. However, we did not find an association between *THBD* rs1042580 AG/GG genotypes and mortality in dialysis patients. Furthermore, we did not find an important interaction between *THBD* rs1042580 and factor V Leiden and between *THBD* rs1042580 and *PROC* rs1799809.

In contrast to previous studies in sepsis patients, we found no association between the *PROC* rs1799808 and mortality. However, we found that *PROC* rs1799809 was associated with a small increased (hazard ratio 1.2, 95% CI 1.0–1.4) mortality risk. Haplotypes tagged by these SNVs have been associated with decreased survival and increased organ dysfunction in severe sepsis patients [32,33]. An earlier study found that *PROC* rs1799808 was less important in the determination of protein C levels, indicating that the effect on protein C levels was mainly mediated by the *PROC* rs1799809 [15]. Studies in the general population on *PROCR* rs867186, *PROCR* rs2069951, and *PROCR* rs2069952 have been inconsistent in the risk of venous thrombosis [15,16,26] and arterial thrombosis [34,35]. We did not find an association between these SNVs and mortality.

The genotype distribution of *PROC* rs1799809 deviated from Hardy-Weinberg equilibrium in the NECOSAD study and the genotype distribution of *F5* rs6025 (factor V Leiden), *PROC* rs1799808, and *PROCR* rs2069952 were not in Hardy-Weinberg equilibrium in the 4D cohort. It is likely that in diseased populations, such as dialysis patients, selection could have resulted in deviations from Hardy-Weinberg equilibrium.

A potential limitation of our study is that we replicated our results in a dialysis population consisting of hemodialysis patients with diabetes mellitus. For most of the SNVs this was not a problem, since there were no large differences when we restricted the NECOSAD cohort to hemodialysis patients with diabetes mellitus. However, in the 4D-study, we could not investigate the association between mortality and the protein C SNVs in peritoneal dialysis patients and in patients without diabetes mellitus. Furthermore, although we included more than 2000 dialysis patients, our study could be underpowered to detect small differences. In addition, we did not correct for multiple testing, since in this candidate gene study the single nucleotide were chosen based on a priori hypotheses.

In conclusion, our study suggests that factor V Leiden and *PROC* rs1799809 contributes to an increased mortality risk in dialysis patients. This study is the first to investigate the association between protein C pathway SNVs and mortality in large cohorts of dialysis patients.

Acknowledgments

NECOSAD

We thank the patients, investigators and study nurses of the participating dialysis centers and the data managers of the Netherlands Cooperative Study on the Adequacy of Dialysis (NECOSAD) for collection and management of data. NECOSAD was supported in part by unrestricted grants from the Dutch Kidney Foundation. The funding source was involved in neither the collection, interpretation, and analysis of the data nor the decision for the writing and submission of this report for publication. This study was supported by the applied GENomic stratEgies for Treatment and Prevention of Cardiovascular death in Uraemia and End stage REnal disease (GENECURE) project (?www.genecure.eu), a Specific Targeted Research or Innovation Project, funded by the European Commission under the Sixth Framework Programme as FP6-037696.

4D-study

We express our gratitude to all patients who participated in the 4D-study. We thank all investigators and study nurses who took part and contributed to data collection in the 4D-study. (?www.uni-wuerzburg.de/nephrologie)

Author Contributions

Conceived and designed the experiments: GO CD CYV FRR MMH RTK EWB FWD CW MV. Performed the experiments: GO CD CYV HLV PHR MMH WM. Analyzed the data: GO CD CYV MV. Contributed reagents/materials/analysis tools: GO CD CYV HLV FRR PHR MMH WM WHO RTK EWB FWD CW MV. Wrote the paper: GO CD CYV HLV FRR PHR MMH WM WHO RTK EWB FWD CW MV.

References

1. Mosnier LO, Zlokovic BV, Griffin JH (2007) The cytoprotective protein C pathway. Blood 109: 3161–3172.
2. Bertina RM, Koeleman BP, Koster T, Rosendaal FR, Dirven RJ, et al. (1994) Mutation in blood coagulation factor V associated with resistance to activated protein C. Nature 369: 64–67.
3. Joyce DE, Gelbert L, Ciaccia A, DeHoff B, Grinnell BW (2001) Gene expression profile of antithrombotic protein c defines new mechanisms modulating inflammation and apoptosis. J Biol Chem 276: 11199–11203.
4. Cheng T, Liu D, Griffin JH, Fernandez JA, Castellino F, et al. (2003) Activated protein C blocks p53-mediated apoptosis in ischemic human brain endothelium and is neuroprotective. Nat Med 9: 338–342.

5. Domotor E, Benzakour O, Griffin JH, Yule D, Fukudome K, et al. (2003) Activated protein C alters cytosolic calcium flux in human brain endothelium via binding to endothelial protein C receptor and activation of protease activated receptor-1. Blood 101: 4797–4801.
6. Mosnier LO, Griffin JH (2003) Inhibition of staurosporine-induced apoptosis of endothelial cells by activated protein C requires protease-activated receptor-1 and endothelial cell protein C receptor. Biochem J 373: 65–70.
7. Riewald M, Petrovan RJ, Donner A, Mueller BM, Ruf W (2002) Activation of endothelial cell protease activated receptor 1 by the protein C pathway. Science 296: 1880–1882.
8. Branson HE, Katz J, Marble R, Griffin JH (1983) Inherited protein C deficiency and coumarin-responsive chronic relapsing purpura fulminans in a newborn infant. Lancet 2: 1165–1168.
9. Allaart CF, Poort SR, Rosendaal FR, Reitsma PH, Bertina RM, et al. (1993) Increased risk of venous thrombosis in carriers of hereditary protein C deficiency defect. Lancet 341: 134–138.
10. Bernard GR, Vincent JL, Laterre PF, LaRosa SP, Dhainaut JF, et al. (2001) Efficacy and safety of recombinant human activated protein C for severe sepsis. N Engl J Med 344: 699–709.
11. Folsom AR, Rosamond WD, Shahar E, Cooper LS, Aleksic N, et al. (1999) Prospective study of markers of hemostatic function with risk of ischemic stroke. The Atherosclerosis Risk in Communities (ARIC) Study Investigators. Circulation 100: 736–742.
12. Auro K, Alanne M, Kristiansson K, Silander K, Kuulasmaa K, et al. (2007) Combined effects of thrombosis pathway gene variants predict cardiovascular events. PLoS Genet 3: e120.
13. de Jager DJ, Grootendorst DC, Jager KJ, van Dijk PC, Tomas LM, et al. (2009) Cardiovascular and noncardiovascular mortality among patients starting dialysis. JAMA 302: 1782–1789.
14. Smith NL, Hindorff LA, Heckbert SR, Lemaitre RN, Marciante KD, et al. (2007) Association of genetic variations with nonfatal venous thrombosis in postmenopausal women. JAMA 297: 489–498.
15. Pomp ER, Doggen CJ, Vos HL, Reitsma PH, Rosendaal FR (2009) Polymorphisms in the protein C gene as risk factor for venous thrombosis. Thromb Haemost 101: 62–67.
16. Uitte de Willige S, Van Marion V, Rosendaal FR, Vos HL, de Visser MC, et al. (2004) Haplotypes of the EPCR gene, plasma sEPCR levels and the risk of deep venous thrombosis. J Thromb Haemost 2: 1305–1310.
17. Bezemer ID, Bare LA, Doggen CJ, Arellano AR, Tong C, et al. (2008) Gene variants associated with deep vein thrombosis. JAMA 299: 1306–1314.
18. van Dijk PC, Jager KJ, de Charro F, Collart F, Cornet R, et al. (2001) Renal replacement therapy in Europe: the results of a collaborative effort by the ERA-EDTA registry and six national or regional registries. Nephrol Dial Transplant 16: 1120–1129.
19. Wanner C, Krane V, Marz W, Olschewski M, Mann JF, et al. (2005) Atorvastatin in patients with type 2 diabetes mellitus undergoing hemodialysis. N Engl J Med 353: 238–248.
20. Verduijn M, Jager KJ, Zoccali C, Dekker FW (2011) Genetic association studies: discovery of the genetic basis of renal disease. Nephron Clin Pract 119: c236–c239.
21. Kenet G, Sadetzki S, Murad H, Martinowitz U, Rosenberg N, et al. (2000) Factor V Leiden and antiphospholipid antibodies are significant risk factors for ischemic stroke in children. Stroke 31: 1283–1288.
22. Ye Z, Liu EH, Higgins JP, Keavney BD, Lowe GD, et al. (2006) Seven haemostatic gene polymorphisms in coronary disease: meta-analysis of 66,155 cases and 91,307 controls. Lancet 367: 651–658.
23. Heijmans BT, Westendorp RG, Knook DL, Kluft C, Slagboom PE (1998) The risk of mortality and the factor V Leiden mutation in a population-based cohort. Thromb Haemost 80: 607–609.
24. Pabinger I, Vossen CY, Lang J, Conard J, Garcia-Dabrio MC, et al. (2012) Mortality and inherited thrombophilia: results from the European Prospective Cohort on Thrombophilia. J Thromb Haemost 10: 217–222.
25. Allon M, Zhang L, Maya ID, Bray MS, Fernandez JR (2012) Association of factor v gene polymorphism with arteriovenous graft failure. Am J Kidney Dis 59: 682–688.
26. Saposnik B, Reny JL, Gaussem P, Emmerich J, Aiach M, et al. (2004) A haplotype of the EPCR gene is associated with increased plasma levels of sEPCR and is a candidate risk factor for thrombosis. Blood 103: 1311–1318.
27. Tveit DP, Hypolite IO, Hshieh P, Cruess D, Agodoa LY, et al. (2002) Chronic dialysis patients have high risk for pulmonary embolism. Am J Kidney Dis 39: 1011–1017.
28. Casserly LF, Reddy SM, Dember LM (2000) Venous thromboembolism in end-stage renal disease. Am J Kidney Dis 36: 405–411.
29. Feldman HI, Kobrin S, Wasserstein A (1996) Hemodialysis vascular access morbidity. J Am Soc Nephrol 7: 523–535.
30. Girndt M, Heine GH, Ulrich C, Kohler H (2007) Gene polymorphism association studies in dialysis: vascular access. Semin Dial 20: 63–67.
31. Knoll GA, Wells PS, Young D, Perkins SL, Pilkey RM, et al. (2005) Thrombophilia and the risk for hemodialysis vascular access thrombosis. J Am Soc Nephrol 16: 1108–1114.
32. Walley KR, Russell JA (2007) Protein C -1641 AA is associated with decreased survival and more organ dysfunction in severe sepsis. Crit Care Med 35: 12–17.
33. Chen QX, Wu SJ, Wang HH, Lv C, Cheng BL, et al. (2008) Protein C -1641A/-1654C haplotype is associated with organ dysfunction and the fatal outcome of severe sepsis in Chinese Han population. Hum Genet 123: 281–287.
34. Ireland H, Konstantoulas CJ, Cooper JA, Hawe E, Humphries SE, et al. (2005) EPCR Ser219Gly: elevated sEPCR, prothrombin F1+2, risk for coronary heart disease, and increased sEPCR shedding in vitro. Atherosclerosis 183: 283–292.
35. Reiner AP, Carty CL, Jenny NS, Nievergelt C, Cushman M, et al. (2008) PROC, PROCR and PROS1 polymorphisms, plasma anticoagulant phenotypes, and risk of cardiovascular disease and mortality in older adults: the Cardiovascular Health Study. J Thromb Haemost 6: 1625–1632.

Urine Osmolarity and Risk of Dialysis Initiation in a Chronic Kidney Disease Cohort – a Possible Titration Target?

Max Plischke[1], Maria Kohl[2], Lise Bankir[3], Sascha Shayganfar[4], Ammon Handisurya[1], Georg Heinze[2], Martin Haas[1]*

1 Division of Nephrology and Dialysis, Department of Internal Medicine III, Medical University Vienna, Vienna, Austria, **2** Section for Clinical Biometrics, Center of Medical Statistics, Informatics and Intelligent Systems, Medical University of Vienna, Vienna, Austria, **3** INSERM UMRS 1138, Equipe 2, Centre de Recherche des Cordeliers, Paris, France, **4** Division of Cardiology, Pulmonology, and Vascular Medicine, Medical Faculty, University Hospital Düsseldorf, Düsseldorf, Germany

Abstract

Background: Increasing evidence is linking fluid intake, vasopressin suppression and osmotic control with chronic kidney disease progression. Interestingly, the association between urine volume, urine osmolarity and risk of dialysis initiation has not been studied in chronic kidney disease patients before.

Objective: To study the relationship between urine volume, urine osmolarity and the risk of initiating dialysis in chronic kidney disease.

Design: In a retrospective cohort analysis of 273 patients with chronic kidney disease stage 1–4 we assessed the association between urine volume, urine osmolarity and the risk of dialysis by a multivariate proportional sub-distribution hazards model for competing risk data according to Fine and Gray. Co-variables were selected via the purposeful selection algorithm.

Results: Dialysis was reached in 105 patients over a median follow-up period of 92 months. After adjustment for age, baseline creatinine clearance, other risk factors and diuretics, a higher risk for initiation of dialysis was found in patients with higher urine osmolarity. The adjusted sub-distribution hazard ratio for initiation of dialysis was 2.04 (95% confidence interval, 1.06 to 3.92) for each doubling of urine osmolarity. After 72 months, the estimated adjusted cumulative incidence probabilities of dialysis were 15%, 24%, and 34% in patients with a baseline urine osmolarity of 315, 510, and 775 mosm/L, respectively.

Conclusions: We conclude that higher urine osmolarity is associated with a higher risk of initiating dialysis. As urine osmolarity is a potentially modifiable risk factor, it thus deserves further, prospective research as a potential target in chronic kidney disease progression.

Editor: Kathrin Eller, Medical University of Graz, Austria

Funding: Maria Kohl (statistician) was supported by the European Community's Seventh Framework Programme, grant number 241544. The funders had no role in study design, data collection and analysis, decision to publish, or preparation of the manuscript. Maria Kohl was involved in study design, analysis, and preparation of the manuscript. Mortality data, obtained via Statistics Austria, was payed for using the authors' departments (Department of Internal Med. III, Division of Nephrology and Dialysis, Medical University Vienna) research budget, which is not tied to any external funding institution. As this was a retrospective study, other expenses (laboratory, etc) were fully covered by routine patient care at the authors' outpatient department.

Competing Interests: The authors have declared that no competing interests exist.

* E-mail: martin.haas@meduniwien.ac.at

Introduction

Medicinal use of water in chronic kidney disease (CKD) has gained research interest lately [1], as established efforts to retard CKD progression remain far from satisfactory [2]. Epidemiological data associating fluid intake or urine volume with GFR decline in humans have not been fully conclusive [3–7]. Nonetheless, there is increasing evidence linking fluid intake, vasopressin suppression and osmotic control with CKD and ADPKD progression [8–12]. Kidney excretion is adjusted according to water and dietary solute intake, as well as water and solute losses by lungs, skin, and the gastrointestinal tract. The required urine volume can be determined by dividing the daily osmolar excretion, to maintain the body's solute content at steady state, by the maximal urine osmolality, with failing kidneys losing capacity to concentrate urine maximally. As such, water intake required to achieve comparable urinary solute dilution varies considerably between individuals. [1]

Interestingly, median 24-hour urine osmolality is greater than that of plasma in humans, suggesting continuous antidiuretic action [13], which has been associated with renal function decline [10]. Consequentially, Wang et al. recently devised a quantitative method to determine the amount of water needed on a case-by-case basis to achieve a mean urine osmolality equivalent to that of plasma [13]. Relationships between urine osmolarity (given as mosm/L compared to mosm/kg H_2O for osmolality) and GFR decline have been described in two studies [3,7] with contrasting results. We were interested in studying urine volume and urine osmolarity in terms of harder endpoints in chronic kidney disease. Thus we set out to study these variables in terms of risk of initiating dialysis, with death as a competing event.

Subjects and Methods

Patients

All patients attending our nephrology outpatient department between 1 January 2000 and 31 December 2002 were included in a single-centre cohort study. The study baseline was defined as one year after the first visit, while the time period between the first visit and baseline was defined as the run-in phase. Baseline demographic data for each patient were collected from outpatient files including medication, co-morbidities, and the nature of renal disease. A minimum of two visits, with 24-hour urine samples taken before and after baseline, were defined as inclusion criteria. Exclusion criteria were a reported urine volume less than 500 ml/d or a creatinine clearance below 15 ml/min (CKD 5). The mean of all measurements taken during the run-in phase (median: 5 [25th–75th percentiles: 3–8]) was used as the baseline value for each parameter.

The primary endpoint of the study was time to dialysis, with death as the competing event. Mortality data and data on the initiation of dialysis until 31 December 2008 were obtained from Statistics Austria (the national statistics institution) and the Austrian Dialysis and Transplantation Registry (ÖDTR), respectively. Patients starting dialysis had no loss of follow-up according to ÖDTR. Because of a possible relocation of a patient to a country other than Austria, a minor loss of follow-up for mortality data from Statistics Austria cannot be excluded.

Ethics Statement

This was a retrospective study making use of data already collected during routine patient care at our outpatient department. The processing and analysis of data was done after anonymization. Therefore no informed consent was requested from patients. This approach was reviewed and approved by the local ethics committee (Ethikkomission Medizinische Universität Wien).

Laboratory data

Standard 24-hour urine samples of the patients were analysed in regard of proteinuria, creatinine, sodium, urea nitrogen, and potassium levels, in accordance with routinely used methods at our central laboratory (Clinical Institute of Medical and Chemical Laboratory Diagnostics, Medical University of Vienna). On the day of each visit, serum samples were analysed for creatinine, sodium, potassium, glucose and urea nitrogen levels in accordance with routine methods.

After conversion of glucose and urea nitrogen from mg/dl in mmol/L the estimated urine osmolarity (U_{osm}) (mosm/L) was calculated as follows:

$$Uosm = 2 \times (UNa + UK) + Uurea$$

Estimated plasma osmolarity (P_{osm}) (mosm/L) was calculated as follows:

$$Posm = 2 \times (PNa + PK) + Purea + Pglu\cos e$$

U_{Na}, U_K, and U_{urea} are the concentrations of sodium, potassium and urea in the urine (all in mmol/L), and P_{Na}, P_K, P_{urea}, and $P_{glucose}$ are the concentrations of sodium, potassium, urea and glucose in plasma (in mmol/L).

Statistical analysis

Continuous variables were described by medians (25th to 75th percentiles), and compared between groups using Wilcoxon's rank sum tests. Correlations between continuous variables were assessed by Spearman's rank correlation coefficient. For further analysis, osmolarity, proteinuria and creatinine clearance were log-base-2 transformed because of the skewed distributions of these variables. To describe intra- versus inter-individual variance of urine osmolarity, we conducted a variance component analysis including all run-in urine osmolarity values that were available for each patient using a mixed model with patients as levels of a random factor. The outcome variable was time to dialysis, with death as the competing event. Patients who were alive without dialysis at the time of their last visit were censored. Absolute event rates were computed as the number of events divided by the total follow-up time for all patients. Observations with missing values were not used in the calculated models. We described the distribution of time to dialysis using cumulative incidence functions, and compared groups using Gray's test [14].

Due to the established relationship between baseline creatinine clearance and risk of initiating dialysis/ESRD, and the known progressive loss in urine concentration ability with decreasing renal function [1], it seemed important to introduce creatinine clearance as an adjustment factor in all further analyses.

We fitted two multivariate proportional sub-distribution hazards models for competing risk data according to Fine and Gray [15] in order to assess the effect of urine osmolarity or volume on the risk for initiating dialysis. In these models, we considered osmolarity or urine volume and included those variables that either proved significant in a multivariate model ($P<0.10$) or changed the log hazard ratio of osmolarity or urine volume by more than 15% when those variables were excluded from the analyses (purposeful selection algorithm) [16]. We assumed that any variable not selected would have no relevant impact on our conclusions. All variables listed in Table 1 (except 24-hour proteinuria, 24-hour osmolar excretion and 24-hour sodium excretion) were considered as potential confounders. Results from multivariate competing risk regression were described by means of sub-distribution hazard ratios (SHR) and 95% confidence intervals (95% CI), and by computing and visualising estimated cumulative incidence curves at specific covariate values. As urine osmolarity and creatinine clearance were log-base-2 transformed, their SHR correspond to each doubling of these variables. We checked for significant pairwise interactions of variables and for time-dependent effects by including interactions with follow-up time. Non-linear effects were assessed by the method of fractional polynomials [17]. For sensitivity analysis, we also estimated a cause-specific (death-censored) Cox regression model. The R-software, version 2.12 (www.r-project.org), was used for statistical analysis.

Results

Baseline data

Three hundred and seventy-two patients were examined for eligibility. After applying all inclusion and exclusion criteria, a total of 273 patients (56% male) with CKD class 1-4 and a median age of 56 years (42 to 67 years) were confirmed eligible and included in the study (**Table 1**). Median creatinine clearance was 48 (30 to 79) ml/min. Kidney disease was unknown in 46% of the patients; the

Table 1. Demographic and clinical characteristics of all patients at baseline, and in the subgroups of CKD patients stages 1-3a (creatinine clearance ≥45 ml/min) and stage 3b-4 (creatinine clearance ≥15 and <45 ml/min).

	Total	CKD 1-3a	CKD 3b-4
	(n = 273)	(n = 141)	(n = 132)
Age (years)	56 (42–67)	50 (37–61)	59 (46–71)
Male	153 (56%)	87 (62%)	66 (50%)
BMI	26 (23–30)	26 (23–30)	26 (23–30)
CCl (ml/min)	48 (30–79)	78 (60–105)	30 (25–35)
MAP (mmHg)	97 (93–102)	97 (93–103)	98 (94–102)
P_{osm} (mosm/L)	308 (302–315)	303 (300–308)	313 (308–318)
Urine analysis			
Proteinuria (g/L)	0.87 (0.24–2.34)	0.76(0.21–2.34)	1.01 (0.26–2.31)
Proteinuria 24 h (g/24 h)	2.05 (0.53–5.63)	1.72 (0.53–5.2)	2.21 (0.57–6.12)
Volume (ml/24 h)	2220 (1935–2871)	2157 (1839–2700)	2325 (2000–3000)
U_{osm} (mosm/L)	510 (414–622)	607 (477–740)	445 (370–519)
Osmolar excretion (mosm/24 h)	1200 (930–1412)	1309 (1091–1636)	1018 (810–1254)
Sodium (mmol/L)	84 (68–104)	96 (75–116)	75 (61–93)
Sodium excretion (mmol/24 h)	201 (141–251)	215 (167–265)	181 (134–234)
Underlying kidney disease			
Polycystic kidney disease	18 (7%)	6 (4%)	12 (9%)
Diabetic nephropathy	20 (7%)	7 (5%)	13 (10%)
Glomerular disease	98 (36%)	73 (52%)	25 (19%)
Other	11 (4%)	4 (3%)	7 (5%)
Unknown	126 (46%)	51 (36%)	75 (57%)
Comorbidities			
Chronic heart failure	8 (3%)	3 (2%)	5 (4%)
Diabetes mellitus	59 (23%)	23 (18%)	36 (27%)
Liver cirrhosis (child C)	0 (0%)	0 (0%)	0 (0%)
Medication			
ACEI/AT-II Blocker	216 (85%)	111 (85%)	105 (84%)
Diuretics	120 (47%)	45 (35%)	75 (60%)
Beta-blocker	119 (47%)	47 (36%)	72 (58%)
Non-dihydropyridine CCB	39 (15%)	21 (16%)	18 (14%)

Abbreviations: BMI, body mass index; CCl, creatinine clearance; MAP, mean arterial pressure; P_{osm}, plasma osmolarity; U_{osm}, urine osmolarity; ACEI/AT-II, angiotensin converting enzyme/angiotensin II receptor antagonist; CCB, calcium channel blocker. Values are given as median (Q1-Q3), if not stated otherwise.

remaining patients had mainly polycystic kidney disease, different forms of glomerulonephritis, or diabetic nephropathy (Table 1). Nearly all patients received antihypertensive drugs with an effect on protein excretion, such as inhibitors of the renin angiotensin aldosterone system, non-dihydropyridine calcium channel blockers, or beta-blockers.

There was a significant inverse correlation between average run-in 24-hour urine volume and average run-in urine osmolarity ($R = -0.45$; $P < 0.001$). Urine osmolarity was significantly higher in men than in women (522 [446 to 629] vs. 458 [385 to 596] mosm/L; $P < 0.01$), in patients without diuretics (520 [422 to 679] vs. 490 [408 to 577] mosm/L; $P < 0.05$), and in patients without beta-blocker therapy (526 [429 to 673] vs. 463 [392 to 557] mosm/L; $P < 0.01$). Urine osmolarity and creatinine clearance were positively correlated ($R = 0.6$, $p < 0.01$). The total variance for run-in urine osmolarity was 45253; the intra-individual variance was about one fourth ($\sigma 2 = 11349$), i.e., random fluctuation within a patient explained 25% of the total variance, while the inter-individual variance component explained about 75% of the total variance. One patient was missing data for proteinuria, and 20 patients each were missing data for diuretics and beta-blocker therapy.

Follow-up

Median follow-up until death or censoring was 92 (76 to 95) months. End-stage renal disease developed in 105 patients (39%).

Thirty-eight patients (14%) died on dialysis and 35 patients (13%) died with functioning kidneys.

The absolute event rate for ESRD was 0.07/year. Event rates were 0.05/year for patients with mild to moderate chronic kidney disease (CKD stage 1–3, creatinine clearance ≥30 ml/min), and 0.22/year for those with severe CKD (stage 4, creatinine clearance 15–29 ml/min).

Urine osmolarity and risk of initiating dialysis

Univariate analysis, without adjustment for baseline creatinine clearance (see correlation above), suggested a higher cumulative incidence of dialysis in patients with lower-than-median urine osmolarities ($p<0.01$). Multivariate competing risk regression analysis, with death as the competing risk, adjusted for age, creatinine clearance, proteinuria, type of underlying renal disease, beta-blocker and diuretic therapies, showed that a higher urine osmolarity was associated with a higher risk of initiating dialysis (**Table 2**).

Based on this model, we estimated the adjusted cumulative incidence probabilities of dialysis for patients with three different urine osmolalities (10th, 50th and 90th percentile), assuming average values for all other covariates. A constant and stepwise significant increase was seen in patients with low (315 mosm/L), intermediate (510 mosm/L), and high (775 mosm/L) baseline urine osmolarity (**Figure 1**; $p<0.05$). At 72 months, the estimated cumulative incidence probabilities of dialysis in these patients were 15%, 24% and 34%, respectively. Lower baseline creatinine clearance, higher baseline protein excretion, the type of underlying renal disease, and treatment with diuretics were also independently associated with a higher risk of dialysis (Table 2). No significant interactions of urine osmolarity with other variables in the model were found. There was no evidence of time-dependent effects or a non-linear effect of urine osmolarity or any other metric covariate. The cause-specific Cox model yielded a similar result for the adjusted effect of urine osmolarity (cause-specific hazard ratio 2.19, 95% CI 1.21 to 3.95).

Urine volume and risk of initiating dialysis

There was a significant inverse association between average 24-hour urine volume and average urine osmolarity ($R = -0.46$; $P<0.01$). Therefore, we did not adjust for urine osmolarity in the multivariate regression analysis for urine volume. In this model, higher protein excretion, lower creatinine clearance, and the underlying renal disease but not urine volume were associated with a higher risk of dialysis (**Table 3**).

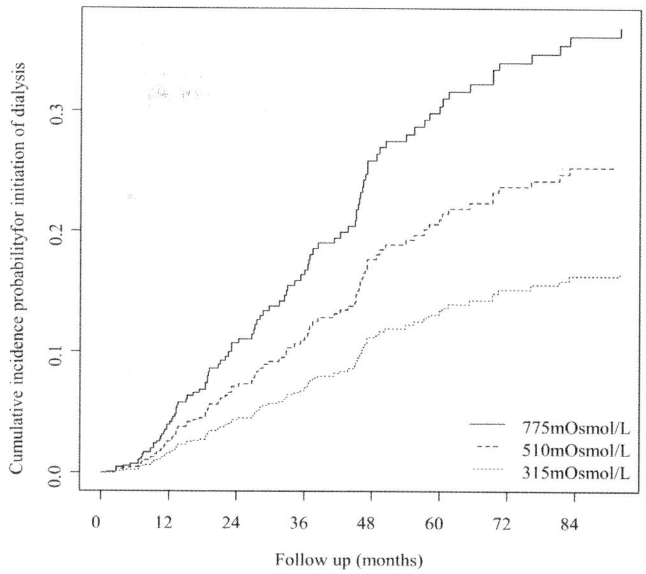

Figure 1. Cumulative incidence probabilities of dialysis initiation for different baseline urine osmolarities. Cumulative incidence probabilities of dialysis initiation for a baseline urine osmolarity of 315, 510 or 775 mosm/L (10th, 50th, and 90th percentile), estimated from the proportional sub-distribution hazards model. Given the estimated adjusted subdistribution hazard ratio (SHR) of 2.04 ($p = 0.033$) per doubling of urine osmolarity, the SHRs comparing patients with 775 mosm/L or 315 mosm/L to patients with 510 mosm/L were 1.54 (95%CI:1.03 to 2.28) or 0.61 (95%CI: 0.39 to 0.96), respectively.

Discussion

The present study demonstrates an independent, positive relationship between urine osmolarity and risk of initiating dialysis in a cohort of CKD patients stage 1 through 4. Competing risk models were adjusted for age, creatinine clearance, proteinuria, type of underlying renal disease, beta-blocker and diuretic therapies.

Two published studies have described relationships between 24-h urine osmolarity and GFR change over time. Hebert et al. reported a significant inverse relationship between baseline urine osmolarity and GFR decline in non-polycystic kidney disease patients (subgroup of full cohort), adjusted for diet, blood pressure and body surface area. Adjusting for additional covariates such as baseline GFR or diuretics use failed to result in statistically

Table 2. The independent effect of urine osmolarity, age, protein excretion, kidney function, renal disease and different drugs, on the risk of initiating dialysis in the competing risk regression analysis.

	SH Ratio	95% confidence interval		p-value
Urine osmolarity (per doubling)	2.04	1.06	3.92	0.03
Age (per decade)	0.87	0.74	1.02	0.08
Proteinuria (per doubling)	1.85	1.60	2.13	<0.001
Creatinine clearance (per doubling)	0.15	0.09	0.23	<0.001
Renal disease (PKD vs. other renal diseases)	3.44	1.73	6.81	<0.001
Beta-blocker therapy (yes vs. no)	1.54	0.97	2.43	0.07
Diuretic therapy (yes vs. no)	1.62	1.03	2.55	0.04

Abbreviations: SH Ratio, subdistribution hazard ratio; PKD, polycystic kidney disease

Table 3. The independent effect of urine volume, age, protein excretion, kidney function, renal disease and different drugs, on the risk of of initiating dialysis in the competing risk regression analysis.

	SH Ratio	95% confidence interval		p-value
Urine volume (per 0.5 L/d)	1.05	0.92	1.20	0.49
Age (per decade)	0.90	0.77	1.05	0.18
Proteinuria (per doubling)	1.79	1.54	2.07	<0.001
Creatinine clearance (per doubling)	0.20	0.13	0.30	<0.001
Renal disease (PKD vs. other renal diseases)	3.76	1.92	7.34	<0.001
Beta-blocker therapy (yes vs. no)	1.58	0.98	2.54	0.06
Diuretic therapy (yes vs. no)	1.59	0.99	2.54	0.05

Abbreviations: SH Ratio, subdistribution hazard ratio; PKD, polycystic kidney disease

significant models. Other models were calculated for follow-up urine osmolarities (collected after the study baseline; thus, not fully comparable) and did stay significant after further adjustments. [3] Torres et al. in turn suggested that higher baseline 24-h Uosm was associated with higher GFR decline across time in a cohort of ADPKD patients. [7]

The association between urine osmolarity and the risk of initiating dialysis, a stronger marker for end stage renal disease, has not been previously investigated. Our data thus adds to the existing evidence. The data is in line with Torres et al. suggesting a faster renal function decline in patients with higher urine osmolarity. Our cohort appeared to have the highest urine osmolarity with a median of 510 (IQR: 414–622) mosm/L versus a mean of 368±159 mosm/L (Torres et al.), and a mean of 270 to 334 mosm/L (depending on protein diet group and polycystic kidney disease status) (Hebert et al.). It is therefore conceivable that lowering urine osmolarity below a specific threshold might be harmful to the kidney as well. A recent study addressing the association between sodium excretion, an important part of total urine osmolarity, and end-stage renal disease in patients with type 1 diabetes mellitus showed an inverse association with end stage renal disease [18]. Furthermore, a U-shaped curve was described for sodium excretion and mortality, such that subjects with the highest and the lowest sodium excretion had the highest mortality, partly supporting the hypothesis of low urine osmolarity being associated with harmful effects. Interestingly, in the univariate versus the multivariable analysis the strong effect of impaired renal function seems to obscure the positive correlation of osmolarity with the incidence of ESRD. Adjusting for creatinine clearance reveals this relationship. We conclude that among patients with equal renal function those with higher osmolarity values are more likely to progress to ESRD than those with lower osmolarity values in our cohort.

As described in the methods, estimated urine osmolarity was calculated from urine sodium, potassium and urea concentrations in 24 hour urine samples. These are the dominant solutes in the urine (plus the anions associated with sodium and potassium). Other solutes represent less than 10% of total urinary solutes (in the absence of glucosuria). Thus, estimated urine osmolarity is often used as an approximation of true osmolarity. Regarding the difference between osmolality (in mosm/kg H_2O) and osmolarity (in mosm/L), it is negligible in our study because the density of urine is very close to that of pure water in the range of values considered here. Other authors have used estimated urine osmolarity in several studies. [3,19]

Several authors have studied urine volume and GFR decline. Opposed to the prevailing view that water is beneficial in CKD, Hebert et al. reported higher GFR decline in higher urine volume quartiles. However, multivariable adjustment seemed to diminish the association.[1,3] In support of Hebert et al., Wang et al. found a weak, but significant association between higher urine volume and GFR decline.[4] A large study by Clark et al. showed a relationship between higher urine volume and lower rate of eGFR decline, which stayed significant after multivariable adjustment. [5] Another large study reported worse kidney function in individuals with a lower self-reported fluid intake [6]; however, neither urine volume nor urine osmolarity were evaluated. It has been suggested that lower mean baseline GFR in cohorts of Hebert et al. and Wang et al., which is associated with alterations in water metabolism, might explain these paradoxical findings. With falling GFR, the ability to concentrate urine to osmolalities greater than that of plasma is progressively lost. [1] As such, in contrast to the general population, solute excretion and urine volume are closely interrelated in severe chronic kidney disease [20,21]. In our study we did not find a significant relationship between urine volume and a higher risk of dialysis. The rather weak association between urine volume and 24-hour urine osmolarity in the present study suggests that, in contrast to patients with severe kidney failure, urine concentration by vasopressin was still effective in the vast majority of the patients.

Stimulation of vasopressin secretion is supposed to be the cause of the more rapid decline of kidney function in patients with a high urine osmolality. Vasopressin exerts a range of different effects and interacts through the three receptors V1a, V2 and V1b [22]. The antidiuretic effect is mainly mediated by the V2 receptor and includes increased tubular permeability for water and urea, and stimulation of ENaC-mediated sodium reabsorption [22]. Chronic administration of vasopressin in rats was shown to increase renal blood flow, glomerular filtration rate, and renal mass [23–25]. Vice versa, prevention of hyperfiltration in 5/6 nephrectomised rats by chronic inhibition of vasopressin secretion led to less glomerular sclerosis, less interstitial fibrosis and slower progression of renal failure [8,9,26]. However, precise plasma levels of vasopressin are difficult to obtain. Furthermore, non-detectable changes of vasopressin lead to a broad range of different urine osmolalities [22].

The optimal range of urine osmolality is difficult to define. Studies in normal rats and healthy humans have shown that urine concentration above an osmolarity of about 300 mosm/L induces a significant hyperfiltration [22,27]. In accordance with these findings we registered the lowest risk of initiation dialysis in patients with a urine osmolarity of a similar range. On the other hand we cannot rule out that urine osmolarity values below those in our cohort range might worsen the risk of renal function decline as suggested by the cohort of Hebert et al. (see above).

Either increasing fluid intake or decreasing the intake of osmolytes could achieve a reduction of urine osmolality. A recently published formula could be used to estimate the quantity of fluid needed to achieve a urine osmolality equivalent to that of plasma [13]. An alternative approach might be the use of vaptans, which suppress vasopressin activity by antagonistic binding to the VP receptors. Recently a protective effect of dual V1a/V2 blockade on the progression of CKD has been reported in rats [28]. A similar effect has been shown in diabetic rats, where the rise in albuminuria was prevented by a V2 antagonist [29].

Our study is limited by its design. As an observational cohort study can only prove associations and not causality, it remains to be proven in a prospective trial that changing urine osmolarity indeed has a positive effect on rate of renal function decline in CKD, before any therapeutic recommendation can be made. Furthermore, our study cohort showed a high event rate for ESRD, which might be explained by the cohort's relatively high baseline proteinuria. Thus, it is not clear if the study results are applicable to CKD populations with different demographics. Nonetheless, our study further strengthens the link between urine osmolarity and renal function decline by establishing a relationship with risk of dialysis initiation. In addition to the hard end-point of ESRD, a long follow-up period, the use of baseline variables issued from several measurements over a 1 year run-in phase reducing the impact of possible occasional sampling errors, and the application of competing risk analysis techniques strengthen the conclusions of this study.

While it is indisputable that, in the presence of a competing risk such as death, cumulative incidence curves are the method of choice rather than conventional Kaplan-Meier estimates, there is some controversy as to whether the standard cause-specific (death-censored) Cox regression analysis or the proportional sub-distribution hazards (Fine-Gray) model should be used to obtain adjusted hazard ratios. We decided to use the latter because it directly models differences in cumulative incidences and permits the investigator to predict the cumulative incidence of ESRD based on the covariate values of a patient. This would not have been possible when using the cause-specific Cox model. Our competing risk analysis using the Fine-Gray model mirrors more precisely the association between a covariate and the cumulative incidence of ESRD in patients at high risk of death during the observation period. Our observation that urine osmolarity might be positively associated with the risk for ESRD is robust as regards the type of analysis used, as results of the cause-specific Cox model were very similar.

In conclusion, we demonstrate that higher urine osmolarity is independently associated with a higher risk of initiating dialysis in a cohort of patients with CKD stage 1 to 4. Modifying urine osmolarity by dietary counselling or pharmaceutical interventions might evolve into a further treatment option in ESRD.

Author Contributions

Conceived and designed the experiments: MP MK LB GH MH. Performed the experiments: SS AH. Analyzed the data: MP MK LB GH MH. Contributed reagents/materials/analysis tools: MP MK GH MH. Wrote the paper: MP MK LB GH MH.

References

1. Wang CJ, Grantham JJ, Wetmore JB (2013) The medicinal use of water in renal disease. Kidney Int 84: 45–53.
2. Bankir L, Bouby N, Ritz E (2013) Vasopressin: a novel target for the prevention and retardation of kidney disease? Nat Rev Nephrol 9: 223–239.
3. Hebert LA, Greene T, Levey A, Falkenhain ME, Klahr S (2003) High urine volume and low urine osmolality are risk factors for faster progression of renal disease. Am J Kidney Dis 41: 962–971.
4. Wang X, Lewis J, Appel L, Cheek D, Contreras G, et al. (2006) Validation of creatinine-based estimates of GFR when evaluating risk factors in longitudinal studies of kidney disease. J Am Soc Nephrol 17: 2900–2909.
5. Clark WF, Sontrop JM, Macnab JJ, Suri RS, Moist L, et al. (2011) Urine volume and change in estimated GFR in a community-based cohort study. Clin J Am Soc Nephrol 6: 2634–2641.
6. Strippoli GF, Craig JC, Rochtchina E, Flood VM, Wang JJ, et al. (2011) Fluid and nutrient intake and risk of chronic kidney disease. Nephrology (Carlton) 16: 326–334.
7. Torres VE, Grantham JJ, Chapman AB, Mrug M, Bae KT, et al. (2011) Potentially modifiable factors affecting the progression of autosomal dominant polycystic kidney disease. Clin J Am Soc Nephrol 6: 640–647.
8. Bouby N, Bachmann S, Bichet D, Bankir L (1990) Effect of water intake on the progression of chronic renal failure in the 5/6 nephrectomized rat. Am J Physiol 258: F973–979.
9. Sugiura T, Yamauchi A, Kitamura H, Matsuoka Y, Horio M, et al. (1999) High water intake ameliorates tubulointerstitial injury in rats with subtotal nephrectomy: possible role of TGF-beta. Kidney Int 55: 1800–1810.
10. Meijer E, Bakker SJ, de Jong PE, Homan van der Heide JJ, van Son WJ, et al. (2009) Copeptin, a surrogate marker of vasopressin, is associated with accelerated renal function decline in renal transplant recipients. Transplantation 88: 561–567.
11. Meijer E, Bakker SJ, Halbesma N, de Jong PE, Struck J, et al. (2010) Copeptin, a surrogate marker of vasopressin, is associated with microalbuminuria in a large population cohort. Kidney Int 77: 29–36.
12. Nagao S, Nishii K, Katsuyama M, Kurahashi H, Marunouchi T, et al. (2006) Increased water intake decreases progression of polycystic kidney disease in the PCK rat. J Am Soc Nephrol 17: 2220–2227.
13. Wang CJ, Creed C, Winklhofer FT, Grantham JJ (2011) Water prescription in autosomal dominant polycystic kidney disease: a pilot study. Clin J Am Soc Nephrol 6: 192–197.
14. Gray RJ (1988) A class of K-sample tests for comparing the cumulative incidence of a competing risk. The annals of statistics: 1141–1154.
15. Fine JP, Gray RJ (1999) A proportional hazards model for the subdistribution of a competing risk. Journal of the American statistical association: 496–509.
16. Hosmer DW, Lemeshow S, May S (2008) Applied Survival Analysis: Regression Modeling of Time to Event Data. Chickester, UK: Wiley.
17. Royston P, Altman DG (1994) Regression using fractional polynomials of continuous covariates: parsimonious parametric modelling. Applied Statistics: 429–467.
18. Thomas MC, Moran J, Forsblom C, Harjutsalo V, Thorn L, et al. (2011) The association between dietary sodium intake, ESRD, and all-cause mortality in patients with type 1 diabetes. Diabetes Care 34: 861–866.
19. Perucca J, Bouby N, Valeix P, Bankir L (2007) Sex difference in urine concentration across differing ages, sodium intake, and level of kidney disease. Am J Physiol Regul Integr Comp Physiol 292: R700–705.
20. Feinfeld DA, Danovitch GM (1987) Factors affecting urine volume in chronic renal failure. Am J Kidney Dis 10: 231–235.
21. Luft FC, Fineberg NS, Sloan RS, Hunt JN (1983) The effect of dietary sodium and protein on urine volume and water intake. J Lab Clin Med 101: 605–610.
22. Bankir L (2001) Antidiuretic action of vasopressin: quantitative aspects and interaction between V1a and V2 receptor-mediated effects. Cardiovasc Res 51: 372–390.
23. Bouby N, Ahloulay M, Nsegbe E, Dechaux M, Schmitt F, et al. (1996) Vasopressin increases glomerular filtration rate in conscious rats through its antidiuretic action. J Am Soc Nephrol 7: 842–851.
24. Gellai M, Silverstein JH, Hwang JC, LaRochelle FT Jr., Valtin H (1984) Influence of vasopressin on renal hemodynamics in conscious Brattleboro rats. Am J Physiol 246: F819–827.
25. Bankir L, Bouby N, Trinh-Trang-Tan MM (1991) Vasopressin-dependent kidney hypertrophy: role of urinary concentration in protein-induced hypertrophy and in the progression of chronic renal failure. Am J Kidney Dis 17: 661–665.
26. Bouby N, Fernandes S (2003) Mild dehydration, vasopressin and the kidney: animal and human studies. Eur J Clin Nutr 57 Suppl 2: S39–46.
27. Anastasio P, Cirillo M, Spitali L, Frangiosa A, Pollastro RM, et al. (2001) Level of hydration and renal function in healthy humans. Kidney Int 60: 748–756.
28. Perico N, Zoja C, Corna D, Rottoli D, Gaspari F, et al. (2009) V1/V2 Vasopressin receptor antagonism potentiates the renoprotection of renin-angiotensin system inhibition in rats with renal mass reduction. Kidney Int 76: 960–967.
29. Bardoux P, Bruneval P, Heudes D, Bouby N, Bankir L (2003) Diabetes-induced albuminuria: role of antidiuretic hormone as revealed by chronic V2 receptor antagonism in rats. Nephrol Dial Transplant 18: 1755–1763.

The Association of Uremic Toxins and Inflammation in Hemodialysis Patients

Heng-Jung Hsu[1,2], Chiung-Hui Yen[3], I-Wen Wu[1], Kuang-Hung Hsu[4], Chih-Ken Chen[5], Chiao-Yin Sun[1], Chia-Chi Chou[1], Chun-Yu Chen[1], Chi-Jen Tsai[1], Mai-Szu Wu[6,7]*, Chin-Chan Lee[1]*

1 Division of Nephrology, Chang Gung Memorial Hospital, Keelung, Taiwan, **2** The Graduate Institute of Clinical Medical Sciences, Chang Gung University Medical College, Taoyuan School of Medicine, Taoyuan, Taiwan, **3** Department of Pediatrics, Taipei Medical University Hospital, Taipei, Taiwan, **4** Laboratory of Epidemiology, Department of Health Care Management, Chang Gung University, Taoyuan, Taiwan, **5** Division of Psychiatry, Chang Gung Memorial Hospital, Keelung, Taiwan, **6** Division of Nephrology, Taipei Medical University Hospital, Taipei, Taiwan, **7** Department of Internal Medicine, Taipei Medical University, Taipei, Taiwan

Abstract

Background: Cardiovascular disease is the leading cause of mortality in hemodialysis patients and is associated with chronic inflammation. Elevation of uremic toxins, particular protein-bound uremic toxins, is a possible cause of hyper-inflammation in hemodialysis patients. But the association between uremic toxins and inflammatory markers in hemodialysis is still unclear.

Methods: We conducted a cross-sectional study to evaluate the association of the serum uremic toxins and inflammatory markers in hemodialysis patients.

Results: The uremic toxins were not associated with inflammatory markers- including high sensitivity C-reactive protein, IL(Interleukin) -1β, IL-6, tumor necrosis factor-α. In multiple linear regression, serum levels of total *p*-cresol sulfate (*PCS*) were independently significantly associated with serum total indoxyl sulfate (IS) (standardized coefficient: 0.274, $p<0.001$), and co-morbidity of diabetes mellitus (DM) (standardized coefficient: 0.342, $p<0.001$) and coronary artery disease (CAD) (standardized coefficient: 0.128, $p=0.043$). The serum total *PCS* levels in hemodialysis with co-morbidity of DM and CAD were significantly higher than those without co-morbidity of DM and CAD (34.10±23.44 vs. 16.36±13.06 mg/L, $p<0.001$). Serum levels of total IS was independently significantly associated with serum creatinine (standardized coefficient: 0.285, $p<0.001$), total *PCS* (standardized coefficient: 0.239, $p=0.001$), and synthetic membrane dialysis (standardized coefficient: 0.139, $p=0.046$).

Conclusion: The study showed that serum levels of total PCS and IS were not associated with pro-inflammatory markers in hemodialysis patients. Besides, serum levels of total *PCS* were independently positively significantly associated with co-morbidity of CAD and DM.

Editor: Francesca D'Addio, San Raffaele Hospital, Italy

Funding: This study was supported by grants from the Chang Gung Memorial Hospital Research Fund (CMRPG260363). The funders had no role in study design, data collection and analysis, decision to publish, or preparation of the manuscript.

Competing Interests: The authors have declared that no competing interests exist.

* Email: maiszuwu@gmail.com (MSW); leefang@adm.cgmh.org.tw (CCL)

Introduction

End stage renal disease (ESRD) patients had higher cardiovascular disease (CVD)-related and all-cause mortality. Hyper-inflammation in hemodialysis patients results in CVD [1,2]. Pro-inflammatory cytokines are crucial to the inflammation associated with malnutrition and atherosclerosis in ESRD. Furthermore, it has been shown that high sensitivity C-reactive protein (hs-CRP) is elevated in patients with chronic kidney disease (CKD).

Uremic toxins can be classified into small water soluble uremic toxins, middle molecule uremic toxins, and protein bound uremic toxins. Due to substantial albumin binding, current dialysis modality could provide adequate removal of small water soluble uremic toxins and partial removal of middle molecule uremic toxins, but difficult in protein-bound uremic toxins [3]. *P*-cresol sulfate (*PCS*) and indoxyl sulfate (IS) are protein-bound uremic toxins and were associated with endothelial dysfunction also immune dysregulation in renal disease [4,5]. The cytokines' clearance decreases as well as the chronic renal failure stage increases. Many inflammatory cytokines are classified between the uremic toxins in particular tumor necrosis factor (TNF)- α, Interleukin(IL)-6, IL-1β are considered middle molecules as well as β2 microglobulin [6]. However, the exact association between uremic toxins and inflammation in ESRD patients is still not fully understood. Hence, we conducted the cross-sectional study to evaluate the association between uremic toxins and inflammatory markers.

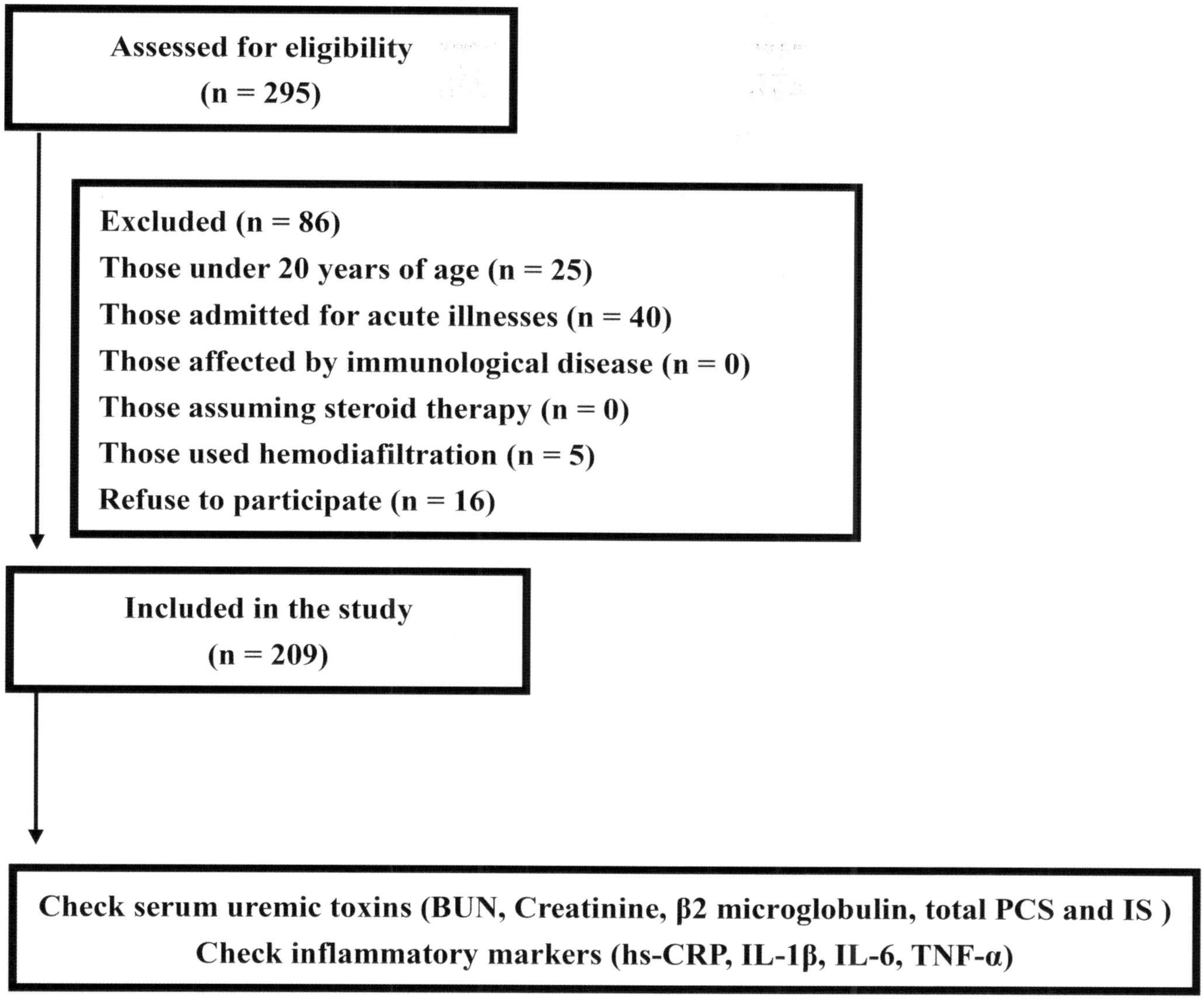

Figure 1. Flow chart indicates patient enrolment.

Subjects and Methods

Patients

We conducted a cross-sectional study at the dialysis center of the Chang Gung Memorial Hospital, Keelung, Taiwan, enrolling 295 chronic hemodialysis patients who had been undergoing regular hemodialysis for more than 6 months. Excluded from the study were those patients who were under 20 years of age, admitted for acute illnesses, using hemodiafiltration, affected by immunologic disease, assuming steroid therapy, and had declined participation (Figure 1). All patients had been receiving a standardized hemodialysis regimen: dialysate flow, 500 mL/min; blood flow, 250–300 mL/min, duration of dialysis per session, 4 h; and, thrice-weekly hemodialysis. We screened the serum uremic toxins (blood urea nitrogen (BUN), creatinine, β2 microglobulin, total *P*CS and IS, and inflammatory markers (hs-CRP, IL-1β, IL- 6, TNF- α) in the study patients. The uremic toxins and cytokines were checked during the normal hemodialysis week. The information about dialysis membrane type, vascular access type, anticoagulation type, and angiotensin converting enzyme inhibitor (ACEI)/angiotensin II type 1 receptor blocker (ARB) assuming was recorded. All written informed consent for participation in the study was obtained from participants. This study complies with the Declaration of Helsinki and was approved by the Ethics Committee of the Institutional Review Board at Chang Gung Memorial Hospital.

Measurement of the serum concentrations of total IS and PCS

To determine total IS and *P*CS serum levels, serum samples were deproteinized by adding 3 parts methanol to 1 part serum.

Table 1. Baseline characteristics of study patients.

Characteristics	All patients N = 209
Age (years)	58.2±13.8
Male (%)	99 (47.4)
Smoking (%)	37 (17.7)
Diabetes (%)	75 (35.9)
CAD (%)	38 (18.2)
CHF (%)	43 (20.6)
PAOD (%)	26 (12.4)
COPD (%)	17 (8.1)
Stroke (%)	20 (9.6)
Cancer (%)	18 (8.6)
Dialysis vintage (months)	67.2±54.8
Body mass index (kg/m^2)	23.3±3.9
nPCR (g/kg/day)	1.14±0.34
Cardiothoracic ratio (%)	0.50±0.07
Residual renal function (mL/min)	0.12±0.22
High flux dialysis (%)	137 (65.6)
Synthetic membrane (%)	160 (76.6%)
Vascular access	
AVF (%)	152 (72.7%)
AVG (%)	30 (14.4%)
Tunneled cuffed Catheter (%)	27 (12.9%)
ACEI/ARB use (%)	72 (34.4%)
Heparin use (%)	160 (76.6%)

Notes: Values are expressed as mean ± SD or total number (percent).
Abbreviations: CAD, coronary artery disease; CHF, congestive heart failure; PAOD, peripheral arterial occlusive disease; COPD, chronic obstructive pulmonary disease; nPCR, normalized protein catabolic rate; AVF, Arterial venous fistula; AVG, Arterial venous graft; ACEI, angiotensin converting enzyme inhibitor; ARB, angiotensin II type 1 receptor blocker.

Table 2. Biochemical and dialysis-related parameters of study patients.

Characteristics	All patients N = 209
Albumin (g/dL)	3.8±0.39
Hemoglobin (g/dL)	10.4±1.5
Calcium (mg/dL)	9.4±0.9
Phosphate (mg/dL)	5.2±1.8
Cholesterol (mg/dL)	177.1±47.7
Kt/V	1.67±0.36
URR (%)	0.74±0.07
BUN (mg/dL)	69.8±22.2
Creatinine (mg/dL)	10.8±2.7
β2 microglobulin (ng/mL)	28.3±11.5
i-PTH (pg/mL)	380.7±558.2
Total IS (mg/L)	36.70±16.74
Total *PCS* (mg/L)	21.25±17.81
hs-CRP (mg/L)	10.8±25.9
IL-1β (ng/L)	1.37±0.83
IL-6 (ng/L)	3.68±3.89
TNF-α (ng/L)	16.67±66.28

Abbreviations: URR, urea reduction rate; BUN, blood urea nitrogen; i-PTH, intact parathyroid hormone; IS, indoxyl sulfate; *PCS*: *p*-cresol sulfate; hs-CRP, high sensitive C-reactive protein; IL-1β, interleukin- 1 beta; IL-6, interleukin 6; TNF-α, tumor necrosis factor- alpha.

All analyses were performed using a Waters Acquity Ultra Performance Liquid Chromatography (UPLC) system (Milford, MA, USA).

Statistical Analysis

Continuous variables were expressed as means ± standard deviations. For normally distributed continuous variables, a two-tailed Student's unpaired *t*-test was employed to evaluate the differences between the means. The differences between groups of categorical variables were analyzed by the χ^2 test or Fisher's exact test. To examine the relationship between IS/*PCS* and other variables, Pearson's correlation test was used. To identify independent associations, stepwise multiple regression analysis was used, and co-variants selection based on univariate analysis with variables with $p<0.1$ were selected. We considered $p<0.05$ statistically significant. All analyses were performed using SPSS version 17.0 for Windows.

Results

Study subjects

The mean age of the patients (99 men and 110 women) was 58.2±13.8 years old; while the mean duration of dialysis was 67.2±54.8 months (table 1). There were 75 (36% of the total study patients) diabetic patients in our study and all were type 2 diabetes mellitus (DM). All patients used anti-coagulation agents with 76.6% patients (n = 160) using heparin whereas 23.4% patients (n = 49) using low-molecular-weight heparin. There were 72.7% patients (n = 152) used arterial venous fistula as hemodialysis access. The prevalence of ACEI/ARB use in study patients was 34.4%. The biochemical and dialysis related parameters were shown in table 2. The serum levels of total IS and total *PCS* in the study patients were 36.70±16.74 and 21.25±17.81 mg/L, respectively.

Relationship between hemodialysis type, uremic toxins, and inflammatory markers

The associations among hemodialysis type, uremic toxins, and inflammatory markers are shown in table 3. Vascular access type was not significantly associated with uremic toxins and inflammatory markers. Hemodialysis synthetic membrane use was significantly associated with serum total IS (correlation coefficient: 0.195, $p<0.001$). High flux dialysis was also significantly associated with serum total IS (correlation coefficient: 0.159, $p = 0.024$). However, hemodialysis synthetic membrane or high flux dialysis was not associated with inflammatory markers- hs-CRP, IL-1β, IL-6, and TNF-α. In protein-bound uremic toxins, serum IS was positively associated with serum total *PCS* (correlation coefficient: 0.292, $p<$ 0.001). However, these was no association between serum IS and inflammatory markers- hs-CRP, IL-1β, IL-6, and TNF-α. Serum

Table 3. The correlations between hemodialysis type, uremic toxins, and inflammatory markers.

	Vascular access	Synthetic membrane use	High flux dialysis	Total IS	Total *PCS*	hs-CRP	IL-1β	IL-6	TNF-α
Vascular access	—	−0.125	−0.101	−0.122	−0.083	−0.093	−0.046	0.049	−0.043
Synthetic membrane use	−0.125	—	0.865***	0.195***	−0.029	−0.060	−0.016	−0.106	−0.082
High flux dialysis	−0.101	0.865***	—	0.159**	−0.052	−0.028	0.005	−0.065	0.089
Total IS (mg/L)	−0.122	0.195***	0.159**	—	0.292***	−0.011	0.013	−0.062	−0.062
Total *PCS* (mg/L)	−0.083	−0.029	−0.052	0.292***	—	0.039	−0.102	0.074	0.093
hs-CRP (mg/L)	−0.093	−0.060	−0.028	−0.011	0.039	—	−0.033	0.407***	0.264***
IL-1β (ng/L)	−0.046	−0.016	0.005	0.013	−0.102	−0.033	—	0.004	−0.022
IL-6 (ng/L)	0.049	−0.106	−0.065	−0.062	0.074	0.407***	0.004	—	0.478***
TNF-α (ng/L)	−0.043	−0.082	0.089	−0.062	0.093	0.264***	−0.022	0.478***	—

**p* value<0.1.
** *p* value<0.05.
****p* value<0.01.
Abbreviations: IS, indoxyl sulfate; *PCS*: *p*-cresol sulfate; hs-CRP, high sensitive C-reactive protein; IL-1β, interleukin −1 beta; IL-6, interleukin 6; TNF-α, tumor necrosis factor- alpha.

PCS was positive associated with serum total IS and not associated with inflammatory markers- hs-CRP, IL-1β, IL-6, and TNF-α. In the inflammatory markers, serum hs-CRP was positively associated with serum IL-6 and TNF-α. Serum IL-6 was positively associated with serum hs-CRP and TNF-α. However, IL-1β was not associated with other inflammatory markers - hs-CRP, IL-6, and TNF-α.

Factors associated with serum levels of total PCS

In order to cognize the factor associated with serum levels of total *PCS*, univariate correlation analysis was performed first. The univariate analysis revealed that the total *PCS* levels were positively associated with the presence of DM (correlation coefficient: 0.322, $p<0.001$), coronary artery disease (CAD) (correlation coefficient: 0.213, $p=0.003$), stroke (correlation coefficient: 0.172, $p=0.017$), and serum levels of BUN (correlation coefficient: 0.173, $p=0.014$) and hemoglobin (correlation coefficient: 0.169, $p=0.017$) (table 4). Besides, there was a positive association between the serum levels of total *PCS* and IS (correlation coefficient: 0.292, $p<0.001$). There was also a trend of partial positive association between presence of peripheral arterial occlusive disease (PAOD) and serum total *PCS*. However, inflammatory cytokine levels were not significantly associated with the serum total *PCS* levels. Stepwise multiple regression analysis revealed that the presence of DM and CAD, and the serum levels of total IS were independent factors associated with the serum total *PCS* levels after adjustment of age, gender, and factors that significant in univariate analysis (comorbidity of PAOD and stroke, serum levels of BUN and hemoglobin). Besides, there was a trend of positive association between presence of stroke and serum total *PCS* after multiple regression analysis. Co-morbidity of PAOD lost the trend of association with the serum total *PCS* levels after multiple regression analysis.

Factors associated with serum levels of total PCS according to age

To assess the association between age, uremic toxins and co-morbidity, the study patients were grouped into older patients (Age ≥59 years old) and younger patients (Age <59 years old) by median age. In older patient group, serum total *PCS* levels were positively associated with co-morbidity of DM, CAD, stroke and serum levels of total IS (table 5). However, presence of DM (standardized coefficient: 0.399, $p<0.001$), stroke (standardized coefficient: 0.190, $p=0.034$) and serum total IS (standardized coefficient: 0.266, $p=0.003$) were independent factors associated with serum total *PCS* after multiple regression analysis. In younger patient group, serum total *PCS* levels were positively associated with presence of PAOD, and serum BUN and total IS. After multiple regression analysis, co-morbidity of PAOD (standardized coefficient: 0.260, $p=0.008$) and serum total IS levels (standardized coefficient: 0.315, $p=0.001$) were independent factors associated with serum total *PCS*.

Factors associated with serum levels of total IS

The analysis revealed that the total IS levels were positively associated with male gender (correlation coefficient: 0.153, $p=0.029$), serum levels of BUN (correlation coefficient: 0.143, $p=0.041$), creatinine (correlation coefficient: 0.311, $p<0.001$), and total *PCS* levels (correlation coefficient: 0.292, $p<0.001$) (table 6). Moreover, the serum total IS levels were also strongly associated with synthetic membrane use (correlation coefficient:

Table 4. Factors associated with serum total *p*-cresol sulfate.

Variable	Units	Univariate Correlation (correlation coefficient)	*p*	Multiple regression analysis (standardized coefficients; Beta)	*p*
Age	1 year	0.120	0.090*	-	-
Male vs female	-	0.126	0.075*	-	-
Smoking (yes vs no)	-	0.094	0.195	-	-
diabetes (yes vs no)	-	0.322	<0.001***	0.342	<0.001***
CAD (yes vs no)	-	0.213	0.003**	0.128	0.043**
CHF (yes vs no)	-	0.048	0.508	-	-
PAOD (yes vs no)	-	0.137	0.058*	-	-
COPD (yes vs no)	-	0.112	0.121	-	-
Stroke (yes vs no)	-	0.172	0.017**	0.117	0.075*
Cancer (yes vs no)	-	−0.107	0.139	-	-
Dialysis vintage	1 month	−0.045	0.530	-	-
Body mass index	1 kg/m^2	0.018	0.795	-	-
nPCR	1 g/kg/day	0.070	0.342	-	-
CT ratio	1%	0.067	0.379	-	-
BUN	1 mg/dL	0.173	0.014**	-	-
Creatinine	1 mg/dL	0.085	0.232	-	-
Hemoglobin	1 g/dL	0.169	0.017**	-	-
Albumin	1 g/dL	0.057	0.420	-	-
hs-CRP	1 mg/L	−0.035	0.631	-	-
Calcium	1 mg/dL	−0.079	0.263	-	-
Phosphate	1 mg/dL	0.015	0.838	-	-
i-PTH	1 pg/mL	−0.078	0.274	-	-
IL-1β	1 ng/L	−0.102	0.169	-	-
IL-6	1 ng/L	0.074	0.426	-	-
TNF-α	1 ng/L	0.093	0.197	-	-
Total IS	1 mg/L	0.292	<0.001***	0.274	<0.001***
Kt/V		−0.086	0.251	-	-
URR	1%	−0.077	0.297	-	-
High Flux dialysis (yes vs no)-		−0.023	0.425	-	-

Abbreviations: CAD, coronary artery disease; CHF, congestive heart failure; PAOD, peripheral arterial occlusive disease; COPD, chronic obstructive pulmonary disease; nPCR, normalized protein catabolic rate; CT ratio, cardiothoracic ratio; BUN, blood urea nitrogen; hs-CRP, high sensitive C- reactive protein; i-PTH, intact parathyroid hormone; IL-1β, interleukin −1 beta; IL-6, interleukin 6; TNF-alpha, tumor necrosis factor-alpha; IS, indoxyl sulfate; URR, urea reduction rate.
*: *p* value<0.1.
**: *p* value<0.05.
***: *p* value<0.01.

0.195, $p<0.001$) and high flux dialysis (correlation coefficient: 0.159, $p<0.001$). There was also a trend of partial positive association between presence of CAD and serum total IS. Then stepwise multiple regression analysis revealed that synthetic membrane use (standardized coefficient: 0.139, $p=0.046$) and serum levels of creatinine (standardized coefficient: 0.285, $p<0.001$) and total *PCS* (standardized coefficient: 0.239, $p=0.001$) were independent factors associated with the serum total IS levels. Inflammatory markers including hs-CRP and cytokine levels were not associated with the serum total IS levels. Co-morbidity of CAD, PAOD, and stroke was also not independently associated with the serum total IS levels.

Factors associated with serum levels of total IS according to age

In older patient group (Age ≥59 years old), serum total IS levels were positively associated with serum creatinine and total *PCS* (table 7). Serum total *PCS* levels (standardized coefficient: 0.224, $p=0.021$) were independent factors associated with serum total IS after multiple regression analysis. In younger patient group (Age < 59 years old), serum total IS levels were positively associated with male gender, and serum levels of creatinine and total *PCS*, and synthetic membrane use. After multiple regression analysis, only serum total *PCS* (standardized coefficient: 0.274, $p=0.004$) and synthetic membrane use (standardized coefficient: 0.241, $p=0.012$) were independent factors associated with serum total IS.

Table 5. Factors associated with serum total *p*-cresol sulfate according to age.

Variable	Units	Univariate Correlation (correlation coefficient)	*p*	Multiple regression analysis (standardized coefficients; Beta)	*p*
All patients					
Age	1 year	0.120	0.090*	-	-
Male vs female	-	0.126	0.075*	-	-
diabetes (yes vs no)	-	0.322	<0.001***	0.342	<0.001***
CAD (yes vs no)	-	0.213	0.003**	0.128	0.043**
PAOD (yes vs no)	-	0.137	0.058*	-	-
Stroke (yes vs no)	-	0.172	0.017**	0.117	0.075*
BUN	1 mg/dL	0.173	0.014**	-	-
Hemoglobin	1 g/dL	0.169	0.017**	-	-
Total IS	1 mg/L	0.292	<0.001***	0.274	<0.001***
Older patients by Median (Age ≥59 years old) (N = 105)					
Male vs female	-	0.141	0.157	-	-
diabetes (yes vs no)	-	0.405	<0.001***	0.399	<0.001***
CAD (yes vs no)	-	0.248	0.013**	-	-
PAOD (yes vs no)	-	0.060	0.553	-	-
Stroke (yes vs no)	-	0.269	0.007***	0.190	0.034*
BUN	1 mg/dL	0.180	0.070*	-	-
Hemoglobin	1 g/dL	0.171	0.086*	-	-
Total IS	1 mg/L	0.249	0.012**	0.266	0.003***
Younger patients by Median (Age <59 years old) (N = 104)					
Male vs female	-	0.116	0.253	-	-
diabetes (yes vs no)	-	0.154	0.140	-	-
CAD (yes vs no)	-	0.099	0.346	-	-
PAOD (yes vs no)	-	0.259	0.012**	0.260	0.008***
Stroke (yes vs no)	-	−0.010	0.923	-	-
BUN	1 mg/dL	0.203	0.044**	-	-
Hemoglobin	1 g/dL	0.147	0.147	-	-
Total IS	1 mg/L	0.355	<0.001***	0.315	0.001***

Abbreviations: CAD, coronary artery disease; PAOD, peripheral arterial occlusive disease; BUN, blood urea nitrogen; IS, indoxyl sulfate.
*: *p* value<0.1.
**: *p* value<0.05.
***: *p* value<0.01.

Comparison of serum levels of total PCS in hemodialysis patients with comorbidity of DM and CAD or not

Due to co-morbidity of DM was independently associated with serum levels of total *PCS*. The baseline characteristics and also biochemical and dialysis-related parameters were also analysis according to the presence or absence of DM (table 8 and table 9). Those hemodialysis patients with DM were older, shorter dialysis vintage, with more cigarette smoking, higher prevalence of co-morbidity of CAD, PAOD, stroke, and lower serum level of creatinine, intact parathyroid hormone (i-PTH), Kt/V and urea reduction rate (URR). Besides, higher serum levels of total *PCS* were noted in those patients with diabetes than those without diabetes (DM patients vs. non DM patients: 29.36±21.59 vs. 17.38±13.77 mg/L, $p<0.001$). Furthermore, previous multiple linear regression analysis showed that comorbidity of CAD was also independently significantly associated with serum total *PCS*. The serum levels of total *PCS* were also compared between those patients with comorbidity of CAD or not. Those patients with comorbidity of CAD had higher serum levels of total *PCS* than those without CAD (CAD patients vs. non CAD patients: 29.94±21.02 vs. 19.97±16.75 mg/L, $p = 0.003$) (data also not shown in table). In order to configure out the association of serum total *PCS* and comorbidity of DM and CAD, patients were divided into four groups: those with comorbidity of DM and CAD; with comorbidity of DM but no CAD; with comorbidity of CAD but not DM; with comorbidity of neither DM nor CAD. We compared the serum total *PCS* levels between those four groups of patients. In hemodialysis patients with DM, the serum levels of *PCS* in those patients with CAD (n = 19) were higher than patients without CAD (n = 56) though without significance (34.10±23.44

Table 6. Factors associated with serum total indoxyl sulfate levels.

Variable	Units	Univariate Correlation (correlation coefficient)	*p*	Multiple regression analysis (standardized coefficients; Beta)	*p*
Age	1 year	0.001	0.988	-	-
Male vs female	-	0.153	0.029**	-	-
Smoking (yes vs no)	-	0.072	0.319	-	-
diabetes (yes vs no)	-	−0.096	0.182	-	-
CAD (yes vs no)	-	0.132	0.067*	-	-
CHF (yes vs no)	-	−0.048	0.507	-	-
PAOD (yes vs no)	-	−0.005	0.944	-	-
COPD (yes vs no)	-	−0.331	0.669	-	-
Stroke (yes vs no)	-	−0.080	0.264	-	-
Cancer (yes vs no)	-	−0.090	0.210	-	-
Dialysis vintage	1 month	−0.032	0.647	-	-
Body mass index	1 kg/m^2	0.005	0.940	-	-
nPCR	1 g/kg/day	0.014	0.852	-	-
CT ratio	1%	−0.072	0.345	-	-
BUN	1 mg/dL	0.143	0.041**	-	-
Creatinine	1 mg/dL	0.311	<0.001***	0.285	<0.001***
Hemoglobin	1 g/dL	0.127	0.070*	-	-
Albumin	1 g/dL	0.119	0.091*	-	-
hs-CRP	1 mg/L	−0.139	0.050*	-	-
Calcium	1 mg/dL	0.027	0.701	-	-
Phosphate	1 mg/dL	0.026	0.713	-	-
i-PTH	1 pg/mL	0.083	0.239	-	-
IL-1β	1 ng/L	0.013	0.859	-	-
IL-6	1 ng/L	−0.062	0.498	-	-
TNF-α	1 ng/L	−0.062	0.392	-	-
Total *PCS*	1 mg/L	0.292	<0.001 ***	0.239	0.001***
Kt/V		−0.031	0.674	-	-
URR	1%	0.003	0.969	-	-
Synthetic membrane use (yes vs no)	-	0.195	<0.001***	0.139	0.046*
High Flux dialysis (yes vs no)	-	0.159	<0.001***	-	-

Abbreviations: CAD, coronary artery disease; CHF, congestive heart failure; PAOD, peripheral arterial occlusive disease; COPD, chronic obstructive pulmonary disease; nPCR, normalized protein catabolic rate; CT ratio, cardiothoracic ratio; BUN, blood urea nitrogen; hs-CRP, high sensitive C- reactive protein; i-PTH, intact parathyroid hormone; IL-1β, interleukin - 1 beta; IL-6, interleukin 6; TNF-alpha, tumor necrosis factor-alpha; *PCS*, *p*-cresol sulfate; URR, urea reduction rate.
*: *p* value<0.1.
**: *p* value<0.05.
***: *p* value<0.01.

vs. 27.60±20.83 mg/L, $p = 0.297$) (figure 2). In hemodialysis patients without DM, the serum levels of *PCS* in those patients with CAD (n = 19) were significantly higher than those patients without CAD (n = 115) (24.68±16.80 vs. 16.36±13.06 mg/L, $p = 0.028$). The serum levels of *PCS* in those patients with DM but not CAD (n = 56) were significantly higher than those neither DM nor CAD (n = 115) (27.60±20.83 vs. 16.36±13.06 mg/L, $p < 0.001$). Besides, serum levels of total *PCS* in those patients with DM but not CAD (n = 56) were higher than those with CAD but not DM (n = 19): (27.60±20.83 vs. 24.68±16.80 mg/L, $p = 0.620$) though without significance. Moreover, serum levels of total *PCS* in those patients with DM and CAD (n = 19) were significantly higher than those with neither DM nor CAD (n = 115): (34.10±23.44 vs. 16.36±13.06 mg/L, $p < 0.001$).

Comparison of serum levels of total IS in hemodialysis patients with comorbidity of DM and CAD or not

The serum levels of total IS were compared between those patients with comorbidity of DM or not. Those hemodialysis patients with comorbidity of DM and those without diabetes had

Table 7. Factors associated with serum total indoxyl sulfate according to age.

Variable	Units	Univariate Correlation (correlation coefficient)	*p*	Multiple regression analysis (standardized coefficients; Beta)	*p*
All patients					
Age	1 year	0.001	0.988	-	-
Male vs female	-	0.153	0.029**	-	-
CAD (yes vs no)	-	0.132	0.067*	-	-
PAOD (yes vs no)	-	−0.005	0.944	-	-
Stroke (yes vs no)	-	−0.080	0.264	-	-
BUN	1 mg/dL	0.143	0.041**	-	-
Creatinine	1 mg/dL	0.311	<0.001***	0.285	<0.001***
Hemoglobin	1 g/dL	0.127	0.070*	-	-
Albumin	1 g/dL	0.119	0.091*	-	-
hs-CRP	1 mg/L	−0.139	0.050*	-	-
Total *PCS*	1 mg/L	0.292	<0.001 ***	0.239	0.001***
Synthetic membrane use (yes vs no)	-	0.195	<0.001***	0.139	0.046*
High Flux dialysis (yes vs no)	-	0.159	<0.001***	-	-
Older patients by Median (Age ≥59 years old) (N = 105)					
Male vs female	-	0.001	0.995	-	-
CAD (yes vs no)	-	0.093	0.356	-	-
PAOD (yes vs no)	-	−0.002	0.987	-	-
Stroke (yes vs no)	-	−0.058	0.563	-	-
BUN	1 mg/dL	0.096	0.336	-	-
Creatinine	1 mg/dL	0.258	0.009***	-	-
Hemoglobin	1 g/dL	0.064	0.520	-	-
Albumin	1 g/dL	0.126	0.204	-	-
hs-CRP	1 mg/L	0.010	0.920	-	-
Total *PCS*	1 mg/L	0.249	0.012**	0.224	0.021**
Synthetic membrane use (yes vs no)	-	0.106	0.286	-	-
Younger patients by Median (Age <59 years old) (N = 104)					
Male vs female	-	0.300	0.002***	-	-
CAD (yes vs no)	-	0.180	0.082*	-	-
PAOD (yes vs no)	-	−0.010	0.926	-	-
Stroke (yes vs no)	-	−0.110	0.290	-	-
BUN	1 mg/dL	0.186	0.063*	-	-
Creatinine	1 mg/dL	0.381	<0.001***	-	-
Hemoglobin	1 g/dL	0.172	0.088*	-	-
Albumin	1 g/dL	0.119	0.239	-	-
hs-CRP	1 mg/L	−0.072	0.486	-	-
Total *PCS*	1 mg/L	0.355	<0.001 ***	0.274	0.004***
Synthetic membrane use (yes vs no)	-	0.309	0.002 ***	0.241	0.012**

Abbreviations: CAD, coronary artery disease; PAOD, peripheral arterial occlusive disease; BUN, blood urea nitrogen; hs-CRP, high sensitive C- reactive protein; *PCS*, *p*-cresol sulfate.
*: p value<0.1.
**: p value<0.05.
***: p value<0.01.

similar levels of total IS (DM patients vs. non DM patients: 35.19±14.60 vs. 38.49±17.54 mg/L, $p = 0.182$). Furthermore, the serum levels of total IS were also compared between those patients with comorbidity of CAD or not. Those patients with comorbidity of CAD had higher serum levels of total IS than those without CAD although without significance (CAD patients vs. non

Table 8. Baseline characteristics according to the presence or absence of diabetes mellitus.

Characteristics	No diabetic N = 134	Diabetic N = 75	*p*
Age (years)	57.0±15.2	61.1±10.8	0.046*
Male (%)	60 (44)	39 (52)	0.299
Smoking (%)	18 (13)	19 (25)	0.013*
CAD (%)	17 (13)	21 (28)	0.011*
CHF (%)	23 (17)	20 (27)	0.16
PAOD (%)	11 (8)	15 (20)	0.021*
COPD (%)	8 (6)	9 (12)	0.164
Stroke (%)	7 (5)	13 (17)	0.007*
Cancer (%)	13 (10)	5 (7)	0.381
Dialysis vintage (months)	82.0±73.4	42.0±35.2	<0.001*
Body mass index (kg/m^2)	23.2±3.6	23.6±4.1	0.683
nPCR (g/kg/day)	1.18±0.29	1.15±0.27	0.66
Cardiothoracic ratio (%)	0.49±0.07	0.51±0.06	0.058
Residual renal function (mL/min)	0.11±0.18	0.13±0.29	0.755
High flux dialysis (%)	93 (69)	44 (59)	0.107
Synthetic membrane (%)	93(74)	51(68)	0.377
Vascular access			0.152
AVF (%)	89 (71)	60 (80)	
AVG (%)	17 (14)	10 (13)	
Catheter (%)	20 (16)	5 (7)	
ACEI/ARB use (%)	42 (33)	29 (39)	0.444
Heparin use (%)	93 (74%)	61 (81)	0.223

Notes: Values are expressed as mean ± SD or total number (percent).
*: *p* value<0.05.
Statistical significance based on Chi-square test for categorical variables or *t*-test for continuous variables.
Abbreviations: CAD, coronary artery disease; CHF, congestive heart failure; PAOD, peripheral arterial occlusive disease; COPD, chronic obstructive pulmonary disease; nPCR, normalized protein catabolic rate; AVF, Arterial venous fistula; AVG, Arterial venous graft; ACEI, angiotensin converting enzyme inhibitor; ARB, angiotensin II type 1 receptor blocker.

CAD patients: 41.86±14.82 vs. 36.25±16.81 mg/L, $p = 0.067$) (data also not shown in table). In order to configure out the association of serum total IS and comorbidity of DM and CAD, patients were also divided into four groups: those with comorbidity of DM and CAD; with comorbidity of DM but no CAD; with comorbidity of CAD but not DM; with comorbidity of neither DM nor CAD. In hemodialysis patients with DM, the serum levels of total IS in those patients with CAD (n = 19) were higher than patients without CAD (n = 56) (38.90±10.86 vs. 33.74±15.68 mg/L, $p = 0.181$) (figure 3). In hemodialysis patients without DM, the serum levels of total IS in those patients with CAD (n = 19) were higher than those patients without CAD (n = 115) (45.55±18.36 vs. 37.44±17.26 mg/L, $p = 0.084$). The serum levels of total IS in those patients with DM but not CAD (n = 56) were lower than those with neither DM nor CAD (n = 115) (33.74±15.68 vs. 37.44±17.26 mg/L, $p = 0.196$). Besides, serum levels of total IS in those patients with DM but not CAD (n = 56) were significantly lower than those with CAD but not DM (n = 19): (33.74±15.68 vs. 45.55±18.36 mg/L, $p = 0.014$). Moreover, serum levels of total IS in those patients with DM and CAD (n = 19) were lower than those CAD but not DM (n = 19): (38.90±10.86 vs. 45.55±18.36 mg/L, $p = 0.185$). Furthermore, previous univariate analysis found that serum levels of IS were associated with high flux dialysis. Biochemical and dialysis-related parameters were also compared between those patients with high flux and low flux dialysis. Those patients with high flux dialysis had higher serum levels of BUN, creatinine, hemoglobin, albumin, total IS, and URR (table 10).

Discussion

The mechanism of inflammation and higher CVD in ESRD patients under hemodialysis is multifactorial. Uremic toxins were considered one of possible cause to induce inflammation and CVD. In this study, the uremic toxins including small soluble, middle molecular, and protein-bound uremic toxins were all evaluated. The result showed that there was no significant association between above uremic toxins and inflammatory markers (hs-CRP, IL-1β, IL-6, and TNF-α). Furthermore, the serum levels of *PCS* were significantly higher in DM and CAD patients.

Table 9. Biochemical and dialysis-related parameters according to the presence or absence of diabetes mellitus.

Characteristics	No diabetic	Diabetic	*p*
	N = 134	N = 75	
BUN (mg/dL)	70.8±24.1	68.8±18.7	0.55
Creatinine (mg/dL)	11.3±2.8	10.0±2.3	0.001*
Hemoglobin (g/dL)	10.5±1.6	10.3±1.3	0.271
Albumin (g/dL)	3.8±0.4	3.8±0.4	0.319
hs-CRP (mg/L)	9.3±19.7	9.8±16.3	0.432
Calcium (mg/dL)	9.5±1.0	9.4±0.9	0.316
Phosphate (mg/dL)	5.1±1.8	5.3±1.7	0.39
Cholesterol (mg/dL)	174.2±35.6	184.0±63.8	0.165
i-PTH (pg/mL)	447.6±667.6	260.6±307.3	0.025*
IL-1β (ng/L)	1.38±0.85	1.39±0.84	0.989
IL-6 (ng/L)	3.69±4.74	3.93±2.26	0.761
TNF-α (ng/L)	15.06±70.38	19.70±62.73	0.645
Total indoxyl sulfate (mg/L)	38.49±17.54	35.19±14.60	0.182
Total *p*-cresol sulfate (mg/L)	17.38±13.77	29.36±21.59	<0.001*
Kt/V	1.71±0.37	1.59±0.34	0.033*
URR (%)	0.75±0.074	0.72±0.07	0.006*

*: *p* value<0.05.
Statistical significance based on *t*-test for continuous variables.
Abbreviations: BUN, blood urea nitrogen; hs-CRP, high sensitive C-reactive protein; i-PTH, intact parathyroid hormone; IL-1β, interleukin −1 beta; IL-6, interleukin 6; TNF-alpha, tumor necrosis factor-alpha; URR, urea reduction rate.

Malnutrition, inflammation, atherosclerosis syndrome is associated with an exceptionally high mortality rate in ESRD patients [2]. Elevations of several inflammatory markers including CRP, IL-6, and TNF-alpha were reported to be associated with mortality in ESRD patients undergoing hemodialysis or peritoneal dialysis [7,8,9,10]. Although the causes of elevated serum levels of pro-inflammatory cytokines in ESRD patients are not well understood, reduced renal clearance of cytokines, accumulation of advanced glycation end-products (AGE), hyperhomocysteinemia [11], dialysis procedure- related inflammation [12], and unrecognized persistent infection were considered to induce the inflammation in ESRD patients. Uremic toxins, especially protein-bound uremic toxins, are also considered to cause inflammation [13,14]. Protein-bound uremic toxins cannot be easily removed during dialysis procedure not matter HD or PD. In vitro studies had shown that *p*- cresol had toxic potential to endothelium. Clinical studies also showed significant association between serum *PCS* and CVD in CKD and ESRD patients [15,16,17,18,19]. Lee et al. found significant association between serum levels of free IS and IL-6 in peritoneal dialysis patients. But no significant association between serum levels of total IS and CRP, IL-6, and IL-10 was noted [20]. However, few studies exploded the association between uremic toxins and pro-inflammatory markers in hemodialysis patients. The study evaluated the uremic toxins including serum BUN, creatinine, β2 microglobulin, total *PCS*, and IS with association of pro-inflammatory cytokines in hemodialysis patients. The result showed lack association of uremic toxins and pro-inflammatory markers. Possible explanation is that inflammation induced by uremic toxins is transiently or focally, which cannot be observed by our study design. It is also possible that *PCS* directed induced atherosclerosis without via the cytokine and inflammation. The mechanism needs more studies to evaluate the close connection between total *PCS* and atherosclerosis in ESRD patients.

It is very interesting that serum total *PCS* was significantly associated with comorbidity of DM and also CAD. The exact connection between co-morbidity of DM, CAD, and serum total *PCS* was unclear. Because of the study design does not allow to establish any causal relationship between variable above that were examined. However, some working hypothesis can be considered. Possible hypotheses are that those patients with co-morbidity of CAD and DM had some particular factors that influence the levels of *PCS* production. But lots of evidences suggested that higher levels of *PCS* induced CAD by causing the deleterious effect on the endothelium. So the relationship between serum levels of total *PCS* and comorbidity of CAD could be understood and solved. But the association between serum total *PCS* and co-morbidity of DM is still unknown. Similarly, Meijers et al. also showed significant higher total and free *PCS* in hemodialysis patients with DM than non- DM [15]. Whether this is related to particular dietary habits is not clear. Indeed, protein intake is a limiting factor for the production by gut resident bacteria of *p* cresol. However, we can reasonable exclude this hypothesis because we did not observe any statistically significant difference among the study patients with DM or not in the serum albumin, BMI, and nPCR. Residual renal function and high flux hemodialysis were also important factors to determine protein-bound uremic toxins [21,22]. However, the residual renal function and high flux dialysis

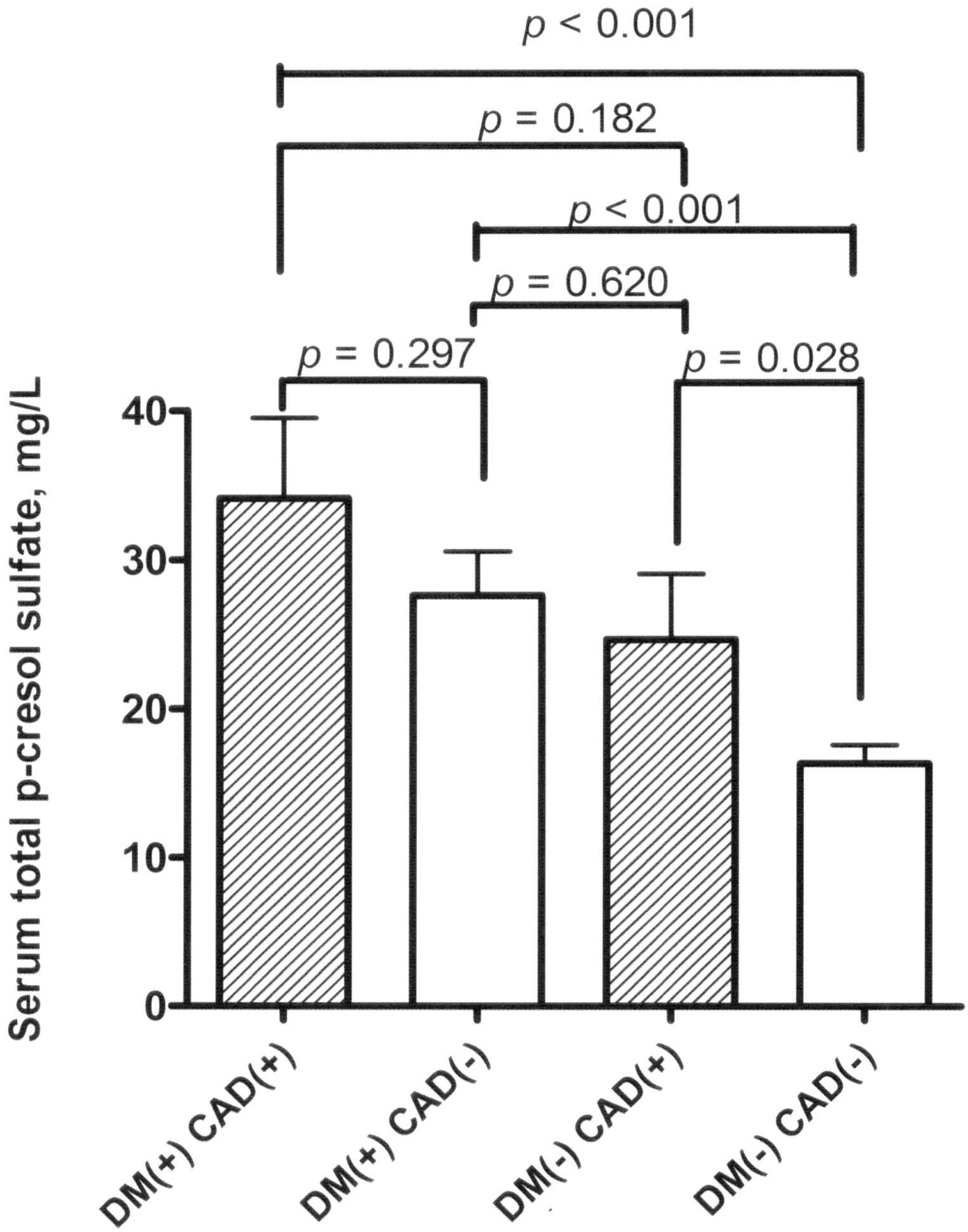

Figure 2. The serum levels of total *p*-cresol sulfate in hemodialysis patients with or without diabetes mellitus (DM) and coronary artery disease (CAD).

use ratio did not significant between DM and non-DM patients (table 8). Another possible explanation is that patients with diabetes have a significant risk of developing severe constipation often due to dysfunction of the autonomic nervous system [23]. Some evidences suggests diabetic patients had altered colonic protein fermentation [24]. *P*-cresol was generated by the intestinal flora and then conjugated to *p*-cresol sulfate in the intestinal wall and to *p*-cresylglucuronide in the liver [3]. When bowel movement decreased due to autonomic dysfunction in DM patients, more gut formation and production of *PCS* may happen.

In hemodialysis patients with DM, although the difference was not prominent significance, there was a trend that the serum levels of total p-cresol sulfate were higher in those patients with co-morbidity of CAD than those without CAD. These result indicated that higher serum total PCS may be associated with CAD even in these high CVD risk patients (diabetic hemodialysis patients). The reason of no significance may be due to small

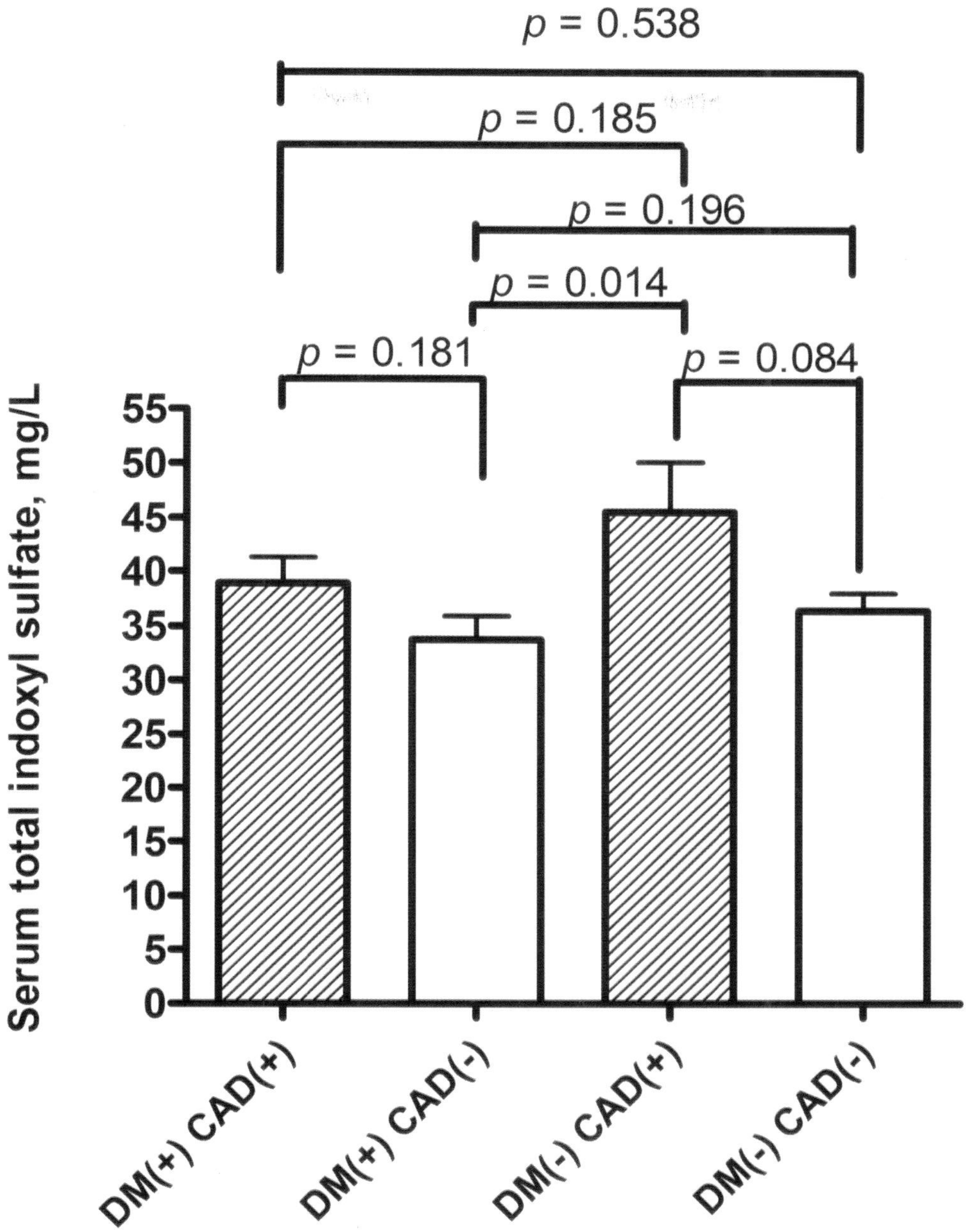

Figure 3. The serum levels of total indoxy sulfate in hemodialysis patients with or without diabetes mellitus (DM) and coronary artery disease (CAD).

patient number (patients with DM & CAD: n = 19 vs. DM without CAD: n = 56). In hemodialysis patients without DM, the serum levels of total *p*-cresol sulfate were significantly higher in those patients with co-morbidity of CAD than those without CAD. The results suggested that particular dietary habit or colonic protein fermentation in those HD patients may develop coronary artery disease no matter in DM or non-DM patients. In stratified analysis by age, serum levels of total *PCS* were independently significantly associated with comorbidity of stroke in older patients. But serum levels of total *PCS* was independently significantly associated with co-morbidity of PAOD in younger patients. All these results showed that serum total levels of *PCS* were highly associated with atherosclerosis-related disease such as CAD, stroke, and PAOD in CKD patients with hemodialysis. But the association between the serum levels of total IS and co-morbidity of CAD, stroke, and PAOD is lacking in the study. Some studies found that serum levels of IS in hemodialysis patients is associated with markers related to atherosclerosis [4]. Because of the controversial results,

Table 10. Biochemical and dialysis-related parameters according to high flux or low flux dialysis.

Characteristics	High flux N=136	Low Flux N=70	p
BUN (mg/dL)	72.7±21.7	64.3±22.3	0.009*
Creatinine (mg/dL)	11.5±2.6	9.6±2.4	<0.001*
Hemoglobin (g/dL)	10.7±1.6	10.0±1.2	0.003*
Albumin (g/dL)	3.9±0.4	3.8±0.4	0.008*
hs-CRP (mg/L)	8.9±19.1	10.0±16.1	0.695
Calcium (mg/dL)	9.5±0.9	9.2±0.9	0.018
Phosphate (mg/dL)	5.3±1.7	5.0±1.9	0.387
Cholesterol (mg/dL)	173.2±49.3	184.5±43.9	0.103
i-PTH (pg/mL)	422.5±646.8	299.5±311.6	0.134
IL-1β (ng/L)	1.38±0.86	1.37±0.78	0.943
IL-6 (ng/L)	3.50±3.64	4.03±4.34	0.478
TNF-α (ng/L)	21.03±80.74	8.75±21.67	0.211
Total indoxyl sulfate (mg/L)	38.60±15.94	33.00±17.75	0.024*
Total *p*-cresol sulfate (mg/L)	20.59±18.47	22.52±16.53	0.466
Kt/V	1.67±0.33	1.68±0.41	0.892
URR (%)	0.75±0.06	0.74±0.08	0.006*

*: p value<0.05.
Statistical significance based on t-test for continuous variables.
Abbreviations: BUN, blood urea nitrogen; hs-CRP, high sensitive C-reactive protein; i-PTH, intact parathyroid hormone; IL-1β, interleukin −1 beta; IL-6, interleukin 6; TNF-alpha, tumor necrosis factor-alpha; URR, urea reduction rate.

the exact association between serum levels of IS and atherosclerosis-related comorbidity in CKD patients need further evaluation.

The study had several limitations. The free-form *PCS* and IS levels were not checked. Furthermore, the mechanism of the higher total-form *PCS* in the DM patients could not be determined. However, this is an important study to evaluate the pro-inflammatory cytokines and protein-bound uremic toxins in hemodialysis patients. In addition, this study found that serum total *PCS* levels were significantly higher in hemodialysis patients with comorbidity of CAD and DM than those without co-morbidity of DM and CAD. This gave us the clue that development of CVD in hemodialysis patients with co-morbidity of DM maybe associated higher total *PCS* due to particular dietary habits and also DM-related alternation in colonic protein fermentation. Besides, due to the constraints of this study design (cross-sectional design), we are not able to provide a powerful evidence for the correlation between serum levels of IS or *PCS* with survival. However, Wang et al. had found association between high total *p*-cresol sulfate and major adverse cardiac events in CKD patients [25]. Wu et al. also showed that serum free *p*-cresol sulfate levels predict cardiovascular and all-cause mortality in elderly hemodialysis patients [17]. All of the results strongly proved the association between cardiovascular disease- related clinical outcome and serum levels of *PCS* in CKD patients.

In conclusion, the study showed that uremic toxins including total *PCS* and IS were not associated with pro-inflammatory markers in ESRD patients with hemodialysis. Besides, serum levels of total *PCS* was independently significantly associated with co-morbidity of CAD and DM.

Author Contributions

Analyzed the data: HJH CHY IWW KHH. Contributed reagents/materials/analysis tools: CKC CYS CCC. Wrote the paper: HJH MSW CCL. Participated in data interpretation: CYC CJT.

References

1. Collins AJ, Kasiske B, Herzog C, Chen SC, Everson S, et al. (2003) Excerpts from the United States Renal Data System 2003 Annual Data Report: atlas of end-stage renal disease in the United States. Am J Kidney Dis 42: A5–7, S1–230.
2. Pecoits-Filho R, Lindholm B, Stenvinkel P (2002) The malnutrition, inflammation, and atherosclerosis (MIA) syndrome – the heart of the matter. Nephrol Dial Transplant 17 Suppl 11: 28–31.
3. Martinez AW, Recht NS, Hostetter TH, Meyer TW (2005) Removal of P-cresol sulfate by hemodialysis. J Am Soc Nephrol 16: 3430–3436.
4. Raff AC, Meyer TW, Hostetter TH (2008) New insights into uremic toxicity. Curr Opin Nephrol Hypertens 17: 560–565.
5. De Smet R, Dhondt A, Eloot S, Galli F, Waterloos MA, et al. (2007) Effect of the super-flux cellulose triacetate dialyser membrane on the removal of non-protein-bound and protein-bound uraemic solutes. Nephrol Dial Transplant 22: 2006–2012.
6. Vanholder R, De Smet R, Glorieux G, Argiles A, Baurmeister U, et al. (2003) Review on uremic toxins: classification, concentration, and interindividual variability. Kidney Int 63: 1934–1943.
7. Zimmermann J, Herrlinger S, Pruy A, Metzger T, Wanner C (1999) Inflammation enhances cardiovascular risk and mortality in hemodialysis patients. Kidney Int 55: 648–658.
8. Yeun JY, Levine RA, Mantadilok V, Kaysen GA (2000) C-Reactive protein predicts all-cause and cardiovascular mortality in hemodialysis patients. Am J Kidney Dis 35: 469–476.
9. Kimmel PL, Phillips TM, Simmens SJ, Peterson RA, Weihs KL, et al. (1998) Immunologic function and survival in hemodialysis patients. Kidney Int 54: 236–244.
10. Bologa RM, Levine DM, Parker TS, Cheigh JS, Serur D, et al. (1998) Interleukin-6 predicts hypoalbuminemia, hypocholesterolemia, and mortality in hemodialysis patients. Am J Kidney Dis 32: 107–114.

11. Cianciolo G, La Manna G, Coli L, Donati G, D'Addio F, et al. (2008) 5-methyltetrahydrofolate administration is associated with prolonged survival and reduced inflammation in ESRD patients. Am J Nephrol 28: 941–948.
12. Stefoni S, Coli L, Cianciolo G, Donati G, Dalmastri V, et al. (2003) In vivo evaluation of cellular and inflammatory response to a new polyethersulfone membrane. Contrib Nephrol: 68–79.
13. Glorieux G, Cohen G, Jankowski J, Vanholder R (2009) Platelet/Leukocyte activation, inflammation, and uremia. Semin Dial 22: 423–427.
14. Ito S, Higuchi Y, Yagi Y, Nishijima F, Yamato H, et al. (2013) Reduction of indoxyl sulfate by AST-120 attenuates monocyte inflammation related to chronic kidney disease. J Leukoc Biol 93: 837–845.
15. Meijers BK, Bammens B, De Moor B, Verbeke K, Vanrenterghem Y, et al. (2008) Free p-cresol is associated with cardiovascular disease in hemodialysis patients. Kidney Int 73: 1174–1180.
16. Liabeuf S, Barreto DV, Barreto FC, Meert N, Glorieux G, et al. (2010) Free p-cresylsulphate is a predictor of mortality in patients at different stages of chronic kidney disease. Nephrol Dial Transplant 25: 1183–1191.
17. Wu IW, Hsu KH, Hsu HJ, Lee CC, Sun CY, et al. (2012) Serum free p-cresyl sulfate levels predict cardiovascular and all-cause mortality in elderly hemodialysis patients a prospective cohort study. Nephrol Dial Transplant 27: 1169–1175.
18. Meijers BK, Claes K, Bammens B, de Loor H, Viaene L, et al. (2010) p-Cresol and cardiovascular risk in mild-to-moderate kidney disease. Clin J Am Soc Nephrol 5: 1182–1189.
19. Amabile N, Guerin AP, Leroyer A, Mallat Z, Nguyen C, et al. (2005) Circulating endothelial microparticles are associated with vascular dysfunction in patients with end-stage renal failure. J Am Soc Nephrol 16: 3381–3388.
20. Lee CT, Kuo CC, Chen YM, Hsu CY, Lee WC, et al. (2010) Factors associated with blood concentrations of indoxyl sulfate and p-cresol in patients undergoing peritoneal dialysis. Perit Dial Int 30: 456–463.
21. Brunet P, Dou L, Cerini C, Berland Y (2003) Protein-bound uremic retention solutes. Adv Ren Replace Ther 10: 310–320.
22. Marquez IO, Tambra S, Luo FY, Li Y, Plummer NS, et al. (2011) Contribution of residual function to removal of protein-bound solutes in hemodialysis. Clin J Am Soc Nephrol 6: 290–296.
23. Welch AC (2003) Constipation & diabetes. Constipation can affect up to 60 percent of people with diabetes. Some treatments may work better than others. Which ones are right for you? Diabetes Forecast 56: 65–66.
24. Todesco T, Zamboni M, Armellini F, Bissoli L, Turcato E, et al. (1993) Plasma acetate levels in a group of obese diabetic, obese normoglycemic, and control subjects and their relationships with other blood parameters. Am J Gastroenterol 88: 751–755.
25. Wang CP, Lu LF, Yu TH, Hung WC, Chiu CA, et al. (2013) Associations among chronic kidney disease, high total p-cresylsulfate and major adverse cardiac events. J Nephrol 26: 111–118.

Survival on Home Dialysis

Mark R. Marshall[1,2,3]*, Rachael C. Walker[4,5], Kevan R. Polkinghorne[3,6,7], Kelvin L. Lynn[8]

1 Faculty of Medical and Health Sciences, University of Auckland, Auckland, New Zealand, **2** Department of Renal Medicine, Counties Manukau District Health Board, Auckland, New Zealand, **3** Australia and New Zealand Dialysis and Transplant Registry (ANZDATA), The Royal Adelaide Hospital, Adelaide, South Australia, Australia, **4** Renal Department, Hawke's Bay District Health Board, Hastings, New Zealand, **5** Sydney School of Public Health, University of Sydney, Sydney, New South Wales, Australia, **6** Department of Nephrology, Monash Medical Centre, Clayton, Victoria, Australia, **7** Departments of Medicine and Epidemiology and Preventive Medicine, Monash University, Clayton, Victoria, Australia, **8** Kidney Health New Zealand, Christchurch, New Zealand

Abstract

Background: New Zealand (NZ) has a high prevalence of both peritoneal dialysis (PD) and home haemodialysis (HD) relative to other countries, and probably less selection bias. We aimed to determine if home dialysis associates with better survival than facility HD by simultaneous comparisons of the three modalities.

Methods: We analysed survival by time-varying dialysis modality in New Zealanders over a 15-year period to 31-Dec-2011, adjusting for patient co-morbidity by Cox proportional hazards multivariate regression.

Results: We modelled 6,419 patients with 3,254 deaths over 20,042 patient-years of follow-up. Patients treated with PD and facility HD are similar; those on home HD are younger and healthier. Compared to facility HD, home dialysis (as a unified category) associates with an overall 13% lower mortality risk. Home HD associates with a 52% lower mortality risk. PD associates with a 20% lower mortality risk in the early period (<3 years) that is offset by a 33% greater mortality risk in the late period (>3 years), with no overall net effect. There was effect modification and less observable benefit associated with PD in those with diabetes mellitus, co-morbidity, and in NZ Maori and Pacific People. There was no effect modification by age or by era.

Conclusion: Our study supports the culture of home dialysis in NZ, and suggests that the extent and duration of survival benefit associated with early PD may be greater than appreciated. We are planning further analyses to exclude residual confounding from unmeasured co-morbidity and other sociodemographic factors using database linkage to NZ government datasets. Finally, our results suggest further research into the practice of PD in NZ Maori and Pacific People, as well as definitive study to determine the best timing for switching from PD in the late phase.

Editor: Emmanuel A. Burdmann, University of Sao Paulo Medical School, Brazil

Funding: The Royal Australasian College of Physicians Foundation funded this study through a Jacquot Research Establishment Award to M.M. The funders had no role in study design, data collection and analysis, decision to publish, or preparation of the manuscript.

Competing Interests: The authors have read the journal's policy and have the following conflicts: M.M. has received honoraria as an advisor to Abbott Australia Pty Ltd. and travel grants from Roche Products NZ Ltd., Novartis NZ Ltd., and Fresenius Medical Care–Asia-Pacific Pty Ltd. K.L.L. has received travel grants from Roche Products NZ Ltd and Fresenius Medical Care–Asia-Pacific Pty Ltd. This does not alter the authors' adherence to all the PLOS ONE policies on sharing data and materials.

* E-mail: mrmarshall@middlemore.co.nz

Introduction

In New Zealand (NZ), there is general consensus that dialysis at home is preferred to dialysis at medical facilities for clinically appropriate people with end-stage kidney disease (ESKD) [1]. This is driven by clinical, patient-centred and health delivery considerations. Research and cumulative clinical experience both point to better survival and patient experience for those dialysing at home compared to those dialysing in facilities [2–6]. Economic evaluations consistently demonstrate lower cost for home dialysis compared to facility dialysis [7,8]. Driven by these factors, there has been a longstanding culture of promoting home dialysis in NZ, resulting in a prevalence that is higher than all but one of the other Organisation for Economic Co-operation and Development (OECD) nations [9].

Globally, there is a resurgence of interest in home dialysis, driven by the identifiable benefits and also the need for cost containment in the context of unstable global economic conditions [10–12]. A key issue for those promoting home dialysis is the validity and extent of the assertion of better outcomes with home dialysis. This assertion is founded on a range of observational analyses that are biased by a number of issues, the most significant being selection bias. In this regard, NZ is a valuable setting for repeating these analyses, due to its uniquely high prevalence of both home HD and PD. This situation usually translates to improved internal validity through less selection bias, and provides sufficient statistical power to allow simultaneous comparisons of all modalities including home HD. In addition, NZ is a economically developed nation with results that are reasonably generalizable. In this research, we address the following clinical question: In a country such as NZ, is home dialysis independently associated with better survival than facility haemodialysis (HD), accounting for patient characteristics?

Table 1. Clinical characteristics of the inception cohort.

Variable		Study Cohort	Excluded Cohort with Missing Data
Number		6,419	64
Age	Years	59.2 (49.3, 68.1)	60.6 (51.5, 66.1)
Gender	Male	3,838 (59.2)	40 (62.5)
	Female	2,581 (40.2)	24 (37.5)
Ethnicity	NZ European-&-Other	2,921 (45.5)	30 (46.9)
	NZ Maori	2,053 (32)	28 (43.8)
	Asian	378 (5.9)	1 (1.6)
	Pacific People	1,067 (16.6)	5 (7.8)
Late referral*		1,486 (23.1)	26 (35.9)
eGFR*	mL/min/1.73 m^2	6.2 (4.3, 8.8)	4.7 (0,7.5)
Smoking*		1,073 (16.7)	11 (17.2)
Diabetes Mellitus*	Type 1	220 (3.4)	3 (4.7)
	Type 2	2,997 (46.7)	36 (56.3)
Primary renal	Glomerulonephritis/Other	2,797 (43.6)	22 (34.4)
Disease	Hypertension/Ischemic	743 (11.6)	13 (20.3)
	Diabetic nephropathy	2,879 (44.9)	29 (45.3)
Co-morbid disease	Coronary artery	2,422 (37.7)	30 (46.9)
at baseline	Peripheral vascular*	1,528 (23.8)	27 (42.2)
	Cerebrovascular	893 (13.8)	13 (20.3)
	Lung	1,111 (17.3)	17 (26.6)
Co-morbid disease	Coronary artery	2,871 (44.7)	32 (50)
at end of follow-up	Peripheral vascular*	1,850 (28.8)	29 (45.3)
	Cerebrovascular	1,068 (16.6)	13 (20.3)
	Lung	1,279 (19.9)	18 (28.1)
Body mass index*	kg/m^2	28.1 (24.2, 3.8)	33.3 (25.5, 36.4)

***Note*:** Continuous variables are shown as median (25th, 75th percentile); categorical variables are shown are number (percentage). For the excluded cohort with missing data, the sum of patients within each category equals the number of patients of within this cohort who have data pertaining to that category.
*$P<0.05$ for study cohort versus excluded cohort with missing data.

We present analyses in a restricted cohort of New Zealanders from the Australian and New Zealand Dialysis and Transplant Registry (ANZDATA) Registry which has prospectively collected data on ESKD patients in these countries since 1963 (www.anzdata.org.au). We compare survival over a 15-year period between those treated with home dialysis and those treated with facility HD, adjusting for measured patient risk factors such as age and co-morbidity.

Methods

Study Design

We performed a cohort study, using an as-treated framework ("did the exposure that the patient actually receive affect mortality?"), as opposed to an intention-to-treat framework ("did exposure that the patient initially receive affect mortality, irrespective of subsequent changes that occurred along the way?") [13]. The study protocol was reviewed and approved by the National (NZ) Health and Disability Ethics Committee (IORG0000895) and the Counties Manukau Institutional Review Board, and the need for patient consent waived under the provisions for retrospective audit and observational study.

Participants and Data Source

The ANZDATA Registry collects data on all ESKD patients from every dialysis centre in Australia and NZ. ESKD patients are defined as those with a diagnosis of chronic kidney disease, and for whom renal replacement therapy is intended to be an indefinite treatment. Until 2004, data collection rounds occurred at 6-monthly intervals (31 March and 30 September). Since 2004, rounds have occurred annually (31 December). Details of the structure and methods of the registry have been reported elsewhere [14].

We created an inception cohort of adult ESKD patients ($\geq$18 years at dialysis inception), whose first episode renal replacement therapy occurred after 1-Jan-1997 in NZ. Prevalent patients at the start of the period of observation were not included, a measure which avoids lead time bias, and immortal time bias. Patients were followed through their entire patient journey until death or 31-December-2011, whichever occurred first. Censoring was at the time of kidney transplantation, return of renal function or loss to follow-up.

Primary Exposure and Outcome Variables

The primary exposure in this study is time-varying dialysis modality. The exposure of 'facility HD' was defined as dialysis in a

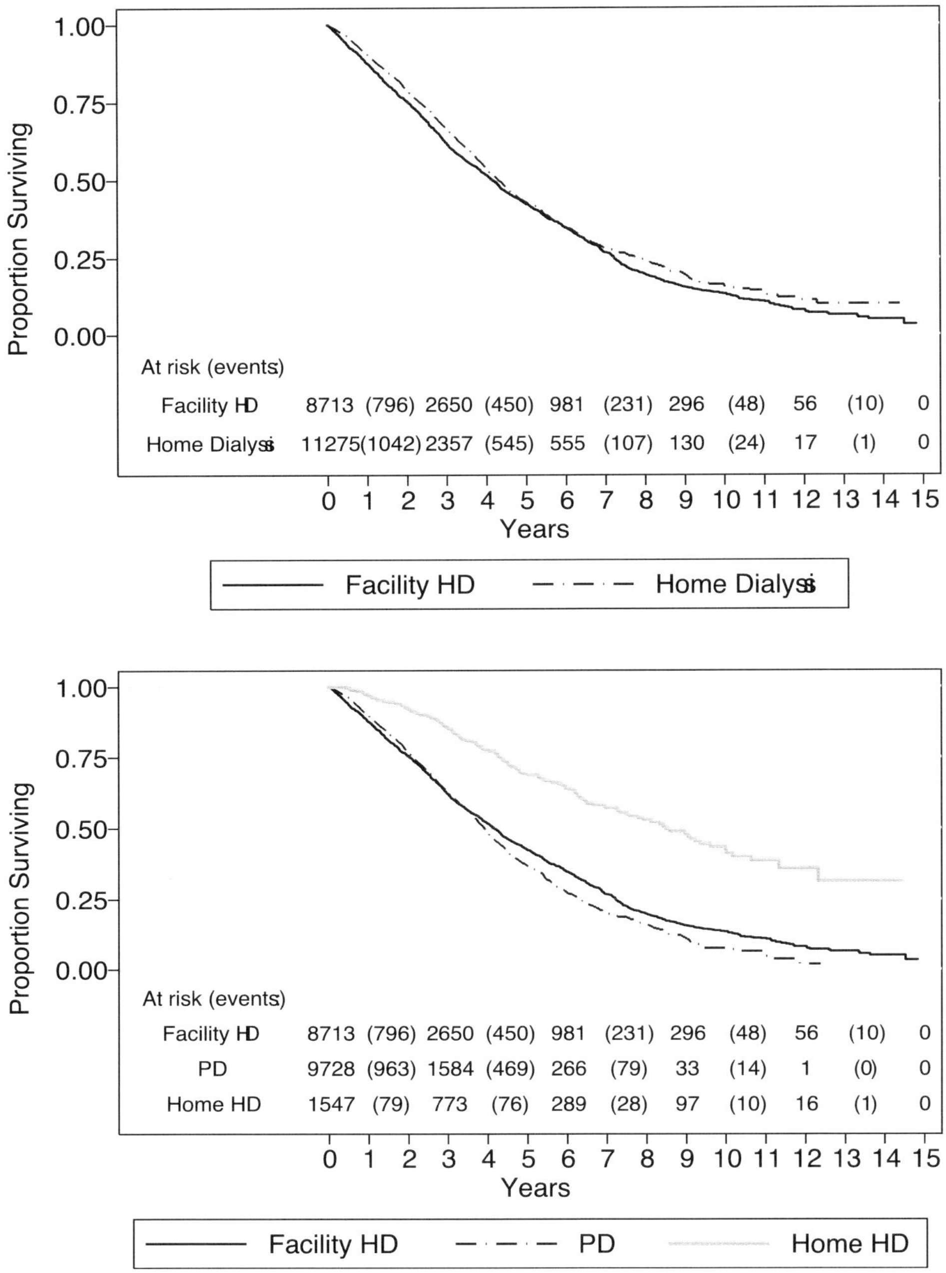

Figure 1. Kaplan Meier estimates of survival. Abbreviations: HD, haemodialysis; PD, peritoneal dialysis.

dependent fashion at a staffed hospital or satellite dialysis HD unit, and the exposure of 'home dialysis' was defined as dialysis in an independent fashion in an unstaffed setting using either HD or peritoneal dialysis (PD). Home dialysis was further analysed in separate categories of PD or home HD. We did not further subcategorize HD modalities as being frequent or extended hours: a previous study in Australia and NZ has shown mortality benefit with home HD and its related characteristics, but not with frequent/extended operating characteristics per se [4].

The primary outcome was patient mortality, based upon details provided by the treating nephrologist.

Data Measurement and Quantitative Variables

We adjusted for known patient-related risk factors collected in the ANZDATA Registry: age, gender, ethnicity, primary kidney disease, estimated glomerular filtration rate (eGFR) [15], late referral for nephrology pre-dialysis care (<3 months before dialysis inception), diabetes mellitus (none, type 1, type 2), body mass index (BMI), medical co-morbidity (coronary artery disease, peripheral vascular disease, cerebrovascular disease, chronic lung disease), smoking, plasma hemoglobin, and year of dialysis inception to account for any secular variation. We did not include serum calcium/phosphate, since these data have only been collected since 1 October 2003. Medical co-morbidity was

Table 2. Clinical characteristics of the study cohort at modality inception.

Variable		Facility Hemodialysis	Peritoneal Dialysis	Home Hemodialysis	Home Dialysis
Number		8.713	9,728	1,547	11,275
Age*#	Years	57.3 (47.6, 65.9)	59.8 (50.2, 68.5)	50.7 (41.5, 59.3)	58
Gender*#	Male	5,258 (60.3)	5,412 (55.6)	1,061 (68.6)	6,473 (57.4)
	Female	3,455 (39.7)	4,316 (44.4)	486 (31.4)	4,802 (42.6)
Ethnicity*#	NZ European-&-Other	3, 169 (36.4)	4,590 (47.2)	748 (48.4)	5,338 (47.3)
	NZ Maori	3,068 (35.2)	3,309 (34)	542 (35)	3,3851 (34.2)
	Asian	465 (5.3)	611 (6.3)	57 (3.7)	688 (5.9)
	Pacific People	2,011 (23.08)	1,218 (12.5)	200 (12.9)	1,418 (12.6)
Late referral*#		2,310 (26.5)	2,293 (23.6)	290 (18.8)	2,583 (22.9)
eGFR*#	mL/min/1.73 m^2	5.8 (4.1, 8.2)	6.5 (4.5, 9.1)	5.7 (3.8, 7.6)	6.4 (4.4, 8.9)
Smoking		1,537 (17.6)	1,672 (17.2)	264 (17.1)	1,936 (17.2)
Diabetes Mellitus*#	Type 1	246 (2.8)	404 (4.3)	46 (2.8)	450 (4.0)
	Type 2	4,378 (50.3)	4,381 (45)	537 (34.7)	4,918 (43.6)
Primary renal*#	Glomerulonephritis/Other	3,694 (42.4)	4,106 (42.2)	918 (59.3)	5,024 (44.6)
Disease	Hypertension/Ischemic	846 (9.71)	1,259 (12.9)	127 (8.2)	1,386 (12.3)
	Diabetic nephropathy	4,173 (47.9)	4.363 (44.9)	502 (32.5)	4,865 (43.1)
Co-morbid disease	Coronary artery*#	3,521 (40.5)	3,950 (40.6)	453 (29.3)	4,403 (39.1)
at baseline	Peripheral vascular*	2,236 (25.7)	2,645 (27.2)	232 (15)	2,877 (25.5)
	Cerebrovascular*	1,251 (14.4)	1,538 (15.8)	108 (7)	1,646 (14.6)
	Lung*#	1,713 (19.7)	1,684 (17.3)	231 (14.9)	1,915 (17.0)
Co-morbid disease	Coronary artery*#	4,118 (47.3)	4,573 (47)	550 (35.6)	5,123 (45.4)
at end of follow-up	Peripheral vascular*	2,633 (30.2)	3,151 (32.4)	298 (19.3)	3,449 (30.6)
	Cerebrovascular*	1,454 (16.7)	1,848 (19)	136 (8.8)	1,984 (17.6)
	Lung*#	1,965 (22.6)	1,894 (19.5)	277 (17.9)	2,171 (19.3)
Body mass index*	kg/m^2	29.0 (24.8, 34.2)	27.3 (24, 31.1)	29.7 (25.4, 36.9)	27.6 (24.1, 31.6)

***Note*:** Continuous variables are shown as median (25th, 75th percentile); categorical variables are shown are number (percentage).
*P<0.05 for facility versus home.
#P<0.05 for facility versus peritoneal dialysis versus home hemodialysis.
Patients may be classified in multiple modality categories due to multiple exposures over the duration of their follow-up.

modeled as time-varying, according to presence or absence at the point of each modality change.

Statistical Methods

We constructed exposure-outcome models for survival using Cox proportional hazards regression. For all comparative analyses of mortality risk by modality, we modeled facility HD as the reference category. In the first set of analyses, we compared facility HD with home dialysis, and in the second set we compared facility HD with PD and home HD separately. Modality was modelled as time varying, and handled by episode-splitting within patients, assuming a constant hazard rate within time periods of modality.

We used two and three way interaction terms in the main-effects models to test effect modification by age, ethnicity, comorbidity, BMI, the presence and type of diabetes mellitus, and year of dialysis inception. We chose these interactions as being clinically plausible, on the basis of both published literature as well as cumulative clinical experience. Interactions were assessed using the two-tailed Wald test P values as a guide to selecting interaction terms for testing, with significance within the model using the likelihood ratio test (P value <0.05). Where effect modification was evinced, separate models were developed in each subgroup.

Continuous co-variates such as age and BMI were modeled as quantiles in order to avoid the assumption of linear relationships. We removed co-variates from the multivariate model in a backward stepwise fashion beginning with the co-variate with the highest P value from two-tailed Wald tests of the individual coefficients, using the partial likelihood ratio test to compare the new reduced model with the older larger. We based final confounder selection upon both biological plausibility and contribution to the comprehensibility of the model, and also the significance of the co-variate within the model as assessed by the two-tailed partial likelihood ratio test P value at a level of <0.2 when jointly adjusted for other covariates.

The findings of this study are largely expected and confirmatory, although there are novel findings. We re-iterate that our facility HD and PD populations were very balanced in terms of demographics and co-comorbidity, and that very few studies in the literature report outcomes that compare all three dialysis modalities (facility HD, PD and home HD). In our study, there are sufficient data-points for us to estimate the effects of facility HD and home HD separately, and treat the exposures separately. As such, our data allow us demonstrate the extended duration of the survival advantage with PD compared to facility HD, with perhaps more confidence than other investigators. In addition, this

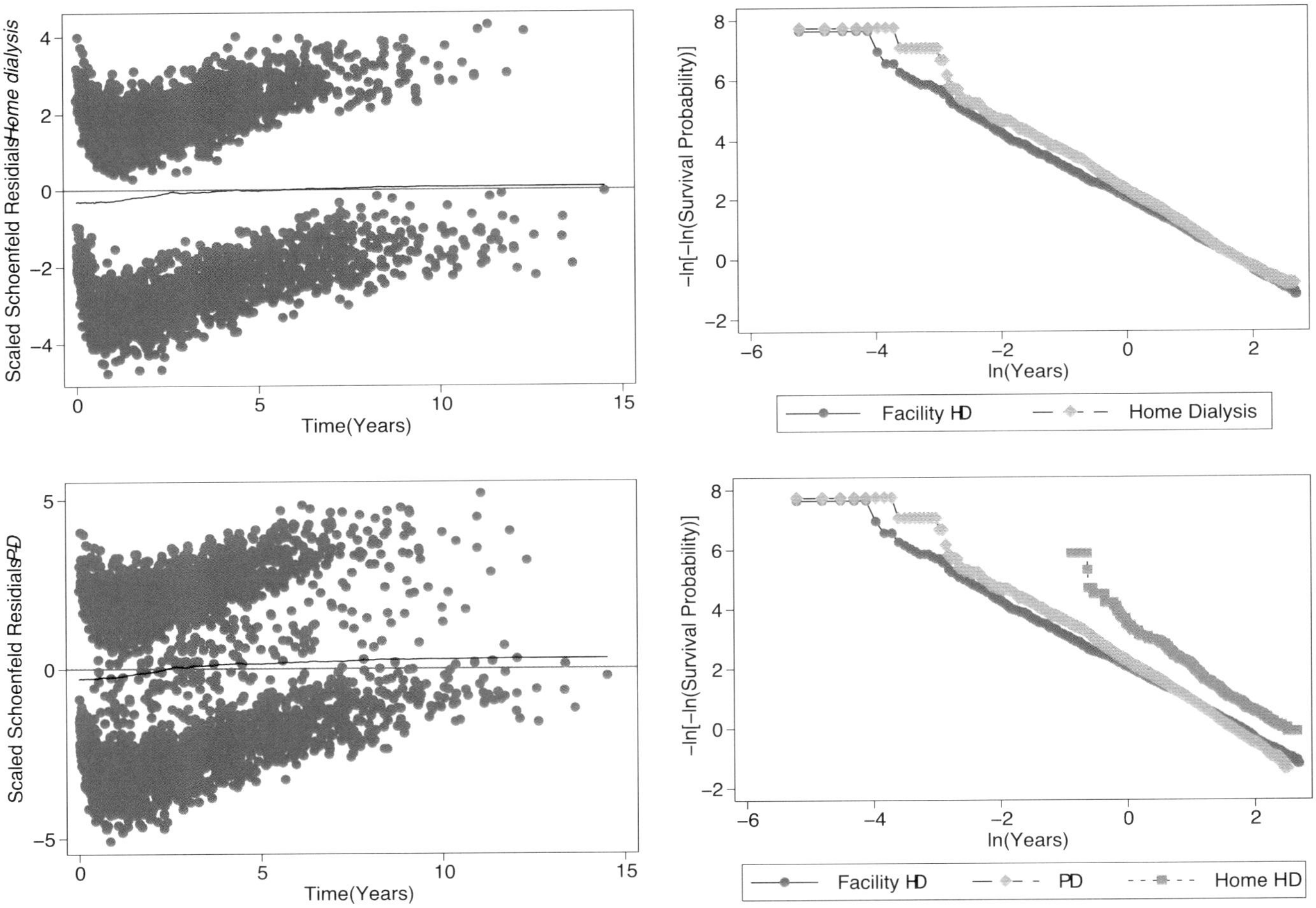

Figure 2. Time dependence of effects Illustrated using -ln [-ln(survival)] versus ln(analysis time) plots (left) and scaled Schoenfeld residuals plots (right). Plots for facility HD versus home dialysis are in the top panels, and for facility HD versus PD and home HD on the bottom.

also allows us to directly compare PD (10880 records, 3738 patients, 1525 failures) with home HD (1942 records, 1942 patients, 194 failures) as sub-modalities of home dialysis. In our study, it is clear that home HD is associated with the lowest mortality risk of the home modalities, even within the first 3 years: the a hazard ratio for death (95% confidence intervals) with home HD is 0.52 (0.41–0.65) compared to PD in the early period.

We included a gamma distributed shared frailty, using the center of initial dialysis treatment as the group. This procedure adds a random effect to model heterogeneity of effect across defined groups, and accounts in this case for the 'treatment-by-centre' interaction. We included a shared frailty in the final model based upon significance at a level of <0.05 as assessed by the two-tailed partial likelihood ratio test.

The assumption for proportional hazards for the final models was assessed formally by the use of scaled Schoenfeld residuals, and visually by -ln [-ln(survival)] versus ln(analysis time) plots for modality, adjusted for confounders. We assessed overall goodness of fit visually by comparing plots of Kaplan-Meier observed survival curves to the Cox predicted curves for modality.

Where necessary, comparisons between groups were made using the Student's t-test, Mann–Whitney U or Kruskal–Wallis tests, or chi-square test as appropriate.

Statistical significance to associations was attributed to findings if the two-tailed P value was <0.05.

We used Stata Intercooled MP/11.2 for analyses (StataCorp, www.stata.com).

Results

Participants and Outcome Data

We identified an inception cohort of 6483 adult patients with 3298 deaths over 20,123 patient-years follow-up. There were 6419 with 3254 deaths over 20,042 patient-years of follow-up with sufficient data for modelling: Table 1 summarizes the inception and study cohorts. Of note, those with missing data had a higher probability of being late referrals with a low eGFR at dialysis inception, active smokers, and diabetes mellitus. Of the modelled deaths, 52% were due to cardiovascular causes, 14% due to infectious causes, and the remainder due to treatment withdrawal, cancer and other causes.

Descriptive Data

Table 2 summarizes patient characteristics of the study cohort at modality inception (the point of commencement of dialysis modality). In this table only, some patients are classified in multiple modality categories according to their time-varying exposure over the period of observation, although for Table 1 and all analyses of mortality by modality every patient is "counted" only once. Patients treated with facility HD and PD had comparable demographics and co-morbidity. Compared to those treated with

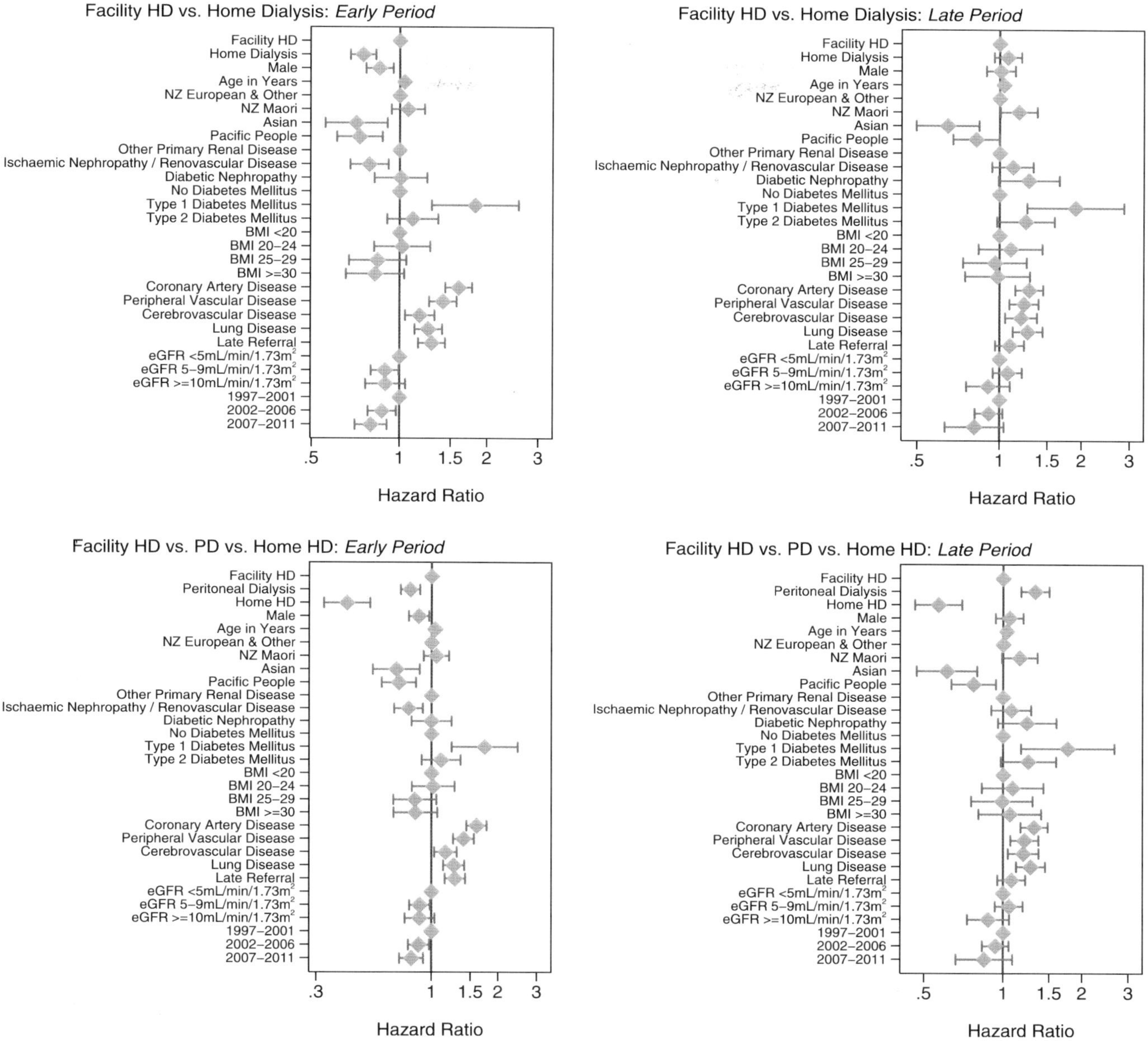

Figure 3. Hazard ratios for mortality from the main effects model comparing facility HD versus home dialysis (top panels) and facility HD versus PD and home HD (bottom panels), fully adjusted for the confounders listed in Table 2 (the markers represent point estimates, and the whiskers 95% confidence intervals). Estimates of effect for follow-up<3years are on the left ("Early period"); corresponding estimates for follow-up>3years are on the right ("Late period"). Abbreviations: BMI, body mass index; eGFR, estimated glomerular filtration rate; HD, haemodialysis; NZ, New Zealand; PD, peritoneal dialysis.

facility HD or PD, however, patients on home HD were younger, more likely to have ESKD secondary to single-organ (e.g. glomerulonephritis) rather than systemic disease, and less likely to have diabetes mellitus or medical co-morbidity.

Kaplan Meier estimates of survival by modality are illustrated in Figure 1. The unadjusted median (interquartile range) survival for all patients in the study sample is 4.27 (4.12, 4.38) years. The corresponding values for those on facility HD and home dialysis are 4.16 (2.05, 7.23) and 4.30 (2.35, 7.79) years. The corresponding values for PD and home HD are 3.92 (2.11, 6.34) and 8.49 (4.30, −) years.

Main Results

In the first set of analyses, we compared facility HD to home dialysis. In the second set of analyses, we compared facility HD with PD and home HD separately. All comparative results of mortality risk by modality are reported as hazard ratios relative to the reference category of facility HD.

Initial modelling demonstrated loss of proportional hazards for the variable home dialysis ($P = 0.0021$) and with the second set analyses confirming this for those on PD ($P<0.00005$) but not those treated with home HD ($P = 0.36$). Further modelling of the interaction between modality and time on dialysis show that both home dialysis and PD interacted with time at all levels up to and including 3 years (lower risk before, with higher risk of death after

Table 3. Time dependency of treatment effects, fully adjusted for the co-variates listed in Table 2.

Modality	Time Interaction Term	Time on Dialysis	Before	During	After
				Hazard ratio for mortality (95% CI)	
Home dialysis	Continuous/ linear	1 year	0.68 (0.58–0.80)*		1.47 (1.23–1.47)**
	Continuous/ linear	2 years	0.80 (0.70–0.87)*		1.33 (1.14–1.53)**
	Continuous/ linear	3 years	0.81 (0.74–0.89)*		1.36 (1.17–1.57)**
	Category	0–1 years		1.0	
	Category	1–2 years		1.29 (1.00–1.61)#	
	Category	2–3 years		1.25 (0.98–1.57)	
	Category	≥3 years		1.57 (1.30–1.90)#	
Peritoneal dialysis	Continuous/ linear	1 year	0.70 (0.60–0.82)*		1.64 (1.37–1.96)**
	Continuous/ linear	2 years	0.83 (0.74–0.93)*		1.47 (1.27–1.71)**
	Continuous/ linear	3 years	0.87 (0.79–0.96)*		1.54 (1.33–1.80)**
	Category	0–1 years		1.0	
	Category	1–2 years		1.35 (1.01–1.70)#	
	Category	2–3 years		1.32 (1.00–1.67)	
	Category	≥3 years		1.84 (1.51–2.24)#	

* $P<0.05$ versus facility HD.
** $P<0.05$ versus hazard ratio during earlier period.
#$P<0.05$ versus the baseline category of 0–1 years.
The interaction between modality and time is explored as a linear function of time on dialysis, and also a categorical one. Only results for home dialysis and PD are shown; home HD is not included since we did not identify any time dependency of effect. When modeling the treatment effect as a linear function of time, the point estimates in the later period indicate the additional change in effect during that period. For instance, the point estimates for home dialysis indicate a 19% reduction in mortality risk in the first 3 years, offset by an further 36% increase in relative risk in the period after three years for a total 10% increase in risk in the later period; explicitly, $(1-1.36)*(1-0.81)+0.81 = 0.10$. When modeling the treatment effect as a categorical function of time, the point estimates in the later period indicate the further change in effect during that period relative to the baseline category, in this case 0–1 years.

each time period compared to facility dialysis, see Table 3 and Figure 2). On this basis, we estimated main and interaction effects models for follow-up periods of <3 years (referred to hereafter as the "early" period) and >3 years (the "late" period).

The results of the first set of analyses (comparing facility HD to home dialysis) are illustrated and tabulated in Figure 3 (top panels) and Table 4. Overall, there is a 13% lower mortality risk associated with home dialysis. However, the presence and extent of this effect varies over time: it is most marked in the early period and not apparent in the late period.

The results of the second set of analyses (comparing facility HD with PD and home HD separately) are provided in Figure 3 (bottom panels) and Table 5. Overall, there is no difference in mortality risk between PD and facility HD, although there is a 20% lower mortality risk associated with PD in the early period that is offset by a 33% greater mortality risk in the late period. Overall, there is a 52% lower mortality risk associated with home HD, with no significant variation of the presence and extent of this effect over time.

Two-way and Three-way Interactions

In the first set of analyses, the effect of modality on mortality risk is not modified within subcategories of patient age, ethnicity, BMI, and year of dialysis inception. There is, however, notable modification of effect among patients with medical comorbidity. As per Table 4, the mortality risk associated with home dialysis and facility HD is similar in the early period in these groups, with an actual reversal of effect in those with type 2 diabetes mellitus in the late period: in these patients, there is a 28% higher mortality risk associated with home dialysis compared to facility HD. In the first set of analyses, there are no three-way interactions of statistical significance.

In the second set of analyses, the effect of modality on mortality risk is not modified within subcategories of patient age and BMI. There is minor modification of effect by the presence of medical comorbidity and by year of dialysis inception, although the results among subcategories of comorbidity and year are not materially different from those in the overall population. There is, however, notable modification of effect by ethnicity, and the presence and type of diabetes mellitus.

For PD, NZ European-&-Other patients as well as those without type 2 diabetes mellitus have a lower associated mortality risk compared to facility HD in the early period, and no difference in the late period. In NZ Maori and Pacific People and those with type 2 diabetes mellitus, there is no difference in mortality risk between PD and facility HD in the early period, and a higher mortality risk associated with PD in the late period.

For home HD, there is only minor modification of effect by most of these factors, although this may be due to the low statistical power in this group. Notwithstanding, there may be important modification of effect by ethnicity: in Pacific People,

Table 4. Overall population conditional effects of modality on mortality, and interaction effects, fully adjusted for the co-variates in Table 2.

		Follow-up	Home Dialysis
			Hazard ratio for mortality (95% CI)
Total population		Overall	0.87 (0.81–0.94)*
		<3 years	0.75 (0.68–0.83)*
		>3 years	1.07 (0.96–1.21)
Comorbidity#	Absent	Overall	0.78 (0.67–0.90)*
		<3 years	0.64 (0.52–0.78)*
		>3 years	1.07 (0.85–1.35)
	Present	Overall	0.93 (0.85–1.01)
		<3 years	0.81 (0.72–0.91)*
		>3 years	1.08 (0.94–1.23)
Diabetes mellitus#	Absent	Overall	0.74 (0.66–0.83)*
		<3 years	0.65 (0.56–0.75)*
		>3 years	0.91 (0.77–1.09)
	Type 1	Overall	0.48 (0.29–0.78)*
		<3 years	0.38 (0.20–0.73)*
		>3 years	0.66 (0.32–1.33)
	Type 2	Overall	1.04 (0.94–1.16)
		<3 years	0.92 (0.80–1.05)
		>3 years	1.28 (1.10–1.50)*

*P values <0.05 relative to reference modality.
#P values <0.05 for interaction.
In the home dialysis, the primary exposure was defined as either PD or home HD. Facility HD is the reference modality.

there is no difference in mortality risk between home HD and facility HD.

In the second set of analyses, there is a single three-way interaction of borderline statistical significance, between subcategories of ethnicity and year of dialysis inception. Exploration of this interaction within these subcategories produced results that are not materially different from those in the overall population (data not shown).

Discussion

Our study generally supports the clinical and organizational culture of promoting home dialysis in NZ. Our main observations are from models that are fully adjusted for patient risk factors such as patient age and co-morbidity: 1) compared to facility HD, home dialysis is independently associated with improved overall survival; (2) compared to facility HD and PD, home HD is associated with the best overall survival; and (3) compared to facility HD, PD is associated with equivalent overall survival.

Our results comparing home HD and facility HD are consistent with those in the literature, including those found in a previous study of an Australian and NZ cohort: home HD has equivalent or better overall survival compared to facility HD and PD [4,16–28]. We did not identify any modification of effect by time on dialysis or patient characteristics, with reasonable allowance for the reduced statistical power within this small group. In contrast, only some of our results comparing PD and facility HD are consistent with those in the literature, with particular differences around statistical interactions in our models. Traditionally, the effect of PD on survival is modified by time on dialysis [29–33], era [34], diabetes mellitus [4,29–31,33,35–40], age [4,29–31,33,35,36,40], BMI [32,39,41–43] and co-morbidity [37,38]. The points of difference in our study are 1) the longer duration (3 years) of early relative survival advantage with PD than is usually described; 2) stable rather than improving relative survival with PD over time; 3) the absence of any modification of effect by age or BMI; and 4) the modification of effect by ethnicity.

The duration of early survival advantage with PD in our study was found to be longer than the 1–2 years usually identified by other investigators [29–32], and this finding persists in a variety of sensitivity analyses as shown in Table 2. The decreasing comparative survival with PD over time is usually attributed to diminishing residual renal function, changing peritoneal function with generally decreasing ultrafiltration capacity, and the use of central venous catheters early in the course of those starting dialysis with HD. It is likely that these factors are also present in our study population. The longer duration of early survival advantage in our study probably arises in part from the separation of home HD from facility HD in our analysis. This is different from the customary approach of all but one of the analysis in the literature, which traditionally compares PD with all HD, considering facility and home HD together irrespective of setting. Our approach allows for the correct handling of facility HD, modelling clinical outcomes that are more realistic than they might otherwise appear when facility HD is combined with home HD, which is the customary practice in most previous research. Our findings raise the possibility that the extent and duration of survival benefit associated with early PD may in fact be underestimated in the literature.

In our study, we were not able to identify secular improvements in relative survival over time. Such improvements have been noted

Table 5. Overall population conditional effects of modality on mortality, and interaction effects, fully adjusted for the co-variates in Table 2.

			Peritoneal Dialysis	Home Hemodialysis
			Hazard ratio for mortality (95% CI)	
Total Population			0.98 (0.90–1.06)	0.48 (0.41–0.56)*
		follow-up<3 years	0.80 (0.72–0.88)*	0.41 (0.32–0.53)*
		follow-up>3 years	1.33 (1.17–1.50)*	0.57 (0.46–0.70)*
Ethnicity#	NZ European-&-Other	Overall	0.80 (0.71–0.90)*	0.34 (0.26–0.43)*
		follow-up<3 years	0.66 (0.57–0.76)*	0.28 (0.19–0.40)*
		follow-up>3 years	1.14 (0.93–1.38)	0.44 (0.31–0.61)*
	NZ Maori	Overall	1.15 (1.00–1.31)*	0.60 (0.48–0.76)*
		follow-up<3 years	1.04 (0.87–1.24)	0.61 (0.43–0.88)*
		follow-up>3 years	1.31 (1.07–1.61)*	0.60 (0.45–0.81)*
	Asian	Overall	1.00 (0.69–1.45)	0.61 (0.18–2.00)
		follow-up<3 years	0.72 (0.44–1.17)	0.54 (0.07–4.16)
		follow-up>3 years	1.29 (0.75–2.20)	0.45 (0.11–1.90)
	Pacific People	Overall	1.31 (1.06–1.63)*	0.81 (0.50–1.38)
		follow-up<3 years	1.01 (0.75–1.36)	0.91 (0.43–1.92)
		follow-up>3 years	1.87 (1.36–2.58)*	0.74 (0.35–1.57)
Comorbidity#	Absent	Overall	0.87 (0.74–1.02)	0.48 (0.37–0.63)*
		follow-up<3 years	0.68 (0.55–0.83)*	0.45 (0.30–0.66)*
		follow-up>3 years	1.37 (1.07–1.75)*	0.59 (0.40–0.86)*
	Present	Overall	1.02 (0.93–1.12)	0.48 (0.40–0.58)*
		follow-up<3 years	0.86 (0.76–0.96)*	0.39 (0.29–0.54)*
		follow-up>3 years	1.34 (1.16–1.54)*	0.57 (0.44–0.73)*
Diabetes mellitus#	Absent	Overall	0.85 (0.76–0.96)*	0.37 (0.29–0.47)*
		follow-up<3 years	0.69 (0.59–0.81)*	0.34 (0.24–0.49)*
		follow-up>3 years	1.16 (0.96–1.40)	0.41 (0.30–0.56)*
	Type 1	Overall	0.48 (0.29–0.80)*	0.44 (0.19–1.03)
		follow-up<3 years	0.42 (0.22–0.82)*	0.20 (0.04–0.90)*
		follow-up>3 years	0.62 (0.29–1.33)	0.92 (0.35–2.46)
	Type 2	Overall	1.15 (1.03–1.29)*	0.64 (0.52–0.80)*
		follow-up<3 years	0.95 (0.83–1.09)	0.60 (0.41–0.81)*
		follow-up>3 years	1.54 (1.30–1.82)*	0.70 (0.53–0.94)*
Year of dialysis Inception#	1997–2001	Overall	1.00 (0.87–1.13)	0.49 (0.39–0.62)*
		follow-up<3 years	0.71 (0.59–0.86)*	0.49 (0.33–0.71)*
		follow-up>3 years	1.43 (1.18–1.72)*	0.50 (0.36–0.68)*
	2002–2006	Overall	0.98 (0.87–1.11)*	0.51 (0.40–0.65)*
		follow-up<3 years	0.81 (0.69–0.96)*	0.43 (0.29–0.63)*
		follow-up>3 years	1.25 (1.04–1.49)*	0.60 (0.44–0.81)*
	2007–2011	Overall	0.86 (0.72–1.03)*	0.39 (0.26–0.62)*
		follow-up<3 years	0.79 (0.65–0.96)*	0.28 (0.16–0.50)*
		follow-up>3 years	1.47 (0.86–2.51)	0.96 (0.44–2.08)

*P values <0.05 relative to reference modality.
#P values <0.05 for interaction.
Conventional facility HD is the reference modality.

for of PD patients in particular, albeit mostly in the United States where there is a particularly low prevalence of PD [44,45]. It is likely that this has arisen from improvements to care over time, and such improvements are usually considered to include the introduction of disconnect systems, a shift from CAPD to APD, and the penetration of icodextrin and biocompatible dialysis solutions. There have been similar changes in NZ: the percentages of those APD, icodextrin and biocompatible dialysis solutions in close to zero in 1996 and 44%, 46%, 3% respectively in 2011. However, as stated, these changes have not been associated with the expected improvement in patient survival. This raises the possibility that improved outcomes for PD patients reported in the literature are less the result of technical advances, and perhaps more the result of increased experience and improved clinical care in regions where exposure to PD is low. In NZ, there is already longstanding experience with PD among the NZ nephrology community, and is likely to translate into stable practices based on a large amount of cumulative clinical knowledge and heuristics.

We did not identify any differences in early survival benefit associated with PD across subpopulations of patient age. In other studies in the literature, age probably functions as a marker of frail phenotype with increased (unmeasured) medical co-morbidity. We speculate that ethnicity may be functioning similarly in our study. However, ethnicity may also be exerting an effect through other unmeasured factors, such as socioeconomic status (lower status which is known to influence the technical success of dialysis at home [46,47]), and also perhaps rurality (greater rurality is known to increase uptake of PD in those with poor access to facility dialysis and reluctance to relocate, irrespective of whether or not they are marginal or even frankly inappropriate for PD [48,49]). Notwithstanding, the relatively poorer survival of NZ Maori and Pacific People on PD warrants further study, and perhaps an augmented clinical approach if findings are confirmed.

There will always be controversy as to the underlying reason for the better survival observed on home HD. On the one hand, there are no high quality (clinical trial) data showing that dialyses in the home environment in itself influences mortality. Using this reasoning, the observation of better survival should be ascribed to differences in the treatment itself (home HD being prescribed and delivered in a way that better manages fluid overload and uremia), or in the patients who undergo the treatment (home dialysis patients having unmeasured associated factors that result in better survival). On the other hand, there are consistent observational data showing better survival on home dialysis, with studies demonstrating that this is not entirely explained by age, measured co-morbidity, or the dialysis prescription [4]. Our own opinion is that there is a causal relationship between the home setting and better survival, probably mediated by greater adherence to dialysis, medication, fluid restriction, and lifestyle measures [7,50–54]. It is plausible that these factors are also enablers to higher quality dialysis therapy, explaining the lower reported rates of technical and infectious events that is observed with home versus facility HD in the NZ setting [4,55]. We are unable to explore these factors currently due to lack of appropriate data in the ANZDATA Registry. However, we are planning further analyses using database linkage to routinely collected NZ government datasets, with a view to reducing unmeasured confounding in our analyses by including domiciliary/social circumstances, socioeconomic deprivation, primary and secondary healthcare utilization, and medication prescription as co-variates. Notwithstanding, it is our opinion that the observed benefit of home HD arises in part from an enhanced culture of self-care with identified benefits as described.

Our results support an early survival advantage for PD, and the paradigm of a "PD first" policy which is under consideration in some parts of NZ. Our results also suggest the pressing need for study to determine optimal timing for switching modalities from PD to HD, which is surprisingly poorly researched given the importance of the issue. Timely transition from PD to HD in the late phase is associated with better survival, as is the avoidance of transition to PD after an unplanned start on HD in the early phase [56–58]. Our research suggests an appropriately powered randomized controlled trial, allocating patients to a switch from PD to HD at different pre-determined intervals, with appropriate collection of clinical and biochemical information from which to develop criteria and decision support systems.

As is the case for all observational studies, associations do not prove causality. Our study is likely to be limited by ascertainment error in the recording of co-morbidity, residual confounding from the limited collection of co-morbidity, and lack of socioeconomic, medication, and biochemical data in the analyses. Notwithstanding, our study supports the widespread adoption of home dialysis in NZ, and a drive to further increase home dialysis in that country. The immediate next steps for our research team include the following initiatives. We are planning further analyses in the NZ dialysis population that (i) incorporate additional measures of patients' socioeconomic and functional status from data lonkage with government datasets, and (ii) address the variable and interchangeable exposure of patients in this country to HDF and frequent/extended HD during the course of their modality experience.

Acknowledgments

The ANZDATA Registry exists because of the tireless work of the nephrology community throughout Australia and New Zealand in collecting the information.

Author Contributions

Conceived and designed the experiments: MRM RCW KLL. Performed the experiments: MRM KRP. Analyzed the data: MRM KRP. Contributed reagents/materials/analysis tools: MRM KRP. Wrote the paper: MRM RCW KRP KLL.

References

1. Lynn KL, Buttimore AL (2005) Future of home haemodialysis in Australia and New Zealand. Nephrology (Carlton) 10: 231–233.
2. McGregor D, Buttimore A, Robson R, Little P, Morton J, et al. (2000) Thirty years of universal home dialysis in Christchurch. N Z Med J 113: 27–29.
3. Blagg CR (2005) Home haemodialysis: 'home, home, sweet, sweet home!'. Nephrology (Carlton) 10: 206–214.
4. Marshall MR, Hawley CM, Kerr PG, Polkinghorne KR, Marshall RJ, et al. (2011) Home hemodialysis and mortality risk in Australian and New Zealand populations. Am J Kidney Dis 58: 782–793.
5. Wyld M, Morton RL, Hayen A, Howard K, Webster AC (2012) A systematic review and meta-analysis of utility-based quality of life in chronic kidney disease treatments. PLoS Med 9: e1001307.
6. Dale PL, Hutton J, Elgazzar H (2008) Utility of health states in chronic kidney disease: a structured review of the literature. Curr Med Res Opin 24: 193–206.
7. Mowatt G, Vale L, MacLeod A (2004) Systematic review of the effectiveness of home versus hospital or satellite unit hemodialysis for people with end-stage renal failure. Int J Technol Assess Health Care 20: 258–268.
8. Mowatt G, Vale L, Perez J, Wyness L, Fraser C, et al. (2003) Systematic review of the effectiveness and cost-effectiveness, and economic evaluation, of home versus hospital or satellite unit haemodialysis for people with end-stage renal failure. Health Technol Assess 7: 1–174.
9. National Institutes of Health, National Institute of Diabetes and Digestive and Kidney Diseases (2012) U.S. Renal Data System, USRDS 2012 Annual Data Report: Atlas of Chronic Kidney Disease and End-Stage Renal Disease in the United States.
10. Chan CT, Lok CE (2009) Why not home dialysis? Adv Chronic Kidney Dis 16: 158–159.
11. Golper TA, Guest S, Glickman JD, Turk J, Pulliam JP (2011) Home Dialysis in the new USA Bundled Payment Plan: Implications and Impact. Peritoneal Dialysis International 31: 12–16.
12. Thodis ED, Oreopoulos DG (2011) Home dialysis first: a new paradigm for new ESRD patients. J Nephrol 24: 398–404.
13. Vonesh E, Schaubel D, Hao W, Collins A (2000) Statistical methods for comparing mortality among ESRD pateints: Examples of regional/international variations. Kidney Int 57: S19–S27.
14. The Australia and New Zealand Dialysis and Transplant Registry. Adelaide, Australia: ANZDATA Registry.

15. Levey AS, Bosch JP, Lewis JB, Greene T, Rogers N, et al. (1999) A more accurate method to estimate glomerular filtration rate from serum creatinine: a new prediction equation. Modification of Diet in Renal Disease Study Group. Ann Intern Med 130: 461–470.
16. Mailloux LU, Bellucci AG, Mossey RT, Napolitano B, Moore T, et al. (1988) Predictors of survival in patients undergoing dialysis. American Journal of Medicine 84: 855–862.
17. Mailloux LU, Bellucci AG, Napolitano B, Mossey T, Wilkes BM, et al. (1994) Survival estimates for 683 patients starting dialysis from 1970 through 1989: Identification of risk factors for survival. Clinical Nephrology 42: 127–135.
18. Mailloux LU, Kapikian N, Napolitano B, Mossey RT, Bellucci AG, et al. (1996) Home hemodialysis: patient outcomes during a 24-year period of time from 1970 through 1993. Adv Ren Replace Ther 3: 112–119.
19. Prowant B, Nolph KD, Dutton S, et al. (1983) Actuarial analysis of patient survival and dropout with various end-stage renal disease therapies. American Journal of Kidney Diseases 3: 27–31.
20. Saner E, Nitsch D, Descoeudres C, Frey FJ, Uehlinger DE (2005) Outcome of home haemodialysis patients: a case-cohort study. Nephrol Dial Transplant 20: 604–610.
21. Weller JM, Port FK, Swartz RD, Ferguson CW, Williams GW, et al. (1982) Analysis of survival of end-stage renal disease patients. Kidney Int 21: 78–83.
22. Williams GW, Weller JM, Ferguson CW, Forsythe SB, Wu SC (1983) Survival of endstage renal disease patients: age-adjusted differences in treatment outcomes. Kidney Int 24: 691–693.
23. Woods JD, Port FK, Stannard D, Blagg CR, Held PJ (1996) Comparison of mortality with home hemodialysis and center hemodialysis: a national study. Kidney Int 49: 1464–1470.
24. Rubin J, Barnes T, Bower J (1985) Morbidity and mortality in CAPD and home hemodialysis: One Center's five-year experience. ASAIO Journal 8: 22–27.
25. Rubin J, Barnes T, Burns P, et al. (1983) Comparison of home hemodialysis to continuous ambulatory peritoneal dialysis. Kidney International 23: 51–56.
26. Rubin J, Hsu H, Bower J (1989) Survival on dialysis therapy: One center's experience. American Journal of the Medical Sciences 297: 80–90.
27. Grant AC, Rodger RSC, Howie CA, Junor BJR, Briggs JD, et al. (1992) Dialysis at home in the west of Scotland: A comparison of hemodialysis and continuous ambulatory peritoneal dialysis in age- and sex-matched controls. Peritoneal Dialysis International 12: 365–368.
28. Nitsch D, Steenkamp R, Tomson CR, Roderick P, Ansell D, et al. (2011) Outcomes in patients on home haemodialysis in England and Wales, 1997–2005: a comparative cohort analysis. Nephrol Dial Transplant 26: 1670–1677.
29. Heaf JG, Lokkegaard H, Madsen M (2002) Initial survival advantage of peritoneal dialysis relative to haemodialysis. Nephrol Dial Transplant 17: 112–117.
30. Termorshuizen F, Korevaar JC, Dekker FW, Van Manen JG, Boeschoten EW, et al. (2003) Hemodialysis and peritoneal dialysis: comparison of adjusted mortality rates according to the duration of dialysis: analysis of The Netherlands Cooperative Study on the Adequacy of Dialysis 2. J Am Soc Nephrol 14: 2851–2860.
31. Jaar BG, Coresh J, Plantinga LC, Fink NE, Klag MJ, et al. (2005) Comparing the risk for death with peritoneal dialysis and hemodialysis in a national cohort of patients with chronic kidney disease. Ann Intern Med 143: 174–183.
32. McDonald SP, Marshall MR, Johnson DW, Polkinghorne KR (2009) Relationship between dialysis modality and mortality. J Am Soc Nephrol 20: 155–163.
33. Schaubel DE, Morrison HI, Fenton SS (1998) Comparing mortality rates on CAPD/CCPD and hemodialysis. The Canadian experience: fact or fiction? Perit Dial Int 18: 478–484.
34. Vonesh EF, Snyder JJ, Foley RN, Collins AJ (2004) The differential impact of risk factors on mortality in hemodialysis and peritoneal dialysis. Kidney Int 66: 2389–2401.
35. Vonesh EF, Snyder JJ, Foley RN, Collins AJ (2006) Mortality studies comparing peritoneal dialysis and hemodialysis: what do they tell us? Kidney Int Suppl: S3–11.
36. Collins AJ, Hao W, Xia H, Ebben JP, Everson SE, et al. (1999) Mortality risks of peritoneal dialysis and hemodialysis. Am J Kidney Dis 34: 1065–1074.
37. Ganesh SK, Hulbert-Shearon T, Port FK, Eagle K, Stack AG (2003) Mortality differences by dialysis modality among incident ESRD patients with and without coronary artery disease. J Am Soc Nephrol 14: 415–424.
38. Stack AG, Molony DA, Rahman NS, Dosekun A, Murthy B (2003) Impact of dialysis modality on survival of new ESRD patients with congestive heart failure in the United States. Kidney Int 64: 1071–1079.
39. Stack AG, Murthy BV, Molony DA (2004) Survival differences between peritoneal dialysis and hemodialysis among "large" ESRD patients in the United States. Kidney Int 65: 2398–2408.
40. Winkelmayer WC, Glynn RJ, Mittleman MA, Levin R, Pliskin JS, et al. (2002) Comparing mortality of elderly patients on hemodialysis versus peritoneal dialysis: a propensity score approach. J Am Soc Nephrol 13: 2353–2362.
41. Abbott KC, Glanton CW, Trespalacios FC, Oliver DK, Ortiz MI, et al. (2004) Body mass index, dialysis modality, and survival: analysis of the United States Renal Data System Dialysis Morbidity and Mortality Wave II Study. Kidney Int 65: 597–605.
42. Snyder JJ, Foley RN, Gilbertson DT, Vonesh EF, Collins AJ (2003) Body size and outcomes on peritoneal dialysis in the United States. Kidney Int 64: 1838–1844.
43. Inrig JK, Sun JL, Yang Q, Briley LP, Szczech LA (2006) Mortality by dialysis modality among patients who have end-stage renal disease and are awaiting renal transplantation. Clin J Am Soc Nephrol 1: 774–779.
44. Churchill DN, Thorpe KE, Vonesh EF, Keshaviah PR (1997) Lower probability of patient survival with continuous peritoneal dialysis in the United States compared with Canada. Canada-USA (CANUSA) Peritoneal Dialysis Study Group. J Am Soc Nephrol 8: 965–971.
45. Vonesh EF, Moran J (1999) Mortality in end-stage renal disease: a reassessment of differences between patients treated with hemodialysis and peritoneal dialysis. J Am Soc Nephrol 10: 354–365.
46. Sanabria M, Munoz J, Trillos C, Hernandez G, Latorre C, et al. (2008) Dialysis outcomes in Colombia (DOC) study: a comparison of patient survival on peritoneal dialysis vs hemodialysis in Colombia. Kidney Int Suppl: S165–172.
47. Xu R, Han Q-F, Zhu T-Y, Ren Y-P, Chen J-H, et al. (2012) Impact of Individual and Environmental Socioeconomic Status on Peritoneal Dialysis Outcomes: A Retrospective Multicenter Cohort Study. PLoS ONE 7: e50766.
48. Rodriguez RA (2012) Dialysis and mortality: does it matter where you live? Clin J Am Soc Nephrol 7: 1055–1057.
49. Tonelli M, Hemmelgarn B, Culleton B, Klarenbach S, Gill JS, et al. (2007) Mortality of Canadians treated by peritoneal dialysis in remote locations. Kidney Int 72: 1023–1028.
50. Christensen AJ, Smith TW, Turner CW, Holman JM, Jr., Gregory MC (1990) Type of hemodialysis and preference for behavioral involvement: interactive effects on adherence in end-stage renal disease. Health Psychol 9: 225–236.
51. Kraus M, Burkart J, Hegeman R, Solomon R, Coplon N, et al. (2007) A comparison of center-based vs. home-based daily hemodialysis for patients with end-stage renal disease. Hemodial Int 11: 468–477.
52. Polaschek N (2007) Client attitudes towards home dialysis therapy. Edtna-Erca Journal 33: 20–24.
53. Christensen AJ, Smith TW, Turner CW, Holman JM, Jr., Gregory MC, et al. (1992) Family support, physical impairment, and adherence in hemodialysis: an investigation of main and buffering effects. J Behav Med 15: 313–325.
54. Snyder WL (1977) Factors affecting adherence to diet and medication orders by hemodialysis patients. Abstracts of Hospital Management Studies 14: 18102 PA: 18167p.
55. McGregor DO, Buttimore AL, Lynn KL, Nicholls MG, Jardine DL (2001) A comparative study of blood pressure control with short in-center versus long home hemodialysis. Blood Purification 19: 293–300.
56. Lameire N, Van Biesen W, Vanholder R (2000) The role of peritoneal dialysis as first modality in an integrative approach to patients with end-stage renal disease. Perit Dial Int 20 Suppl 2: S134–141.
57. Van Biesen W, Vanholder RC, Veys N, Dhondt A, Lameire NH (2000) An evaluation of an integrative care approach for end-stage renal disease patients. J Am Soc Nephrol 11: 116–125.
58. Boissinot L, Landru I, Cardineau E, Zagdoun E, Ryckelycnk JP, et al. (2013) Is transition between peritoneal dialysis and hemodialysis really a gradual process? Perit Dial Int 33: 391–397.

Effect of Dialysis Initiation Timing on Clinical Outcomes: A Propensity-Matched Analysis of a Prospective Cohort Study

Jeonghwan Lee[1,2], Jung Nam An[3], Jin Ho Hwang[4], Yong-Lim Kim[2,5], Shin-Wook Kang[2,6], Chul Woo Yang[2,7], Nam-Ho Kim[2,8], Yun Kyu Oh[2,3], Chun Soo Lim[2,3], Yon Su Kim[2,9], Jung Pyo Lee[2,3]*

1 Department of Internal Medicine, Hallym University Hangang Sacred Heart Hospital, Seoul, Korea, **2** Clinical Research Center for End Stage Renal Disease (CRC for ESRD), Daegu, Korea, **3** Department of Internal Medicine, Seoul National University Boramae Medical Center, Seoul, Korea, **4** Department of Internal Medicine, Chung-Ang University Medical Center, Seoul, Korea, **5** Department of Internal Medicine, Kyungpook National University School of Medicine, Daegu, Korea, **6** Department of Internal Medicine, Yonsei University College of Medicine, Seoul, Korea, **7** Department of Internal Medicine, The Catholic University of Korea College of Medicine, Seoul, Korea, **8** Department of Internal Medicine, Chonnam National University Medical School, Gwangju, Korea, **9** Department of Internal Medicine, Seoul National University Hospital, Seoul National University College of Medicine, Seoul, Korea

Abstract

Background: Controversy persists regarding the appropriate initiation timing of renal replacement therapy for patients with end-stage renal disease. We evaluated the effect of dialysis initiation timing on clinical outcomes. Initiation times were classified according to glomerular filtration rate (GFR).

Methods: We enrolled a total of 1691 adult patients who started dialysis between August 2008 and March 2013 in a multicenter, prospective cohort study at the Clinical Research Center for End Stage Renal Disease in the Republic of Korea. The patients were classified into the early-start group or the late-start group according to the mean estimated GFR value, which was 7.37 ml/min/1.73 m^2. The primary outcome was patient survival, and the secondary outcomes were hospitalization, cardiovascular events, vascular access complications, change of dialysis modality, and peritonitis. The two groups were compared before and after matching with propensity scores.

Results: Before propensity score matching, the early-start group had a poor survival rate ($P<0.001$). Hospitalization, cardiovascular events, vascular access complications, changes in dialysis modality, and peritonitis were not different between the groups. A total of 854 patients (427 in each group) were selected by propensity score matching. After matching, neither patient survival nor any of the other outcomes differed between groups.

Conclusions: There was no clinical benefit after adjustment by propensity scores comparing early versus late initiation of dialysis.

Editor: Emmanuel A. Burdmann, University of Sao Paulo Medical School, Brazil

Funding: This study was supported by a grant from the Korea Healthcare Technology R& D Project, Ministry for Health and Welfare, Republic of Korea (A102065). The funders had no role in study design, data collection and analysis, decision to publish, or preparation of the manuscript.

Competing Interests: The authors have declared that no competing interests exist.

* Email: nephrolee@gmail.com

Introduction

Chronic kidney disease (CKD) is a major public health problem, and the number of patients requiring dialysis for end-stage renal disease (ESRD) has been increasing rapidly around the world [1]. In 2011, the prevalence of dialysis patients in the United States was 430,273 (0.2% of the general population), and the rate of ESRD cases per million population reached 1,901 [2]. Medical expenditures for patients with ESRD in the United States reached $49.3 billion in 2011, and ESRD patients accounted for 6.3% of total Medicare costs. Most cases of ESRD are complicated, with various comorbidities, and are associated with poor health outcomes. In the United States, ESRD patients were reported to have a residual life expectancy of 6.2 years [2]. According to two large population cohort studies in Canada and Taiwan, patients aged 55 years with stage 5 CKD or who were on dialysis had life expectancies of 5.6 and 12.0 years and cardiovascular mortality rates of 58% and 71%, respectively [3–5]. Adequate dialysis therapy can relieve the burden of painful uremic symptoms and improve overall survival [6–8]. Therefore, it is important to initiate dialysis therapy at the appropriate time to prevent fatal uremic complications and improve patient survival.

However, controversy persists regarding the optimal timing for dialysis initiation. There is a conventional belief that delaying dialysis until the patient's eGFR falls below 6 ml/min/1.73 m^2

was potentially dangerous and that starting dialysis early could improve the nutritional status and survival of ESRD patients through increased uremic solute clearance, particularly in patients with diabetes or high comorbidities [9]. According to data from the United States Renal Data System (USRDS), the proportion of patients who started dialysis at an eGFR greater than 10 ml/min/1.73 m^2 had been steadily increasing up to 2009, reaching 54% of the patient population [10]. However, several observational and meta-analysis studies reported that early initiation of dialysis is associated with certain harmful clinical outcomes [11–14]. To date, there has been only one prospective, randomized, controlled study (the Initiating Dialysis Early and Late Trial; IDEAL study) on dialysis initiation time and patient survival. This study reported that planned early initiation of dialysis was not associated with improvements in either survival or clinical outcomes [15]. Recent guidelines reflecting the results of the IDEAL study emphasize that the eGFR, based on serum creatinine levels, should not be the only factor used to guide dialysis initiation time and recommend that dialysis should be preferentially deferred until the development of uremic symptoms or complications [16–18].

Clinical outcomes and mortality rates among patients initiating dialysis are known to differ according to the demographic characteristics of race or ethnicity [19]. Asian advanced CKD patients have lower mortality and cardiovascular morbidity than Caucasians despite a faster decline in GFR and a higher incidence of renal replacement therapy [20–22]. However, clinical evidence on dialysis initiation time and associated clinical outcomes is insufficient among non-Caucasian populations. Although there are a few retrospective, observational studies on dialysis initiation timing among Asian ESRD patients [23–27], single-center designs and/or insufficient adjustments in multivariate analyses attributable to limited data collection from retrospective designs make the results of these studies difficult to generalize to all populations. In the IDEAL study, most of the patients (70%) enrolled were Caucasian, and only 9.2% were Asian. Here, we aimed to compare the survival and other clinical outcomes of patients starting dialysis for ESRD according to initiation time in a Korean prospective cohort study using propensity score-matching analysis.

Methods

Study Participants

We enrolled adult patients (≥20 years old) who were started on maintenance dialysis for ESRD between August 2008 and March 2013 through an ongoing cohort study (Clinical Research Center for End Stage Renal Disease, CRC for ESRD) in South Korea. The CRC for ESRD is a nationwide, multi-center, web-based, prospective cohort of CKD patients who have started dialysis (clinicaltrial.gov NCT00931970) [28]. The CRC for ESRD cohort began to register ESRD patients on dialysis in July 2008, and 31 hospitals in South Korea are currently participating. All of the patients were informed about the study and participated voluntarily with written consent. The study was approved by the institutional review board at each center. [The Catholic University of Korea, Bucheon St. Mary's Hospital; The Catholic University of Korea, Incheon St. Mary's Hospital; The Catholic University of Korea, Seoul St. Mary's Hospital; The Catholic University of Korea, St. Mary's Hospital; The Catholic University of Korea, St. Vincent's Hospital; The Catholic University of Korea, Uijeongbu St. Mary's Hospital; Cheju Halla General Hospital; Chonbuk National University Hospital; Chonnam National University Hospital; Chung-Ang University Medical Center; Chungbuk National University Hospital; Chungnam National University Hospital; Dong-A University Medical Center; Ewha Womans University Medical Center; Fatima Hospital; Gachon Medical School Gil Medical Center; Inje University Busan Paik Hospital; Kyungpook National University Hospital; Kwandong University College of Medicine, Myongji Hospital; National Health Insurance Corporation Ilsan Hospital; National Medical Center; Busan National University Hospital; Samsung Medical Center; Seoul National University Boramae Medical Center; Seoul National University Hospital; Seoul National University, Bundang Hospital; Yeungnam University Medical Center; Yonsei University, Severance Hospital; Yonsei University, Gangnam Severance Hospital; Ulsan University Hospital; Wonju Christian Hospital (in alphabetical order)]. All of the investigators conducted this study in accordance with the guidelines of the 2008 Declaration of Helsinki.

After the last enrollments in March 2013, participants were followed until October 2013 to observe at least 6-month mortality and clinical outcomes. Patients whose creatinine levels were missing at the time of dialysis initiation were excluded. Patients were categorized into the early-start group or the late-start group according to whether their eGFR was greater or less than the mean eGFR value at the start of dialysis. The eGFR was calculated using CKD-Epidemiology Collaboration (CKD-EPI) equations [29]. The modified Charlson co-morbidity index (mCCI) was calculated for each patient at the initiation of dialysis. The mCCI was developed to predict one-year mortality, and it has been validated in ESRD patients [30,31].

Clinical Outcomes

The primary outcome was all-cause mortality after the start of dialysis. The secondary outcomes included first hospitalization, cardiovascular events, changes in dialysis modality, vascular complications in hemodialysis patients, and peritonitis in peritoneal dialysis patients. Hospitalization was defined as admission for at least 24 hours, excluding diagnostic work-ups for transplantation. Cardiovascular events included clinical events requiring admission for ischemic heart disease, congestive heart failure, arrhythmia, or cerebrovascular disease. Changes in dialysis modality included shift from hemodialysis to peritoneal dialysis or vice versa. Vascular complications included vascular events requiring angioplasty, surgical intervention, or changes in vascular catheters for hemodialysis. Peritonitis was defined as the presence of the following conditions: 1) signs and symptoms of peritoneal inflammation; and 2) a peritoneal effluent white blood cell count greater than 100 cells/mm^3 and a neutrophil percentage greater than 50%.

Statistical Analysis

The propensity scores, which were calculated from the logistic regression models, represent the probability of being assigned to either an early or a late dialysis initiation. Through the matching procedure for propensity scores, the early- and late-start groups showed similar distributions of propensity scores, indicating that the differences in covariates between the two groups were minimized. We matched propensity scores one by one using nearest neighbor methods, no replacement, and 0.2 caliper width. The characteristics of both the early- and late-start groups were compared before and after propensity score matching.

Continuous variables are expressed as the mean and standard deviation, and categorical variables are presented as frequencies with percentages. Continuous variables were compared using a t-test, and categorical variables were compared using the Chi-square test or Fisher's exact tests. Survival was compared using Kaplan-Meier curve and log-rank test. IBM SPSS software (version 21.0) was used in all descriptive and survival analysis, and R software (version 2.14.2) was used in the propensity score matching. A two-tailed P value <0.05 was considered statistically significant.

Results

Patient Characteristics

Initially, among the 4770 patients retrieved from the CRC for ESRD database, 2991 dialysis patients who had started dialysis before cohort registration were excluded (Figure 1). In addition, 88 patients without information on serum creatinine levels and/or eGFR at the time of dialysis initiation were excluded from the analysis. Ultimately, a total of 1691 adult patients who started maintenance dialysis for ESRD were enrolled. Patients were classified into the early-start group (eGFR greater than the mean value) or late-start group (eGFR less than the mean value) based on the mean value of eGFR at the start of dialysis, which was 7.372 ml/min/1.73 m^2.

The patients' clinical and laboratory characteristics are compared and summarized in Table 1. The mean age was 56.6±14.3 years old, and 61.4% of the patients were male. Patients with diabetes as a primary cause of renal disease comprised 51.2% of the study population. Most of the patients (71.1%) received hemodialysis as the modality for renal replacement therapy. Before propensity score matching, 1051 patients were in the late-start group, and 640 patients were in the early-start group. Considering all of the participants, the mean eGFR values were 11.2±8.1 ml/min/1.73 m^2 in the early-start group and 5.0±1.4 ml/min/1.73 m^2 in the late-start group. In the early-start group, the patients were older (58.8±14.4 vs. 55.3±14.0 years old, P<0.001), and diabetic kidney disease (59.7% vs. 46.8%) was more common. A total of 69.6% of the patients in the early-start group received

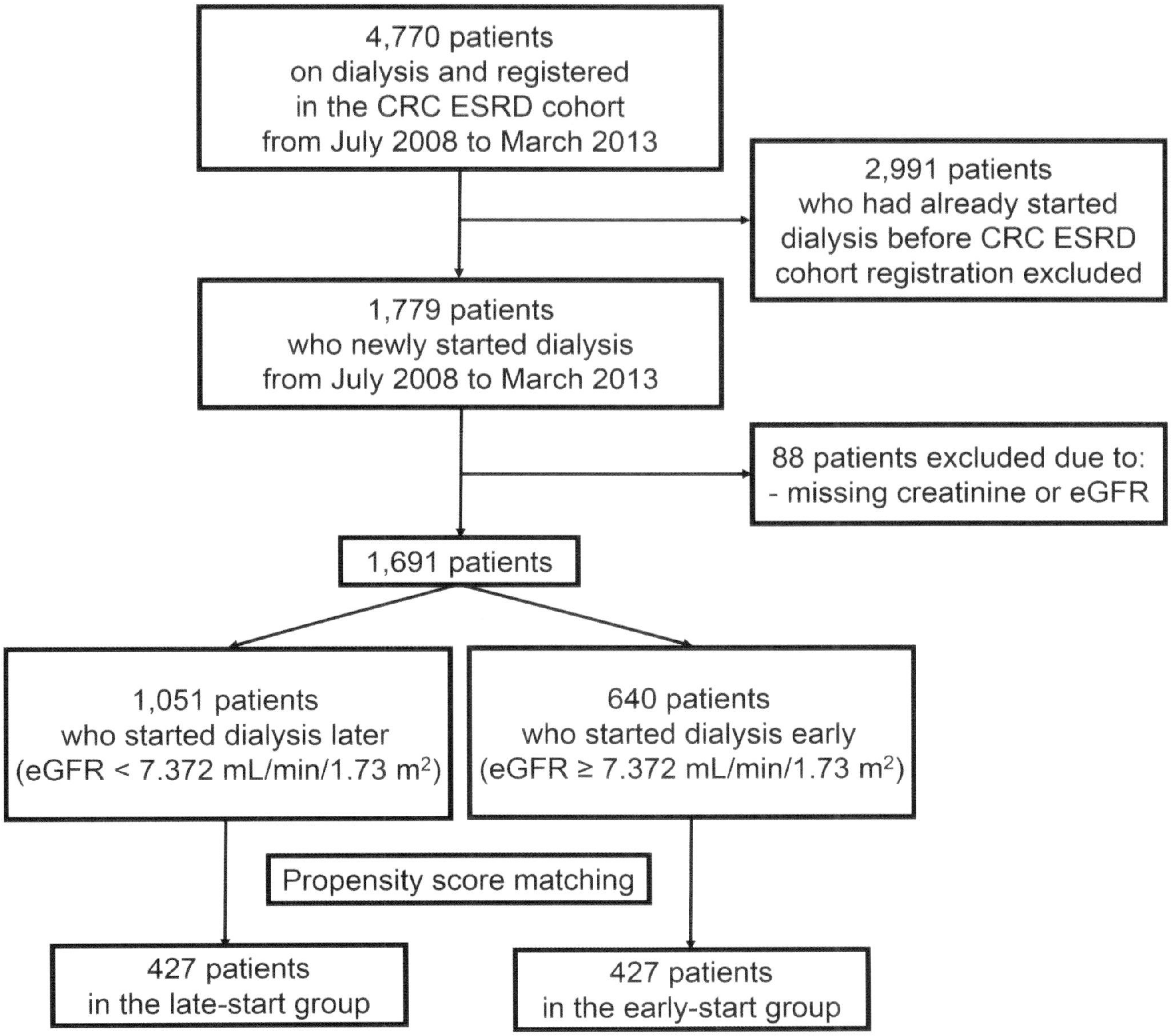

Figure 1. Flow chart of study enrollment. Between August 2008 and March 2013, 1069 dialysis patients with end-stage renal disease were initially enrolled. After propensity score matching, 854 patients remained in the final analysis.

Table 1. Patient characteristics before and after propensity score matching.

Variables	Before PSM				After PSM			
	Late Start (N = 1051)	Early Start (N = 640)	P	Standardized Difference	Late Start (N = 427)	Early Start (N = 427)	P	Standardized Difference
Age (years old)	55.3±14.0	58.8±14.4	<0.001	0.227	57.6±13.1	57.4±14.3	0.853	−0.012
Sex (male)	609 (57.9%)	430 (67.2%)	<0.001	−0.227	264 (61.8%)	272 (63.7%)	0.571	−0.040
Primary renal disease			<0.001	−0.254			0.339	−0.059
Diabetes	488 (46.8%)	377 (59.7%)			240 (56.2%)	244 (57.1%)		
Hypertension	187 (17.9%)	83 (13.2%)			57 (13.3%)	68 (15.9%)		
Glomerulonephritis	180 (17.3%)	58 (9.2%)			63 (14.8%)	44 (10.3%)		
Other	114 (10.9%)	59 (8.4%)			37 (8.7%)	38 (8.9%)		
Unknown	74 (7.1%)	54 (8.6%)			30 (7.0%)	33 (7.7%)		
Type of dialysis			0.266	0.070			0.653	−0.030
Hemodialysis	758 (72.1%)	444 (69.6%)			298 (69.8%)	304 (71.2%)		
Peritoneal dialysis	293 (27.9%)	194 (30.4%)			129 (30.2%)	123 (28.8%)		
Systolic BP (mmHg)	142.6±24.1	139.6±22.6	0.015		142.9±23.0	140.3±23.0	0.108	
Diastolic BP (mmHg)	78.9±14.8	76.3±13.6	0.001		78.2±14.5	77.4±14.0	0.409	
BMI (kg/m^2)	23.2±3.5	23.0±3.4	0.380	−0.055	23.2±3.3	23.1±3.5	0.742	−0.023
Charlson comorbidity index	4.69±2.25	5.80±2.66	<0.001	0.402	5.27±2.29	5.32±2.53	0.734	0.021
WBC (/mm^3)	5790±3924	5212±3956	0.004	−0.149	5319±3986	5450±3891	0.625	0.033
Hemoglobin (g/dL)	8.7±2.5	9.6±4.7	<0.001	0.178	9.1±3.3	9.2±1.5	0.510	0.023
Calcium (md/dL)	7.7±3.1	8.1±3.0	0.010	0.130	8.1±4.6	8.2±3.6	0.729	0.031
Phosphorus (md/dL)	6.2 ±2.8	4.6±2.6	<0.001	−0.597	4.9±1.3	4.8±1.3	0.209	−0.041
Uric acid (md/dL)	8.8±5.0	7.2±2.6	<0.001	−0.600	7.8 ±2.0	7.7 ±2.6	0.519	−0.040
Albumin (g/dL)	3.4±0.6	3.2±0.6	<0.001	−0.216	3.3±0.6	3.3±0.6	0.481	−0.046
Creatinine (md/dL)	10.45±5.91	5.35±1.35	<0.001		9.19±3.24	5.49±1.26	<0.001	
eGFR* (ml/min/1.73 m^2)	5.0±1.4	11.2±8.1	<0.001		5.5±1.2	10.4±4.9	<0.001	
Ferritn (ng/ml)	308.4 ±500.2	327.6 ±401.0	0.458		281.8±431.0	318.8±372.6	0.222	
Cholesterol (mg/dL)	159.5±48.5	155.4±51.6	0.120		158.3 ±48.6	156.4±48.3	0.578	
hsCRP (mg/L)	4.0±16.4	6.9±20.5	0.004		5.9±23.5	4.4±12.4	0.261	
iPTH (pg/mL)	300.4±255.6	200.0±198.0	<0.001		269.8±228.2	210.3±210.9	0.001	
Use of vitamin D	188 (17.9%)	62 (9.7%)	<0.001		67 (15.7%)	44 (10.3%)	0.025	
Use of phosphate binders	575 (54.7%)	288 (45.0%)	<0.001		233 (54.6%)	211 (49.4%)	0.212	
Single-pool Kt/V†	1.33±0.47	1.24±0.55	0.047		1.33±0.40	1.23±0.59	0.121	
Weekly Kt/V‡	2.47±1.02	2.59±1.38	0.735		2.79±1.02	2.83±1.32	0.994	

BMI, body mass index; iPTH, intact PTH; PSM, propensity score-matching; WBC, white blood cell count.
*Levels of eGFR were calculated using the CKD-EPI equation.
†Single-pool Kt/V was measured in patients with hemodialysis.
‡Weekly Kt/V was measured in patients with peritoneal dialysis.

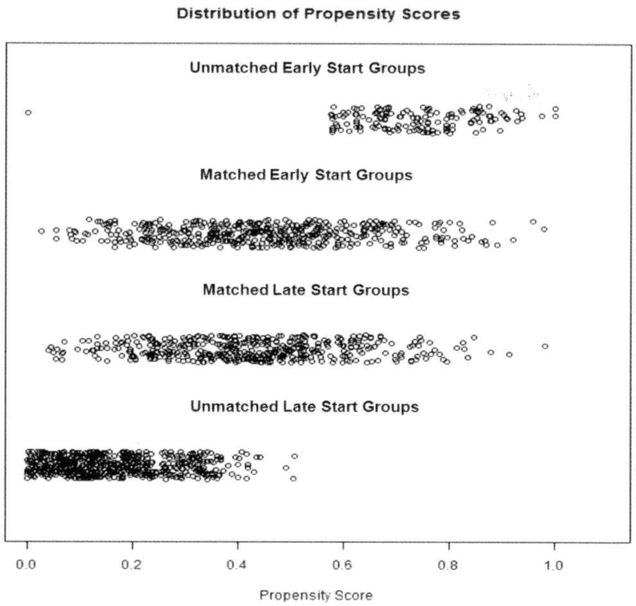

Figure 2. Distribution of propensity scores before and after propensity score matching. The propensity scores of unmatched patients were significantly different between the early- and late-start groups. The propensity scores of matched patients were almost the same between groups.

hemodialysis as the first modality of dialysis, whereas 30.4% of the patients started with peritoneal dialysis. The mCCI was higher in the early-start group. Systolic and diastolic blood pressure, serum phosphorus, uric acid, albumin, intact parathyroid hormone (iPTH), and high-sensitive C-reactive protein (hsCRP) levels, use of vitamin D or phosphate binders were lower, and hemoglobin and calcium levels were higher in the early-start group. The adequacy of hemodialysis (single-pool Kt/V) was slightly lower in the early-start group of hemodialysis patients, but the weekly Kt/V of peritoneal dialysis was not different between the two groups.

Propensity Matching of Cohort

We performed a logistic regression analysis to obtain propensity scores for dialysis initiation timing using the following covariates: age, sex, primary renal disease, type of dialysis, body mass index, mCCI, hemoglobin level, calcium level, phosphorus level, uric acid level, albumin level, and comorbidities. After propensity score matching, 854 patients (427 in each group) remained. The distributions of propensity scores before and after matching are illustrated in Figure 2. In the propensity score-matched participants, almost all of the baseline parameters, including age, sex, primary renal disease, type of dialysis, systolic and diastolic blood pressure, body mass index, mCCI, hemoglobin levels, serum calcium, phosphorus, uric acid, glucose, albumin, hsCRP levels, and adequacy of dialysis (single-pool Kt/V in hemodialysis patients and weekly Kt/V in peritoneal dialysis patients) were similar between the groups. The propensity scores of the matched patients were almost the same between the early- and late-start groups.

Survival and Clinical Outcomes

The patients' survival rates are shown in Figure 3. Before propensity score matching, the early-start group had a worse survival rate ($P<0.001$). Hospitalization ($P=0.195$), cardiovascular events ($P=0.352$), vascular access complications ($P=0.158$), changes in dialysis modality ($P=0.660$), and peritonitis ($P=0.833$) were not different between the groups (Figure S1). After matching, patient survival, hospitalization, cardiovascular events, vascular access complications, change of dialysis modality, and peritonitis were not different between the groups.

Subgroup analyses of all-cause mortality were performed in the propensity score-matched cohort, and the hazard ratio of starting dialysis early is illustrated in Figure 4 using a Cox proportional analysis. The hazard associated with starting dialysis early was not elevated in any subgroups except patients with diabetes. In patients with diabetes, the hazard associated with an early-start to dialysis was significantly greater (HR 2.024, 95% CI 1.025–3.996).

The causes of mortality are listed in Table 2. The distributions of the mortality causes were not different before ($P=0.817$) and after ($P=0.521$) propensity score matching. In propensity score-matched participants, mortality rates from cardiovascular events ($P=0.630$), cerebrovascular accidents ($P=0.659$), infections

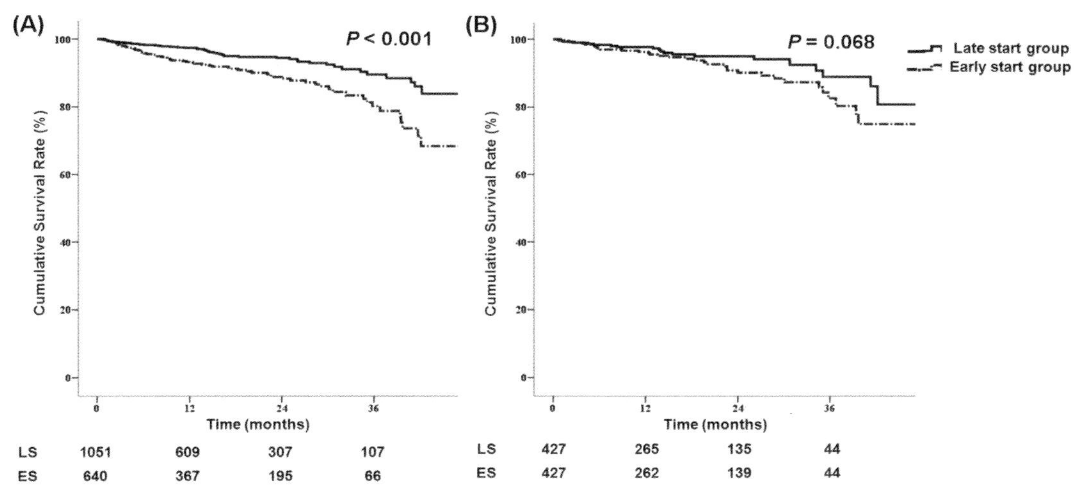

Figure 3. Kaplan-Meier patient survival curve for the timing of dialysis initiation. (A) Before matching, the patients in the early start group had poor survival. (B) After propensity score matching, patients in the early- and late-start groups showed no differences in survival.

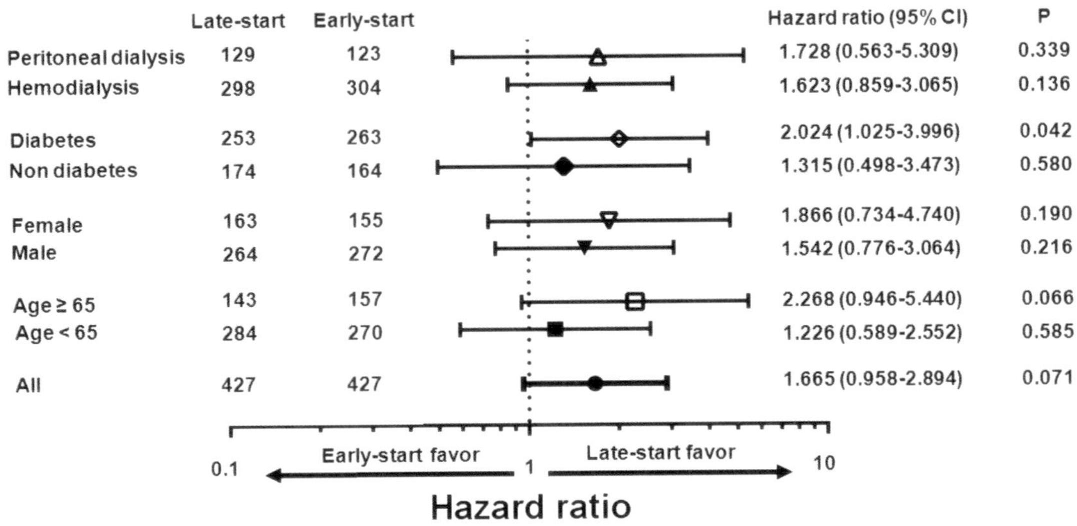

Figure 4. Hazard ratio (HR) for mortality of early dialysis initiation using a Cox proportional analysis in the propensity score-matched cohort. The hazard of early dialysis initiation was not elevated in any subgroup except patients with diabetes. In patients with diabetes, the hazard of early dialysis initiation was significantly greater (HR 2.024, 95% CI 1.025–3.996).

(P = 0.783), and malignancies (P = 0.984) were not different between the early- and late-start groups. Cardiovascular events, including acute myocardial infarction, arrhythmia, cardiac arrest, valvular heart disease, and congestive heart failure, were the leading causes of mortality.

Discussion

We evaluated the effects of early dialysis initiation on all-cause mortality and other clinical outcomes using a propensity score-matching analysis in an Asian prospective cohort study. Before matching, the early-start group seemed to have poorer survival than the late-start group. However, after matching, these differences in survival disappeared, and there were no significant differences in all-cause mortality or other clinical outcomes.

Comparing the entire cohort of participants, the early start-group was older than the late-start group. In addition, the proportions of male patients and cases of diabetic kidney disease were greater in the early-start group. The mCCI was also higher in the early-start group. Although systolic and diastolic blood pressure levels were lower and hemoglobin levels were higher in the early-start group, serum albumin levels were lower in the early-start group. In summary, except for residual renal function, the demographic and laboratory parameters were worse in the early-start group. It is possible that the patients in the early-start group initiated dialysis earlier because they had more complications due to ESRD. The high burden of comorbidities in the early-start group might have been the principal cause of poor survival before matching. Indeed, after adjusting for these confounding factors using propensity score-matching methods, survival and clinical outcomes were comparable between groups.

Although the proportion of early dialysis initiation remained stable between 2009 and 2011 in the United States, the percentage of patients who started dialysis early had grown steadily until 2009, up to 54% [10]. A worldwide trend toward early dialysis initiation had been supported by the belief that increased solute clearance could improve patient survival and clinical outcomes. Prolonged uremia can decrease appetite and evoke anorexia, poor oral intake, and malnutrition [32]. Several studies had shown that decreased eGFR values at the time of dialysis initiation were closely associated with poor nutritional status and mortality [33–37]. In addition, there had been concern that delaying dialysis might fail to prevent fatal uremic complications, including severe

Table 2. Causes of patient mortality.

Causes of mortality	All participants (N = 1691)			PS-matched participants (N = 854)		
	All participants	**Late-start (N = 1051)**	**Early-start (N = 640)**	**PS-matched participants**	**Late-start (N = 427)**	**Early-start (N = 427)**
Cardiovascular events	34 (29.6%)	17 (33.3%)	17 (26.6%)	16 (29.1%)	7 (33.3%)	9 (26.5%)
Cerebrovascular events	7 (6.1%)	2 (3.9%)	5 (7.8%)	5 (9.1%)	2 (9.5%)	3 (8.8%)
Infections	30 (26.1%)	15 (29.4%)	15 (23.4%)	13 (23.6%)	6 (28.6%)	7 (20.6%)
Malignancies	7 (6.1%)	3 (5.9%)	4 (6.3%)	2 (3.6%)	1 (4.8%)	1 (2.9%)
Other	22 (19.1%)	8 (15.7%)	14 (21.9%)	10 (18.2%)	1 (4.8%)	9 (26.5%)
Unknown	15 (13.0%)	6 (11.8%)	9 (14.1%)	9 (16.4%)	4 (19.0%)	5 (14.7%)

hyperkalemia, uncontrolled hypertension, pulmonary edema, pericarditis, and encephalopathy. In fact, before the IDEAL study, clinical guidelines had permitted early dialysis initiation for an eGFR of over 10 ml/min/1.73 m^2 if there were relevant uremic symptoms or evidence of malnutrition [38–41]. In the United States, reflecting these guidelines, the mean eGFR at dialysis initiation increased from 8.1 ml/min/1.73 m^2 in 1997 to 10.8 ml/min/1.73 m^2 in 2007 [42]. However, the association between low eGFR at the time of dialysis initiation and poor survival cannot be used as direct evidence justifying early dialysis initiation. Almost studies reporting the benefit of early dialysis initiation were of a retrospective observational design, and the adjustments made for demographic factors and comorbid conditions were insufficient [33,34,43,44]. In addition, the possibility of lead-time bias in the studies favoring early dialysis initiation should be considered. A survival benefit of early dialysis initiation could result from the statistical misinterpretation of the fact that patients had merely started dialysis early, rather than that they actually lived longer. Korevaar et al. reported that the survival benefit of 2.5 months in the patients with early dialysis initiation was overwhelmed by the effect of delaying dialysis approximately 4.1 months in the patients with late dialysis initiation [45].

Notably, contrary to general expectations, recent observational studies have shown that early dialysis initiation was irrelevant to survival benefits or even associated with poor clinical outcomes [11,14,26,46–50]. Starting dialysis early can expose ESRD patients to dialysis-associated complications [51]. The decline in residual renal function can progress at a rapid pace, even after dialysis [52]. Dialysis therapy can also result in protein loss and aggravate nutritional status in ESRD patients [53]. Catheter- or access site-related peritoneal or bloodstream infections are increased in patients undergoing dialysis [54]. These factors can thus collectively contribute to the poor survival and negative clinical outcomes of patients with early dialysis initiation. Although there have been several lines of evidence supporting the harmful effects of early dialysis initiation, there is still a debate as to whether a high eGFR itself is the main cause of poor outcomes in patients with early dialysis initiation. Most eGFR equations are based on serum creatinine levels, so there is a possibility of overestimating the eGFR in cases of low serum creatinine levels due to low muscle mass or fluid overload [55]. Beddhu et al. reported that high eGFR values were closely associated with increased mortality, but high creatinine clearance was not [56]. In addition, survivor bias can overestimate the risk of early dialysis initiation due to the limitations of observational studies. Patients who had died before initiating dialysis were excluded from the analyses of observational studies, and the number of such patients is likely to be higher in the late-start group. Therefore, those who start dialysis later may collectively comprise a healthier group. Crew et al. minimized the lead-time and survivor bias through the enrollment of patients before the initiation of dialysis and analyzed clinical outcomes after the eGFR reached approximately 20 ml/min/1.73 m^2. This work demonstrated that patients who initiated dialysis early or late did not exhibit differences in survival [57]. Lastly, patients who had a high burden of uremic symptoms and/or comorbidities are likely to start dialysis earlier. It is known that patients who are older, male, or who had diabetes, low body mass index, high comorbidities with cardiovascular complications, or poor functional status are likely to start dialysis earlier [48,58–60]. These high risk comorbidities and demographic factors can aggravate survival and other clinical outcomes in patients with early dialysis initiation. Several investigations reported that the risk of early dialysis initiation decreased after multivariate adjustments for demographic factors, laboratory data, and comorbidities [46,48]. Bao et al. investigated that high mortality was closely associated with frailty, including slowness or weakness, exhaustion, and low physical activity and found that the risks associated with early dialysis initiation disappeared after adjustment for frailty [61]. A recent meta-analysis showed that an early start to dialysis was associated with increased mortality and that patients with older age, diabetes, and high comorbidities seemed to start dialysis earlier [12]. The results of our study before matching are similar to the results of these studies. Patients in the early-start group of the present study were older and had more comorbidities, including diabetes. The poor survival of these patients disappeared after matching the covariates.

To date, only one randomized, controlled study has evaluated the association between dialysis initiation time and survival [15]. In the IDEAL study, Cooper et al. allocated ESRD patients to planned dialysis initiation at an eGFR greater than 10 ml/min/1.73 m^2 or conventional dialysis initiation at an eGFR less than 7 ml/min/1.73 m^2. There were no differences in survival, complications, or quality of life between the two groups. Although the actual difference in eGFR between the two groups was only approximately 2 ml/min/1.73 m^2, the patients in the late-start group could begin dialysis approximately 6 months later than those in the early-start group. When the participants in the IDEAL study were analyzed separately by dialysis modality, more adverse events associated with fluids and electrolytes were observed in the late hemodialysis group, and more patients who had been randomized to peritoneal dialysis switched to hemodialysis; however, early dialysis initiation did not provide survival or other clinical benefits [62,63]. It is difficult to generalize the results of the IDEAL study to all patients preparing for dialysis because the patients enrolled in the IDEAL study were almost all Caucasians and relatively well prepared for ESRD, with low rates of temporary vascular access and a high proportion of peritoneal dialysis. In addition, there was a high incidence of cross-over from the late dialysis group to the early dialysis group. However, the results of the IDEAL study clearly indicate that early dialysis initiation is not unconditionally beneficial for patients with ESRD and that the late initiation strategy can delay dialysis initiation for a proportion of well-prepared patients. The results of our study are consistent with those of the IDEAL study in that neither early nor late initiation of dialysis based on eGFR values was associated with mortality or clinical outcomes. Reflecting the results of recent investigations, newer guidelines recommend delaying dialysis and addressing relevant clinical signs or symptoms rather than instituting dialysis therapy solely based on eGFR values [16–18].

This study has several limitations. First, because this study is an observational cohort study beginning at the time of dialysis initiation, the possibility of survivor bias still exists. This factor can favor late dialysis initiation. In addition, because all patients enrolled were Asian, the results of this study cannot easily be generalized to all ESRD patients, as the prognosis and clinical outcomes of ESRD patients are well known to be closely associated with demographic factors and comorbid conditions. However, this study still has an advantage in that it is the only prospective and well-matched cohort study in Asian ESRD patients using propensity score-matching analysis. After matching, almost all variables, including age and comorbidities, became similar between the early- and late-start groups, except for variables associated with residual renal function. Because demographic factors, comorbid conditions, and laboratory parameters converged after matching, the possibility of bias, including lead-time bias, is minimized. In addition, because there was a substantial difference in eGFR between the groups (approximately

5 ml/min/1.73 m^2), the effects of early dialysis initiation could be explored with confidence.

We evaluated the effects of dialysis initiation timing based on eGFR on clinical outcomes using propensity score-matching analysis. Early dialysis initiation did not improve patient survival or other clinical outcomes, including hospitalization, cardiovascular events, vascular access complications, changes in dialysis modality, or peritonitis. It is appears that, rather than the eGFR at the initiation timing of dialysis, a patient's health status, including age, sex, physical activity, and comorbidities, has a greater impact on clinical outcomes in patients initiating dialysis. Although the optimal time for dialysis initiation remains controversial, dialysis initiation should not be determined based on eGFR values alone. Residual renal function, comorbidities, and uremic symptoms should be considered before starting dialysis.

Acknowledgments

A portion of this work was selected for a poster presentation, which was presented at Kidney Week 2013 at the American Society of Nephrology Annual Meeting on November 9 at the Georgia World Congress Center in Atlanta, GA. We express our gratitude to all of the participants and investigators of the cohort study (Clinical Research Center for End Stage Renal Disease, CRC for ESRD) in South Korea.

Author Contributions

Conceived and designed the experiments: JPL. Performed the experiments: JL YLK SWK CWY NHK YKO CSL YSK JPL. Analyzed the data: JL JNA JHH JPL. Contributed reagents/materials/analysis tools: YLK YKO CSL YSK JPL. Contributed to the writing of the manuscript: JL JPL.

References

1. Zhang QL, Rothenbacher D (2008) Prevalence of chronic kidney disease in population-based studies: systematic review. BMC Public Health 8: 117.
2. Collins AJ, Foley RN, Chavers B, Gilbertson D, Herzog C, et al. (2014) US Renal Data System 2013 Annual Data Report. Am J Kidney Dis 63: A7.
3. Gansevoort RT, Correa-Rotter R, Hemmelgarn BR, Jafar TH, Heerspink HJ, et al. (2013) Chronic kidney disease and cardiovascular risk: epidemiology, mechanisms, and prevention. Lancet 382: 339–352.
4. Wen CP, Cheng TY, Tsai MK, Chang YC, Chan HT, et al. (2008) All-cause mortality attributable to chronic kidney disease: a prospective cohort study based on 462293 adults in Taiwan. Lancet 371: 2173–2182.
5. Turin TC, Tonelli M, Manns BJ, Ravani P, Ahmed SB, et al. (2012) Chronic kidney disease and life expectancy. Nephrol Dial Transplant 27: 3182–3186.
6. Chandna SM, Da Silva-Gane M, Marshall C, Warwicker P, Greenwood RN, et al. (2011) Survival of elderly patients with stage 5 CKD: comparison of conservative management and renal replacement therapy. Nephrol Dial Transplant 26: 1608–1614.
7. Joly D, Anglicheau D, Alberti C, Nguyen AT, Touam M, et al. (2003) Octogenarians reaching end-stage renal disease: cohort study of decision-making and clinical outcomes. J Am Soc Nephrol 14: 1012–1021.
8. Carson RC, Juszczak M, Davenport A, Burns A (2009) Is maximum conservative management an equivalent treatment option to dialysis for elderly patients with significant comorbid disease? Clin J Am Soc Nephrol 4: 1611–1619.
9. Rosansky S, Glassock RJ, Clark WF (2011) Early start of dialysis: a critical review. Clin J Am Soc Nephrol 6: 1222–1228.
10. Rosansky SJ, Clark WF (2013) Has the yearly increase in the renal replacement therapy population ended? J Am Soc Nephrol 24: 1367–1370.
11. Crews DC, Scialla JJ, Liu J, Guo H, Bandeen-Roche K, et al. (2014) Predialysis health, dialysis timing, and outcomes among older United States adults. J Am Soc Nephrol 25: 370–379.
12. Pan Y, Xu XD, Guo LL, Cai LL, Jin HM (2012) Association of early versus late initiation of dialysis with mortality: systematic review and meta-analysis. Nephron Clin Pract 120: c121–131.
13. Susantitaphong P, Altamimi S, Ashkar M, Balk EM, Stel VS, et al. (2012) GFR at initiation of dialysis and mortality in CKD: a meta-analysis. Am J Kidney Dis 59: 829–840.
14. Stel VS, Dekker FW, Ansell D, Augustijn H, Casino FG, et al. (2009) Residual renal function at the start of dialysis and clinical outcomes. Nephrol Dial Transplant 24: 3175–3182.
15. Cooper BA, Branley P, Bulfone L, Collins JF, Craig JC, et al. (2010) A randomized, controlled trial of early versus late initiation of dialysis. N Engl J Med 363: 609–619.
16. Nesrallah GE, Mustafa RA, Clark WF, Bass A, Barnieh L, et al. (2014) Canadian Society of Nephrology 2014 clinical practice guideline for timing the initiation of chronic dialysis. CMAJ 186: 112–117.
17. KDIGO (2013) KDIGO clinical practice guideline for the evaluation and management of chronic kidney disease. Kidney Int Suppl 3: 1–150.
18. Tattersall J, Dekker F, Heimburger O, Jager KJ, Lameire N, et al. (2011) When to start dialysis: updated guidance following publication of the Initiating Dialysis Early and Late (IDEAL) study. Nephrol Dial Transplant 26: 2082–2086.
19. Arce CM, Goldstein BA, Mitani AA, Winkelmayer WC (2013) Trends in relative mortality between Hispanic and non-Hispanic whites initiating dialysis: a retrospective study of the US Renal Data System. Am J Kidney Dis 62: 312–321.
20. Derose SF, Rutkowski MP, Crooks PW, Shi JM, Wang JQ, et al. (2013) Racial differences in estimated GFR decline, ESRD, and mortality in an integrated health system. Am J Kidney Dis 62: 236–244.
21. Conley J, Tonelli M, Quan H, Manns BJ, Palacios-Derflingher L, et al. (2012) Association between GFR, proteinuria, and adverse outcomes among White, Chinese, and South Asian individuals in Canada. Am J Kidney Dis 59: 390–399.
22. Barbour SJ, Er L, Djurdjev O, Karim M, Levin A (2010) Differences in progression of CKD and mortality amongst Caucasian, Oriental Asian and South Asian CKD patients. Nephrol Dial Transplant 25: 3663–3672.
23. Chang JH, Rim MY, Sung J, Ko KP, Kim DK, et al. (2012) Early start of dialysis has no survival benefit in end-stage renal disease patients. J Korean Med Sci 27: 1177–1181.
24. Oh KH, Hwang YH, Cho JH, Kim M, Ju KD, et al. (2012) Outcome of early initiation of peritoneal dialysis in patients with end-stage renal failure. J Korean Med Sci 27: 170–176.
25. Yamagata K, Nakai S, Iseki K, Tsubakihara Y, Committee of Renal Data Registry of the Japanese Society for Dialysis Therapy (2012) Late dialysis start did not affect long-term outcome in Japanese dialysis patients: long-term prognosis from Japanese Society for Dialysis Therapy Registry. Ther Apher Dial 16: 111–120.
26. Hwang SJ, Yang WC, Lin MY, Mau LW, Chen HC (2010) Impact of the clinical conditions at dialysis initiation on mortality in incident haemodialysis patients: a national cohort study in Taiwan. Nephrol Dial Transplant 25: 2616–2624.
27. Shiao CC, Huang JW, Chien KL, Chuang HF, Chen YM, et al. (2008) Early initiation of dialysis and late implantation of catheters adversely affect outcomes of patients on chronic peritoneal dialysis. Perit Dial Int 28: 73–81.
28. Kim do H, Kim M, Kim H, Kim YL, Kang SW, et al. (2013) Early referral to a nephrologist improved patient survival: prospective cohort study for end-stage renal disease in Korea. PLoS One 8: e55323.
29. Levey AS, Stevens LA, Schmid CH, Zhang YL, Castro AF 3rd, et al. (2009) A new equation to estimate glomerular filtration rate. Ann Intern Med 150: 604–612.
30. Charlson ME, Pompei P, Ales KL, MacKenzie CR (1987) A new method of classifying prognostic comorbidity in longitudinal studies: development and validation. J Chronic Dis 40: 373–383.
31. Hemmelgarn BR, Manns BJ, Quan H, Ghali WA (2003) Adapting the Charlson Comorbidity Index for use in patients with ESRD. Am J Kidney Dis 42: 125–132.
32. Fouque D, Kalantar-Zadeh K, Kopple J, Cano N, Chauveau P, et al. (2008) A proposed nomenclature and diagnostic criteria for protein-energy wasting in acute and chronic kidney disease. Kidney Int 73: 391–398.
33. Liu H, Peng Y, Liu F, Xiao H, Chen X, et al. (2008) Renal function and serum albumin at the start of dialysis in 514 Chinese ESRD in-patients. Ren Fail 30: 685–690.
34. Cooper BA, Aslani A, Ryan M, Ibels LS, Pollock CA (2003) Nutritional state correlates with renal function at the start of dialysis. Perit Dial Int 23: 291–295.
35. Pupim LB, Kent P, Caglar K, Shyr Y, Hakim RM, et al. (2002) Improvement in nutritional parameters after initiation of chronic hemodialysis. Am J Kidney Dis 40: 143–151.

36. Churchill DN (1997) An evidence-based approach to earlier initiation of dialysis. Am J Kidney Dis 30: 899–906.
37. Hakim RM, Lazarus JM (1995) Initiation of dialysis. J Am Soc Nephrol 6: 1319–1328.
38. Hemodialysis Adequacy 2006 Work Group (2006) Clinical practice guidelines for hemodialysis adequacy, update 2006. Am J Kidney Dis 48 Suppl 1: S2–90.
39. Peritoneal Dialysis Adequacy Work Group (2006) Clinical practice guidelines for peritoneal dialysis adequacy. Am J Kidney Dis 48 Suppl 1: S98–129.
40. Kelly J, Stanley M, Harris D, Caring for Australians with Renal Impairment (2005) The CARI guidelines. Acceptance into dialysis guidelines. Nephrology (Carlton) 10 Suppl 4: S46–60.
41. European Best Practice Guidelines Expert Group on Hemodialysis (2002) Section I. Measurement of renal function, when to refer and when to start dialysis. Nephrol Dial Transplant 17 Suppl 7: 7–15.
42. O'Hare AM, Choi AI, Boscardin WJ, Clinton WL, Zawadzki I, et al. (2011) Trends in timing of initiation of chronic dialysis in the United States. Arch Intern Med 171: 1663–1669.
43. Traynor JP, Simpson K, Geddes CC, Deighan CJ, Fox JG (2002) Early initiation of dialysis fails to prolong survival in patients with end-stage renal failure. J Am Soc Nephrol 13: 2125–2132.
44. Tang SC, Ho YW, Tang AW, Cheng YY, Chiu FH, et al. (2007) Delaying initiation of dialysis till symptomatic uraemia is it too late? Nephrol Dial Transplant 22: 1926–1932.
45. Korevaar JC, Jansen MA, Dekker FW, Jager KJ, Boeschoten EW, et al. (2001) When to initiate dialysis: effect of proposed US guidelines on survival. Lancet 358: 1046–1050.
46. Clark WF, Na Y, Rosansky SJ, Sontrop JM, Macnab JJ, et al. (2011) Association between estimated glomerular filtration rate at initiation of dialysis and mortality. CMAJ 183: 47–53.
47. Rosansky SJ, Eggers P, Jackson K, Glassock R, Clark WF (2011) Early start of hemodialysis may be harmful. Arch Intern Med 171: 396–403.
48. Lassalle M, Labeeuw M, Frimat L, Villar E, Joyeux V, et al. (2010) Age and comorbidity may explain the paradoxical association of an early dialysis start with poor survival. Kidney Int 77: 700–707.
49. Sawhney S, Djurdjev O, Simpson K, Macleod A, Levin A (2009) Survival and dialysis initiation: comparing British Columbia and Scotland registries. Nephrol Dial Transplant 24: 3186–3192.
50. Kazmi WH, Gilbertson DT, Obrador GT, Guo H, Pereira BJ, et al. (2005) Effect of comorbidity on the increased mortality associated with early initiation of dialysis. Am J Kidney Dis 46: 887–896.
51. Wright S, Klausner D, Baird B, Williams ME, Steinman T, et al. (2010) Timing of dialysis initiation and survival in ESRD. Clin J Am Soc Nephrol 5: 1828–1835.
52. Jansen MA, Hart AA, Korevaar JC, Dekker FW, Boeschoten EW, et al. (2002) Predictors of the rate of decline of residual renal function in incident dialysis patients. Kidney Int 62: 1046–1053.
53. Mehrotra R, Duong U, Jiwakanon S, Kovesdy CP, Moran J, et al. (2011) Serum albumin as a predictor of mortality in peritoneal dialysis: comparisons with hemodialysis. Am J Kidney Dis 58: 418–428.
54. Nguyen DB, Lessa FC, Belflower R, Mu Y, Wise M, et al. (2013) Invasive methicillin-resistant Staphylococcus aureus infections among patients on chronic dialysis in the United States, 2005–2011. Clin Infect Dis 57: 1393–1400.
55. Grootendorst DC, Michels WM, Richardson JD, Jager KJ, Boeschoten EW, et al. (2011) The MDRD formula does not reflect GFR in ESRD patients. Nephrol Dial Transplant 26: 1932–1937.
56. Beddhu S, Samore MH, Roberts MS, Stoddard GJ, Ramkumar N, et al. (2003) Impact of timing of initiation of dialysis on mortality. J Am Soc Nephrol 14: 2305–2312.
57. Crews DC, Scialla JJ, Boulware LE, Navaneethan SD, Nally JV Jr, et al. (2014) Comparative effectiveness of early versus conventional timing of dialysis initiation in advanced CKD. Am J Kidney Dis 63: 806–815.
58. van de Luijtgaarden MW, Noordzij M, Tomson C, Couchoud C, Cancarini G, et al. (2012) Factors influencing the decision to start renal replacement therapy: results of a survey among European nephrologists. Am J Kidney Dis 60: 940–948.
59. Streja E, Nicholas SB, Norris KC (2013) Controversies in timing of dialysis initiation and the role of race and demographics. Semin Dial 26: 658–666.
60. Slinin Y, Guo H, Li S, Liu J, Morgan B, et al. (2014) Provider and care characteristics associated with timing of dialysis initiation. Clin J Am Soc Nephrol 9: 310–317.
61. Bao Y, Dalrymple L, Chertow GM, Kaysen GA, Johansen KL (2012) Frailty, dialysis initiation, and mortality in end-stage renal disease. Arch Intern Med 172: 1071–1077.
62. Collins J, Cooper B, Branley P, Bulfone L, Craig J, et al. (2011) Outcomes of patients with planned initiation of hemodialysis in the IDEAL trial. Contrib Nephrol 171: 1–9.
63. Johnson DW, Wong MG, Cooper BA, Branley P, Bulfone L, et al. (2012) Effect of timing of dialysis commencement on clinical outcomes of patients with planned initiation of peritoneal dialysis in the IDEAL trial. Perit Dial Int 32: 595–604.

Hemodynamics and Function of Resistance Arteries in Healthy Persons and End Stage Renal Disease Patients

Morten K. Borg[1], Per Ivarsen[2], Emil Brøndum[1], Johan V. Povlsen[2], Christian Aalkjær[1]*

1 Department of Biomedicine, Aarhus University, Aarhus, Denmark, **2** Department of Renal Medicine, Aarhus University Hospital and Department of Clinical Medicine, Faculty of Health, Aarhus University, Aarhus, Denmark

Abstract

Introduction: Cardiovascular disease is the leading cause of death in patients with end stage renal disease (ESRD). The vasodilator mechanisms in small resistance arteries are in earlier studies shown to be reduced in patients with end stage renal disease. We studied whether endothelium dependent vasodilatation were diminished in ESRD patients and the interaction between the macro- and microcirculation.

Methods: Eleven patients with ESRD had prior to renal transplant or insertion of peritoneal dialysis catheter measured pulse wave velocity. During surgery, a subcutaneous fat biopsy was extracted. Resistance arteries were then dissected and mounted on a wire myograph for measurements of dilator response to increasing concentrations of acetylcholine after preconstriction with noradrenaline. Twelve healthy kidney donors served as controls.

Results: Systolic blood pressure was elevated in patients compared to the healthy controls; no difference in the concentration of asymmetric dimethyl arginine was seen. No significant difference in the endothelium dependent vasodilatation between patients and controls was found. Correlation of small artery properties showed an inverse relationship between diastolic blood pressure and nitric oxide dependent vasodilatation in controls. Pulse pressure was positively correlated to the total endothelial vasodilatation in patients. A negative association between S-phosphate and endothelial derived hyperpolarisation-like vasodilatation was seen in resistance arteries from controls.

Conclusion: This study finds similar vasodilator properties in kidney patients and controls. However, correlations of pulse pressure and diastolic blood pressure with resistance artery function indicate compensating measures in the microcirculation during end stage renal disease.

Editor: Emmanuel A Burdmann, University of Sao Paulo Medical School, Brazil

Funding: The study was funded by the P Carl Petersen Foundation and the Danish Kidney Association. The funders had no role in study design, data collection and analysis, decision to publish, or preparation of the manuscript.

Competing Interests: The authors have declared that no competing interests exist.

* E-mail: ca@fi.au.dk

Introduction

Cardiovascular disease (CVD) is overrepresented in patients with reduced kidney function, and the risk increases with declining kidney function, why CVD is the major cause of death in patients with end stage renal disease (ESRD) [1]. Both arterial stiffness and small artery structural and functional alterations are involved in the pathophysiology leading to changes in the cardiovascular system, but the mechanisms responsible are not fully elucidated.

Arterial stiffness, defined as decreased ability and degree of the conductive arteries to absorb the pulse pressure is related to mortality in dialysis and non-dialysis patients [2,3]. The degree of arterial stiffness can be estimated by measuring pulse pressure, pulse wave velocity (PWV) or augmentation index (AI). The mechanisms inducing stiffening of the conductive arteries are complex and include both non-renal risk factors e.g. smoking, diabetes, hypertension and renal risk factors such as calcification, increased plasma concentration of asymmetric dimethylarginine (ADMA), inflammation and oxidative stress [4,5].

The function of the large arteries' viscoelasticity reduces the pulsative pressure and flow that results from the intermittent ventricular ejection, securing a stabile pressure and flow at the level of small arteries. When stiffness increases, an augmentation of the pulse wave is present because of changes in the timing and size of reflection. This might induce damage and change the functionality of the vascular microcirculation as it is exposed to a higher pulsative pressure and flow.

Endothelium-dependent vasodilatation occurs via three main pathways; cyclooxygenase (COX) products, nitric oxide (NO) and endothelium-derived hyperpolarisation (EDH) [6]. Endothelium-dependent vasodilatation in the large arteries from ESRD patients has been examined with forearm blood flow measurements and shown to be associated with an impairment of the vasodilator properties due to a defect in the NO-pathway [7]. Similar results have been obtained in brachial artery, where shear stress induced vasodilatation in ESRD patients was found attenuated at maximal shear stress [8]. The diminished vasodilator function in the macro circulation of ESRD patients, measured as post-ischemic reactive hyperemia, is associated with increased all-cause mortality [9].

Investigations of the micro circulation (the resistance arteries) of ESRD patients show no difference from similar arteries from healthy controls when comparing morphology and sensitivity to vasoconstrictors [10]. Endothelium independent vasodilatation is also found unchanged, whereas studies examining the endothelium dependent vasodilatation have yielded different results, as resistance arteries from ESRD patients have shown to have a reduced relaxation to acetylcholine (ACh) [11]. This appears to be due to a defect in the NO-pathway [12], while another study shows that the EDHF-response is attenuated, but only when using bradykinin as the agonist and not ACh [13].

In this study we wanted to evaluate differences in vascular function in arteries from patients with ESRD and normal controls and to study the interaction between the macro- and micro-circulation. Especially we wanted to test whether endothelium dependent vasodilatation was diminished in ESRD patients with well controlled blood pressure.

Materials and Methods

Study population

Eleven patients with ESRD were enrolled in the study. Nine had living related donor renal transplant and two insertion of peritoneal dialysis catheter. Patients included were above 18 years of age. Exclusion criteria were persisting cardiac arrhythmias, severe congestive heart failure, reduced pulmonary function, severe psychiatric disease, acute infection and leg-amputation. Five patients were treated with peritoneal dialysis (vintage 252 days (101-568) median (range)); four with hemodialysis (vintage 769 days (14-1201)) and two were not on dialysis. Patient's kidney diseases were glomerulonephritis (n = 5), adult polycystic kidney disease (n = 2), obstructive nephropathy (n = 2), type 1 diabetes mellitus (n = 1) and vasculitis (n = 1). No patient had diabetes mellitus as comorbidity. Nine out of eleven were treated with antihypertensive medication. Two were treated with angiotensin converting enzyme inhibitors, four with angiotensin receptor blockade, six with calcium antagonists, four with beta-blockers, six with diuretics, ten with erythropoietin analogs and one with statins.

The majority of patients were cardiovascular assessed as part of the pre-transplantation assessment or ESRD regular control with echocardiography, coronary angiogram and CT scans of the iliac arteries. All investigation was performed in the year before the study and none had any cardiovascular event between the cardiovascular assessment and transplantation. All patients had an echocardiography; ten had normal ejection fraction (EF) while one patient had an EF of 40%. One of the patients had indication of a light aortastenosis and five patients had light left ventricular hypertrophy. Nine patients had a coronary angiogram; seven patients had normal coronary arteries, one had earlier coronary by-pass and one had some calcification but no stenosis. Seven had a CT scan of the iliac arteries; five had no calcification, 2 had mild to moderate calcification. Cholesterol was measured in six patients, with a mean value of 4.9 mmol/l. Inflammatory profile were assessed with c-reactive protein in ten of eleven patients prior to surgery; all values were less than 10 mg/l.

Twelve kidney donors with no preexisting medical conditions or drug intake served as healthy controls. Before surgery the kidney recipients received 2 days of immunosuppressive therapy consisting of 0.2 mg/kg tacrolimus, 1.5 g mycophenolat mofetil acid and 20 mg prednisolone. The study was performed in accordance with the Declaration of Helsinki. Protocol and consent forms were approved by the local research Ethics Committee (Central Denmark Region), and all participants gave written informed consent before inclusion.

Protocol

Participant's body weight, height and blood pressure were measured and hemodynamic data were calculated the day before surgery. Patient's type of dialysis, vintage, underlying condition and drug intake were obtained from medical records. Blood samples were taken on the day of surgery. During surgery a 2×3 cm biopsy containing skin and subcutaneous fat was removed from the abdominal wall with scalpel without the use of diathermy.

Microvascular function

Subcutaneous fat biopsies were immediately after extraction placed in 5°C physiological salt solution (PSS), transported to the lab where 2 mm long segments of arteries were isolated and mounted on two stainless steel wires (40 μm diameter) in the organ baths of a 4-channel wire myograph (model 610M, Danish Myo Technology (DMT), Aarhus, Denmark) or in a double channel myograph (model 410A, DMT) for isometric force measurement. The myograph contained PSS at 37°C, continuously bubbled with a gas mixture containing 5% $CO_2$and 21% O_2 in a nitrogen based gas to keep pH at 7.4 at all times. Upon mounting, the arteries were left 20 min to equilibrate before stepwise stretching, characterizing the elastic properties as described by Mulvany and Halpern [14]. Experiments were conducted at 90% of L_{100} (defined as the circumference of the relaxed artery exposed to a transmural pressure of 100 mmHg). Viability of the arteries was tested using 10 μM noradrenaline (NA) twice before beginning the experiments. The arteries were preconstricted with 3 μM NA and subsequent relaxation using increasing concentrations of the endothelium-dependent vasodilator ACh. The experiment were repeated after incubation (20 min) with first the COX-inhibitor indomethacin (3 μM) and then the combination of the NOS inhibitor L-NAME (100 μM) and indomethacin.

To ensure that the endothelium was viable no artery was submitted to more than 3 endothelium-dependent relaxation curves and were left resting for 20 minutes between curves during incubation.

The composition of PSS was (mM): NaCl 119, KCl 4.7, KH_2PO_4 1.18, $MgSO_4$ 1.17, $NaHCO_3$ 25, $CaCl_2$ 1.6, EDTA 0.026, and glucose 5.5. The chemicals were obtained from Sigma (St.Louis, MO, USA). Indomethacin was dissolved in ethanol, the other chemicals in distilled water.

Hemodynamics

Cardiac output (CO) was measured by rebreathing technique in a closed system containing a gas mixture of sulfahexafloride and nitrous oxide in a mixture of oxygen and nitrogen (Innocor, Denmark). Rebreathing was performed in the sitting position during 15 s with a breathing rate of 14–16 min^{-1} and a volume of 1.8 l after a rest of at least 10 min [15]. Gas was sampled continuously from the mouthpiece and analyzed online on an infrared gas analyzer. Pulmonary blood flow (PBF) was calculated from uptake rate of nitrous oxide into the blood. The first two or three breaths were excluded from analysis if the total lung volume measured by sulfahexafloride indicated incomplete gas mixture. In the majority of patients without pulmonary arterio-venous shunt PBF equals CO [16,17]. In contrast in patients with pulmonary shunt, the shunt fraction is calculated and added to PBF to get CO. The shunt fraction is calculated from the oxygen concentration [18]. The calculations were performed assuming that the gasses were mixed completely and that the equilibration of gasses between alveoli and capillary was rapid and that lung flow was constant. Systolic blood pressure (SBP) and diastolic blood pressure (DBP) were measured by an automatic device connected to the Innocor. Systemic vascular resistance index (SVRi) was calculated as: (Mean arterial blood pressure – central venous pressure)/Cardiac output and indexed to body surface by Innocor. The measurement was performed twice, and the mean values were used in data analysis.

PWV and AI were measured in the supine position after 10 min of rest. Carotid–femoral PWV was measured with SphygmoCor, AtCor Medical, Texas, US, using the integral software.

Augmentation pressure was calculated as the difference between the second and first systolic peaks, and AI was calculated as the augmentation pressure expressed as percentage of pulse pressure. AI was measured for aorta. All of the measurements were made in duplicate by one trained study nurse, and the mean values were used in the subsequent analysis.

Biochemistry

Asymmetric dimethyl arginine (ADMA) was measured using ELISA (DLD Diagnostika GmbH, Germany). All other biochemistry was analysed at the Department of Clinical Biochemistry, Aarhus University Hospital. EGFR was calculated from the 4 point MDRD formula.

Statistics

Data in figures are presented as mean ± SEM, in tables as mean ± SEM or median (range). Concentration-response curves to ACh are given as percentage relaxation of the pre-constriction to NA. EC_{50} values are calculated by non-linear regression for variable slope for each vessel and presented as the negative logarithmic value in mol/L (pEC50). NO dependent response was calculated as the difference between EC_{50} values of indomethacin and indomethacin/L-NAME curves respectively (ΔpEC_{50}). Mean pEC_{50}, ΔpEC_{50} and baseline characteristics on patients were compared using unpaired student's *t*-test. Associations between variables were calculated using Pearson's correlation. $P<0.05$ were considered significant. All statistical analyses were performed with GraphPad Prism (v. 4.03 GraphPad Software Inc., CA, US)

Results

Study population

Kidney function was significant lower in ESRD patient, as expected. Age, weight and BMI were similar, whereas systolic, but not diastolic, blood pressure was significantly elevated in ESRD patients (Table 1), despite antihypertensive treatment. Blood hemoglobin concentration was decreased in ESRD patients, whereas no significant difference in ADMA concentration was found.

Microvascular function

Relaxation of subcutaneous resistance arteries with ACh was not significantly different between ESRD patients and controls (Figure 1A). Both maximal relaxation and pEC50 were comparable (maximal relaxation: 84±4% vs. 90±2%, p = 0.22; pEC50: 7.06±0.12 vs. 6.97±0.06, p = 0.52).

The EDH-like relaxation was recorded after blockade of eNOS and COX (Figure 1B). The maximal relaxation and sensitivity to ACh was similar between the two groups (maximal relaxation: 68±5% vs. 66±5%, p = 0.82; pEC50: 6.39±0.17 vs. 6.15±0.21, p = 0.38).

The NO-dependent vasodilatation was calculated as ΔpEC_{50} for concentration response curves incubated with indomethacin and indomethacin + L-NAME respectively (figure 2). No

Table 1. Baseline characteristics for end stage renal disease (ESRD) patients and healthy controls.

Variable	ESRD (n = 11)	Controls (n = 12)
Sex (male/female)	6/5	4/8
Age (years)	51(19–85)	54(36–70)
S-Creatinine (µmol/mL)	806±82*	68±3
eGFR (mL/min/1,73 m²)	6.7±0.7*	87.5±4.2
Systolic blood pressure (mmHg)	130±2*§	119±4#
Diastolic blood pressure (mmHg)	78±3§	76±2#
Pulse pressure (mmHg)	52±3§	43±4#
Weight (kg)	73.2±3.2§	75.9±3.8#
BMI (kg/m²)	24.6±1.2§	26.2±0.9#
Hemoglobin (mmol/L)	7.2±0.3*	8.2±0.2
S-Calcium-ion (mmol/L)	1.18±0.03	1.22±0.02
S-Phosphate (mmol/l)	1.87±0.10*	1.14±0.03
S-PTH (pmol/l)	24.9±5.1	NA
Albuminuria (g/day)	3.38±1.30*§	0±0
ADMA (µmol/L)	0.78±0.04§	0.72±0.02

Data are mean±SEM, except for age which is median (range); * $p<0.05$, § n = 10, # n = 11.

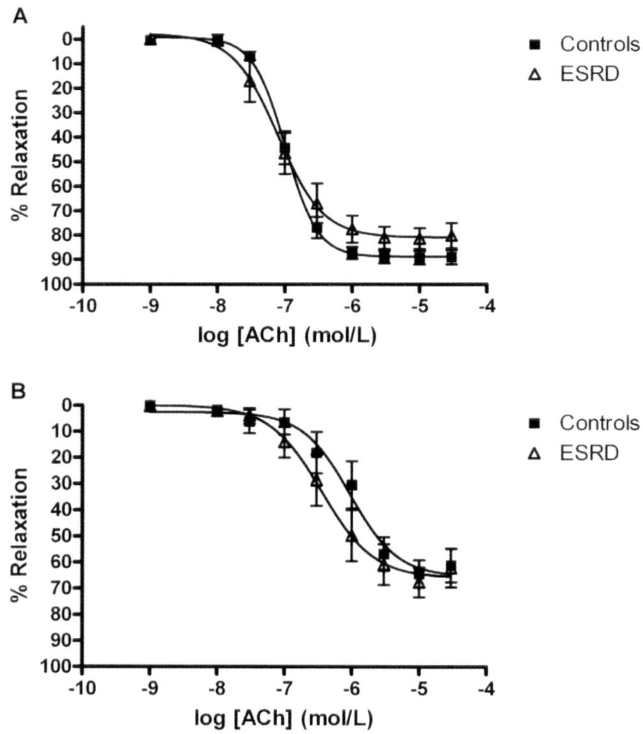

Figure 1. Concentration-response relaxation curves to acetylcholine in arteries from healthy controls and patients with end stage renal disease. A: Endothelium dependent vasodilatation; p = ns. B: Endothelium-derived hyperpolarisation-like relaxation in the presence of indomethacin and L-NAME; p = ns.

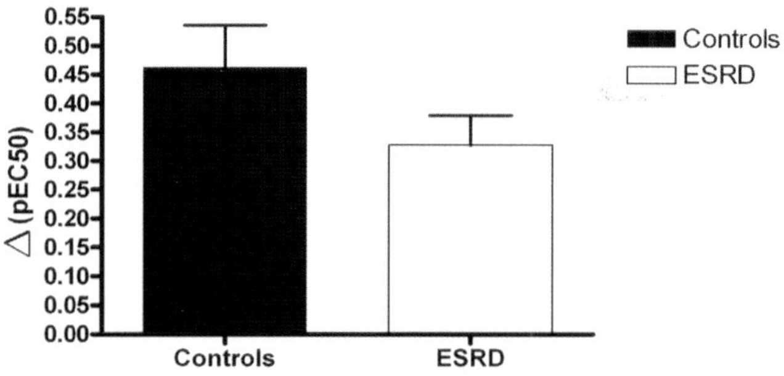

Figure 2. Nitric oxide dependent-response, calculated as the difference between pEC_{50}-values of concentration response curves incubated with indomethacin and indomethacin/L-NAME respectively – ΔpEC_{50}; controls (n = 10), ESRD (n = 11); p = 0.15.

significant difference between ESRD and controls was found (ΔpEC_{50} was 0.33±0.05 vs. 0.46±0.07, ESRD and controls, respectively, p = 0.15).

To assess whether three concentration response curves to acetylcholine can be obtained, time control experiments were performed. Three concentration response curves, with 20 minutes of rest in between, were conducted; without use of any blocking agent (figure 3). As seen there was no deterioration in the response to acetylcholine with time.

Hemodynamics

PWV and SVRi were not significantly different in the two groups, while AI was lower in the ESRD group (table 2), which was not expected. This was probably because of small sample size.

Associations between micro- and macrovascular functions

DBP was inversely related to the NO-dependent vasorelaxation in controls (r = −0.59; p<0.05) (figure 4). The inverse relation was not significant in ESRD (r = −0.44; p = 0.10).

Pulse pressure was positively correlated to ACh induced vasodilatation in ESRD (r = 0.81; p<0.01), this was not the case in control subjects (r = −0.17; p = 0.31) (figure 5).

Table 2. Hemodynamics in patients with end stage renal disease (ESRD) and healthy controls.

Variable	ESRD (n = 5)	Controls (n = 12)
Pulse wave velocity (m/s)	11.38±3.33§	7.11±0.39#
Augmentation index (%)	122±7*	154±9#
Cardiac output index (L/min/m²)	3.58±0.42*	2.79±0.14
SVR index (mmHg/(L/min)/m²)	28.05±2.99	32.58±1.40

Systemic vascular resistance (SVR).
Data are mean±SEM; * p<0.05; § n = 4; # n = 10.

Correlation of ADMA and NO-response showed a trend in controls (figure 6), although not statistically significant (r = 0.49; p = 0.07), whereas no trend was seen in ESRD (r = 0.01; p = 0.97).

As expected S-phosphate levels were different in the two groups. A negative association was found between S-phosphate and EDH-like response in controls(r = −0.66; p<0.05), but not in ESRD (r = −0.30; p = 0.18) (figure 7).

Cardiac output and vasodilatation were inversely related in controls (figure 8), higher cardiac output resulted in a diminished vasorelaxation (r = −0.50; p = 0.05). While no relation was present in ESRD (r = 0.76; p = 0.12).

Discussion

In the present study, we evaluated micro- and macrovascular differences in ESRD patients and healthy controls and for the first time correlated these findings. The ESRD patients had little comorbidity and well controlled blood pressure. In the microvascular function no significant different response to endothelium dependent vasodilatation was seen between ESRD and healthy controls. In the macrovascular arteries a significant higher SBP was present in the ESRD patients. Micro- and macrovascular function was correlated, DBP and the NO-dependent vasorelaxation was inversely related in controls. Pulse pressure was positively correlated to endothelial vasodilatation in ESRD and interestingly a negative correlation between S-phosphate and EDH-like response was found in controls.

The microvascular endothelial dependent vasodilator response to ACh has earlier been shown to be diminished in ESRD, while attempts to determine the affected pathway, has yielded diverging

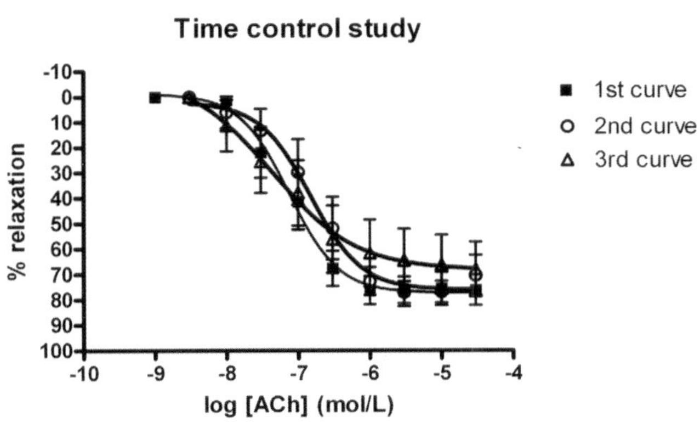

Figure 3. Time control experiments; three consecutive concentration response curves, with 20 minutes of rest in between, without use of blocker.

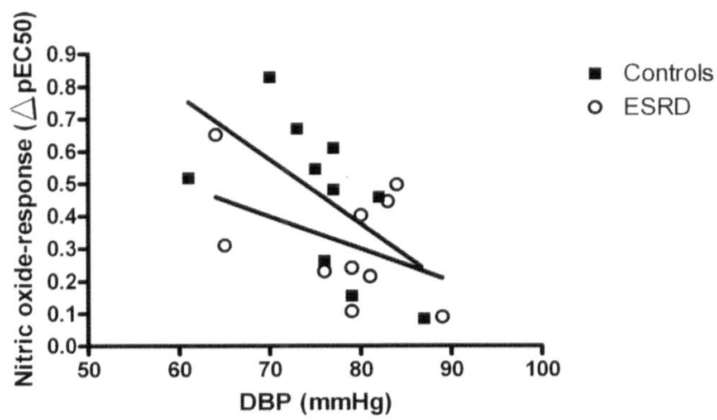

Figure 4. Association between diastolic blood pressure and nitric oxide-response (ΔpEC_{50}) in controls (r = −0.59; p<0.05) and ESRD (r = −0.44; p = 0.10), Pearson one-tailed correlation.

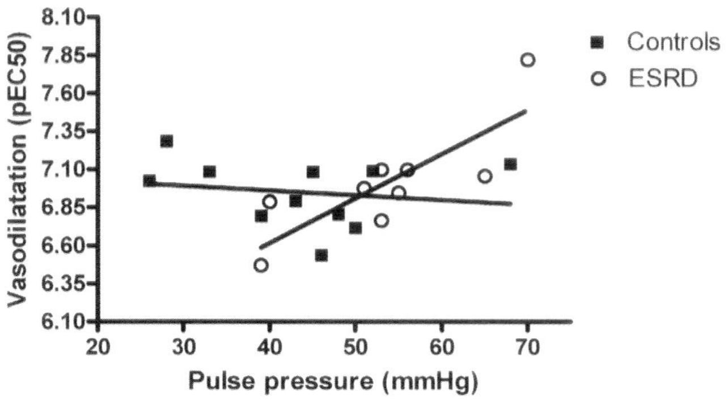

Figure 5. Association between pulse pressure and vasodilatation (pEC_{50}) in controls ($r = -0.17$; $p = 0.31$) and ESRD ($r = 0.81$; $p < 0.01$), Pearson one-tailed correlation.

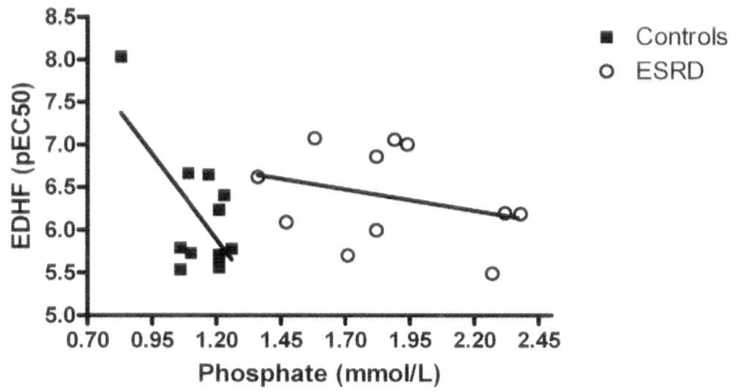

Figure 7. Association between S-Phosphate and EDH-like relaxation (pEC_{50}) in controls ($r = -0.66$; $p < 0.05$) and ESRD ($r = -0.30$; $p = 0.18$), Pearson one-tailed correlation.

results [11–13]. In our study a similar vasodilator response to ACh was found, both under control conditions and after inhibition of NOS and COX dependent pathways. The earlier studies suggested that the ACh induced vasodilatation is diminished in ESRD patients [11]; others have confirmed this and suggested that the affected pathway is NOS dependent [12] or involves EDH-like relaxation [13]. Luksha et al. [13] found that only bradykinin-induced EDH-like relaxation was reduced, while ACh-induced EDH-like relaxation was similar in the two groups. Hence parts of our results differ from earlier studies. The diverging results must rely on a complex mixture of a different period of exposure to the uremic milieu, patients' age, physical form, pharmacological treatment, dialysis and blood pressure levels while the experimental setup seems comparable. The lack of a significant difference in resistance artery function in the two groups is consistent with the similar SVRi in the two groups.

Our patients have substantial lower blood pressure than the patients in the aforementioned papers. Since diastolic hypertension is known to cause an attenuated ACh induced vasorelaxation in the resistance arteries [19], the possibility of normal endothelial function in resistance arteries of ESRD patients with well controlled blood pressures seems feasible. We found a negative association between diastolic blood pressure and NO-response in controls (figure 4), while this was not statistically significant in ESRD. This further suggests a greater role of high blood pressure in the attenuation of endothelial function in resistance arteries than the uremia per se. The similar ADMA levels in patients and controls additionally suggest a relative low exposure to the uremic toxicity indicating well treated dialysis patients. This contrasts with the patients used in the previous studies [12,13] where ADMA levels were significantly increased.

Interestingly we found a positive correlation between pulse pressure and micro-vascular vasodilatation in ESRD patients, which was not present in control subjects. This indicates that higher pulse pressure, which could translate into arterial stiffness, generates a process in the microcirculation that increases the vasodilator properties. Knowing that our patients are well treated in terms of blood pressure and with exposure to uremic toxins, we can speculate, that with longer exposure to renal deficiency, this compensation reaches its maximum and instead diminishing of the vasodilatation starts, as shown in other studies [11–13].

As expected the pulse wave velocity was increased in the ESRD population [20] – although in our study not statistically significant. At the same time cardiac output was higher possibly as a consequence of a reduced hemoglobin level.

Interestingly, we showed that the EDH-like response in healthy controls is dependent on the S-phosphate level, with a decreased vasodilator response with higher S-phosphate, even within the normal range of S-phosphate. We believe that further studies in this field are required to finally establish this correlation. Interestingly is has recently been shown that incubating resistance vessels from both healthy controls and patients with chronic kidney disease with a higher concentration of phosphate decrease the endothelium dependent vasodilatation [21]. The same group

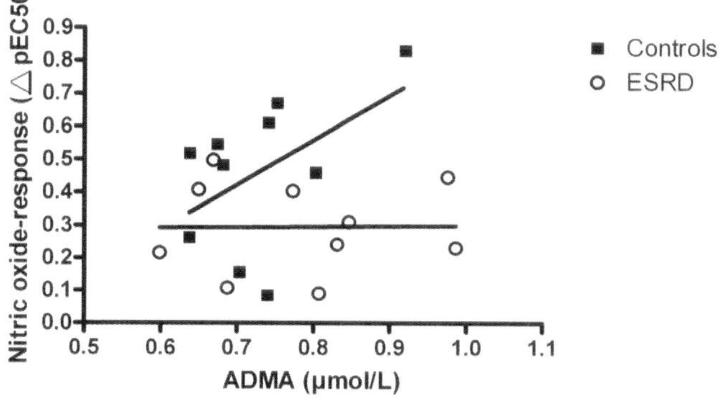

Figure 6. Association between ADMA and NOS dependent relaxation (ΔpEC_{50}) in controls ($r = 0.49<$; $p = 0.07$) and ESRD ($r = 0.01$; $p = 0.97$), Pearson one-tailed correlation.

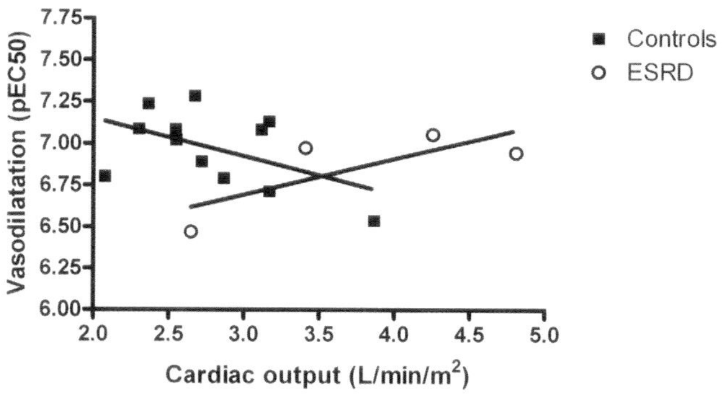

Figure 8. Association between cardiac output and vasodilatation (pEC_{50}) in controls ($r = -0.50$; $p = 0.05$) and ESRD ($r = 0.76$; $p = 0.12$), Pearson one-tailed correlation.

has shown that loading healthy people with phosphate reduces flow-mediated dilatation, indicating impaired endothelial function. After loading, S-phosphate was still within normal range [21]. Other studies have shown that FGF23, which might be an indicator of dietary phosphate load [22] is related to a reduced flow-mediated dilatation [23]. Our data indicates that the level of S-phosphate might affect the vasorelaxation.

When assessing cardiac output and sensitivity of resistance arteries to ACh, opposing associations were seen in controls and ESRD (figure 8). This could suggest that in healthy subjects, better vasodilator capacity in the resistance arteries is associated with a lower cardiac output, which could translate into diminished workload on the heart in the long term, and subsequent a lower risk of cardiac failure.

Study limitation

The sample size of study groups was relatively small which possess a risk of committing type II errors and overinterpretation of the correlations. The majority of patients was receiving kidney transplants, and was therefore with less comorbidity than most patients in dialysis. This could explain why we see little difference between healthy controls and kidney patients in some of our assays.

Conclusions

In conclusion this study finds similar vasodilator properties in small resistance arteries of ESRD and control subjects. ESRD patients were well controlled in terms of blood pressure and uremic exposure. However correlations of pulse pressure, diastolic blood pressure and cardiac output with micro-vascular functions, indicate compensating measures in the microcirculation of ESRD patients.

Acknowledgments

The authors wish to thank the included patients and staff at Aarhus University Hospital involved in sample collection. Special thanks to laboratory technician Jørgen Andresen and project nurse Karin Hansen for excellent technical assistance.

Author Contributions

Conceived and designed the experiments: MB PI CA EB JP. Performed the experiments: MB PI CA. Analyzed the data: MB PI CA. Contributed reagents/materials/analysis tools: MB PI CA JP. Wrote the paper: MB PI CA.

References

1. Foley RN, Parfrey PS (1998) Cardiovascular disease and mortality in ESRD. J Nephrol 11: 239–245.
2. Pannier B, Guerin AP, Marchais SJ, Safar ME, London GM (2005) Stiffness of capacitive and conduit arteries: prognostic significance for end-stage renal disease patients. Hypertension 45: 592–596.
3. Blacher J, Guerin AP, Pannier B, Marchais SJ, Safar ME, et al. (1999) Impact of aortic stiffness on survival in end-stage renal disease. Circulation 99: 2434–2439.
4. Mallamaci F, Tripepi G, Cutrupi S, Malatino LS, Zoccali C (2005) Prognostic value of combined use of biomarkers of inflammation, endothelial dysfunction, and myocardiopathy in patients with ESRD. Kidney Int 67: 2330–2337.
5. Tripepi G, Mattace RF, Sijbrands E, Seck MS, Maas R, et al. (2011) Inflammation and asymmetric dimethylarginine for predicting death and cardiovascular events in ESRD patients. Clin J Am Soc Nephrol 6: 1714–1721.
6. Triggle CR, Samuel SM, Ravishankar S, Marei I, Arunachalam G, et al. (2012) The endothelium: influencing vascular smooth muscle in many ways. Can J Physiol Pharmacol 90: 713–738.
7. Passauer J, Pistrosch F, Bussemaker E, Lassig G, Herbrig K, et al. (2005) Reduced agonist-induced endothelium-dependent vasodilation in uremia is attributable to an impairment of vascular nitric oxide. J Am Soc Nephrol 16: 959–965.
8. Verbeke FH, Pannier B, Guerin AP, Boutouyrie P, Laurent S, et al. (2011) Flow-mediated vasodilation in end-stage renal disease. Clin J Am Soc Nephrol 6: 2009–2015.
9. London GM, Pannier B, Agharazii M, Guerin AP, Verbeke FH, et al. (2004) Forearm reactive hyperemia and mortality in end-stage renal disease. Kidney Int 65: 700–704.
10. Aalkjaer C, Pedersen EB, Danielsen H, Fjeldborg O, Jespersen B, et al. (1986) Morphological and functional characteristics of isolated resistance vessels in advanced uraemia. Clin Sci (Lond) 71: 657–663.
11. Morris ST, McMurray JJ, Spiers A, Jardine AG (2001) Impaired endothelial function in isolated human uremic resistance arteries. Kidney Int 60: 1077–1082.
12. Luksha N, Luksha L, Carrero JJ, Hammarqvist F, Stenvinkel P, et al. (2011) Impaired resistance artery function in patients with end-stage renal disease. Clin Sci (Lond) 120: 525–536.
13. Luksha L, Stenvinkel P, Hammarqvist F, Carrero JJ, Davidge ST, et al. (2012) Mechanisms of endothelial dysfunction in resistance arteries from patients with end-stage renal disease. PLoS One 7: e36056.
14. Halpern W, Mulvany MJ (1977) Tension responses to small length changes of vascular smooth muscle cells [proceedings]. J Physiol 265: 21P–23P.
15. Damgaard M, Norsk P (2005) Effects of ventilation on cardiac output determined by inert gas rebreathing. Clin Physiol Funct Imaging 25: 142–147.
16. Friedman M, Wilkins SA Jr, Rothfeld AF, Bromberg PA (1984) Effect of ventilation and perfusion imbalance on inert gas rebreathing variables. J Appl Physiol 56: 364–369.
17. Petrini MF, Peterson BT, Hyde RW (1978) Lung tissue volume and blood flow by rebreathing theory. J Appl Physiol 44: 795–802.
18. Clemensen P, Christensen P, Norsk P, Gronlund J (1994) A modified photo- and magnetoacoustic multigas analyzer applied in gas exchange measurements. J Appl Physiol 76: 2832–2839.
19. Olsen MH, Wachtell K, Aalkjaer C, Devereux RB, Dige-Petersen H, et al. (2001) Endothelial dysfunction in resistance arteries is related to high blood pressure and circulating low density lipoproteins in previously treated hypertension. Am J Hypertens 14: 861–867.
20. Townsend RR, Wimmer NJ, Chirinos JA, Parsa A, Weir M, et al. (2010) Aortic PWV in chronic kidney disease: a CRIC ancillary study. Am J Hypertens 23: 282–289.
21. Abstracts of the 50th ERA-EDTA (European Renal Association-European Dialysis and Transplant Association) Congress. May 18-21, 2013. Istanbul, Turkey. Nephrol Dial Transplant 28 Suppl 1: i1–553.
22. Isakova T, Gutierrez OM, Wolf M (2009) A blueprint for randomized trials targeting phosphorus metabolism in chronic kidney disease. Kidney Int 76: 705–716.
23. Yilmaz MI, Sonmez A, Saglam M, Yaman H, Kilic S, et al. (2013) Longitudinal analysis of vascular function and biomarkers of metabolic bone disorders before and after renal transplantation. Am J Nephrol 37: 126–134.

Course of Symptoms and Health-Related Quality of Life during Specialized Pre-Dialysis Care

Moniek C. M. de Goeij[1]*, Gurbey Ocak[1], Joris I. Rotmans[2], Jan-Willem Eijgenraam[3], Friedo W. Dekker[1], Nynke Halbesma[1]

1 Department of Clinical Epidemiology, Leiden University Medical Center, Leiden, The Netherlands, **2** Department of Nephrology, Leiden University Medical Center, Leiden, The Netherlands, **3** Department of Internal Medicine, Nephrology, Groene Hart Hospital, Gouda, The Netherlands

Abstract

Background: Concerns are present on the limited value of renal function alone in defining the optimal moment to start dialysis. Disease-related symptoms and health-related quality of life (HRQOL) may have additional clinical value in defining this moment, but little is known about how these parameters change during pre-dialysis care. The aims of our study were to describe the course of symptoms and HRQOL during pre-dialysis care and to investigate their association with poor health outcomes.

Methods: In the prospective PREPARE-2 cohort, incident patients starting specialized pre-dialysis care were included when referred to one of the 25 participating Dutch outpatient clinics (2004–2011). In the present analysis, 436 patients with data available on symptoms and HRQOL were included. Clinical data, symptoms (revised illness perception questionnaire), and HRQOL (short form-36 questionnaire; physical and mental summary score) were collected every 6-month interval. A time-dependent Cox proportional hazard model was used to associate symptoms and HRQOL with the combined poor health outcome (i.e. starting dialysis, receiving a kidney transplant, and death).

Results: All symptoms increased, especially fatigue and loss of strength, and both the physical and mental summary score decreased over time, with the most pronounced change during the last 6–12 months of follow-up. Furthermore, each additional symptom (adjusted HR 1.04 (95% CI, 1.00–1.09)) and each 3-point lower physical and mental summary score (adjusted HR 1.04 (1.02–1.06) and 1.04 (1.02–1.06) respectively) were associated with a higher risk of reaching the combined poor health outcome within the subsequent 6 months.

Conclusions: The number of symptoms increased and both the physical and mental HRQOL score decreased during pre-dialysis care and these changes were associated with starting dialysis, receiving a kidney transplant, and death. These results may indicate that symptoms and HRQOL are good markers for the medical condition and disease stage of pre-dialysis patients.

Editor: Olaf M. Dekkers, Leiden University Medical Centre, Netherlands

Funding: This study was supported by a grant from the Dutch Kidney Foundation (SB 110, www.nierstichting.nl), and unrestricted grants from Amgen (www.amgen.nl) and Baxter (www.baxter.nl). The funders had no role in study design, data collection and analysis, decision to publish, or preparation of the manuscript.

Competing Interests: The authors have declared that no competing interests exist.

* E-mail: M.C.M.de_Goeij@lumc.nl

Introduction

A large debate is ongoing about the optimal moment to start with dialysis.[1–5] The last decades there has been a trend towards starting dialysis at higher levels of renal function.[6–9] However, many observational studies[9–18] and the first randomized controlled trial, the Initiating Dialysis Early And Late (IDEAL) study [19], showed no difference in patient survival between early and late initiation of dialysis. In addition, consensus has been reached within the European Renal Best Practice guidelines on the limited value of renal function alone in the decision to start with dialysis. [4] Disease-related symptoms and a low health-related quality of life (HRQOL) are highly present in pre-dialysis patients and therefore may have an added clinical value on top of renal function in this difficult decision.

Symptoms can start appearing when renal function decreases to half of the normal function and continue to rise when renal function further decreases. [20] Furthermore, several cross-sectional studies showed that a low renal function is associated with a low HRQOL[21–23] and that HRQOL is a good predictor for mortality and progression to end-stage renal disease in chronic kidney disease (CKD) patients [24]. However, knowledge is lacking on the specific development of symptoms and HRQOL during pre-dialysis care. Moreover, several guidelines indicating when to start dialysis already take into account the presence of symptoms. [25,26] However, the incorporations of these symptoms into the guidelines are not consistent and specific. Furthermore, both the IDEAL study and some observational studies showed that for the decision to start with dialysis, symptoms were at least as important as renal function.

Table 1. Baseline characteristics for total population and stratified by type of endpoint.

	Total	Combined poor health outcome^	End of follow-up/Other
	(n = 436)	*(n = 284)*	*(n = 152)*
Age (years)	69 (56–76)	68 (54–75)	71 (60–78)
Sex (male, %)	66	67	65
Caucasian (%)	92	93	92
BMI (kg/m^2)*	26.7±5.1	26.8±4.9	26.4±5.6
Smokers/quitters <1 year before inclusion (%)	25	24	26
Primary kidney disease (%)			
Diabetes mellitus	13	12	15
Glomerulonephritis	14	13	15
Renal vascular disease	31	30	31
Interstitial nephropathy	7	7	7
Cystic kidney disease	12	16	5
Multisystem disease	4	4	4
Other	19	18	23
eGFR (ml/min/1.73 m^2)[†]	16.9±6.1	15.2±5.5	20.1±5.8
Proteinuria (g/24 h)[§]	1.0 (0.3–2.2)	1.3 (0.4–2.5)	0.7 (0.2–1.4)
Urea (mmol/l)[•]	22.2±7.0	23.0±6.9	20.4±7.0
Creatinine clearance (ml/min/1.73 m^2)[□]	19.2±7.9	17.3±7.3	23.4±7.7
Systolic blood pressure (mmHg)[Δ]	142±22	143±22	140±23
Hemoglobin (g/dl)**	12.3±1.5	12.2±1.4	12.6±1.6
Potassium (mmol/l)[‡]	4.7±0.6	4.8±0.7	4.7±0.6
Bicarbonate (mmol/l)[••]	23.0±4.0	22.4±3.6	24.3±4.3
Comorbidities (%)			
Cardiovascular disease[□□]	42	41	45
Diabetes Mellitus[ΔΔ]	26	24	30

Median (boundaries of interquartile range) is given for age and proteinuria and mean ± standard deviation is given for all other normally distributed continuous variables.
^Defined as starting dialysis, receiving a kidney transplant, and death.
*Available for 428 patients.
[†]Estimated glomerular filtration rate (eGFR) is calculated with the 4-variable Modification of Diet in Renal Disease formula and available for 379 patients.
[§]Available for 225 patients.
[•]Available for 365 patients.
[□]Creatinine clearance is estimated with the formula creatinine in urine (mmol/24 h) * 700/serum creatinine (μmol/l), normalized per 1.73 m^2 of body surface area and available for 242 patients.
[Δ]Available for 432 patients.
**Available for 378 patients.
[‡]Available for 377 patients.
[••]Available for 223 patients.
[□□]Defined as presence of a cerebrovascular accident, vascular problems, angina pectoris, myocardial infarction, or decompensatio cordis.
[ΔΔ]Present as primary kidney disease or comorbidity.

[3,4,19,27] In the late start group of the IDEAL study, many patients (75.9%) started dialysis earlier than intentioned mainly because of uremia. However, no prospective data is present on which symptoms and what level of HRQOL are important for nephrologists and patients in this decision.

This lack of knowledge supports the need for a descriptive study investigating the precise course of multiple symptoms and HRQOL, both physical and mental, in pre-dialysis patients. Therefore, our first aim was to describe the course of disease-related symptoms and HRQOL during pre-dialysis care (CKD stages IV–V) and our second aim was to investigate whether disease-related symptoms and HRQOL are associated with poor health outcomes.

Methods

Ethics Statement

The study was reviewed and approved by the medical ethics committee of the Leiden University Medical Center. The medical ethics committee or institutional review board (as appropriate) of the other participating centers (see file S1) reviewed and approved the local feasibility of the study. All participants gave their written informed consent prior to study inclusion.

Study Design

The PREdialysis PAtient REcord-2 (PREPARE-2) study is a prospective follow-up study of incident pre-dialysis patients treated in 25 participating Dutch nephrology outpatient clinics in The

Netherlands. Of these outpatient clinics 4 were academic and 21 were peripheral. Patients were included between July 2004 and June 2011, at the start of specialized pre-dialysis care (n = 502). Patients were treated by their nephrologists in a regular scheme according to the treatment guidelines of the Dutch Federation of Nephrology [28], a Dutch guideline partly based on the K/DOQI [26] and KDIGO guidelines [29]. Patients were followed until the start of dialysis, receiving a kidney transplant, death, or censoring. Censoring was defined as: moving to an outpatient clinic not participating in the PREPARE-2 study, recovery of kidney function, refusal of further study participation, lost to follow-up or August 1, 2012 (end of follow-up), whichever came first.

Patients

To be eligible for inclusion, patients had to be at least 18 years of age and the inclusion should take place at the moment of referral to a specialized pre-dialysis outpatient clinic. In practice, this refers to incident pre-dialysis patients with an estimated glomerular filtration rate (eGFR) of less than 20–30 ml/min/ 1.73 m^2. Most of these incident patients have a progressive renal function loss. Patients with a failing kidney transplant were also eligible for inclusion if the transplantation was at least one year ago.

Data Collection

Data on demography, biometry, primary kidney disease, comorbidities, medication use, laboratory values, symptoms, and HRQOL were collected during routine visits to pre-dialysis outpatient clinics. These visits took place at the start of specialized pre-dialysis care, at the moment of reaching one of the study endpoints (throughout text indicated as endpoint) as described previously, and every intermediate 6-month interval. Laboratory data were extracted from the electronic hospital information systems or medical records. Primary kidney disease was classified according to the codes of the European Renal Association-European Dialysis and Transplantation Association. [30] Written questionnaires used to asses symptoms and HRQOL were provided during routine visits at the start of pre-dialysis care, each 6-month interval, and at the moment of reaching an endpoint. Patients were asked to fill it in at home and return the questionnaire as soon as possible. Assistance from medical staff, a family member, or a friend was allowed.

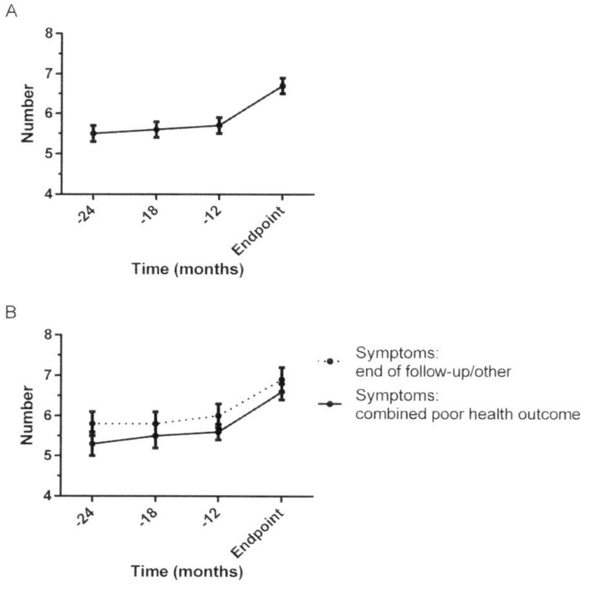

Figure 1. Course of symptoms during pre-dialysis care. The course of the total number of symptoms is presented for the total population (A) and stratified by the type of endpoint reached (combined poor health outcome; dialysis/transplantation/death, or end of follow-up/other endpoint, B). The black and grey dots indicate the mean and the error bars indicate the standard error of the mean (SEM). The time in months before reaching an endpoint is presented on the x-axis (−12 means that the measurement was 7–12 months before reaching an endpoint, −18 means 13–18 months etc). On the y-axis, the mean (SEM) total number of symptoms is presented, which can range from 0 to 12.

Measurements and Definitions

The revised illness perception questionnaire (IPQ-R) [31] was used to assess the onset of symptoms. This questionnaire has been validated [32,33] and is widely used in the field of nephrology [34–36]. The following symptoms from the IPQ-R (12 out of 14 symptoms) are essentially the same as those in the commonly used kidney disease specific quality of life (KDQOL) questionnaire and can be considered as uremia- or disease-related and were therefore included in our analyses [20]; pain, nausea, breathlessness, weight loss, fatigue, stiff joints, wheeziness, headaches, upset stomach, sleep difficulties, dizziness, and loss of strength. These disease-related symptoms are often called uremic symptoms because they are highly present in patients with advanced kidney failure. The onset of these symptoms during pre-dialysis care was defined as answering 'yes' for the first time on the question 'I have experienced this complaint since the beginning of my kidney disease'. HRQOL was assessed with the short form-36 (SF-36) questionnaire [37], a generic validated questionnaire consisting of 36 items that can be divided into 8 subscales. The scores on the individual items within a subscale were summed and transformed to a 0–100 scale, with higher scores indicating a better HRQOL. The 8 subscales can further be divided into two summary measures; physical summary score (consisting of the 4 subscales physical functioning, role functioning physical, bodily pain and general health) and mental summary score (consisting of the 4 subscales vitality, social functioning, role functioning emotional and mental health). Only the two summary measures (unstandardized) were used in our analyses. eGFR and creatinine clearance (CrCl) were used as indicators for renal function. GFR was estimated using the 4-variable Modification of Diet in Renal Disease (MDRD) formula. [38] CrCl was estimated with the following formula: creatinine in urine (mmol/24 h) *700/serum creatinine (μmol/l), and normalized per 1.73 m^2 of body surface area using the formula of Du Bois and Du Bois. [39] The measurement at the moment of reaching an endpoint was defined as follows; the measurement closest to the moment of reaching an endpoint and not measured more than 6 months before this moment.

Outcome

The outcomes for our first aim were the frequencies of all symptoms and the mean physical and mental summary score over time before reaching one of the endpoints. The outcome for our second aim was reaching the combined poor health outcome during follow-up; starting dialysis, receiving a kidney transplant, and death.

Statistical Analyses

The patients who filled in at least one HRQOL questionnaire, including the IPQ-R and the SF-36, during pre-dialysis care

Table 2. Comparison of the presence of symptoms and HRQOL at the start of pre-dialysis care and the moment of reaching an endpoint.

	All			Combined poor health outcome^			End of follow-up/Other		
	(n = 436)			(n = 284)			(n = 152)		
	Start	Endpoint	% onset§	Start	Endpoint	% onset§	Start	Endpoint	% onset§
Symptoms									
Pain	34.0	52.4	27.9	33.4	51.8	27.6	35.1	53.4	28.2
Nausea	29.0	46.8	25.1	30.5	45.4	21.4	26.2	49.3	31.3
Breathlessness	30.6	50.3	28.4	33.2	50.7	26.2	25.7	49.7	32.3
Weight loss	38.7	54.5	25.8	36.2	54.4	28.5	43.4	54.7	20.0
Fatigue	82.5	94.0	65.7	82.5	93.0	60.0	82.5	95.9	76.6
Stiff joints	51.3	67.9	34.1	51.5	65.4	28.7	50.8	72.7	44.5
Wheeziness	25.2	34.8	12.8	24.4	32.1	10.2	26.8	40.0	18.0
Headaches	23.0	37.1	18.3	23.3	36.1	16.7	22.4	39.1	21.5
Upset stomach	30.2	42.9	18.2	32.7	44.6	17.7	25.6	39.7	19.0
Sleep difficulties	37.9	55.3	28.0	39.6	56.3	27.6	34.7	53.5	28.8
Dizziness	33.7	50.3	25.0	34.0	47.4	20.3	33.3	55.8	33.7
Loss of strength	61.1	82.8	55.8	62.3	83.0	54.9	58.9	82.3	56.9
Number (total is 12)	4.8 (0.1)	6.7 (0.2)**	–	4.8 (0.2)	6.6 (0.2)**	–	4.7 (0.2)	6.9 (0.3)**	–
HRQOL									
Physical†	54.4 (1.1)	47.0 (1.3)**	–	53.5 (1.4)	44.6 (1.4)**	–	56.0 (1.9)	51.5 (2.4)	–
Mental†	67.8 (1.0)	58.9 (1.4)**	–	67.3 (1.3)	56.5 (1.5)**	–	68.9 (1.7)	63.4 (2.8)	–

Symptoms are presented as frequencies (%) and the number of symptoms and HRQOL as mean (standard error of the mean).
^Defined as starting dialysis, receiving a kidney transplant, and death.
§The onset of symptoms (%) was calculated as follows: (% endpoint - % start)/(100% - % start).
†The mean physical and mental summary scores in the general Dutch population are 76.3 and 77.9 respectively.
*$p<0.05$, adjusted for eGFR;
**$p<0.005$, adjusted for eGFR, difference between baseline and the moment of reaching an endpoint, obtained with a linear mixed model.

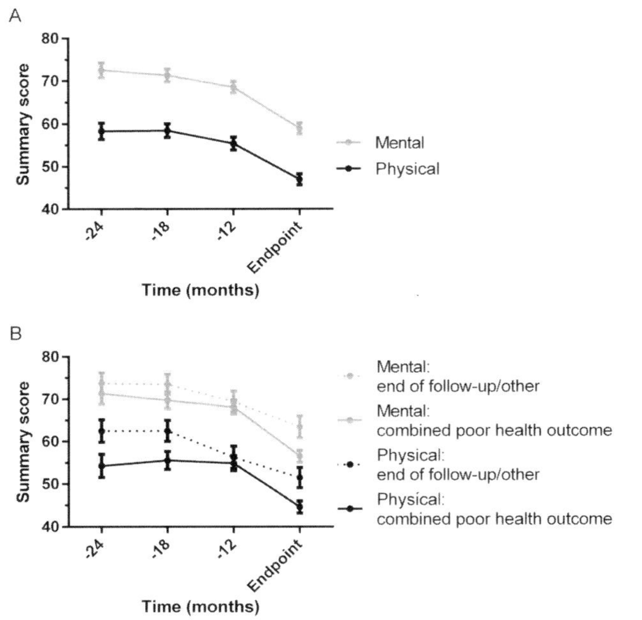

Figure 2. Course of HRQOL during pre-dialysis care. The course of the physical and mental summary score are presented for the total population (A) and stratified by the type of endpoint reached (combined poor health outcome; dialysis/transplantation/death, or end of follow-up/other endpoint, B). The black and grey dots indicate the mean and the error bars indicate the standard error of the mean (SEM). The time in months before reaching an endpoint is presented on the x-axis (−12 means that the measurement was 7–12 months before the moment of reaching an endpoint, −18 means 13–18 months etc). On the y-axis, the mean (SEM) score from the SF-36 questionnaire is presented (separately for the physical and mental summary measure), which can range from 0 to 100.

(n = 436) were included. Baseline characteristics were presented as mean ± standard deviation (SD) for normally distributed variables and as median and boundaries of interquartile range (IQR) for skewed variables. Missing values at baseline and at the moment of reaching an endpoint were imputed (using 20 repetitions) with the method of multiple imputation in PASW/SPSS version 20.0. This is a recommended technique when data is missing at random, in which missing data for a patient are imputed by a value that is predicted by other known characteristics of this patient. [40,41] All characteristics presented in Table 1, all symptoms, and the physical and mental summary score (at baseline and at the moment of reaching an endpoint), follow-up time, and the type of endpoint reached (starting dialysis, receiving a kidney transplant, death, end of follow-up (August 1, 2012), or other endpoint; moving to an outpatient clinic not participating in the PREPARE-2 study, recovery of kidney function, refusal of further study participation, or lost to follow-up) were included in this imputation model. Skewed distributed continuous variables and the follow-up time were logarithmically transformed. The method of multiple imputation was chosen because data being missing completely at random is uncommon in clinical practice and multiple imputation is still a valid method when some data is missing 'not at random' (related to unknown characteristics). [42] At baseline, 100% of the included patients filled in at least a part of the questionnaire and this percentage dropped to 66% at the moment of reaching an endpoint.

To describe the course of symptoms and HRQOL during pre-dialysis care, the frequency of all 12 separate symptoms, the mean (standard error of the mean, SEM) total number of symptoms and the mean (SEM) physical and mental summary score at the start of pre-dialysis care and at the moment of reaching an endpoint were calculated. A linear mixed model was used to investigate the statistical difference between these two time points, adjusted for eGFR. This model takes into account correlations between repeated measurements within the same individual. Second, the mean (SEM) total number of symptoms, physical and mental summary score, eGFR, and CrCl at the moment of reaching an endpoint and the preceding 3 time points were estimated with a linear mixed model. Moreover, on each time point a Pearson's correlation was calculated between eGFR and CrCl and the total number of symptoms, the physical summary score and the mental summary score. Furthermore, we repeated all analyses in the subgroup of patients that started dialysis, received a kidney transplant or died (combined poor health outcome) and in the subgroup of patients that reached the end of follow-up or another type of endpoint.

A time-dependent Cox proportional hazard model was used to investigate the risk of reaching the combined poor health outcome within 6 months. Symptoms were analyzed separate and as a total number. The physical and mental summary score were analyzed in steps of 3 score points (this is considered to be a clinically relevant difference [43]). The analyses were adjusted for the potential confounders age, sex, diabetes mellitus, cardiovascular disease, and time-dependent eGFR.

To test the robustness of our results, five sensitivity analyses were performed. First, a complete case analysis was performed, which is an alternative method for handling missing data. Second, we repeated our analyses subdividing the group of patients who start with dialysis into peritoneal dialysis and hemodialysis, and

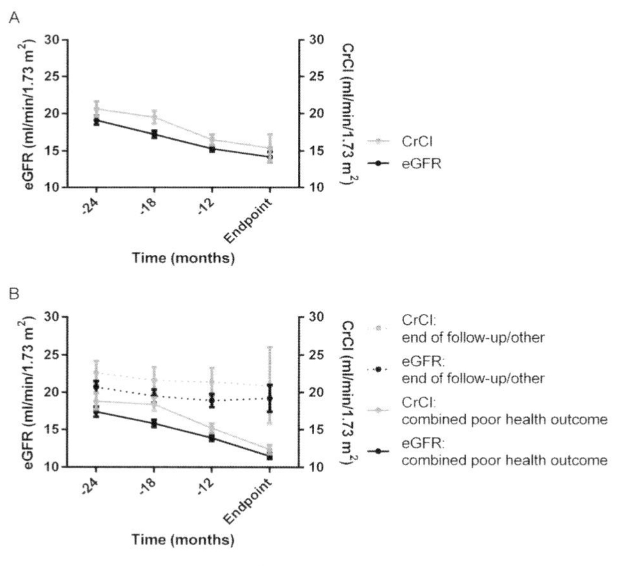

Figure 3. Course of eGFR and CrCl during pre-dialysis care. The course of eGFR and CrCl are presented for the total population (A) and stratified by the type of endpoint reached (combined poor health outcome; dialysis/transplantation/death, or end of follow-up/other endpoint, B). The black and grey dots indicate the mean and the error bars indicate the standard error of the mean (SEM). The time in months before reaching an endpoint is presented on the x-axis (−12 means that the measurement was 7–12 months before the moment of reaching an endpoint, −18 means 13–18 months etc). On the left y-axis, the mean (SEM) eGFR (ml/min/1.73 m^2) is presented, and on the right y-axis the mean (SEM) CrCl (ml/min/1.73 m^2).

subdividing the group of patients reaching another outcome into receiving a kidney transplant, death, end of follow-up, and other endpoint. Third, we performed a time-dependent Cox proportional hazard model with starting dialysis as outcome instead of the combined poor health outcome. Fourth, we repeated our imputation procedure and analyses after defining our measurement at the moment of reaching an endpoint as really measured at that moment, and not in the preceding 6 months. Fifth, we used other available measurements to define weight loss and fatigue at the moment of reaching an endpoint. Weight loss was redefined as >5% of weight lost. Fatigue was redefined as scoring below the Dutch mean normal score on the vitality subscale of the SF-36 questionnaire (score of approximately 70 [44]).

Results

Baseline Characteristics

In total, 502 incident pre-dialysis patients were included in the PREPARE-2 study of whom 436 patients were available for analyses. Table 1 shows that the median (IQR) age of these patients was 69 (56–76) years, 66% were male and the mean ± SD eGFR was 16.9±6.1 ml/min/1.73 m^2. The 66 patients excluded from our analyses were younger, had a lower eGFR and CrCl, experienced more proteinuria and had a higher prevalence of diabetes mellitus.

Description of the Course of Symptoms, HRQOL and Renal Function

In total, 284 of the 436 patients (65%) reached the combined poor health outcome (median follow-up 12.4 (IQR, 5.8–21.0) months), of whom 79% started dialysis, 11% received a kidney transplant, and 10% died. Of the 152 patients that reached another endpoint (median follow-up 30.6 (IQR, 16.1–48.3) months), 33% refused further participation, 11% had a recovered kidney function, 5% moved to another center, 2% were lost to follow-up, and 49% were still in the study. The overall eGFR and CrCl decline (n = 436) were 0.16 (95% confidence interval (CI), 0.11;0.21) and 0.21 (95% CI, 0.10;0.32) ml/min/1.73 m^2/month respectively. The median number of filled in HRQOL questionnaires was 3 (IQR 2–4) and respectively 19%, 26%, and 55% filled in 1, 2, and 3 or more questionnaires during pre-dialysis care. Only the minority were filled in with the assistance of medical staff (1%). Furthermore, 21% were filled in with the assistance of a friend or family member and 78% were filled in without assistance. After imputation all patients had at least 2 complete questionnaires.

At the start of pre-dialysis care, most of the symptoms were already experienced by 20 to 40% of the patients (Table 2). Only the symptoms fatigue, stiff joints, and loss of strength were experienced by more than 50% of the patients. Furthermore, patients with diabetes mellitus or cardiovascular disease (either as primary kidney disease or comorbidity) experienced more symptoms compared to patients without (mean (SEM) total number of symptoms 4.9 (0.2) versus 4.5 (0.2)). The onset of fatigue and loss of strength were the strongest during pre-dialysis care and the onset of wheeziness, headaches, and upset stomach the lowest. The onset of all symptoms was comparable between patients reaching the combined poor health outcome (i.e. dialysis, transplantation, and death) and patients reaching another endpoint (i.e. end of follow-up and other). The mean (SEM) total number of symptoms was 4.8 (0.1) at the start of pre-dialysis care and 6.7 (0.2) at the moment of reaching an endpoint. Figure 1a depicts the course of the total number of symptoms during the last 2 years of pre-dialysis care. The onset of symptoms was most frequent during the last 6 to 12 months before reaching an endpoint, which was comparable between patients reaching the combined poor health outcome and patients reaching another endpoint (Figure 1b). On all four time points, symptoms were not correlated with eGFR or CrCl.

The physical summary score decreased from 54.4 (1.1) at the start of pre-dialysis care to 47.0 (1.3) at the moment of reaching an endpoint (Table 2). The mental summary score decreased from 67.8 (1.0) to 58.9 (1.4). The sharpest decrease was observed during the 6 to 12 months before reaching an endpoint (Figure 2a). After stratification by the type of endpoint reached, during the last 6 months patients who started dialysis, were transplanted, or died (combined poor health outcome) showed a slightly stronger decrease of both the physical and mental summary score than patients reaching the end of follow-up or another endpoint (Figure 2b). On all four time points, no correlation was present with eGFR or CrCl. Figure 3a confirms the gradual decrease of eGFR and CrCl during pre-dialysis care, which was stronger in patients who reached the combined poor health outcome (Figure 3b).

Association of Symptoms and HRQOL with the Combined Poor Health Outcome

The symptoms breathlessness, fatigue, wheeziness, and loss of strength showed the strongest association with reaching the combined poor health outcome (i.e. dialysis, transplantation, and death) within the subsequent 6 months (Table 3, adjusted column). Each additional symptom resulted in a crude 1.02-fold (95% CI, 0.98–1.06) increased risk, which was not statistically significant. Adjustment for potential confounders increased this HR to 1.04 (95% CI, 1.00–1.09). For HRQOL, every 3-point lower physical and mental summary score were associated with a higher risk of reaching the combined poor health outcome within the subsequent 6 months (crude HR 1.03 (95% CI 1.02–1.05) and HR 1.04 (95% CI 1.02–1.05), respectively). The results slightly increased after adjustment for potential confounders (Table 3).

Sensitivity Analyses

All sensitivity analyses - 1.) a complete case analysis, 2.) extensive stratification of the endpoints reached, 3.) using the start of dialysis as outcome (Table 4), 4.) defining the measurement at the moment of reaching an endpoint as really measured at that moment (not in the preceding 6 months), and 5.) redefining fatigue and weight loss - resulted in comparable courses of symptoms and HRQOL over time and similar risk estimates, implying robust results.

Discussion

In our cohort of incident patients on pre-dialysis care, many patients had already experienced symptoms at the start of pre-dialysis care. In addition, the presence of all reported symptoms increased during pre-dialysis care, especially fatigue and loss of strength. HRQOL, defined as the physical and mental summary score, decreased during pre-dialysis care. The sharpest increase of symptoms and decrease of HRQOL was observed during the last 6 to 12 months of pre-dialysis care. These results were supported by the observation that patients who reported a high number of symptoms or a low HRQOL started dialysis, received a kidney transplant, or died (combined poor health outcome) earlier than patients who reported a low number of symptoms or a high HRQOL.

To our knowledge, this is the first study to report the onset of symptoms over time in patients on specialized pre-dialysis care.

Table 3. Association of symptoms and a low HRQOL with the risk of reaching the combined poor health outcome within the subsequent 6 months based on separate time-dependent Cox proportional hazard models.

	HR (95% CI)	Adjusted HR (95% CI)§
	(events/n = 284/436)	*(events/n = 284/436)*
Symptoms		
Pain	1.07 (0.84;1.37)	1.08 (0.84;1.40)
Nausea	1.11 (0.87;1.42)	1.06 (0.81;1.38)
Breathlessness	1.26 (0.99;1.60)	1.26 (0.98;1.62)
Weight loss	0.95 (0.74;1.22)	1.20 (0.93;1.55)
Fatigue	1.18 (0.81;1.73)	1.33 (0.90;1.97)
Stiff joints	0.97 (0.76;1.24)	1.08 (0.83;1.40)
Wheeziness	1.03 (0.79;1.34)	1.23 (0.93;1.63)
Headaches	1.02 (0.78;1.33)	1.18 (0.88;1.59)
Upset stomach	1.16 (0.91;1.49)	1.00 (0.77;1.29)
Sleep difficulties	1.17 (0.92;1.50)	1.12 (0.87;1.43)
Dizziness	0.93 (0.73;1.19)	1.06 (0.83;1.36)
Loss of strength	1.07 (0.82;1.41)	1.25 (0.95;1.65)
Number (per 1 symptom)	1.02 (0.98;1.06)	1.04 (1.00;1.09)
HRQOL		
Physical (per 3 score points)	1.03 (1.02;1.05)**	1.04 (1.02;1.06)**
Mental (per 3 score points)	1.04 (1.02;1.05)**	1.04 (1.02;1.06)**

The HR with its 95% confidence interval (CI) represents the increased risk of reaching the combined poor health outcome (dialysis, transplantation, and death) within the subsequent 6 months in patients with the symptom compared to patients without the symptom present, the increased risk with each additional symptom, and the increased risk with every 3-point lower physical and mental summary score. A decrease of 3 score points is considered to be clinically relevant. [43]
§Adjusted for age, sex, diabetes mellitus, cardiovascular disease, and time dependent eGFR.
*$p<0.05$;
**$p<0.005$.

Our finding that HRQOL, both physical and mental, decreased during pre-dialysis care is in line with other studies.[21–23] These cross-sectional studies demonstrated that HRQOL was highest in the 'healthy' general population, lowest in patients on dialysis, and in between for patients with CKD not on dialysis. However, the results of these studies were not CKD-stage specific and because of the cross-sectional character, the change of HRQOL over time could not be described or associated with the start of dialysis or other poor health outcomes.

Therefore, the major strength of our study is the longitudinal character, instead of a cross-sectional design. This gave us the opportunity to report the course of symptoms and HRQOL over the last years of pre-dialysis care. However, an issue that deserves further attention is that not all consecutive patients starting pre-dialysis care were included in the PREPARE-2 study, only those who were asked and willing to participate, which could have led to selection bias. Unfortunately, it is very difficult to ascertain the direction of this bias. Besides this important issue, some patients reached another endpoint than dialysis, leading to a large diversity of patients at the moment of reaching an endpoint. However, results were comparable between all type of endpoints reached. Another issue that deserves attention is that symptoms were obtained from the IPQ-R. This questionnaire is not primarily designed to assess the longitudinal presence of symptoms and does not include questions about severity. This means that the 'yes' category of the IPQ-R consists of patients having experienced the onset of that symptom a few years ago or just recently. This mixture of onset times in our study could have led to an underestimation of the real risks of reaching the combined poor health outcome. Besides this, symptom burden is a reliable measure, because it shows similar correlations with HRQOL and illness perceptions as symptom severity. [45,46] This might be an indication that once the onset of a symptom has occurred (this onset coincides with a certain threshold of symptom severity) severity has no added value on a persons' mental and physical well-being. Moreover, in answering symptom-related questions in the IPQ-R, patients' perceptions of illness play a major role. [47] The formulation of the question may also influence the response of patients. However, more objective measures of weight loss and fatigue resulted in similar frequencies. Finally, a filled in IPQ-R and SF-36 questionnaire were not available for 66 patients. Therefore, our choice to only analyze patients with at least one filled in questionnaire could have led to selection bias. [41] However, the 66 excluded patients had a slightly worse prognosis than the 436 included patients, so our results may be an underestimation.

Uremia is defined as all the signs and symptoms accompanying advanced kidney failure that cannot be attributed to comorbid disease. The onset of uremia-related signs and symptoms can become present when renal function decreases to half of the normal function (normal eGFR is 100–120 ml/min/1.73 m^2 on the age of 30) and continue to rise when renal function further decreases. [20] This means that uremia-related symptoms mainly become present in patients with CKD stages IV–V. Therefore, the results from our pre-dialysis cohort, showing an increase in symptoms over time and as a consequence a decrease in perceived physical and mental HRQOL, are biologically plausible. Breathlessness, weight loss, fatigue, and wheeziness were the symptoms

Table 4. Association of symptoms and a low HRQOL with the risk of starting dialysis within the subsequent 6 months based on separate time-dependent Cox proportional hazard models.

	HR (95% CI)	Adjusted HR (95% CI)§
	(events/n = 225/436)	*(events/n = 225/436)*
Symptoms		
Pain	1.02 (0.77;1.35)	1.04 (0.78;1.39)
Nausea	1.13 (0.85;1.49)	1.10 (0.81;1.49)
Breathlessness	1.29 (0.98;1.69)	1.28 (0.96;1.71)
Weight loss	1.00 (0.75;1.32)	1.33 (0.99;1.77)
Fatigue	1.25 (0.81;1.94)	1.48 (0.94;2.31)
Stiff joints	0.95 (0.72;1.26)	1.07 (0.80;1.44)
Wheeziness	1.06 (0.79;1.42)	1.29 (0.94;1.78)
Headaches	0.86 (0.63;1.18)	1.08 (0.76;1.53)
Upset stomach	1.08 (0.82;1.43)	0.90 (0.67;1.22)
Sleep difficulties	1.22 (0.92;1.60)	1.17 (0.89;1.55)
Dizziness	0.95 (0.72;1.26)	1.13 (0.86;1.49)
Loss of strength	1.00 (0.74;1.34)	1.20 (0.89;1.64)
Number (per 1 symptom)	1.02 (0.97;1.07)	1.05 (1.00;1.10)
HRQOL		
Physical (per 3 score points)	1.03 (1.01;1.05)**	1.04 (1.02;1.06)**
Mental (per 3 score points)	1.04 (1.02;1.06)**	1.04 (1.02;1.07)**

The HR with its 95% confidence interval (CI) represents the increased risk of starting dialysis within the subsequent 6 months in patients with the symptom compared to patients without the symptom present, the increased risk with each additional symptom, and the increased risk with every 3-point lower physical and mental summary score. A decrease of 3 score points is considered to be clinically relevant. [43].
§Adjusted for age, sex, diabetes mellitus, cardiovascular disease, and time dependent eGFR.
*$p<0.05$;
**$p<0.005$.

most strongly associated with the start of dialysis (Table 4). This finding could indicate that these symptoms were considered the most by nephrologists and patients in the decision to start with dialysis. However, in our cohort data is lacking on whether the decision to start was indeed based on these symptoms. The possible role of breathlessness and wheeziness in the decision to start with dialysis could be explained by the presence of fluid overload. Fluid overload is a main indication to start with dialysis, as is stated in several guidelines [25,26], and breathlessness and wheeziness can be consequences of pulmonary edema.

In conclusion, the presence of all symptoms increase and both physical and mental HRQOL decrease during pre-dialysis care with the sharpest change during the last 6 to 12 months before reaching an endpoint. These descriptive results may indicate that symptoms and both physical and mental HRQOL are good markers for the medical condition and disease stage of pre-dialysis patients, and are therefore good candidates to be used in defining the optimal moment to start with dialysis (or to identify those patients at a high risk of dying). Indeed we found that several symptoms and a lower level of HRQOL were already associated with the start of dialysis, which may indicate that these symptoms were already considered by nephrologists and patients in this decision. However, for each individual we need to know the exact reason for starting dialysis and the survival time on dialysis, to investigate on which specific symptoms and what level of HRQOL this decision should be based. Therefore, in the future, more research should focus on finding clinical signs and symptoms that can help to plan when to start dialysis to increase survival and HRQOL on dialysis. The European EQUAL study [48] will focus on this specific question. Eventually, a clinical decision rule based on all known factors may be a good and helpful tool for nephrologists and patients to make a more evidence based choice when a patient needs to start with dialysis.

Acknowledgments

The authors gratefully thank all patients who participated in the PREPARE-2 study. The nursing staffs of the participating centers, as well as the trial nurses and data managers from the Hans Mak Institute are gratefully acknowledged for collecting the clinical data. We thank the PREPARE-2 Study Group for the data collection and active participation in the study.

Author Contributions

Conceived and designed the experiments: MCMdG GO JIR JWE FWD NH. Analyzed the data: MCMdG FWD NH. Wrote the paper: MCMdG GO JIR JWE FWD NH.

References

1. Krediet RT, Dekker FW (2010) Dialysis: Can plasma creatinine levels guide initiation of dialysis? Nat Rev Nephrol 6: 563–564. nrneph.2010.109 [pii];10.1038/nrneph.2010.109 [doi].
2. Lameire N, Van Biesen W (2010) The initiation of renal-replacement therapy just-in-time delivery. N Engl J Med 363: 678–680. NEJMe1006669 [pii];10.1056/NEJMe1006669 [doi].
3. Stel VS, Jager KJ (2011) Glomerular filtration rate and initiation of dialysis. CMAJ 183: 24–25. cmaj.101636 [pii];10.1503/cmaj.101636 [doi].
4. Tattersall J, Dekker F, Heimburger O, Jager KJ, Lameire N, et al. (2011) When to start dialysis: updated guidance following publication of the Initiating Dialysis Early and Late (IDEAL) study. Nephrol Dial Transplant 26: 2082–2086. gfr168 [pii];10.1093/ndt/gfr168 [doi].
5. Van Biesen W, Vanholder R (2010) When to start chronic dialysis: tunnel vision induced by numbers? Nephrol Dial Transplant 25: 2405–2407. gfq391 [pii];10.1093/ndt/gfq391 [doi].
6. Stel VS, Tomson C, Ansell D, Casino FG, Collart F, et al. (2010) Level of renal function in patients starting dialysis: an ERA-EDTA Registry study. Nephrol Dial Transplant 25: 3315–3325. gfq209 [pii];10.1093/ndt/gfq209 [doi].
7. Rosansky SJ, Clark WF, Eggers P, Glassock RJ (2009) Initiation of dialysis at higher GFRs: is the apparent rising tide of early dialysis harmful or helpful? Kidney Int 76: 257–261. ki2009161 [pii];10.1038/ki.2009.161 [doi].
8. Termorshuizen F, Korevaar JC, Dekker FW, Jager KJ, van Manen JG, et al. (2003) Time trends in initiation and dose of dialysis in end-stage renal disease patients in The Netherlands. Nephrol Dial Transplant 18: 552–558.
9. Clark WF, Na Y, Rosansky SJ, Sontrop JM, Macnab JJ, et al. (2011) Association between estimated glomerular filtration rate at initiation of dialysis and mortality. CMAJ 183: 47–53. cmaj.100349 [pii];10.1503/cmaj.100349 [doi].
10. Beddhu S, Samore MH, Roberts MS, Stoddard GJ, Ramkumar N, et al. (2003) Impact of timing of initiation of dialysis on mortality. J Am Soc Nephrol 14: 2305–2312.
11. Kazmi WH, Gilbertson DT, Obrador GT, Guo H, Pereira BJ, et al. (2005) Effect of comorbidity on the increased mortality associated with early initiation of dialysis. Am J Kidney Dis 46: 887–896. S0272-6386(05)01108-X [pii];10.1053/j.ajkd.2005.08.005 [doi].
12. Lassalle M, Labeeuw M, Frimat L, Villar E, Joyeux V, et al. (2010) Age and comorbidity may explain the paradoxical association of an early dialysis start with poor survival. Kidney Int 77: 700–707. ki201014 [pii];10.1038/ki.2010.14 [doi].
13. Stel VS, Dekker FW, Ansell D, Augustijn H, Casino FG, et al. (2009) Residual renal function at the start of dialysis and clinical outcomes. Nephrol Dial Transplant 24: 3175–3182. gfp264 [pii];10.1093/ndt/gfp264 [doi].
14. Traynor JP, Simpson K, Geddes CC, Deighan CJ, Fox JG (2002) Early initiation of dialysis fails to prolong survival in patients with end-stage renal failure. J Am Soc Nephrol 13: 2125–2132.
15. Hwang SJ, Yang WC, Lin MY, Mau LW, Chen HC (2010) Impact of the clinical conditions at dialysis initiation on mortality in incident haemodialysis patients: a national cohort study in Taiwan. Nephrol Dial Transplant 25: 2616–2624. gfq308 [pii];10.1093/ndt/gfq308 [doi].
16. Wright S, Klausner D, Baird B, Williams ME, Steinman T, et al. (2010) Timing of dialysis initiation and survival in ESRD. Clin J Am Soc Nephrol 5: 1828–1835. CJN.06230909 [pii];10.2215/CJN.06230909 [doi].
17. Rosansky SJ, Eggers P, Jackson K, Glassock R, Clark WF (2011) Early start of hemodialysis may be harmful. Arch Intern Med 171: 396–403. archinternmed.2010.415 [pii];10.1001/archinternmed.2010.415 [doi].
18. Korevaar JC, Jansen MA, Dekker FW, Jager KJ, Boeschoten EW, et al. (2001) When to initiate dialysis: effect of proposed US guidelines on survival. Lancet 358: 1046–1050. S0140-6736(01)06180- [pii];10.1016/S0140-(01)06180-3 [doi].
19. Cooper BA, Branley P, Bulfone L, Collins JF, Craig JC, et al. (2010) A randomized, controlled trial of early versus late initiation of dialysis. N Engl J Med 363: 609–619. NEJMoa1000552 [pii];10.1056/NEJMoa1000552 [doi].
20. Meyer TW, Hostetter TH (2007) Uremia. N Engl J Med 357: 1316–1325. 357/13/1316 [pii];10.1056/NEJMra071313 [doi].
21. Perlman RL, Finkelstein FO, Liu L, Roys E, Kiser M, et al. (2005) Quality of life in chronic kidney disease (CKD): a cross-sectional analysis in the Renal Research Institute-CKD study. Am J Kidney Dis 45: 658–666. S0272638605000053 [pii].
22. Kusek JW, Greene P, Wang SR, Beck G, West D, et al. (2002) Cross-sectional study of health-related quality of life in African Americans with chronic renal insufficiency: the African American Study of Kidney Disease and Hypertension Trial. Am J Kidney Dis 39: 513–524. S0272638602298996 [pii].
23. Chin HJ, Song YR, Lee JJ, Lee SB, Kim KW, et al. (2008) Moderately decreased renal function negatively affects the health-related quality of life among the elderly Korean population: a population-based study. Nephrol Dial Transplant 23: 2810–2817. gfn132 [pii];10.1093/ndt/gfn132 [doi].
24. Tsai YC, Hung CC, Hwang SJ, Wang SL, Hsiao SM, et al. (2010) Quality of life predicts risks of end-stage renal disease and mortality in patients with chronic kidney disease. Nephrol Dial Transplant 25: 1621–1626. gfp671 [pii];10.1093/ndt/gfp671 [doi].
25. European Best Practice Guidelines Expert Group on Hemodialysis, European Renal Association (2002)Section I. Measurement of renal function, when to refer and when to start dialysis. Nephrol Dial Transplant 17 Suppl 7: 7–15.
26. National Kidney Foundation, Kidney Disease Outcomes Quality Initiative (KDOQI) (2002) KDOQI clinical practice guidelines for chronic kidney disease: evaluation, classification, and stratification. Am J Kidney Dis 39: S1–266. S0272638602093563 [pii].
27. Ledebo I, Kessler M, Van Biesen W, Wanner C, Wiecek A, et al. (2001) Initiation of dialysis-opinions from an international survey: Report on the Dialysis Opinion Symposium at the ERA-EDTA Congress, 18 September 2000, Nice. Nephrol Dial Transplant 16: 1132–1138.
28. Dutch Federation of Nephrology (2011) Multidisciplinary guidelines pre-dialysis. Dutch Federation of Nephrology.
29. Kidney Disease: Improving Global Outcomes (KDIGO) (2011) Clinical practice guidelines. KDIGO.
30. European Renal Association, Dialysis and Transplantation Association (ERA/EDTA) Registry (2011) (ERA/EDTA) Registry Annual Report 2009.
31. Moss-Morris R, Weinman J, Petrie KJ, Horne R, Cameron LD, et al. (2002) The revised Illness Perception Questionnaire (IPQ-R). Psychology & Health 17: 1–16.
32. Chilcot J, Norton S, Wellsted D, Farrington K (2012) The factor structure of the Revised Illness Perception Questionnaire (IPQ-R) in end-stage renal disease patients. Psychol Health Med 17: 578–588. 10.1080/13548506.2011.647702 [doi].
33. Pagels A, Soderquist BK, Heiwe S (2012) Evaluating the Illness Perception Questionnaire on patients with chronic kidney disease in Sweden. Scand J Caring Sci 26: 474–484. 10.1111/j.1471-6712.2011.00952.x [doi].
34. Chilcot J, Norton S, Wellsted D, Davenport A, Firth J, et al. (2013) Distinct Depression Symptom Trajectories over the First Year of Dialysis: Associations with Illness Perceptions. Ann Behav Med 45: 78–88. 10.1007/s12160-012-9410-5 [doi].
35. Covic A, Seica A, Gusbeth-Tatomir P, Gavrilovici O, Goldsmith DJ (2004) Illness representations and quality of life scores in haemodialysis patients. Nephrol Dial Transplant 19: 2078–2083. 10.1093/ndt/gfh254 [doi];gfh254 [pii].
36. van Dijk S, Scharloo M, Kaptein AA, Thong MS, Boeschoten EW, et al. (2009) Patients' representations of their end-stage renal disease: relation with mortality. Nephrol Dial Transplant 24: 3183–3185. gfp184 [pii];10.1093/ndt/gfp184 [doi].
37. Ware JE Jr, Sherbourne CD (1992) The MOS 36-item short-form health survey (SF-36). I. Conceptual framework and item selection. Med Care 30: 473–483.
38. Levey AS, Greene T, Kusek JW, Beck G (2000) A simplified equation to predict glomerular filtration rate from serum creatinine. J Am Soc Nephrol 155A.
39. Du Bois D, Du Bois EF (1989) A formula to estimate the approximate surface area if height and weight be known. 1916. Nutrition 5: 303–311.
40. van Buuren S, Boshuizen HC, Knook DL (1999) Multiple imputation of missing blood pressure covariates in survival analysis. Stat Med 18: 681–694. 10.1002/(SICI)1097-0258(19990330)18:6<681::AID-SIM71>3.0.CO;2-R [pii].
41. Donders AR, van der Heijden GJ, Stijnen T, Moons KG (2006) Review: a gentle introduction to imputation of missing values. J Clin Epidemiol 59: 1087–1091. S0895-4356(06)00197-1 [pii];10.1016/j.jclinepi.2006.01.014 [doi].
42. Schafer JL, Graham JW (2002) Missing data: our view of the state of the art. Psychol Methods 7: 147–177.
43. Leaf DE, Goldfarb DS (2009) Interpretation and review of health-related quality of life data in CKD patients receiving treatment for anemia. Kidney Int 75: 15–24. ki2008414 [pii];10.1038/ki.2008.414 [doi].
44. Aaronson NK, Muller M, Cohen PD, Essink-Bot ML, Fekkes M, et al. (1998) Translation, validation, and norming of the Dutch language version of the SF-36 Health Survey in community and chronic disease populations. J Clin Epidemiol 51: 1055–1068. S0895-4356(98)00097-3 [pii].
45. Abdel-Kader K, Unruh ML, Weisbord SD (2009) Symptom burden, depression, and quality of life in chronic and end-stage kidney disease. Clin J Am Soc Nephrol 4: 1057–1064. CJN.00430109 [pii];10.2215/CJN.00430109 [doi].
46. Weisbord SD, Fried LF, Arnold RM, Fine MJ, Levenson DJ, et al. (2005) Prevalence, severity, and importance of physical and emotional symptoms in chronic hemodialysis patients. J Am Soc Nephrol 16: 2487–2494. ASN.2005020157 [pii];10.1681/ASN.2005020157 [doi].
47. Weinman J, Petrie KJ, Moss-Morris R, Horne R (1996) The illness perception questionnaire: a new method for assessing the cognitive representation of illness. Psychol Health 11: 431–435.
48. Jager KJ, Ocak G, Drechsler C, Caskey FJ, Evans M, et al. (2012) The EQUAL study: a European study in chronic kidney disease stage 4 patients. Nephrol Dial Transplant. gfs277 [pii];10.1093/ndt/gfs277 [doi].

Permissions

All chapters in this book were first published in PLOS ONE, by The Public Library of Science; hereby published with permission under the Creative Commons Attribution License or equivalent. Every chapter published in this book has been scrutinized by our experts. Their significance has been extensively debated. The topics covered herein carry significant findings which will fuel the growth of the discipline. They may even be implemented as practical applications or may be referred to as a beginning point for another development.

The contributors of this book come from diverse backgrounds, making this book a truly international effort. This book will bring forth new frontiers with its revolutionizing research information and detailed analysis of the nascent developments around the world.

We would like to thank all the contributing authors for lending their expertise to make the book truly unique. They have played a crucial role in the development of this book. Without their invaluable contributions this book wouldn't have been possible. They have made vital efforts to compile up to date information on the varied aspects of this subject to make this book a valuable addition to the collection of many professionals and students.

This book was conceptualized with the vision of imparting up-to-date information and advanced data in this field. To ensure the same, a matchless editorial board was set up. Every individual on the board went through rigorous rounds of assessment to prove their worth. After which they invested a large part of their time researching and compiling the most relevant data for our readers.

The editorial board has been involved in producing this book since its inception. They have spent rigorous hours researching and exploring the diverse topics which have resulted in the successful publishing of this book. They have passed on their knowledge of decades through this book. To expedite this challenging task, the publisher supported the team at every step. A small team of assistant editors was also appointed to further simplify the editing procedure and attain best results for the readers.

Apart from the editorial board, the designing team has also invested a significant amount of their time in understanding the subject and creating the most relevant covers. They scrutinized every image to scout for the most suitable representation of the subject and create an appropriate cover for the book.

The publishing team has been an ardent support to the editorial, designing and production team. Their endless efforts to recruit the best for this project, has resulted in the accomplishment of this book. They are a veteran in the field of academics and their pool of knowledge is as vast as their experience in printing. Their expertise and guidance has proved useful at every step. Their uncompromising quality standards have made this book an exceptional effort. Their encouragement from time to time has been an inspiration for everyone.

The publisher and the editorial board hope that this book will prove to be a valuable piece of knowledge for researchers, students, practitioners and scholars across the globe.

List of Contributors

Young Ok Kim, Dong Chan Jin, Ho Chul Song, Euy Jin Choi and Chul Woo Yang
Department of Internal Medicine, College of Medicine, The Catholic University of Korea, Seoul, Korea

Hyung Wook Kim
Department of Internal Medicine, College of Medicine, The Catholic University of Korea, Seoul, Korea
St. Vincent's Hospital, Suwon, Korea

Yong Kyun Kim
Department of Internal Medicine, College of Medicine, The Catholic University of Korea, Seoul, Korea
MRC for Cell Death Disease Research Center, The Catholic University of Korea, Seoul, Korea

Su-Hyun Kim
Department of Internal Medicine, College of Medicine, Chung- Ang University, Seoul, Korea

Yong-Lim Kim
Department of Internal Medicine, Kyungpook National University School of Medicine, Daegu, Korea

Yon-Su Kim
Department of Internal Medicine, College of Medicine, Seoul National University, Seoul, Korea,

Shin-Wook Kang
Department of Internal Medicine, College of Medicine, Yonsei University, Seoul, Korea

Nam-Ho Kim
Department of Internal Medicine, Chonnam National University Medical School, Gwangju, Korea

Ulla K. Seidel, Janine Gronewold, Olga Todica and Dirk M. Hermann
Department of Neurology, University Hospital Essen, Essen, Germany

Michaela Volsek, Andreas Kribben and Heike Bruck
Department of Nephrology, University Hospital Essen, Essen, Germany

Chon-Seng Hong
Department of Internal Medicine, Chi-Mei Medical Center, Tainan, Taiwan

Kun-Ming Chung
Department of General Medicine, Chi-Mei Medical Center, Tainan, Taiwan

Po-Chang Huang
Department of Orthopedics Medicine, Chi-Mei Medical Center, Taiwan

Jhi-Joung Wang and Chin-Chen Chu
Department of Medical Research, Chi-Mei Medical Center, Tainan, Taiwan

Chun-Ming Yang
Department of Neurology, Chi-Mei Medical Center, Tainan, Taiwan

Chung-Ching Chio
Department of Neurological Surgery, Chi-Mei Medical Center, Tainan, Taiwan

Fu-Lin Chang
Department of Pharmaceutical Science and Technology, Chung Hwa University of Medical Technology, Tainan, Taiwan

Chih-Chiang Chien
Department of Nephrology, Chi-Mei Medical Center, Tainan, Taiwan
Department of Food Nutrition, Chung Hwa University of Medical Technology, Tainan, Taiwan

Yen-Wen Liu, Wei-Chuan Tsai, Liang-Miin Tsai and Jyh-Hong Chen
Division of Cardiology, Department of Internal Medicine, National Cheng Kung University Hospital, College of Medicine, National Cheng Kung University, Tainan, Taiwan

Chi-Ting Su
Division of Nephrology, Department of Internal Medicine, National Taiwan University Hospital Yun-Lin Branch, Yun-Lin, Taiwan

Yu-Tzu Chang and Junne-Ming Sung
Division of Nephrology, Department of Internal Medicine, National Cheng Kung University Hospital, College of Medicine, National Cheng Kung University, Tainan, Taiwan

Yu-Ru Su
Department of Statistics, National Cheng Kung University, Tainan, Taiwan,

Saprina P. H. Wang
Graduate Institute of Biomedical Engineering, National Cheng Kung University, Tainan, Taiwan,

Chun- Shin Yang
Division of Nephrology, Department of Internal Medicine, Catholic Fu-An Hospital, Yun-Lin, Taiwan

James G. Heaf
Department of Nephrology B, Copenhagen University Hospital at Herlev, Herlev, Denmark,

Sonja Wehberg
Department of Epidemiology, Odense University Hospital, Odense, Denmark

Ran Chen, Bei Wang, Ming-Ming Ma, Yuan Yang and Bo-Wen Zhao
Department of Diagnostic Ultrasound and Echocardiography, Sir Run Run Shaw Hospital, Zhejiang University College of Medicine and Sir Run Run Shaw Institute of Clinical Medicine of Zhejiang University, Hangzhou, China

Xia Wu
Department of Radiology, Sir Run Run Shaw Hospital, Zhejiang University College of Medicine and Sir Run Run Shaw Institute of Clinical Medicine of Zhejiang University, Hangzhou, China

Li-Jun Shen
Department of Ultrasound, The First People's Hospital, Hangzhou Xiao Shan District, Hangzhou, China

Wen Wang and Bo Zhang
Department of Neurosurgery, First Affiliated Hospital of Dalian Medical University, Dalian, PR China

Merel van Diepen and Friedo W. Dekker
Department of Clinical Epidemiology, Leiden University Medical Center, Leiden, the Netherlands

Marielle A. Schroijen and Olaf M. Dekkers
Department of Clinical Epidemiology, Leiden University Medical Center, Leiden, the Netherlands
Department of Endocrinology and Metabolic Diseases, Leiden University Medical Center, Leiden, the Netherlands

Joris I. Rotmans
Department of Nephrology, Leiden University Medical Center, Leiden, the Netherlands

Raymond T. Krediet
Department of Nephrology, Academic Medical Center, Amsterdam, the Netherlands

Elisabeth W. Boeschoten
Hans Mak Institute, Naarden, the Netherlands

Shuo-Chun Weng
Center for Geriatrics and Gerontology, Taichung Veterans General Hospital, Taichung, Taiwan
Division of Nephrology, Department of Internal Medicine, Taichung Veterans General Hospital, Taichung, Taiwan
Institute of Clinical Medicine, National Yang-Ming University, Taipei, Taiwan

Tung-Min Yu
Division of Nephrology, Department of Internal Medicine, Taichung Veterans General Hospital, Taichung, Taiwan

Ming-Ju Wu
Division of Nephrology, Department of Internal Medicine, Taichung Veterans General Hospital, Taichung, Taiwan
Institute of Clinical Medicine, National Yang-Ming University, Taipei, Taiwan
School of Medicine, Chung Shan Medical University, Taichung, Taiwan
School of Medicine, College of Medicine, China Medical University, Taichung, Taiwan

Chi-Hung Cheng
Division of Nephrology, Department of Internal Medicine, Taichung Veterans General Hospital, Taichung, Taiwan
Department of Biotechnology, HungKuang University, Taichung, Taiwan

Kuo-Hsiung Shu
Division of Nephrology, Department of Internal Medicine, Taichung Veterans General Hospital, Taichung, Taiwan
School of Medicine, Chung Shan Medical University, Taichung, Taiwan

Cheng-Hsu Chen
Division of Nephrology, Department of Internal Medicine, Taichung Veterans General Hospital, Taichung, Taiwan
School of Medicine, College of Medicine, China Medical University, Taichung, Taiwan

Der-Cherng Tarng
Institute of Clinical Medicine, National Yang-Ming University, Taipei, Taiwan
Department and Institute of Physiology, National Yang-Ming University, Taipei, Taiwan
Division of Nephrology, Department of Medicine and Immunology Research Center, Taipei Veterans General Hospital, Taipei, Taiwan

Chyong-Mei Chen
Department of Statistics and Informatics Science, Providence University, Taichung, Taiwan

Alden Yuanhong Lai and Haikel Asyraf Lim
Department of Psychology, National University of Singapore, Singapore

Konstadina Griva
Department of Psychology, National University of Singapore, Singapore
Unit of Behavioural Medicine, University College London, London, United Kingdom

Zhenli Yu
Department of Renal Medicine, Khoo Teck Puat Hospital, Singapore

Marjorie Wai Yin Foo
Department of Nephrology, Peritoneal Dialysis Centre, Singapore General Hospital, Singapore

Stanton P. Newman
Unit of Behavioural Medicine, University College London, London, United Kingdom
Health Services Research Group, City University London, London, United Kingdom

Huanhuan Su, Guihua Jiang and Junzhang Tian
Department of Medical Imaging, Guangdong No. 2 Provincial People's Hospital, Guangzhou, PR China

Yingwei Qiu
Department of Medical Imaging, Guangdong No. 2 Provincial People's Hospital, Guangzhou, PR China
Department of Medical Imaging, The First Affiliated Hospital of Gannan Medical University, Ganzhou, PR China

Xiaofei Lv
Departments of Medical Imaging and Interventional Radiology, Cancer Center, Sun Yat-Sen University, Guangzhou, PR China

Cheng Li
Department of Renal Transplantation, Guangdong No. 2 Provincial People's Hospital, Guangzhou, PR China

Ashwani K Gupta and Waseem David
Department of Nephrology, University of Florida-Jacksonville, Jacksonville, Florida, United States of America

Ylenia Ingrasciotta, Janet Sultana, Francesco Giorgianni, Achille Patrizio Caputi, Vincenzo Arcoraci,Domenico Santoro and Gianluca Trifiro`
Department of Clinical and Experimental Medicine, University of Messina, Messina, Italy

Daniele Ugo Tari, Claudio Linguiti and Margherita Perrotta
Caserta Local Health Service, Caserta, Italy

Andrea Nucita
Department of Cognitive Science, Educational and Cultural Studies (CSECS), University of Messina, Messina, Italy

Fabio Pellegrini and Andrea Fontana
Unit of Biostatistics, IRCCS "Casa Sollievo della Sofferenza", San Giovanni Rotondo (FG), Italy

Lorenzo Cavagna
Division of Rheumatology, University and IRCCS Foundation Policlinico S. Matteo, Pavia, Italy

Jiun-Chi Huang
Division of Nephrology, Department of Internal Medicine, Kaohsiung Medical University Hospital, Kaohsiung Medical University, Kaohsiung, Taiwan
Department of Internal Medicine, Kaohsiung Municipal Hsiao-Kang Hospital, Kaohsiung Medical University, Kaohsiung, Taiwan

Szu-Chia Chen and Jer-Ming Chang
Division of Nephrology, Department of Internal Medicine, Kaohsiung Medical University Hospital, Kaohsiung Medical University, Kaohsiung, Taiwan
Department of Internal Medicine, Kaohsiung Municipal Hsiao-Kang Hospital, Kaohsiung Medical University, Kaohsiung, Taiwan
Faculty of Medicine, College of Medicine, Kaohsiung Medical University, Kaohsiung, Taiwan

Ho-Ming Su
Division of Cardiology, Department of Internal Medicine, Kaohsiung Medical University Hospital, Kaohsiung Medical University, Kaohsiung, Taiwan
Department of Internal Medicine, Kaohsiung Municipal Hsiao-Kang Hospital, Kaohsiung Medical University, Kaohsiung, Taiwan
Faculty of Medicine, College of Medicine, Kaohsiung Medical University, Kaohsiung, Taiwan

Chi-Chih Hung
Division of Nephrology, Department of Internal Medicine, Kaohsiung Medical University Hospital, Kaohsiung Medical University, Kaohsiung, Taiwan
Faculty of Medicine, College of Medicine, Kaohsiung Medical University, Kaohsiung, Taiwan

Shang-Jyh Hwang and Hung-Chun Chen
Division of Nephrology, Department of Internal Medicine, Kaohsiung Medical University Hospital, Kaohsiung Medical University, Kaohsiung, Taiwan

Faculty of Renal Care, College of Medicine, Kaohsiung Medical University, Kaohsiung, Taiwan

Shu-Yi Wei
Department of Internal Medicine, Kaohsiung Municipal United Hospital, Kaohsiung, Taiwan
Yuh-Ing Junior College of Health Care & Management, Kaohsiung, Taiwan

Judith Kooiman
Department of Thrombosis and Hemostasis and Department of Nephrology, Leiden University Medical Center, Leiden, Zuid-Holland, The Netherlands

Milan Seth and Hitinder S. Gurm
Department of Internal Medicine, Division of Cardiovascular Medicine, University of Michigan, Ann Arbor, Michigan, United States of America

David Share
Blue Cross Blue Shield of Michigan, Detroit, Michigan, United States of America

Simon Dixon
Beaumont Hospital, Royal Oak, Michigan, United States of America

Fan Yang, Li Zhang, Hao Wu, Hongbin Zou and Yujun Du
Department of Nephrology, The First Bethune Hospital of Jilin University, Jilin, China

Shou-Hsuan Liu, Cheng-Chia Lee, Chan-Yu Lin, Yung-Chang Chen, Ming-Yang Chang, Hsiang-Hao Hsu, Ji-Tseng Fang, Cheng-Chieh Hung, Chih-Wei Yang and Ya-Chung Tian
Kidney Research Center, Department of Nephrology, Lin-Kou Chang Gung Memorial Hospital and Department of Medicine, Chang Gung University, Tao Yuan, Taiwan

Yi-Jung Li, Hsin-Hsu Wu and Cheng-Hao Weng
Kidney Research Center, Department of Nephrology, Lin-Kou Chang Gung Memorial Hospital and Department of Medicine, Chang Gung University, Tao Yuan, Taiwan
Graduate Institute of Clinical Medical Sciences, Chang Gung University, Tao Yuan, Taiwan

Xian-Hui Gao and Guo-Yi Zhang
Laboratory of Preventive Medicine, School of Public Health, Liaoning Medical University, Jinzhou, China

Ying Wang
Department of Toxicology, School of Public Health, Liaoning Medical University, Jinzhou, China

Hui-Ying Zhang
Sleep Monitoring Center, First Affiliated Hospital of Liaoning Medical University, Jinzhou, China

Neelke C. van der Weerd
Department of Nephrology, Academic Medical Center, Amsterdam, The Netherlands
Department of Nephrology, VU Medical Center, Amsterdam, The Netherlands

Menso J. Nubé, Pieter M. ter Wee and Muriel P. C. Grooteman
Department of Nephrology, VU Medical Center, Amsterdam, The Netherlands
Institute for Cardiovascular Research VU Medical Center (ICaR-VU), VU Medical Center, Amsterdam, The Netherlands

E. Lars Penne
Department of Nephrology, VU Medical Center, Amsterdam, The Netherlands
Department of Internal Medicine, Medical Center Alkmaar, Alkmaar, The Netherlands

Peter J. Blankestijn and Albert H. A. Mazairac
Department of Nephrology, University Medical Center Utrecht, Utrecht, The Netherlands

Claire H. Den Hoedt
Department of Nephrology, University Medical Center Utrecht, Utrecht, The Netherlands
Department of Internal Medicine, Maasstad Hospital, Rotterdam, The Netherlands

Marinus A. van den Dorpel
Department of Internal Medicine, Maasstad Hospital, Rotterdam, The Netherlands

Michiel L. Bots
Julius Center for Health Sciences and Primary Care, University Medical Center Utrecht, Utrecht, The Netherlands

Renée Lévesque
Department of Nephrology, Centre Hospitalier de l'Université de Montré al, St-Luc Hospital, Que´bec, Canada

Zhi-Kai Yang, Jie Dong and Hai-Yan Wang
Renal Division, Department of Medicine, Peking University First Hospital, Institute of Nephrology, Peking University, Key Laboratory of Renal Disease, Ministry of Health, Key Laboratory of Renal Disease, Ministry of Education, Beijing, China

Qing-Feng Han and Yue Wang
Department of Nephrology, Peking University Third Hospital, Beijing, China

Tong-Ying Zhu and Chuan-Ming Hao
Department of Nephrology, Huashan Hospital of Fudan University, Shanghai, China

Ye-Ping Ren and Rui Zhang
Department of Nephrology, Second Affiliated Hospital of Harbin Medical University, Heilongjiang, China

Jiang-Hua Chen and Xiao-Hui Zhang
Kidney Disease Center, The First Affiliated Hospital, College of Medicine, Zhejiang University, Hangzhou, China

Hui-Ping Zhao and Mei Wang
Department of Nephrology, Peking University People's Hospital, Beijing, China

Meng-Hua Chen and Na Tian
Department of Nephrology, General Hospital of Ningxia Medical University, Ningxia, China

Carla Y. Vossen, Friedo W. Dekker, Marion Verduijn and Gürbey Ocak
Department of Clinical Epidemiology, Leiden University Medical Center, Leiden, The Netherlands,

Frits R. Rosendaal
Department of Clinical Epidemiology, Leiden University Medical Center, Leiden, The Netherlands
Department of Thrombosis and Haemostasis, Leiden University Medical Center, Leiden, The Netherlands,
Einthoven Laboratory for Experimental Vascular Medicine, Leiden University Medical Center, Leiden, The Netherlands

Christoph Wanner
Department of Medicine, Division of Nephrology, University Hospital, Würzburg, Germany,
Comprehensive Heart Failure Center, University of Wuerzburg, Wuerzburg, Germany

Christiane Drechsler
Department of Medicine, Division of Nephrology, University Hospital, Würzburg, Germany,
Comprehensive Heart Failure Center, University of Wuerzburg, Wuerzburg, Germany,
Institute of Clinical Epidemiology and Biometry, University of Wuerzburg, Wuerzburg, Germany,

Hans L. Vos and Pieter H. Reitsma
Department of Thrombosis and Haemostasis, Leiden University Medical Center, Leiden, The Netherlands,
Einthoven Laboratory for Experimental Vascular Medicine, Leiden University Medical Center, Leiden, The Netherlands

Michael M. Hoffmann
Institute of Clinical Chemistry and Laboratory Medicine, University Medical Center, Freiburg, Germany

Winfried März
Department of Public Health, Social and Preventive Medicine, University of Heidelberg, Mannheim, Germany

Willem H. Ouwehand
Department of Hematology, University of Cambridge and National Health Service Blood and Transplant, Cambridge, United Kingdom
Department of Human Genetics, Wellcome Trust Sanger Institute, Cambridge, United Kingdom

Raymond T. Krediet
Department of Nephrology, Academic Medical Center, Amsterdam, The Netherlands,

Elisabeth W. Boeschoten
Hans Mak Institute, Naarden, The Netherlands

Max Plischke, Ammon Handisurya and Martin Haas
Division of Nephrology and Dialysis, Department of Internal Medicine III, Medical University Vienna, Vienna, Austria

Maria Kohl and Georg Heinze
Section for Clinical Biometrics, Center of Medical Statistics, Informatics and Intelligent Systems, Medical University of Vienna, Vienna, Austria

Lise Bankir
INSERM UMRS 1138, Equipe 2, Centre de Recherche des Cordeliers, Paris, France

Sascha Shayganfar
Division of Cardiology, Pulmonology, and Vascular Medicine, Medical Faculty, University Hospital Düsseldorf, Düsseldorf, Germany

I-Wen Wu,Chiao-Yin Sun, Chia-Chi Chou, Chun-Yu Chen, Chi-Jen Tsai and Chin-Chan Lee
Division of Nephrology, Chang Gung Memorial Hospital, Keelung, Taiwan

Heng-Jung Hsu
Division of Nephrology, Chang Gung Memorial Hospital, Keelung, Taiwan
The Graduate Institute of Clinical Medical Sciences, Chang Gung University Medical College, Taoyuan School of Medicine, Taoyuan, Taiwan

Chiung-Hui Yen
Department of Pediatrics, Taipei Medical University Hospital, Taipei, Taiwan

Kuang-Hung Hsu
Laboratory of Epidemiology, Department of Health Care Management, Chang Gung University, Taoyuan, Taiwan

Chih-Ken Chen
Division of Psychiatry, Chang Gung Memorial Hospital, Keelung, Taiwan

Mai-Szu Wu
Division of Nephrology, Taipei Medical University Hospital, Taipei, Taiwan
Department of Internal Medicine, Taipei Medical University, Taipei, Taiwan

Mark R. Marshall
Faculty of Medical and Health Sciences, University of Auckland, Auckland, New Zealand
Department of Renal Medicine, Counties Manukau District Health Board, Auckland, New Zealand
Australia and New Zealand Dialysis and Transplant Registry (ANZDATA), The Royal Adelaide Hospital, Adelaide, South Australia, Australia

Kevan R. Polkinghorne
Australia and New Zealand Dialysis and Transplant Registry (ANZDATA), The Royal Adelaide Hospital, Adelaide, South Australia, Australia
Department of Nephrology, Monash Medical Centre, Clayton, Victoria, Australia
Departments of Medicine and Epidemiology and Preventive Medicine Monash University, Clayton, Victoria, Australia

Rachael C. Walker
Renal Department, Hawke's Bay District Health Board, Hastings, New Zealand
Sydney School of Public Health, University of Sydney, Sydney, New South Wales, Australia

Kelvin L. Lynn
Kidney Health New Zealand, Christchurch, New Zealand

Jeonghwan Lee
Department of Internal Medicine, Hallym University Hangang Sacred Heart Hospital, Seoul, Korea
Clinical Research Center for End Stage Renal Disease (CRC for ESRD), Daegu, Korea

Yun Kyu Oh, Chun Soo Lim and Jung Pyo Lee
Clinical Research Center for End Stage Renal Disease (CRC for ESRD), Daegu, Korea
Department of Internal Medicine, Seoul National University Boramae Medical Center, Seoul, Korea

Yong-Lim Kim
Clinical Research Center for End Stage Renal Disease (CRC for ESRD), Daegu, Korea
Department of Internal Medicine, Kyungpook National University School of Medicine, Daegu, Korea

Shin-Wook Kang
Clinical Research Center for End Stage Renal Disease (CRC for ESRD), Daegu, Korea
Department of Internal Medicine, Yonsei University College of Medicine, Seoul, Korea,

Chul Woo Yang
Clinical Research Center for End Stage Renal Disease (CRC for ESRD), Daegu, Korea
Department of Internal Medicine, The Catholic University of Korea College of Medicine, Seoul, Korea

Nam-Ho Kim
Clinical Research Center for End Stage Renal Disease (CRC for ESRD), Daegu, Korea
Department of Internal Medicine, Chonnam National University Medical School, Gwangju, Korea

Yon Su Kim
Clinical Research Center for End Stage Renal Disease (CRC for ESRD), Daegu, Korea
Department of Internal Medicine, Seoul National University Hospital, Seoul National University College of Medicine, Seoul, Korea

Jung Nam An
Department of Internal Medicine, Seoul National University Boramae Medical Center, Seoul, Korea

Jin Ho Hwang
Department of Internal Medicine, Chung-Ang University Medical Center, Seoul, Korea,

Morten K. Borg, Emil Brøndum and Christian Aalkjær
Department of Biomedicine, Aarhus University, Aarhus, Denmark,

Per Ivarsen and Johan V.Povlsen
Department of Renal Medicine, Aarhus University Hospital and Department of Clinical Medicine, Faculty of Health, Aarhus University, Aarhus, Denmark

Moniek C. M.de Goeij, Gurbey Ocak, Friedo W. Dekker and Nynke Halbesma
Department of Clinical Epidemiology, Leiden University Medical Center, Leiden, The Netherlands,

Index

Q

R

S

U

V